PRINCIPLES OF
MEDICAL
BIOCHEMISTRY

PRINCIPLES OF MEDICAL BIOCHEMISTRY

3rd EDITION

Gerhard Meisenberg, PhD

Department of Biochemistry
Ross University School of Medicine
Roseau, Commonwealth of Dominica, West Indies

William H. Simmons, PhD

Department of Molecular Pharmacology and Therapeutics
Loyola University School of Medicine
Maywood, Illinois

ELSEVIER
SAUNDERS

ELSEVIER
SAUNDERS

1600 John F. Kennedy Blvd.
Ste 1800
Philadelphia, PA 19103-2899

PRINCIPLES OF MEDICAL BIOCHEMISTRY, THIRD EDITION   ISBN: 978-0-323-07155-0
Copyright © 2012, 2006, 1998 by Saunders, an imprint of Elsevier, Inc.

Notices

International Standard Book Number: 978-0-323-07155-0

Publisher: Madelene Hyde
Managing Editor: Rebecca Gruliow
Publishing Services Manager: Patricia Tannian
Senior Project Manager: Kristine Feeherty
Design Direction: Steve Stave

Printed in the United States of America

Last digit is the print number: 9 8 7 6 5 4 3 2 1

PREFACE

It is rumored that among students embarking on a course of study in the medical sciences, biochemistry is the most common cause of pretraumatic stress disorder: the state of mind into which people fall in anticipation of unbearable stress and frustration. No other part of their preclinical curriculum seems as abstract, shapeless, unintelligible, and littered with irrelevant detail as is biochemistry. This prejudice is understandable. Biochemistry is less intuitive than most other medical sciences. Even worse, it is a vast field with an ever-expanding frontier. From embryonic development to carcinogenesis and drug action, biochemistry is becoming the ultimate level of explanation.

This third edition of *Principles of Medical Biochemistry* is yet another attempt at imposing structure and meaning on the blooming, buzzing confusion of this runaway science. This text is designed for first-year medical students as well as veterinary, dental, and pharmacy students and students in undergraduate premedical programs. Therefore, its aim goes beyond the communication of basic biochemical facts and concepts. Of equal importance is the link between basic principles and medical applications. To achieve this aim, we enhanced this edition with numerous clinical examples that are embedded in the chapters and illustrate the importance of biochemistry for medicine.

Although biochemistry advances at a faster rate than most other medical sciences, we did not match the increased volume of knowledge by an increased size of the book. The day has only 24 hours, the cerebral cortex has only 30 billion neurons, and students have to learn many other subjects in addition to biochemistry. Rather, we tried to be more selective and more concise. The book still is comprehensive in the sense of covering most aspects of biochemistry that have significant medical applications. However, it is intended for day-to-day use by students. It is not a reference work for students, professors, or physicians. It does not contain "all a physician ever needs to know" about biochemistry. This is impossible to achieve because the rapidly expanding science requires new learning, and unlearning of received wisdom, on a continuous basis.

This book is evidently a compromise between the two conflicting demands of comprehensiveness and brevity. This compromise was possible because medical biochemistry is not a random cross-section of the general biochemistry that is taught in undergraduate courses and PhD programs. Biochemistry for the medical professions is "physiological" chemistry: the chemistry needed to understand the structure and functions of the body and their malfunction in disease. Therefore, we paid little attention to topics of abstract theoretical interest, such as three-dimensional protein structures and enzymatic reaction mechanisms, but we give thorough treatments of medically important topics such as lipoprotein metabolism, mutagenesis and genetic diseases, the molecular basis of cancer, nutritional disorders, and the hormonal regulation of metabolic pathways.

FACULTY RESOURCES

An image collection and test bank are available for your use when teaching via Evolve. Contact your local sales representative for more information, or go directly to the Evolve website to request access: http://evolve.elsevier.com.

Gerhard Meisenberg, PhD
William H. Simmons, PhD

CONTENTS

Part THREE
CELL AND TISSUE STRUCTURE 181

Chapter 12
BIOLOGICAL MEMBRANES 182

Chapter 13
THE CYTOSKELETON 198

Chapter 14
THE EXTRACELLULAR MATRIX 212

Part FOUR
MOLECULAR PHYSIOLOGY 231

Chapter 15
PLASMA PROTEINS 232

Chapter 16
EXTRACELLULAR MESSENGERS 261

PRINCIPLES OF
MEDICAL
BIOCHEMISTRY

Part ONE
PRINCIPLES OF MOLECULAR STRUCTURE AND FUNCTION

Chapter 1

INTRODUCTION TO BIOMOLECULES

Biochemistry is concerned with the molecular workings of the body, and the first question we must ask is about the molecular composition of the normal human body. *Table 1.1* lists the approximate composition of the proverbial 75-kg textbook adult. Next to water, **proteins** and **triglycerides** are most abundant. Triglyceride (aka fat) is the major storage form of metabolic energy and is found mainly in adipose tissue. Proteins are of more general importance. They are major elements of cell structures and are responsible for enzymatic catalysis and virtually all cellular functions. **Carbohydrates,** in the form of glucose and the storage polysaccharide glycogen, are substrates for energy metabolism, but they also are covalently linked components of glycoproteins and glycolipids. Soluble **inorganic salts** are present in all intracellular and extracellular fluids, and insoluble salts, most of them related to calcium phosphate, give strength and rigidity to human bones.

This chapter introduces the principles of molecular structure, the types of noncovalent interactions between biomolecules, and the structural features of the major classes of biomolecules.

WATER IS THE SOLVENT OF LIFE

Charles Darwin speculated that life originated in a warm little pond. Perhaps it really was a big warm ocean, but one thing is certain: We are appallingly watery creatures. Almost two thirds of the adult human body is water (see *Table 1.1*). The structure of water is simplicity itself, with two hydrogen atoms bonded to an oxygen atom at an angle of 105 degrees:

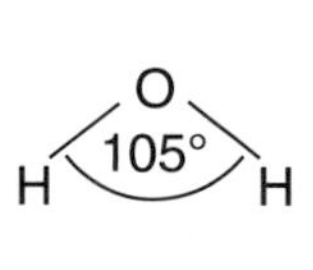

Water is a lopsided molecule, with its binding electron pairs displaced toward the oxygen atom. Thus the oxygen atom has a high electron density, whereas the hydrogen atoms are electron deficient. The oxygen atom has a partial negative charge (δ^-), and the hydrogen atoms have partial positive charges (δ^+). Therefore the water molecule forms an electrical **dipole:**

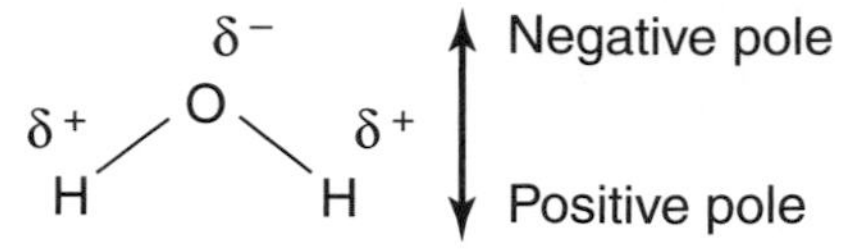

Unlike charges attract each other. Therefore the hydrogen atoms of a water molecule are attracted by the oxygen atoms of other water molecules, forming **hydrogen bonds:**

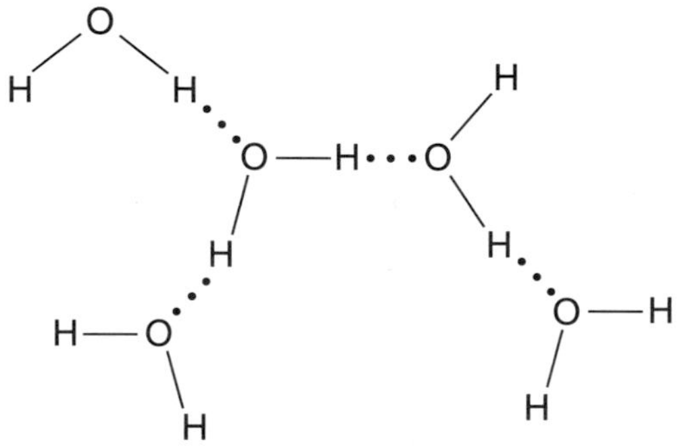

These hydrogen bonds are weak. Only 29 kJ (7 kcal) per mole is needed to break a hydrogen bond in water, whereas 450 kJ (110 kcal) per mole* is required to break a covalent oxygen-hydrogen bond in the water molecule itself. Breaking the hydrogen bonds requires no more than heating the water to 100°C. *The hydrogen bonds determine the physical properties of water,* including its boiling point.

The water in the human body always contains inorganic **cations** (positively charged ions), such as sodium and potassium, and **anions** (negatively charged ions), such as chloride and phosphate. *Table 1.2* lists the typical ionic compositions of intracellular (cytoplasmic) and extracellular (interstitial) fluid. Interestingly, the extracellular fluid has an ionic composition similar to seawater. We carry a warm little pond with us, to provide our cells with their ancestral environment.

Predictably, the cations are attracted to the oxygen atom of the water molecule, and the anions are attracted to the hydrogen atoms. The **ion-dipole interactions** thus formed are the forces that hold the components of soluble salts in solution, as in the case of sodium chloride (table salt):

---

*1 kcal = 4.18 kJ.

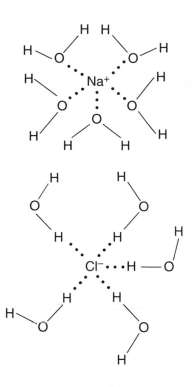

Table 1.1 Approximate Composition of a 75-Kg Adult

Substance	Content (%)
Water	60
Inorganic salt, soluble	0.7
Inorganic salt, insoluble*	5.5
Protein	16
Triglyceride (fat)†	13
Membrane lipids	2.5
Carbohydrates	1.5
Nucleic acids	0.2

*In bones.
†In adipose tissue.

Table 1.2 Typical Ionic Compositions of Extracellular (Interstitial) and Intracellular (Cytoplasmic) Fluids

	Concentration (mmol/L)	
Ion	**Extracellular Fluid**	**Cytoplasm**
Na^+	137	10
K^+	4.7	141
Ca^{2+}	2.4	10^{-4}*
Mg^{2+}	1.4	31
Cl^-	113	4
$HPO_4^{2-}/H_2PO_4^-$	2	11
HCO_3^-	28†	10†
Organic acids, phosphate esters	1.8	100
pH	7.4	6.5–7.5

*Cytoplasmic concentration. Concentrations in mitochondria and endoplasmic reticulum are much higher.
†The lower HCO_3^- concentration in the intracellular space is caused by the lower intracellular pH, which affects the equilibrium:

$$HCO_3^- + H^+ \rightleftharpoons H_2CO_3 \rightleftharpoons CO_2 + H_2O.$$

The calcium phosphates in human bones are not soluble because the **electrostatic interactions** (**"salt bonds"**) between the anions and cations in the crystal structure are stronger than their ion-dipole interactions with water.

WATER CONTAINS HYDRONIUM IONS AND HYDROXYL IONS

Water molecules dissociate reversibly into hydroxyl ions and hydronium ions:

(1) $H_2O + H_2O \rightleftharpoons H_3O^+ + OH^-$
     Hydronium   Hydroxyl
        ion   ion

In pure water, only about one in 280 million molecules is in the H_3O^+ or OH^- form:

(2) $[H_3O^+] = [OH^-] = 10^{-7}$ mol/L

The brackets indicate molar concentrations (mol/L or M). *One mole of a substance is its molecular weight in grams.* Water has a molecular weight close to 18; therefore, 18 g of water is 1 mol. The hydronium ion concentration $[H_3O^+]$ usually is expressed as the **proton concentration** or the **hydrogen ion concentration** $[H^+]$, regardless of the fact that the proton is actually riding on the free electron pair of a water molecule.

In aqueous solutions, the product of proton (hydronium ion) concentration and hydroxyl ion concentration is a constant:

(3) $[H^+] \times [OH^-] = 10^{-14}$ mol²/L²

The proton concentration $[H^+]$, otherwise measured in moles per liter, is more commonly expressed as the **pH value**, defined as the negative logarithm of the hydrogen ion concentration:

(4) $pH = -\log[H^+]$

With *Equations (3)* and *(4)*, the H^+ and OH^- concentrations can be predicted at any given pH value (*Table 1.3*).

The pH value of an aqueous solution depends on the presence of **acids** and **bases**. According to the **Brønsted definition**, in aqueous solutions *an acid is a substance that releases a proton, and a base is a substance that binds a proton.* The prototypical acidic group is the

Table 1.3 Relationship among pH, $[H^+]$, and $[OH^-]$

pH	$[H^+]$*	$[OH^-]$*
4	10^{-4}	10^{-10}
5	10^{-5}	10^{-9}
6	10^{-6}	10^{-8}
7	10^{-7}	10^{-7}
8	10^{-8}	10^{-6}
9	10^{-9}	10^{-5}
10	10^{-10}	10^{-4}

*$[H^+]$ and $[OH^-]$ are measured in mol/L (M).

carboxyl group, which is the distinguishing feature of the organic acids:

Carboxylic acid | Carboxylate anion
(protonated form) | (deprotonated form)

The protonation-deprotonation reaction is reversible; therefore, the carboxylate anion fits the definition of a Brønsted base. It is called the **conjugate base** of the acid.

Amino groups are the major basic groups in biomolecules. In this case, the amine is the base, and the ammonium salt is the conjugate acid:

Amine | Ammonium salt
(deprotonated form) | (protonated form)

Carboxyl groups, phosphate esters, and **phosphodiesters** are the most important acidic groups in biomolecules. They are mainly deprotonated and negatively charged at pH 7. Aliphatic (nonaromatic) **amino groups,** including the primary, secondary, and tertiary amines, are the most important basic groups. They are mainly protonated and positively charged at pH 7.

IONIZABLE GROUPS ARE CHARACTERIZED BY THEIR pK VALUES

The equilibrium of a protonation-deprotonation reaction is described by the **dissociation constant (K_D).** For the reaction

$$R-COOH \rightleftharpoons R-COO^- + H^+$$

the dissociation constant K_D is defined as

$$(5) \quad K_D = \frac{[R-COO^-] \times [H^+]}{[R-COOH]}$$

This can be rearranged to

$$(6) \quad [H^+] = K_D \times \frac{[R-COOH]}{[R-COO^-]}$$

The molar concentrations in this equation are the concentrations observed at equilibrium. Because the hydrogen ion concentration $[H^+]$ is most conveniently expressed as the pH value, *Equation (6)* can be transformed into the negative logarithm:

$$(7) \quad pH = pK - \log \frac{[R-COOH]}{[R-COO^-]}$$

$$= pK + \log \frac{[R-COO^-]}{[R-COOH]}$$

This equation is called the **Henderson-Hasselbalch equation,** and *the pK value is defined as the negative logarithm of the dissociation constant.* The pK value is a property of an ionizable group. If a molecule has more than one ionizable group, then it has more than one pK value.

In the Henderson-Hasselbalch equation, pK is a constant, whereas $[R-COOH]/[R-COO^-]$ changes with the pH. When the pH value equals the pK value, log $[R-COOH]/[R-COO^-]$ must equal zero. Therefore $[R-COOH]/[R-COO^-]$ must equal one: *The pK value indicates the pH value at which the ionizable group is half-protonated.* At pH values below their pK (i.e., high $[H^+]$ or high acidity), ionizable groups are mainly protonated. At pH values above their pK (i.e., low $[H^+]$ or high alkalinity), ionizable groups are mainly deprotonated (*Table 1.4*)

CLINICAL EXAMPLE 1.1: Acidosis

Blood and extracellular fluids have to provide a constant environment for our cells. Physiological levels of inorganic ions have to be maintained, and maintenance of a constant extracellular pH of 7.3 to 7.4 is required. Deviations from the normal pH by as little as 0.5 pH units can be fatal. An abnormally high pH of blood and interstitial fluid is called **alkalosis,** and an abnormally low pH is called **acidosis.** Many pathological processes can lead to alkalosis or acidosis. Acidosis can be caused by metabolic derangements leading to excessive formation of acidic products from nonacidic substrates. For example,

Glucose → Lactic acid
Triglyceride (fat) → β-Hydroxybutyric acid

Some toxins are converted into acids in the human body, causing acidosis. For example,

Methanol → Formic acid

BONDS ARE FORMED BY REACTIONS BETWEEN FUNCTIONAL GROUPS

Most biomolecules contain only three to six different elements out of the 92 that are listed in the periodic table. Carbon (C), hydrogen (H), and oxygen (O) are always present. Nitrogen (N) is present in many biomolecules, and sulfur (S) and phosphorus (P) are present in some. These elements form a limited number of **functional groups,** which determine the physical properties and chemical reactivities of the biomolecules (*Table 1.5*). Many of these functional groups can form bonds through **condensation reactions,** in which two groups join with the release of water (*Table 1.6*). This type of reaction can link small molecules into far larger structures (macromolecules). Bond formation is an endergonic (energy-requiring) process. Therefore the synthesis of macromolecules from small molecules requires metabolic energy.

Table 1.4 Protonation State of a Carboxyl Group and an Amino Group at Different pH Values

	Carboxyl Group		Amino Group	
pH	Percent of Group Protonated (R—COOH)	Percent of Group Deprotonated (R—COO⁻)	Percent of Group Protonated (R—NH₃⁺)	Percent of Group Deprotonated (R—NH₂)
$pK + 3$	0.1	99.9	0.1	99.9
$pK + 2$	1	99	1	99
$pK + 1$	10	90	10	90
pK	50	50	50	50
$pK - 1$	90	10	90	10
$pK - 2$	99	1	99	1
$pK - 3$	99.9	0.1	99.9	0.1

Table 1.5 Functional Groups in Biomolecules

1. Hydrocarbon Groups

—CH₃	Methyl
—CH₂—CH₃	Ethyl
—CH₂—	Methylene
—CH=	Methine

2. Oxygen-Containing Groups

R—OH	Hydroxyl (alcoholic)
—OH	Hydroxyl (phenolic)
C=O	Keto
—C(H)=O	Aldehyde
	Carbonyl
—C(OH)=O	Carboxyl

3. Nitrogen-Containing Groups

—NH₂	Primary amine
NH	Secondary amine
N—	Tertiary amine
—N⁺—	Quaternary ammonium salt

4. Sulfur-Containing Group

—SH	Sulfhydryl group

Cleavage of these bonds by the addition of water is called **hydrolysis.** It is an exergonic (energy-releasing) process that occurs spontaneously, provided it is catalyzed by acids, bases, or enzymes. For example, the digestive enzymes, which catalyze hydrolytic bond cleavages (see Chapter 19), work perfectly well in the lumen of the gastrointestinal tract, where neither adenosine triphosphate (ATP) nor other usable energy sources are available.

Some bonds contain more energy than others. Most ester, ether, acetal, and amide bonds require between 4 and 20 J/mol (1 and 5 kcal/mol) for their formation, and the same amount of energy is released during their hydrolysis. Anhydride bonds and thioester bonds, however, have free energy contents greater than 20 J/mol. They are classified, rather arbitrarily, as **energy-rich bonds.**

ISOMERIC FORMS ARE COMMON IN BIOMOLECULES

The biological properties of molecules are determined not by their composition but by their geometry. **Isomers** are chemically different molecules with identical composition but different geometry. The three different types of isomers are as follows:

1. **Positional isomers** differ in the positions of functional groups within the molecule. Examples include the following:

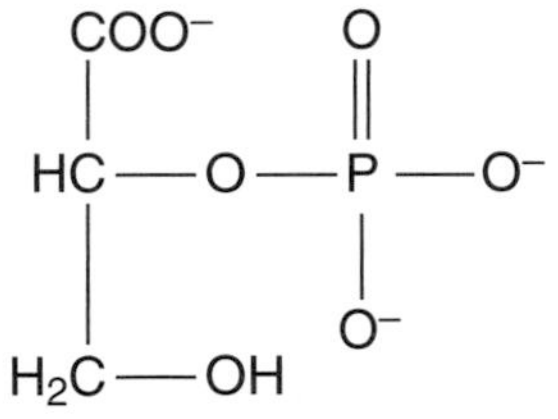

2-Phosphoglycerate 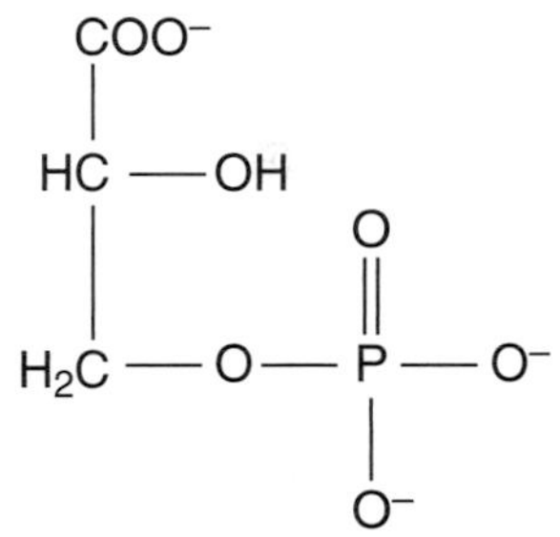   3-Phosphoglycerate

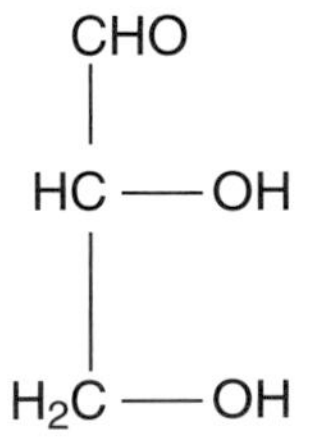

Glyceraldehyde 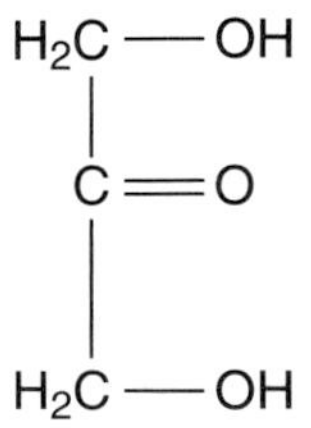   Dihydroxyacetone

2. **Geometric isomers** differ in the arrangement of substituents at a rigid portion of the molecule. A typical example is *cis-trans* isomers of carbon-carbon double bonds:

Table 1.6 Important Bonds in Biomolecules

Bond	Structure	Formed from	Occurs in
Ether	$R_1 - O - R_2$	$R_1 - OH + HO - R_2$	Methyl ethers, some membrane lipids
Carboxylic ester	$R_1 - \overset{\overset{O}{\|\|}}{C} - O - R_2$	$R_1 - \overset{\overset{O}{\|\|}}{C} - OH + HO - R_2$	Triglycerides, other lipids
Acetal	$R_2 - O \quad O - R_3$ $\diagdown C \diagup$ $R_1 \quad H$	$R_2 - O$ $R_1 - \overset{}{C} - OH + HO - R_3$ $\underset{H}{\|}$	Disaccharides, oligosaccharides, and polysaccharides (glycosidic bonds)
Mixed anhydride*	$R - \overset{\overset{O}{\|\|}}{C} - O - \overset{\overset{O^-}{\|}}{\underset{\underset{O}{\|\|}}{P}} - O^-$	$R - \overset{\overset{O}{\|\|}}{C} - OH + HO - \overset{\overset{O^-}{\|}}{\underset{\underset{O}{\|\|}}{P}} - O^-$	Some metabolic intermediates
Phosphoanhydride*	$R - O - \overset{\overset{O^-}{\|}}{\underset{\underset{O}{\|\|}}{P}} - O - \overset{\overset{O^-}{\|}}{\underset{\underset{O}{\|\|}}{P}} - O^-$	$R - O - \overset{\overset{O^-}{\|}}{\underset{\underset{O}{\|\|}}{P}} - OH + HO - \overset{\overset{O^-}{\|}}{\underset{\underset{O}{\|\|}}{P}} - O^-$	Nucleotides; most important: ATP
Phosphate ester	$R - O - \overset{\overset{O^-}{\|}}{\underset{\underset{O}{\|\|}}{P}} - O^-$	$R - OH + HO - \overset{\overset{O^-}{\|}}{\underset{\underset{O}{\|\|}}{P}} - O^-$	Many metabolic intermediates, phosphoproteins
Phosphodiester	$R_1 - O - \overset{\overset{O^-}{\|}}{\underset{\underset{O}{\|\|}}{P}} - O - R_2$	$R_1 - OH + HO - \overset{\overset{O^-}{\|}}{\underset{\underset{O}{\|\|}}{P}} - OH + HO - R_2$	Nucleic acids, phospholipids
Unsubstituted amide	$R - \overset{\overset{O}{\|\|}}{C} - NH_2$	$R - \overset{\overset{O}{\|\|}}{C} - OH + H - \overset{\overset{H}{}}{\underset{\underset{H}{}}{N}}$	Asparagine, glutamine
Substituted amide	$R_1 - \overset{\overset{O}{\|\|}}{C} - \underset{\underset{H}{\|}}{N} - R_2$	$R_1 - \overset{\overset{O}{\|\|}}{C} - OH + H - \underset{\underset{H}{\|}}{N} - R_2$	Polypeptides (peptide bond)
Thioester*	$R_1 - \overset{\overset{O}{\|\|}}{C} - S - R_2$	$R_1 - \overset{\overset{O}{\|\|}}{C} - OH + HS - R_2$	Acetyl-CoA, other "activated" acids
Thioether	$R_1 - S - R_2$	$R_1 - SH + HO - R_2$	Methionine

ATP, Adenosine triphosphate; *CoA*, coenzyme A.
*"Energy-rich" bonds.

cis double bond   *trans* double bond

The two forms are not interconvertible because there is no rotation around the double bond. All substituents (H, R_1, and R_2) are fixed in the same plane. Also, ring systems show geometric isomerism, with substituents protruding over one or the other surface of the ring. Geometric isomers are called **diastereomers.**

3. **Optical isomers** differ in the orientation of substituents around an **asymmetrical carbon:** a carbon with four *different* substituents. If the molecule has only one asymmetrical carbon, the isomers are mirror images. These mirror-image molecules are called **enantiomers.** They are related to each other in the same way as the left hand and the right hand; therefore, optical isomerism is also called **chirality** (from Greek χειρ meaning "hand").

Unlike positional and geometric isomers, which differ in their melting point, boiling point, solubility, and crystal structure, *enantiomers have identical physical and chemical properties.* They can be distinguished only by the direction in which they turn the plane of polarized light. They do, however, differ in their biological properties.

If more than one asymmetrical carbon is present in the molecule, isomers at a single asymmetrical carbon are not mirror images (enantiomers) but are geometric isomers (diastereomers) with different physical and chemical properties.

In the **Fisher projection,** the substituents above and below the asymmetrical carbon face behind the plane of the paper, and those on the left and right face the front. The asymmetrical carbon is in the center of a tetrahedron whose corners are formed by the four substituents. For example,

Plane of
symmetry

CHO   CHO

HO — C — H   H — C — OH

CH₂OH   CH₂OH

L-Glyceraldehyde   D-Glyceraldehyde

COO⁻   COO⁻

H₃⁺N — C — H   H — C — NH₃⁺

CH₃   CH₃

L-Alanine   D-Alanine

PROPERTIES OF BIOMOLECULES ARE DETERMINED BY THEIR NONCOVALENT INTERACTIONS

The functions of biomolecules require interactions with other molecules. Molecules communicate with one another, and, being incapable of speech, they have to communicate by touch. The surfaces of interacting molecules must be complementary, and noncovalent interactions must be formed between them. These interactions are weak. They break up and re-form continuously; therefore,

noncovalent binding is always reversible. We can distinguish five types of noncovalent interaction:

1. **Dipole-dipole interactions** usually come in the form of hydrogen bonds. A hydrogen atom is covalently bound to an electronegative atom such as oxygen or nitrogen. This hydrogen attracts another electronegative atom, either in the same or a different molecule. **Electronegativity** is the tendency of an atom to attract electrons. For the atoms commonly encountered in biomolecules, the rank order of electronegativity is as follows:

$$O > N > S \geq C \geq H$$

Examples:

Hydrogen bond between
ethanol and water

Hydrogen bond between
two peptide bonds

2. **Electrostatic interactions,** or **salt bonds,** are formed between oppositely charged groups:

3. **Ion-dipole interactions** are formed between a charged group and a polarized bond, as in the case of a carboxylate anion and a carboxamide:

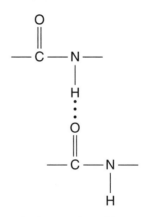

4. **Hydrophobic interactions** hold nonpolar molecules, or nonpolar portions of molecules, together. There is no strong attractive force between such groups. However, an interface between a nonpolar structure and water is thermodynamically unfavorable because it limits the ability of water molecules to form hydrogen bonds with their neighbors. The water molecules are forced to reorient themselves in order to maximize their hydrogen bonds with neighboring water molecules, thereby attaining a more ordered and energetically less favorable state. By clustering together, *nonpolar groups minimize their area of contact with water.*

5. **Van der Waals forces** appear whenever two molecules approach each other (*Fig. 1.1*). A weak attractive force, caused by induced dipoles in the molecules, prevails at moderate distances. However, when the molecules come closer together, an electrostatic repulsion between the electron shells of the approaching groups begins to overwhelm the attractive force. There is an optimal contact distance at which the attractive force is canceled by the repulsive force. Because of van der Waals forces, molecules whose surfaces have complementary shapes tend to bind each other.

Noncovalent interactions determine the biological properties of biomolecules:

● *Water solubility* depends on hydrogen bonds and ion-dipole interactions that the molecules form with water. Charged molecules and those that can form many hydrogen bonds are soluble, and those that have mainly nonpolar bonds, for example, between C and H, are insoluble. If a molecule can exist in charged and uncharged states, the charged form is more soluble.

● *Higher-order structures of macromolecules,* including proteins (see Chapter 2) and nucleic acids (Chapter 6), are formed by noncovalent interactions between portions of the same molecule. Because noncovalent interactions are weak, many of them are needed to hold a protein or nucleic acid in its proper shape.

● *Binding interactions between molecules* are the essence of life. Structural proteins bind each other, metabolic substrates bind to enzymes, gene regulators bind to deoxyribonucleic acid (DNA), hormones bind to receptors, and foreign substances bind to antibodies.

After this review of functional groups, bonds, and noncovalent interactions, the structures of the major classes of biomolecules—triglycerides, carbohydrates, proteins, and nucleic acids—can now be discussed. More details about these structures are presented in later chapters.

TRIGLYCERIDES CONSIST OF FATTY ACIDS AND GLYCEROL

The **triacylglycerols,** better known as **triglycerides** in the medical literature, consist of glycerol and fatty acids. **Glycerol** is a trivalent alcohol:

$$H_2C-OH$$
$$HO-CH$$
$$H_2C-OH$$

Glycerol

Fatty acids consist of a long hydrocarbon chain with a carboxyl group at one end. The typical chain length is between 16 and 20 carbons. For example,

Palmitic acid

Palmitic acid can also be written as

$$H_3C-(CH_2)_{14}-COOH$$

or

COOH

Fatty acids that have only single bonds between carbons are called **saturated fatty acids.** Those with at least

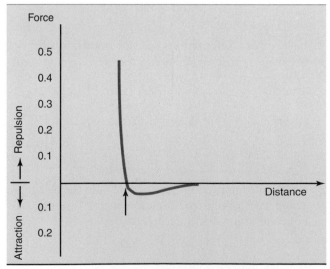

Figure 1.1 Attractive and repulsive van der Waals forces. At the van der Waals contact distance (*arrow*), the opposing forces cancel each other.

one double bond between carbons are called **unsaturated fatty acids**. For example,

$$H_3C - (CH_2)_5 - CH = CH - (CH_2)_7 - COOH$$

Palmitoleic acid

Fatty acids have pK values between 4.7 and 5.0; therefore, they are mainly in the deprotonated ($-COO^-$) form at pH 7.

In the triglycerides, all three hydroxyl groups of glycerol are esterified with a fatty acid, as shown in *Figure 1.2*. The long hydrocarbon chains of the fatty acid residues ensure that *triglycerides are insoluble in water*. In the body, triglycerides minimize contact with water by forming fat droplets.

Collectively, nonpolar biomolecules are called **lipids**. The triglycerides ("fat") are used only as a storage form of metabolic energy, but other lipids serve as structural components of membranes (see Chapter 12) or as signaling molecules (see Chapter 16).

MONOSACCHARIDES ARE POLYALCOHOLS WITH A KETO GROUP OR AN ALDEHYDE GROUP

Monosaccharides are the building blocks of all carbohydrates. They consist of a chain of carbons with a hydroxyl group at each carbon except one. This carbon forms a carbonyl group. **Aldoses** have an aldehyde group, and **ketoses** have a keto group. The length of the carbon chain is variable. For example,

- Triose: three carbons
- Tetrose: four carbons
- Pentose: five carbons
- Hexose: six carbons
- Heptose: seven carbons

D-Glyceraldehyde and dihydroxyacetone are the simplest monosaccharides:

CHO
|
HC — OH
|
H₂C — OH

D-Glyceraldehyde
(an aldotriose)

H₂C — OH
|
C = O
|
H₂C — OH

Dihydroxyacetone
(a ketotriose)

The most important monosaccharide, however, is the aldohexose D-**glucose:**

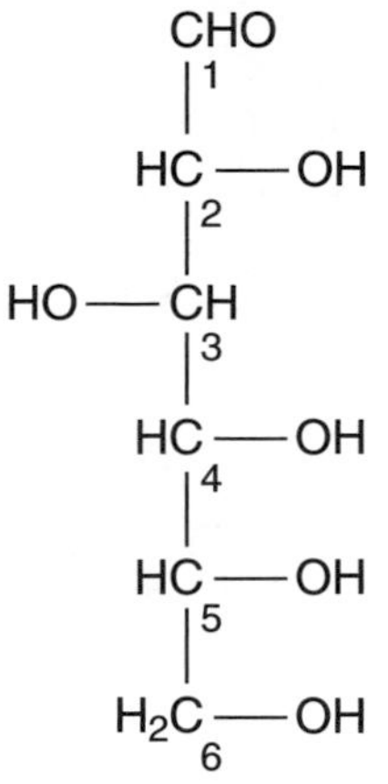

CHO 1
|
HC — OH 2
|
HO — CH 3
|
HC — OH 4
|
HC — OH 5
|
H₂C — OH 6

D-Glucose

The carbons are conveniently numbered, starting with the aldehyde carbon or, for ketoses, the terminal carbon closest to the keto carbon. Carbons 2, 3, 4, and 5 of D-glucose all have four different substituents. These four asymmetrical carbons can form 16 optical isomers. Only one of them is D-glucose. By convention, the "D" in D-glyceraldehyde and D-glucose refers to the orientation of substituents at the asymmetrical carbon farthest removed from the carbonyl carbon (C-2 and C-5, respectively).

Monosaccharides that differ in the orientation of substituents around one of their asymmetrical carbons are called **epimers**. In *Figure 1.3*, for example, D-mannose is a C-2 epimer of glucose, and D-galactose is a C-4 epimer of glucose. *Epimers are diastereomers, not enantiomers*. This means that they have different physical and chemical properties.

MONOSACCHARIDES FORM RING STRUCTURES

Most monosaccharides spontaneously form ring structures in which the aldehyde (or keto) group forms a hemiacetal (or hemiketal) bond with one of the hydroxyl groups. If the ring contains five atoms, it is called a **furanose** ring; if it contains six atoms, it is called a **pyranose** ring. The ring structures are written in either the Fisher projection or the **Haworth projection**, as shown in *Figure 1.4*.

In water, only one of 40,000 glucose molecules is in the open-chain form. When the ring structure forms, carbon 1 of glucose becomes asymmetrical. Therefore two

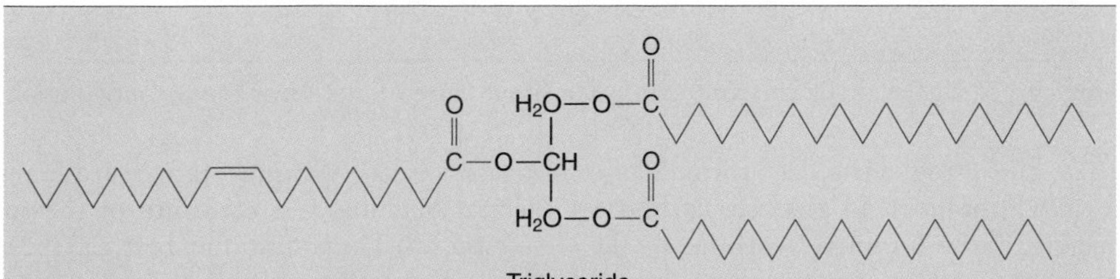

Figure 1.2 Structure of a triglyceride (fat) molecule. Although the ester bonds can form some hydrogen bonds with water, the long hydrocarbon chains of the fatty acids make fat insoluble.

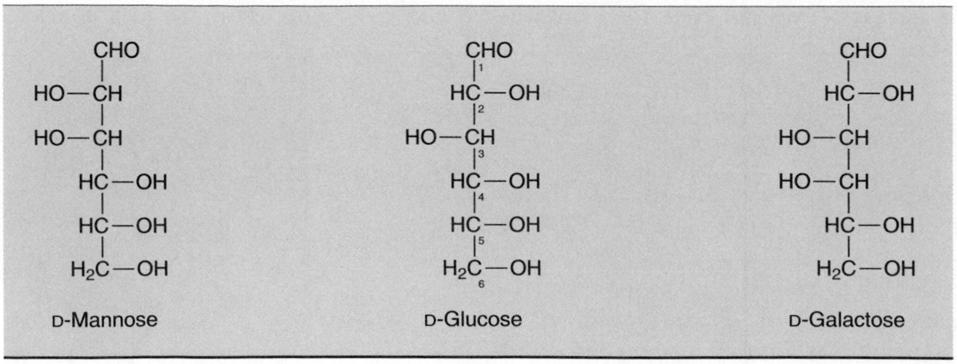

Figure 1.3 D-Mannose and D-galactose are epimers of D-glucose.

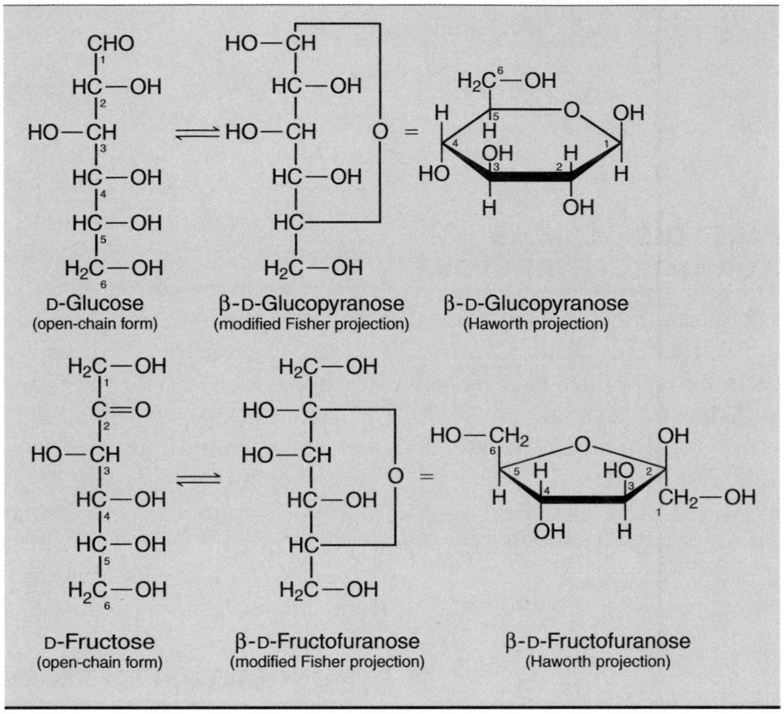

Figure 1.4 Ring structures of the aldohexose D-glucose and the ketohexose D-fructose. The six-member pyranose ring is favored in D-glucose, and the five-member furanose ring is favored in D-fructose.

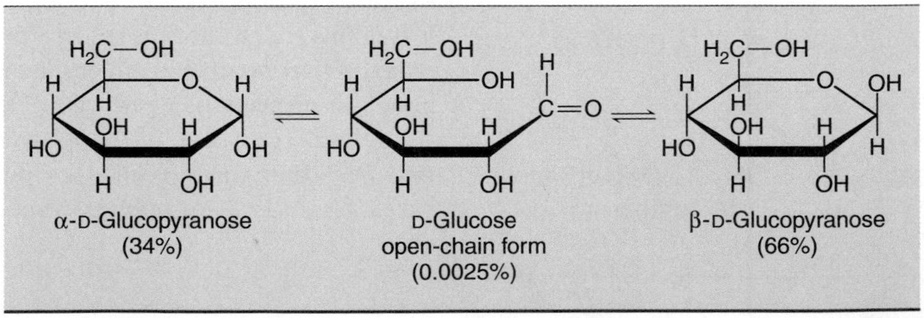

Figure 1.5 Mutarotation of D-glucose. Closure of the ring can occur either in the α- or the β-configuration.

isomers, α-D-glucose and β-D-glucose, can form. These two isomers are called **anomers.** In glucose, carbon 1 (the aldehyde carbon) is the **anomeric carbon.** In the ketoses, the keto carbon (usually carbon 2) is anomeric.

Unlike epimers, which are stable under ordinary conditions, *anomers interconvert spontaneously.* This process is called **mutarotation.** It is caused by the occasional opening and reclosure of the ring, as shown in *Figure 1.5.* The equilibrium between the α- and β-anomers is reached within several hours in neutral solutions, but mutarotation is greatly accelerated in the presence of acids or bases.

COMPLEX CARBOHYDRATES ARE FORMED BY GLYCOSIDIC BONDS

Monosaccharides combine into larger molecules by forming **glycosidic bonds:** acetal or ketal bonds involving the anomeric carbon of one of the participating monosaccharides. The anomeric carbon forms the bond in either the α- or the β-configuration. Once the bond is formed, mutarotation is no longer possible, and the bond is locked in its conformation. For example, the structures of maltose and cellobiose in *Figure 1.6* differ only in the orientation of their 1,4-glycosidic bond.

Structures formed from two monosaccharides are called **disaccharides.** Products with three, four, five, or six monosaccharides are called trisaccharides, tetrasaccharides, pentasaccharides, and hexasaccharides, respectively. **Oligosaccharides** (from Greek Ολιγοσ meaning "a few") contain "a few" monosaccharides, and **polysaccharides** (from Greek πολυσ meaning "many") contain "many" monosaccharides (*Fig. 1.7*).

Carbohydrates can form glycosidic bonds with noncarbohydrates. In **glycoproteins,** carbohydrate is covalently bound to amino acid side chains. In **glycolipids,** carbohydrate is covalently bound to a lipid core. If the sugar binds its partner through an oxygen atom, the bond is called **O-glycosidic;** if the bond is through nitrogen, it is called **N-glycosidic.**

Monosaccharides, disaccharides, and oligosaccharides, commonly known as "sugars," are water soluble because of their high hydrogen bonding potential. Many polysaccharides, however, are insoluble because their large size increases the opportunities for intermolecular interactions. Things become insoluble when the molecules interact more strongly with one another than with the surrounding water.

The carbonyl group of the monosaccharides has reducing properties. *The reducing properties are lost when the carbonyl carbon forms a glycosidic bond.* Of the disaccharides in *Figure 1.6*, only sucrose is not a reducing sugar because both anomeric carbons participate in the glycosidic bond. The other disaccharides have a reducing end and a nonreducing end.

POLYPEPTIDES ARE FORMED FROM AMINO ACIDS

Polypeptides are constructed from 20 different amino acids. All amino acids have a **carboxyl group** and an **amino group,** both bound to the same carbon. This carbon, called the **α-carbon,** also carries a hydrogen atom and a fourth group, the **side chain,** which differs in the 20 amino acids. The general structure of the amino acids can be depicted as follows,

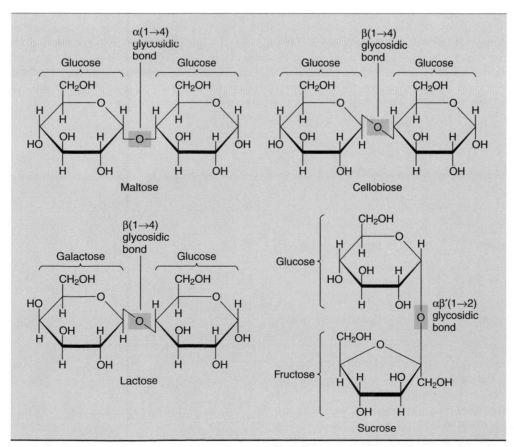

Figure 1.6 Structures of some common disaccharides. By convention, the nonreducing end of the disaccharide is written on the left side and the reducing end on the right side.

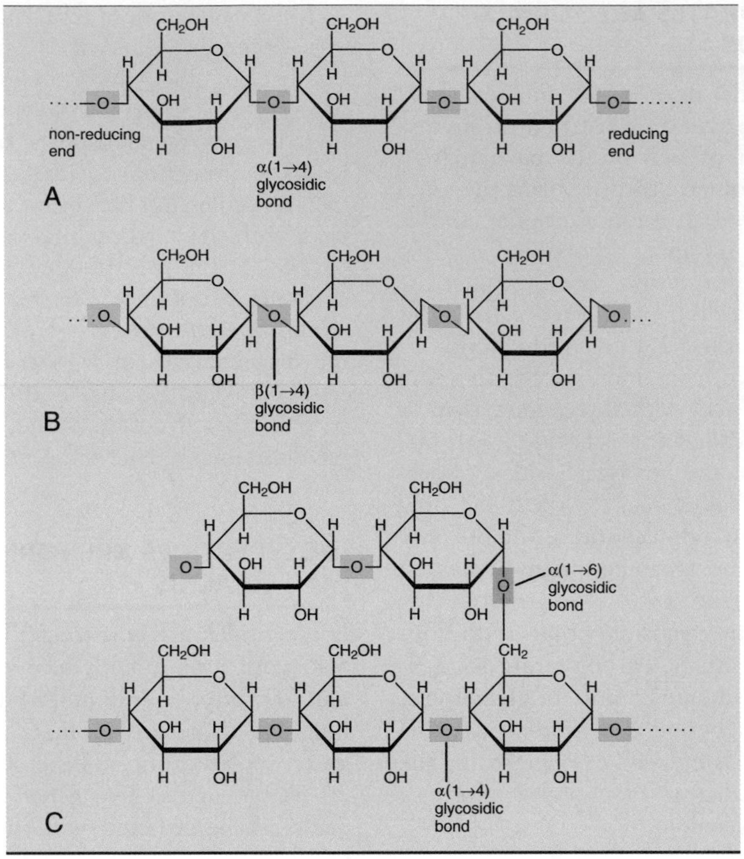

Figure 1.7 Structures of some common polysaccharides. **A,** Amylose is an unbranched polymer of glucose residues in α-1, 4-glycosidic linkage. Together with amylopectin—a branched glucose polymer with a structure resembling glycogen—it forms the starch granules in plants. **B,** Like amylose, cellulose is an unbranched polymer of glucose residues. As a major cell wall constituent of plants, it is the most abundant biomolecule on earth. The marked difference in the physical and biological properties between the two polysaccharides is caused by the presence in cellulose of β-1,4-glycosidic bonds rather than α-1, 4-glycosidic bonds. **C,** Glycogen is the storage polysaccharide of animals and humans. Like amylose, it contains chains of glucose residues in α-1,4-glycosidic linkage. Unlike amylose, however, the molecule is branched. Some glucose residues in the chain form a third glycosidic bond, using their hydroxyl group at carbon 6.

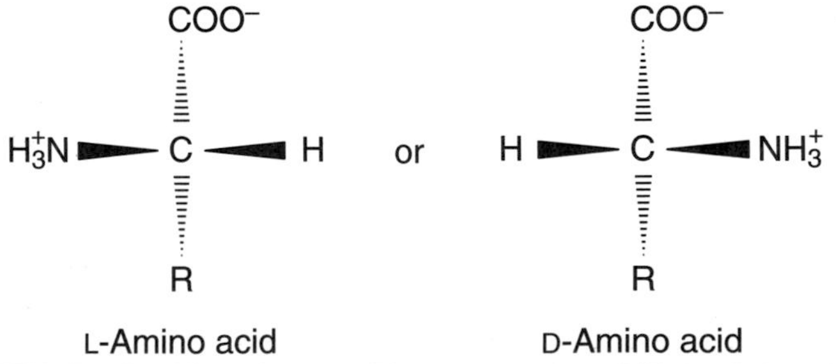

where R (residue) is the variable side chain. The α-carbon is asymmetrical, but of the two possible isomers, only the l-amino acids occur in polypeptides.

Dipeptides are formed by a reaction between the carboxyl group of one amino acid and the amino group of another amino acid. The substituted amide bond thus formed is called the **peptide bond**:

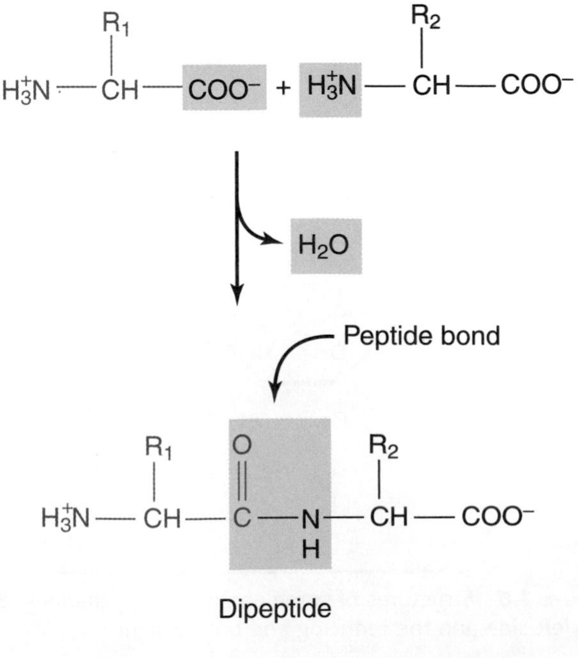

Chains of "a few" amino acids are called **oligopeptides**, and chains of "many" amino acids are called **polypeptides**.

NUCLEIC ACIDS ARE FORMED FROM NUCLEOTIDES

The nucleic acids consist of three kinds of building blocks:

1. A **pentose sugar,** which is ribose in ribonucleic acid (RNA) and 2-deoxyribose in 2-deoxyribonucleic acid (DNA):

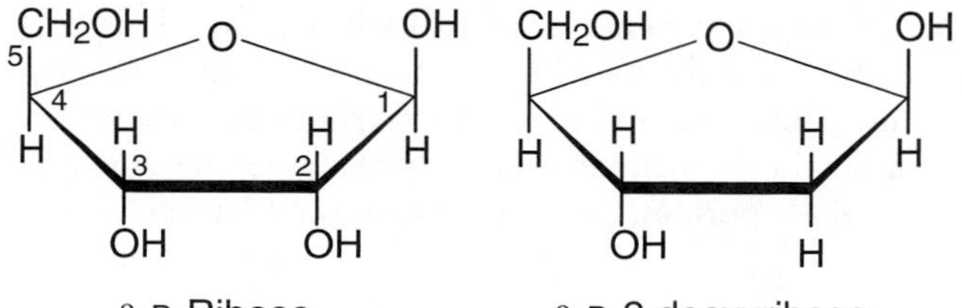

β-D-Ribose   β-D-2-deoxyribose

2. **Phosphate,** which is bound to hydroxyl groups of the sugar.

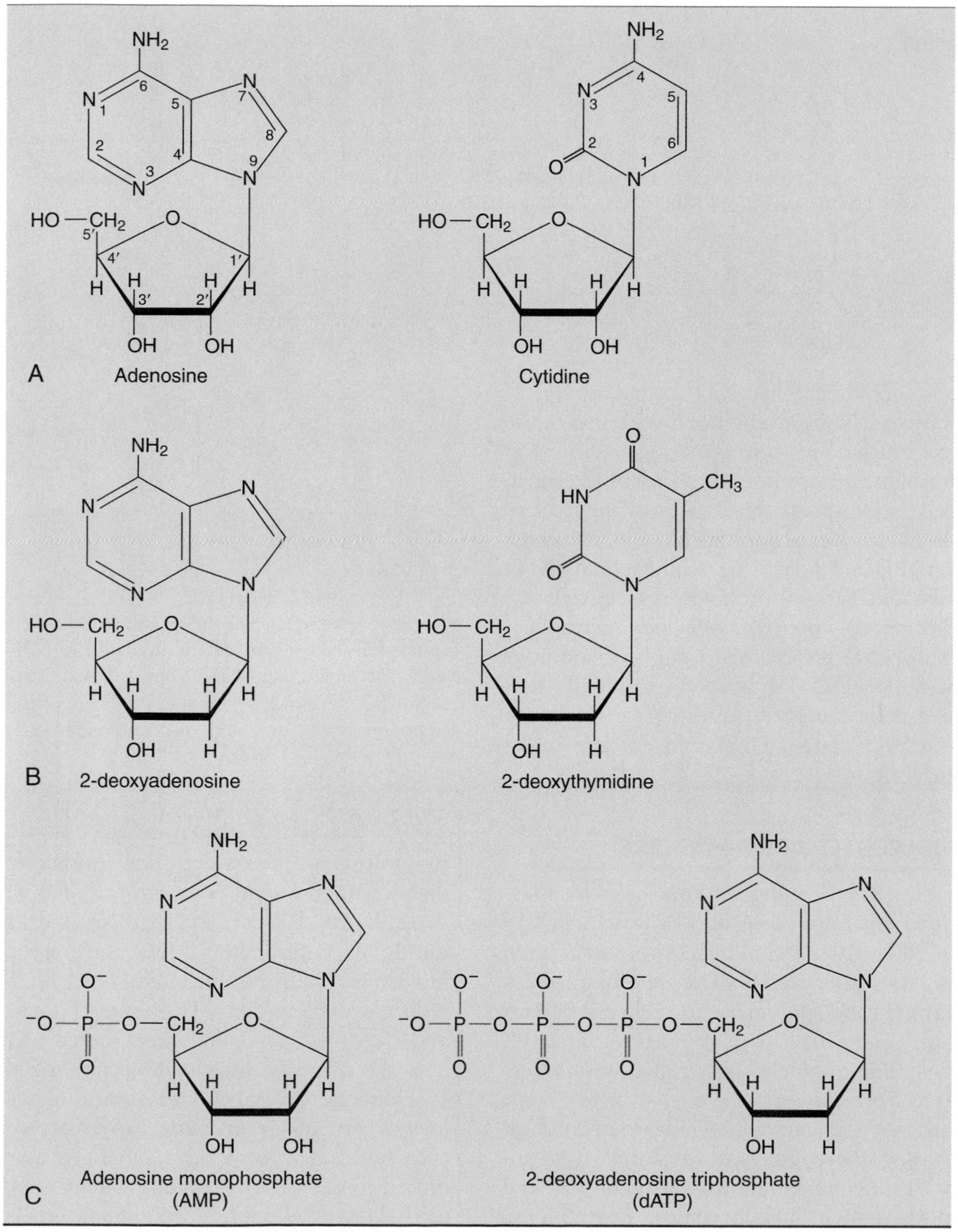

Figure 1.8   Structures of some nucleosides and nucleotides. A prime symbol (′) is used for the numbering of the carbons in the sugar to distinguish it from the numbering of the ring carbons and nitrogens in the bases. **A,** Examples of ribonucleosides. **B,** Examples of deoxyribonucleosides. **C,** Examples of nucleotides.

3. The bases **adenine, guanine, cytosine, uracil** (only in RNA), and **thymine** (only in DNA). Chemically, cytosine, thymine, and uracil are **pyrimidines,** containing a single six-member ring, whereas adenine and guanine are **purines,** consisting of two condensed rings:

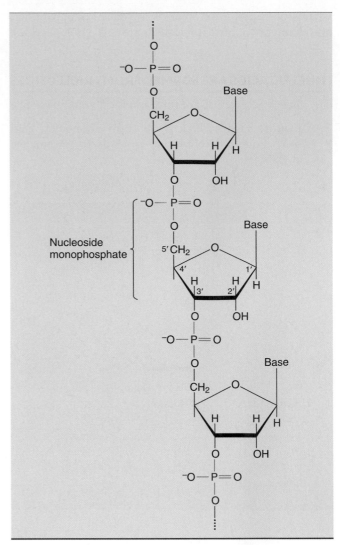

Adenine

Guanine

Cytosine   **Uracil**   **Thymine**

A **nucleoside** is obtained when C-1 of ribose or 2-deoxyribose forms an *N*-glycosidic bond with one of the bases (*Fig. 1.8*). **Nucleotides** consist of sugar, base, and up to three phosphate groups bound to C-5 of the sugar. They are named as phosphate derivatives of the nucleosides. Thus adenosine monophosphate (AMP), adenosine diphosphate (ADP), and adenosine triphosphate (ATP) contain one, two, and three phosphates, respectively.

Nucleic acids are polymers of nucleoside monophosphates. The phosphate group forms a phosphodiester bond between the 5′- and 3′-hydroxyl groups of adjacent ribose or 2-deoxyribose residues (*Fig. 1.9*). Most nucleic acids are very large. DNA can contain many millions of nucleotides.

MOST BIOMOLECULES ARE POLYMERS

The carbohydrates, polypeptides, and nucleic acids illustrate how nature generates molecules of large size and almost infinite diversity by linking simple-structured building blocks into long chains. The macromolecules formed this way are called **polymers** (from Greek πολυσ meaning "many" and Greek μερoσ meaning "part"), whereas their building blocks are called **monomers** (from Greek μoνoσ meaning "single").

Structural diversity is greatest when more than one kind of monomer is used. Polypeptides, for example, are constructed from 20 different amino acids, and DNA and RNA each contains four different bases. Like colored beads in a necklace, these components can be arranged in unique sequences; 20^{100} different sequences are possible for a protein of 100 amino acids, and 4^{100} different sequences are possible for a nucleic acid of 100 nucleotides.

Figure 1.9 Structure of ribonucleic acid (RNA). Deoxyribonucleic acid (DNA) has a similar structure, but it contains 2-deoxyribose instead of ribose. The nucleic acids are polymers of nucleoside monophosphates.

SUMMARY

Biomolecules interact with one another and with water through noncovalent interactions. Their water solubility depends on their ability to form hydrogen bonds or ion-dipole interactions with the surrounding water molecules. Hydrophobic interactions, on the other hand, reduce water solubility. These interactions are reversible, and they are far weaker than the covalent bonds that hold the atoms within the molecules together.

There are several classes of biomolecules. Triglycerides consist of glycerol and three fatty acids linked by ester bonds; carbohydrates consist of monosaccharides linked by glycosidic bonds; proteins consist of amino acids linked by peptide bonds; and nucleic acids consist of nucleoside monophosphates linked by phosphodiester bonds. Polysaccharides, polypeptides, and nucleic acids are polymers: long chains of covalently linked building blocks. Forming the bonds in these large molecules requires metabolic energy, whereas cleavage of the bonds releases energy.

Many biomolecules have ionizable groups. Molecules with free carboxyl groups or covalently bound phosphate carry negative charges at neutral pH, and those with aliphatic (nonaromatic) amino groups carry positive charges. These charges make the molecules water soluble, and they permit the formation of salt bonds with inorganic ions and with other biomolecules. The tendency of an ionizable group to accept or donate protons (positively charged hydrogen ions) is described by its pK value. If the pK value is known, then the percentage of an ionizable group that is in the protonated or deprotonated state at any given pH can be predicted.

QUESTIONS

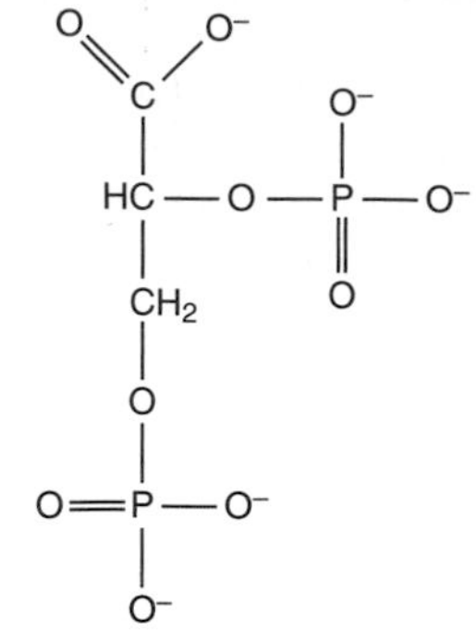

1 **The molecule shown here (2,3-bisphosphoglycerate [BPG]) is present in red blood cells, in which it binds noncovalently to hemoglobin. Which functional groups in hemoglobin can make the strongest noncovalent interactions with BPG at a pH value of 7.0?**

A. Sulfhydryl groups
B. Alcoholic hydroxyl groups
C. Hydrocarbon groups
D. Amino groups
E. Carboxyl groups

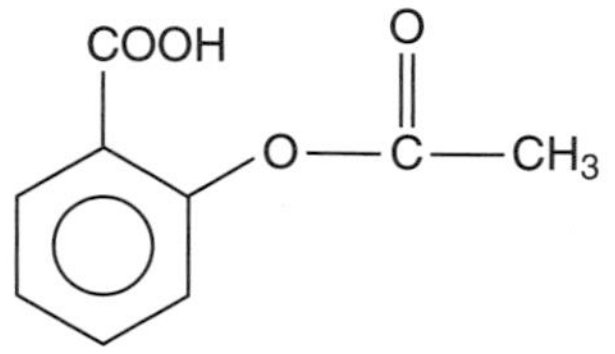

2. **The molecule shown here is acetylsalicylic acid (aspirin). What kind of electrical charge does aspirin carry in the stomach at a pH value of 2 and in the small intestine at a pH value of 7?**

A. Negatively charged in the stomach; positively charged in the intestine
B. Negatively charged both in the stomach and the intestine
C. Uncharged in the stomach; negatively charged in the intestine
D. Uncharged both in the stomach and the intestine
E. Uncharged in the stomach; positively charged in the intestine

3. **Inorganic phosphate, which is a major anion in the intracellular space, has three acidic functions with pK values of 2.3, 6.9, and 12.3, as shown below. In skeletal muscle fibers, the intracytoplasmic pH is about 7.1 at rest and 6.6 during vigorous anaerobic exercise. What does this mean for inorganic phosphate in muscle tissue?**

A. Phosphate molecules absorb protons when the pH decreases during anaerobic exercise.
B. On average, the phosphate molecules carry more negative charges during anaerobic contraction than at rest.
C. Phosphate molecules release protons when the pH decreases during anaerobic exercise.
D. The most abundant form of the phosphate molecule in the resting muscle fiber carries one negative charge.

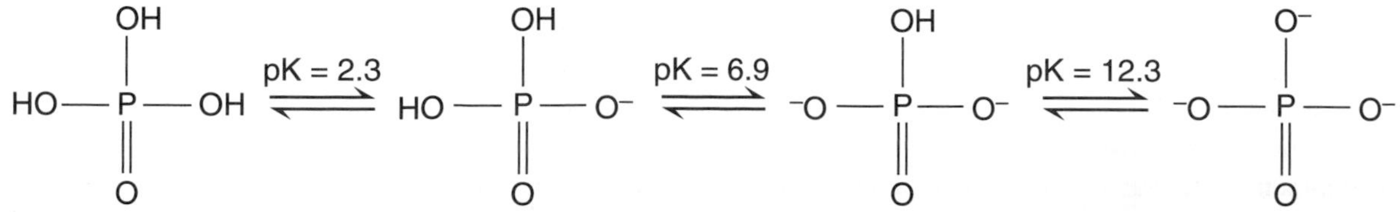

Proteins are the labor force of the cell. Membrane proteins join hands with the fibrous proteins of the cytoplasm and the extracellular matrix to keep cells and tissues in shape, enzyme proteins catalyze metabolic reactions, and DNA-binding proteins regulate gene expression.

Proteins consist of polypeptides: unbranched chains of amino acids with lengths ranging from less than 100 to more than 4000 amino acids. They form complex higher-order structures that are held together by noncovalent interactions, and they can consist of more than one polypeptide. Some proteins can fold into abnormal conformations that cause aggregation. Such abnormal protein aggregates are an important cause of neurodegenerative diseases and other age-related disorders.

This chapter discusses the 20 amino acids that occur in proteins, the noncovalent higher-order structures of proteins, their physical properties, and the diseases related to abnormal protein folding.

AMINO ACIDS ARE ZWITTERIONS

All amino acids have an α-carboxyl group, an α-amino group, a hydrogen atom, and a variable side chain R ("residue") bound to the **α-carbon.** This structure forms two optical isomers:

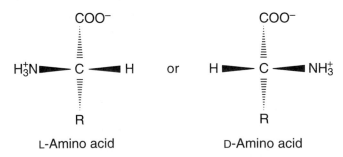

L-Amino acid   D-Amino acid

Only the L-amino acids occur in proteins. D-Amino acids are rare in nature, although they occur in some bacterial products.

The pK of the α-carboxyl group is always close to 2.0, and the pK of the α-amino group is near 9 or 10. The protonation state varies with the pH (*Fig. 2.1*).

At a pH below the pK of the carboxyl group, the amino acid is predominantly a cation; above the pK of the amino group, the amino acid is an anion; and between the two pK values, the amino acid is a **zwitterion** (from German *zwitter* meaning "hermaphrodite"), that is, a molecule carrying both a positive and a negative charge. The **isoelectric point (pI)** is defined as the *pH value at which the number of positive charges equals the number of negative charges.* For a simple amino acid such as alanine, the pI is halfway between the pK values of the two ionizable groups. Note that whereas the pK is the property of an individual ionizable group, the pI is a property of the whole molecule.

The pK values of the ionizable groups are revealed by treating an acidic solution of an amino acid with a strong base or by treating an alkaline solution with a strong acid. *Any ionizable group stabilizes the pH at values close to its pK because it releases protons when the pH in its environment rises, and it absorbs protons when the pH falls.* The **titration curve** shown in *Figure 2.2* has two flat segments that indicate the pK values of the two ionizable groups. In the body, the ionizable groups of proteins and other biomolecules stabilize the pH of the body fluids.

The titration curves of amino acids that have an additional acidic or basic group in the side chain show three rather than two buffering areas. The pI of the acidic amino acids is halfway between the pK values of the two acidic groups, and the pI of the basic amino acids is halfway between the pK values of the two basic groups (*Fig. 2.3*).

AMINO ACID SIDE CHAINS FORM MANY NONCOVALENT INTERACTIONS

The 20 amino acids can be placed in a few major groups (*Fig. 2.4*). Their side chains form noncovalent interactions in the proteins, and some form covalent bonds:

1. **Small amino acids:** Glycine and alanine occupy little space. Glycine, in particular, is found in places where two polypeptide chains have to come close together.

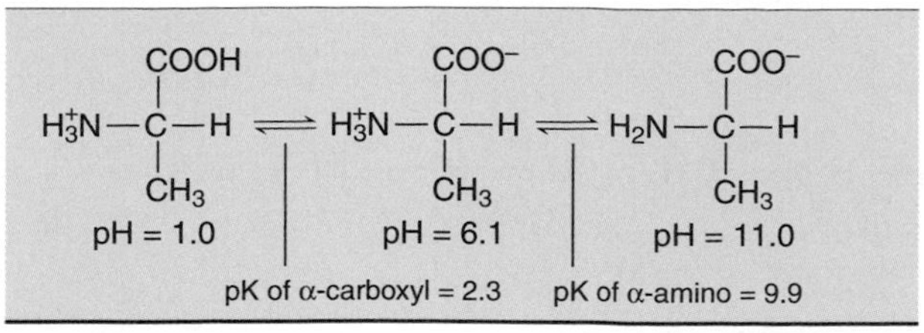

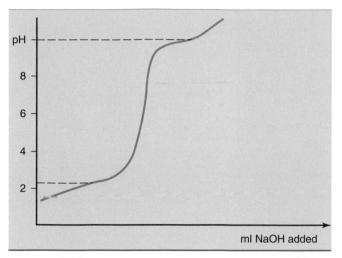

Figure 2.1 Protonation states of the amino acid alanine. The zwitterion is the predominant form in the pH range from 2.3 to 9.9.

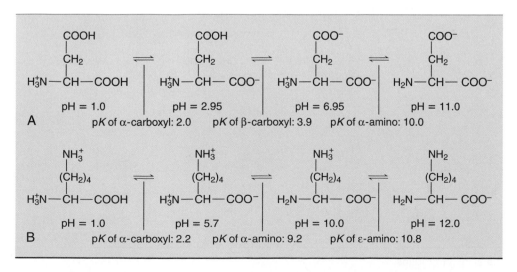

Figure 2.2 Titration curve of the amino acid alanine. The two level segments are caused by the buffering capacity of the carboxyl group (at pH 2.3) and the amino group (at pH 9.9).

2. **Branched-chain amino acids:** Valine, leucine, and isoleucine have hydrophobic side chains.
3. **Hydroxyl amino acids:** Serine and threonine form hydrogen bonds with their hydroxyl group. They also form covalent bonds with carbohydrates and with phosphate groups.

4. **Sulfur amino acids:** Cysteine and methionine are quite hydrophobic, although cysteine also has weak acidic properties. The sulfhydryl (—SH) group of cysteine can form a covalent disulfide bond with another cysteine side chain in the protein.
5. **Aromatic amino acids:** Phenylalanine, tyrosine, and tryptophan are hydrophobic, although the side chains of tyrosine and tryptophan can also form hydrogen bonds. The hydroxyl group of tyrosine can form a covalent bond with a phosphate group.
6. **Acidic amino acids:** Glutamate and aspartate have a carboxyl group in the side chain that is negatively charged at pH 7. The corresponding carboxamide groups in glutamine and asparagine are not acidic but form strong hydrogen bonds. Asparagine is an attachment point for carbohydrate in glycoproteins.
7. **Basic amino acids:** Lysine, arginine, and histidine carry a positive charge on the side chain, although the pK of the histidine side chain is quite low.
8. **Proline amino acid** is a freak among amino acids, with its nitrogen tied into a ring structure as a secondary amino group. Being stiff and angled, it is often found at bends in the polypeptide.

The pK values of the ionizable groups in amino acids and proteins are summarized in *Table 2.1*. Most negative charges in proteins are contributed by the side chains of glutamate and aspartate, and most positive charges are contributed by the side chains of lysine and arginine.

PEPTIDE BONDS AND DISULFIDE BONDS FORM THE PRIMARY STRUCTURE OF PROTEINS

The amino acids in the polypeptides are held together by **peptide bonds**. A **dipeptide** is formed by a reaction between the α-carboxyl and α-amino groups of two amino acids. For example,

Figure 2.3 Prevailing ionization states of the amino acids aspartate **(A)** and lysine **(B)** at different pH values. The isoelectric points of aspartate and lysine are 2.95 and 10.0, respectively.

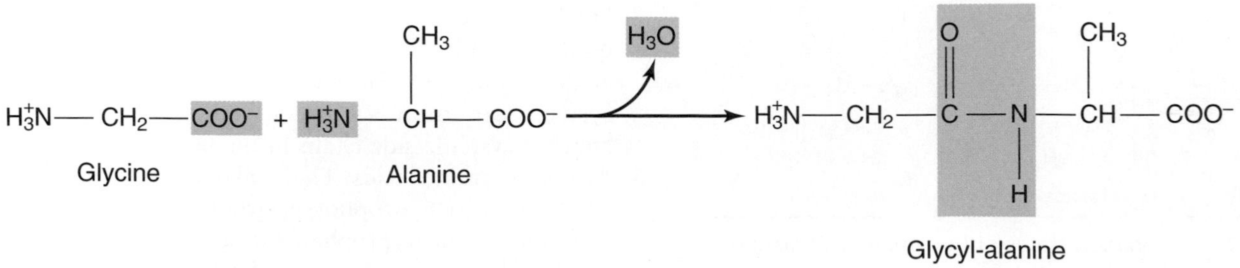

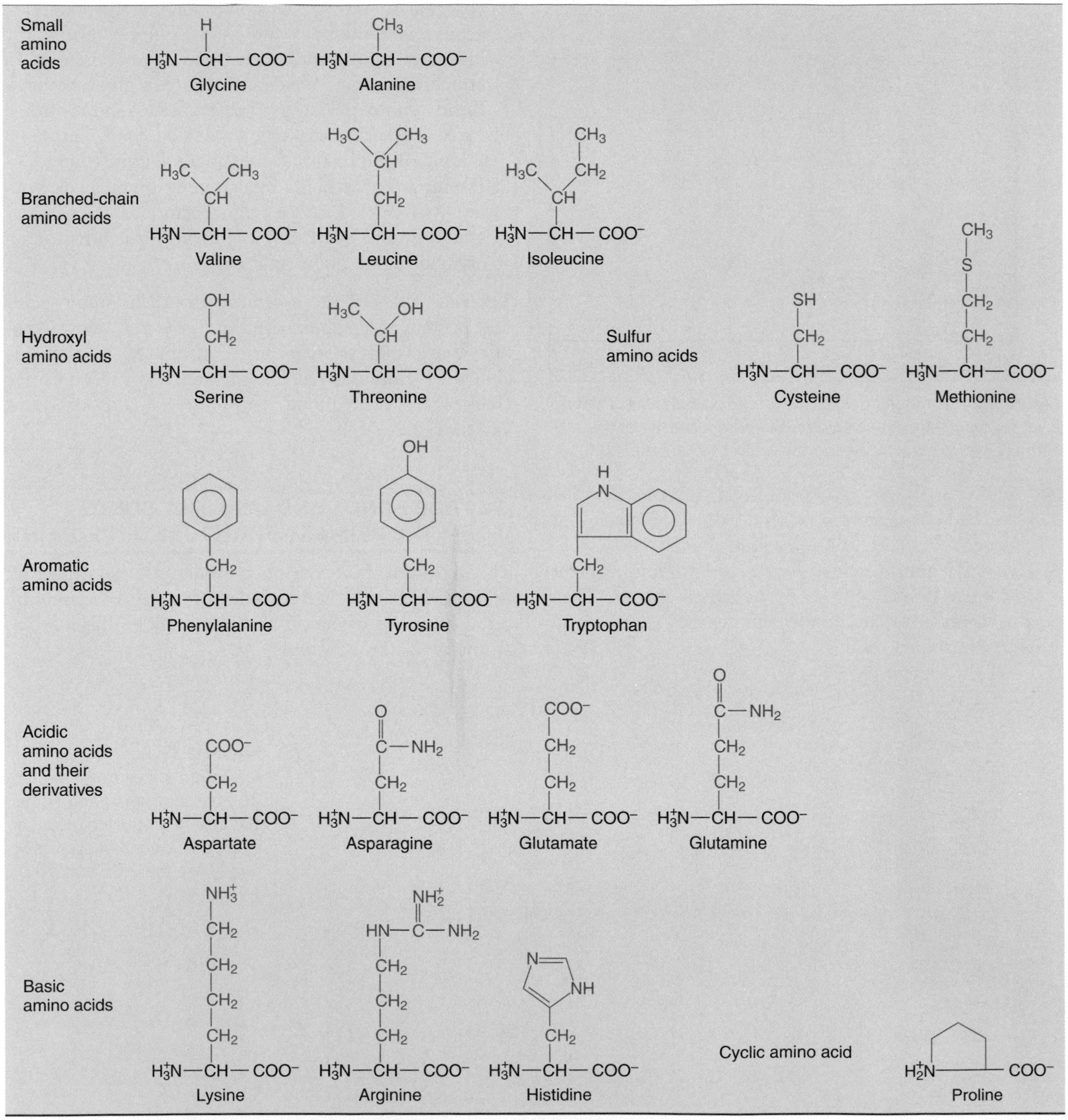

Figure 2.4 Structures of the amino acids in proteins.

Table 2.1 pK Values of Some Amino Acid Side Chains*

Amino Acid	Side Chain		pK
	Protonated Form	**Deprotonated Form**	
Glutamate	$-(CH_2)_2-COOH$	$-(CH_2)_2-COO^-$	4.3
Aspartate	$-CH_2-COOH$	$-CH_2-COO^-$	3.9
Cysteine	$-CH_2-SH$	$-CH_2-S^-$	8.3
Tyrosine	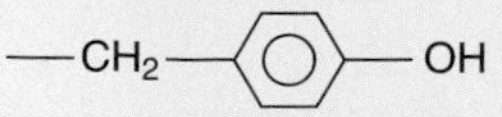 $-CH_2-\bigcirc-OH$	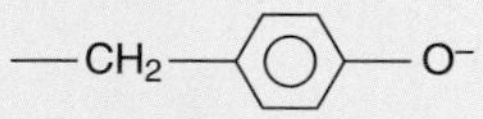 $-CH_2-\bigcirc-O^-$	10.1
Lysine	$-(CH_2)_4-NH_3^+$	$-(CH_2)_4-NH_2$	10.8
Arginine	$-(CH_2)_3-NH-\overset{\overset{NH_2^+}{\|\|}}{C}-NH_2$	$-(CH_2)_3-NH-\overset{\overset{NH}{\|\|}}{C}-NH_2$	12.5
Histidine	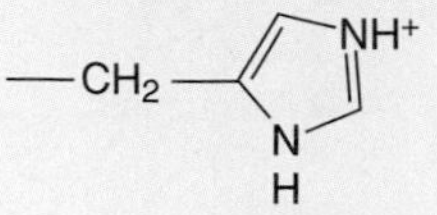 $-CH_2-$ imidazole NH$^+$	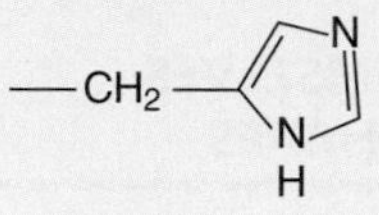 $-CH_2-$ imidazole N	6.0
α-Carboxyl (free amino acid)			1.8–2.4
α-Amino (free amino acid)			≈9.0–10.0
Terminal carboxyl (peptide)			≈3.0–4.5
Terminal amino (peptide)			≈7.5–9.0

*In proteins, the side chain pK values may differ by more than one pH unit from those in the free amino acids.

Adding more amino acids produces **oligopeptides** and finally **polypeptides** (*Fig. 2.5*). Each peptide has an **amino terminus,** conventionally written on the left side, and a **carboxyl terminus,** written on the right side. The peptide bond is not ionizable, but it can form hydrogen bonds. Therefore peptides and proteins tend to be water soluble.

Many proteins contain **disulfide bonds** between the side chains of cysteine residues. They are formed in a reductive reaction in which the two hydrogen atoms of the sulfhydryl groups are transferred to an acceptor molecule:

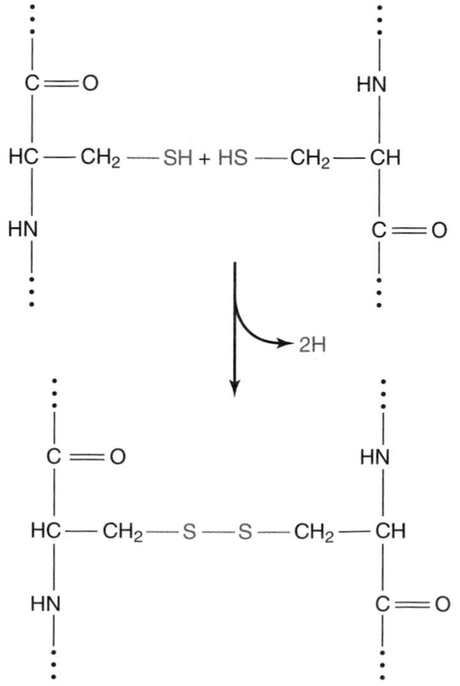

The disulfide bond can be formed between two cysteines in the same polypeptide (intra-chain) or in different polypeptides (inter-chain). The reaction takes place in the endoplasmic reticulum (ER), where secreted proteins and membrane proteins are processed. Therefore *most secreted proteins and membrane proteins have disulfide bonds.* Most cytoplasmic proteins, which do not pass through the ER, have no disulfide bonds.

The enzymatic degradation of disulfide-containing proteins yields the amino acid **cystine:**

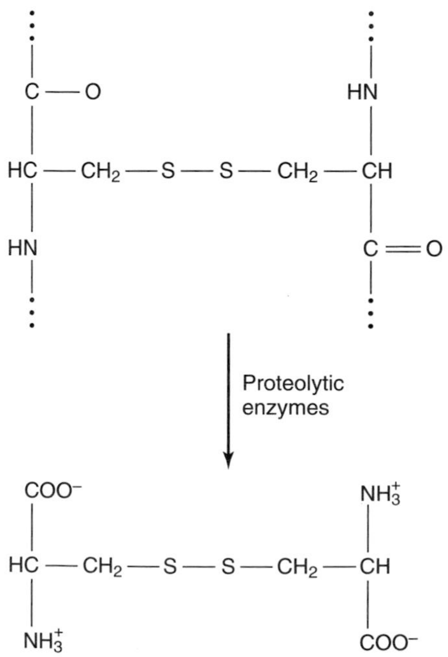

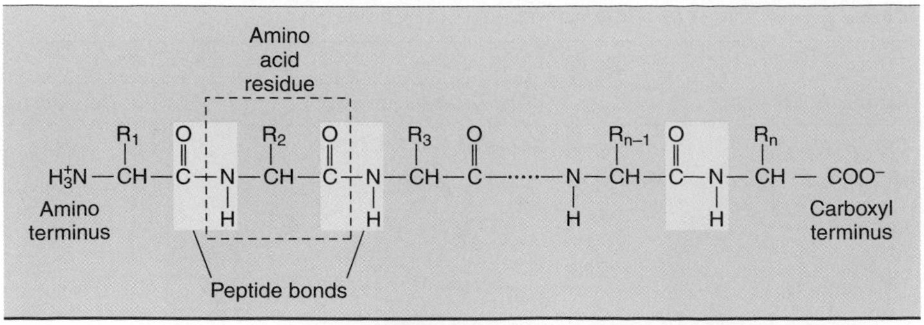

Figure 2.5 Structure of polypeptides. Note the polarity of the chain, with a free amino group at one end of the chain and a free carboxyl group at the opposite end.

The covalent structure of the protein, as described by its amino acid sequence and the positions of disulfide bonds, is called its **primary structure.**

PROTEINS CAN FOLD THEMSELVES INTO MANY DIFFERENT SHAPES

The peptide bond is conventionally written as a single bond, with four substituents attached to the carbon and nitrogen of the bond:

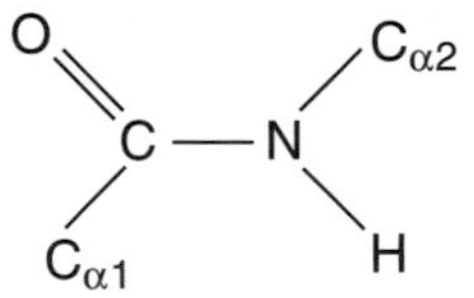

A C—N single bond, like a C—C single bond, should show free rotation. The triangular plane formed by the O=C—Cα1 portion should be able to rotate out of the plane of the Cα2—N—H portion. Actually, however, the peptide bond is a resonance hybrid of two structures:

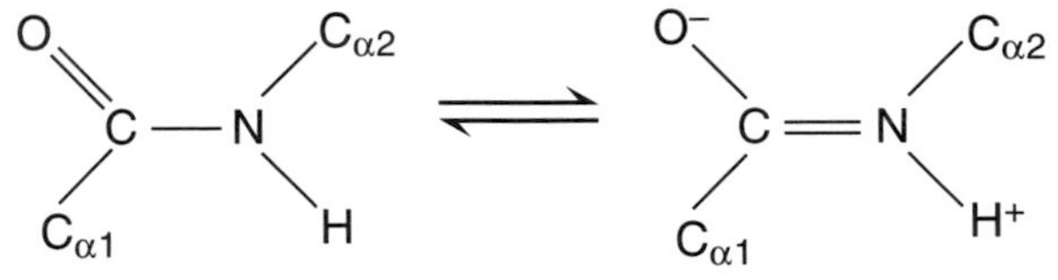

Its "real" structure is between these two extremes. One consequence is that, like C=C double bonds (see Chapters 12 and 23), *the peptide bond does not rotate.* Its four substituents are fixed in the same plane. The two α-carbons are in *trans* configuration, opposite each other.

The other two bonds in the polypeptide backbone, those involving the α-carbon, are "pure" single bonds with the expected rotational freedom. Rotation around the nitrogen—α-carbon bond is measured as the Φ (phi) angle, and rotation around the peptide bond carbon—α-carbon bond as the ψ (psi) angle (*Fig. 2.6*). This rotational freedom turns the polypeptide into a contortionist that can bend and twist itself into many shapes.

Globular proteins have compact shapes. Most are water soluble, but some are embedded in cellular membranes or form supramolecular aggregates, such as the ribosomes. Hemoglobin and myoglobin (see Chapter 3), enzymes

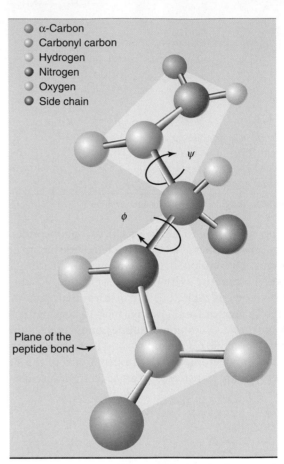

- α-Carbon
- Carbonyl carbon
- Hydrogen
- Nitrogen
- Oxygen
- Side chain

Plane of the peptide bond →

Figure 2.6 Geometry of the peptide bond. The Φ and ψ angles are variable.

(see Chapter 4), membrane proteins (see Chapter 12), and plasma proteins (see Chapter 15) are globular proteins. **Fibrous proteins** are long and threadlike, and most serve structural functions. The keratins of hair, skin, and fingernails are fibrous proteins (see Chapter 13), as are the collagen and elastin of the extracellular matrix (see Chapter 14).

α-HELIX AND β-PLEATED SHEET ARE THE MOST COMMON SECONDARY STRUCTURES IN PROTEINS

A **secondary structure** is a regular, repetitive structure that emerges when all the Φ angles in the polypeptide are the same and all the ψ angles are the same.

Only a few secondary structures are energetically possible.

In the **α-helix** (*Fig. 2.7*), the polypeptide backbone forms a right-handed corkscrew. "Right-handed" refers to the direction of the turn: When the thumb of the right hand pushes along the helix axis, the flexed fingers describe the twist of the polypeptide. The threads of screws and bolts are right-handed, too. The α-helix is very compact. Each full turn has 3.6 amino acid residues, and each amino acid is advanced 1.5 angstrom units (Å) along the helix axis (1 Å $= 10^{-1}$ nm $= 10^{-4}$ μm $= 10^{-7}$ mm). Therefore a complete turn advances by $3.6 \times 1.5 = 5.4$ Å, or 0.54 nm.

The α-helix is maintained by hydrogen bonds between the peptide bonds. Each peptide bond C—O is hydrogen bonded to the peptide bond N—H four amino acid residues ahead of it. Each C—O and each N—H in the main chain are hydrogen bonded. The N, H, and O form a nearly straight line, which is the energetically favored alignment for hydrogen bonds.

The amino acid side chains face outward, away from the helix axis. The side chains can stabilize or destabilize the helix, but they are not essential for helix

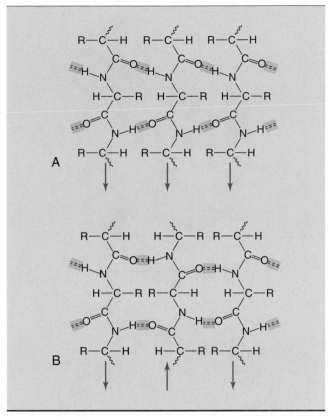

Figure 2.8 Structure of the parallel and antiparallel β-pleated sheets. **A**, The parallel β-pleated sheet. **B**, The antiparallel β-pleated sheet. *Arrows* indicate the direction of the polypeptide chain.

formation. Proline is too rigid to fit into the α-helix, and glycine is too flexible. Glycine can assume too many alternative conformations that are energetically more favorable than the α-helix.

The **β-pleated sheet** (*Fig. 2.8*) is far more extended than the α helix, with each amino acid advancing by 3.5 Å. In this stretched-out structure, *hydrogen bonds are formed between the peptide bond C—O and N—H groups of polypeptides that lie side by side.* The interacting chains can be aligned either parallel or antiparallel, and they can belong either to different polypeptides or to different sections of the same polypeptide. Blanketlike structures are formed when more than two polypeptides participate. The α-helix and β-pleated sheet occur in both fibrous and globular proteins.

GLOBULAR PROTEINS HAVE A HYDROPHOBIC CORE

Many fibrous proteins contain long threads of α-helix or β-pleated sheets, but globular proteins fold themselves into a compact **tertiary structure.** Sections of secondary structure are short, usually less than 30 amino acids in length, and they alternate with irregularly

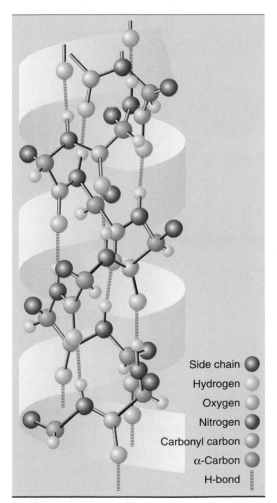

Side chain ⬤
Hydrogen ◯
Oxygen ⬤
Nitrogen ⬤
Carbonyl carbon ◯
α-Carbon ⬤
H-bond ⋮

Figure 2.7 Structure of the α-helix.

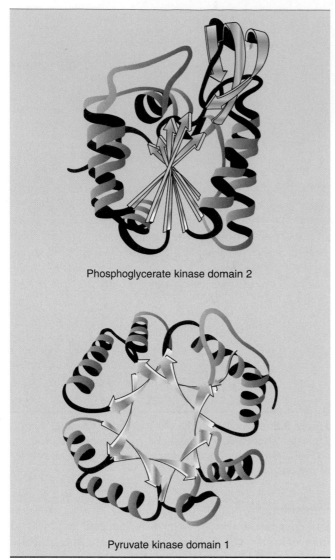

Phosphoglycerate kinase domain 2

Pyruvate kinase domain 1

Figure 2.9 Structures of globular protein domains containing both α-helical *(corkscrew)* and β-pleated sheet *(arrow)* structures. These short sections of secondary structure are separated by nonhelical portions.

folded sequences (*Fig. 2.9*). Unlike the α-helix and β-pleated sheet, *tertiary structures are formed mainly by hydrophobic interactions between amino acid side chains.* These amino acid side chains form a hydrophobic core.

Quaternary structures are defined by the interactions between different polypeptides (**subunits**). Therefore only proteins with two or more polypeptides have a quaternary structure. In some of these proteins, the subunits are held together only by noncovalent interactions, but others are stabilized by inter-chain disulfide bonds.

Glycoproteins contain covalently bound carbohydrate, and **phosphoproteins** contain covalently bound

phosphate. Other nonpolypeptide components can be bound to the protein, either covalently or noncovalently. They are called **prosthetic groups** (*Fig. 2.10*). Many enzymes, for example, contain prosthetic groups that participate as coenzymes in enzymatic catalysis.

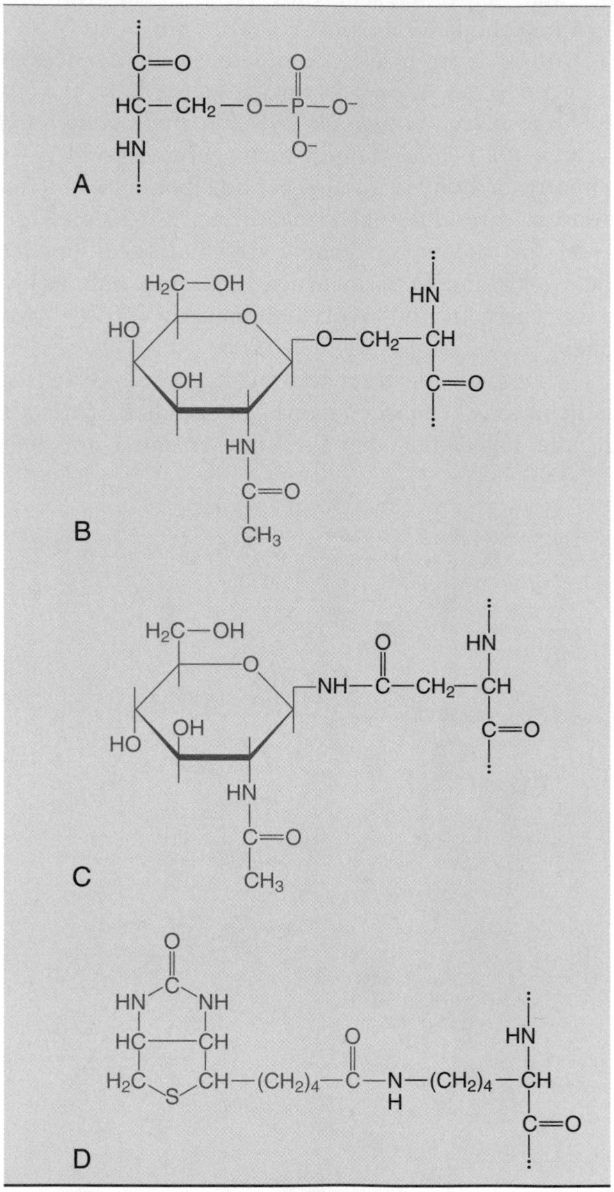

Figure 2.10 Examples of posttranslational modifications in proteins. **A,** A phosphoserine residue. Aside from serine, threonine and tyrosine can form phosphate bonds in proteins. **B,** An *N*-acetylgalactosamine residue bound to a serine side chain. Serine and threonine form *O*-glycosidic bonds in glycoproteins. **C,** An *N*-acetylglucosamine residue bound to an asparagine side chain by an *N*-glycosidic bond. **D,** Some enzymes contain a covalently bound prosthetic group. As a coenzyme (see Chapter 5), the prosthetic group participates in the enzymatic reaction. This example shows biotin, which is bound covalently to a lysine side chain.

PROTEINS LOSE THEIR BIOLOGICAL ACTIVITIES WHEN THEIR HIGHER-ORDER STRUCTURE IS DESTROYED

Peptide bonds can be cleaved by heating with strong acids and bases. Proteolytic enzymes (proteases) achieve the same effect but in a gentle way, as occurs during protein digestion in the stomach and intestine. Disulfide bonds are cleaved by reducing or oxidizing agents:

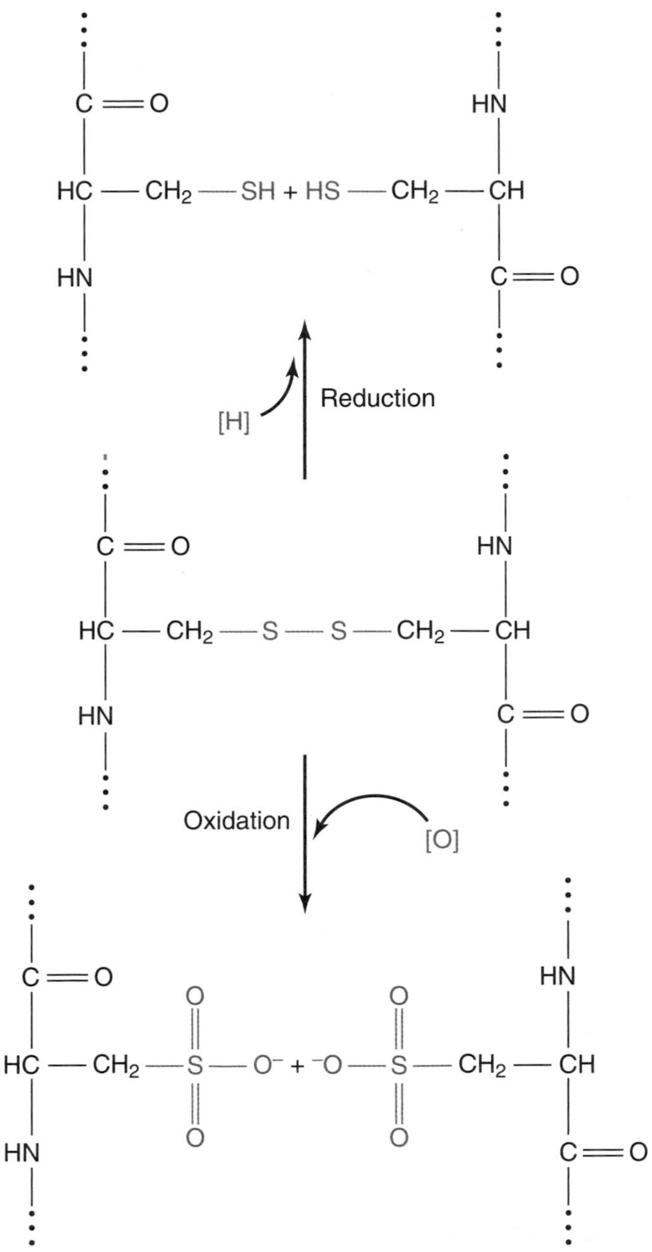

However, the noncovalent interactions are so weak that *the higher-order structure of proteins can be destroyed by heating*. Within a few minutes of being heated above a certain temperature (often between 50°C and 80°C), the higher-order structure collapses into a messy tanglework known as a **random coil**. This process is called **heat denaturation.**

Denaturation destroys the protein's biological properties. Stated another way, *the biological properties of proteins require intact higher-order structures*. Also the physical properties of the protein change dramatically with denaturation. For example, water solubility is lost because the denatured polypeptide chains become irrevocably entangled. Generally, *protein denaturation is irreversible*. A boiled egg does not become unboiled when it is kept in the cold. Only a few simple-structured proteins can be renatured under carefully controlled laboratory conditions.

Not only heat but anything that disrupts noncovalent interactions can denature proteins. Many **detergents** and **organic solvents** denature proteins by disrupting hydrophobic interactions. Being nonpolar, they insert themselves between the side chains of hydrophobic amino acids. Strong **acids** and **bases** denature proteins by changing their charge pattern. In a strong acid, the protein loses its negative charges; in a strong base, it loses its positive charges. This deprives the protein of intramolecular salt bonds. Also, high concentrations of small hydrophilic molecules with high hydrogen bonding potential, such as urea, can denature proteins. They do so by disrupting the hydrogen bonds between water molecules. This limits the extent to which water molecules are forced into a thermodynamically unfavorable "ordered" position at an aqueous-nonpolar interface, weakening the hydrophobic interactions within the protein.

Heavy metal ions (e.g., lead, cadmium, and mercury) can denature proteins by binding to carboxylate groups and, in particular, sulfhydryl groups in proteins. This affinity for functional groups in proteins is one reason for the toxicity of heavy metals.

The fragility of life is appalling. A 6°C rise of the body temperature can be fatal, and the blood pH must never fall below 7.0 or rise above 7.7 for any length of time. These subtle changes in the physical environment do not cleave covalent bonds, but *they disrupt noncovalent interactions*. It is because of the vulnerability of noncovalent higher-order structures that living beings had to evolve homeostatic mechanisms for the maintenance of their internal environment.

THE SOLUBILITY OF PROTEINS DEPENDS ON pH AND SALT CONCENTRATION

Unlike fibrous proteins, most globular proteins are water soluble. Their solubility is affected by the salt concentration. Raising the salt concentration from 0% to 1% or more increases their solubility because the salt ions neutralize the electrical charges on the protein, thereby reducing electrostatic attraction between neighboring protein molecules (*Fig. 2.11, A and B*). Very high salt concentrations, however, precipitate proteins because most of the water molecules become tied up in the hydration shells of the salt ions. Effectively, the salt competes with the protein for the available solvent.

Figure 2.11 Effects of salt and pH on protein solubility. **A,** Protein in distilled water. Salt bonds between protein molecules cause the molecules to aggregate. The protein becomes insoluble. **B,** Protein in 5% sodium chloride (NaCl). Salt ions bind to the surface charges of the protein molecules, thereby preventing intermolecular salt bonds. **C,** The effect of pH on protein solubility. The formation of intermolecular salt bonds is favored at the isoelectric point. At pH values greater or less than the p*I*, the electrostatic interactions between the molecules are mainly repulsive.

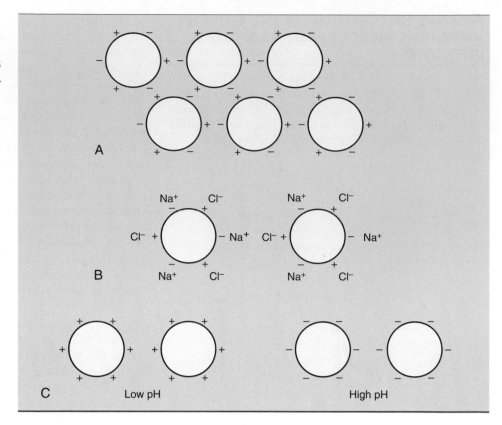

The addition of a water-miscible organic solvent (e.g., ethanol) can precipitate proteins because the organic solvent competes for the available water. Unlike denaturation, precipitation is reversible and does not permanently destroy the protein's biological properties.

The pH value is also important. When the pH is at the protein's p*I*, the protein carries equal numbers of positive and negative charges. This maximizes the opportunities for the formation of intermolecular salt bonds, which glue the protein molecules together into insoluble aggregates or crystals (*Fig. 2.11, A* and *C*). Therefore *the solubility of proteins is minimal at their isoelectric point.*

PROTEINS ABSORB ULTRAVIOLET RADIATION

Proteins do not absorb visible light. Therefore they are uncolored unless they contain a colored prosthetic group, such as the heme group in hemoglobin or retinal in the visual pigment rhodopsin. They do, however, absorb ultraviolet radiation with two absorption maxima. One absorbance peak, at 190 nm, is caused by the peptide bonds. A second peak, at 280 nm, is caused by aromatic amino acid side chains. The peak at 280 nm is more useful in laboratory practice because it is relatively specific for proteins. Nucleic acids, however, have an absorbance peak at 260 nm that overlaps the 280-nm peak of proteins (*Fig. 2.12*).

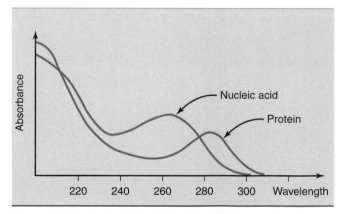

Figure 2.12 Typical ultraviolet absorbance spectra of proteins and nucleic acids. The protein absorbance peak at 280 nm is caused by the aromatic side chains of tyrosine and tryptophan. Nucleic acids absorb at 260 nm because of the aromatic character of their purine and pyrimidine bases.

PROTEINS CAN BE SEPARATED BY THEIR CHARGE OR THEIR MOLECULAR WEIGHT

Dialysis is used in the laboratory to separate proteins from salts and other small contaminants. The protein is enclosed in a little bag of porous cellophane (*Fig. 2.13*). The pores allow salts and small molecules to diffuse out, but the large proteins are retained.

Electrophoresis separates proteins according to their charge-mass ratio, based on their movement in an

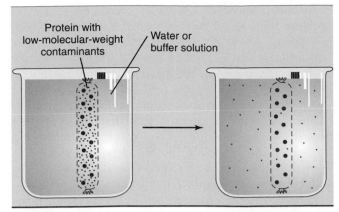

Figure 2.13 Use of dialysis for protein purification. Only small molecules and inorganic ions can pass through the porous membrane.

electrical field. At pH values above the protein's p*I*, the protein carries mainly negative charges and moves to the anode; at pH values below the protein's p*I*, it carries mainly positive charges and moves to the cathode. At the p*I*, the net charge is zero, and the protein stays put.

Electrophoresis on cellulose acetate foil, starch gel, and other carrier materials is the standard method for separation of plasma proteins and detection of abnormal proteins in the clinical laboratory (**Fig. 2.14, A**). When a structurally abnormal protein differs from its normal counterpart by a single amino acid substitution, *the electrophoretic mobility is changed only if the charge pattern is changed.* For example, when a glutamate residue is replaced by aspartate, the electrophoretic mobility remains the same because these two amino acids carry the same charge. However, when glutamate is replaced by an

CLINICAL EXAMPLE 2.1: Hemodialysis

Between 40% and 50% of the blood volume is occupied by blood cells. The remaining fluid, called *plasma*, is a solution containing about 0.9% inorganic ions, 7% protein, and low concentrations of nutrients including 0.1% glucose. Water-soluble waste products such as urea (containing nitrogen from amino acid breakdown) and uric acid (from purine nucleotides) also are present, but their concentrations are low because they are removed continuously by the kidneys. In patients with kidney failure, these waste products accumulate to dangerous levels. The standard treatment is hemodialysis. In this procedure, the patient's blood is passed along semipermeable membranes. The pores in these membranes are small enough to allow the passage of low-molecular-weight waste products (but also salts and nutrients), but plasma proteins and blood cells are retained. The blood is dialyzed not against distilled water (which would lead to a malpractice suit) but against a solution with physiological concentrations of nutrients and inorganic ions.

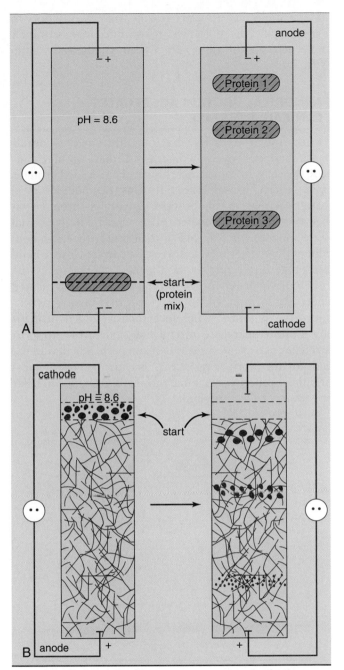

Figure 2.14 Protein separation by electrophoresis. **A,** On a wet cellulose acetate foil, the proteins are separated according to their net change. If an alkaline pH is used, as in this case, the proteins are negatively charged and move to the anode. **B,** Electrophoresis in a cross-linked polyacrylamide gel. Although small molecules can move in the field, larger ones "get stuck" in the gel. Under suitable pH conditions, this method separates on the basis of molecular weight rather than charge.

uncharged amino acid such as valine, one negative charge is removed, and the two proteins can be separated by electrophoresis.

Electrophoresis can be performed in a cross-linked polyacrylamide or agarose gel that impairs the movement of large molecules. At a pH at which all proteins move to the same pole, the molecules are separated mainly by their molecular weight rather than their charge–mass ratio (*Fig. 2.14, B*).

ABNORMAL PROTEIN AGGREGATES CAN CAUSE DISEASE

Ordinarily, proteins that have lost their native conformation are destroyed by proteases, either within or outside the cells. In some cases, however, misfolded proteins arrange into fibrils that are difficult to degrade. A typical pattern is seen in this process. A globular protein that has a rather flexible higher-order structure in its normal state spontaneously refolds into a state with a high content of β-pleated sheet. In some cases, stretches of α-helix rearrange into stretches of β-pleated sheet. Unlike the α-helix, which is strictly intramolecular, the β-pleated sheet can form extended structures that involve two or more polypeptides. Therefore these refolded proteins are prone to aggregate into fibrillar structures with short stretches of β-pleated sheet that run perpendicular to the axis of the fibril (*Fig. 2.15*). Because its histological staining properties resemble those of starch, this fibrillar material is called **amyloid**.

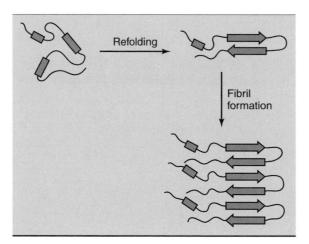

Figure 2.15 Formation of amyloid from a globular protein. In many cases, the α-helical structure *(barrels)* is lost and is replaced by the β-pleated sheet structure *(arrows)*.

Although amyloid is not very toxic and causes no immune response, it can damage the organs in which it deposits. About 20 different diseases are caused by amyloid deposits. In classic cases the amyloid is formed from a secreted protein and accumulates in the extracellular space.

Amyloid can be formed from a number of proteins (*Table 2.2*). One of them is **transthyretin**, a plasma protein whose function is the transport of thyroid hormones and retinol in the blood (see Chapter 15). Transthyretin-derived amyloid in heart, blood vessels, and kidneys is a frequent incidental autopsy finding in people who die after age 80. In severe cases, however, the amyloid causes organ damage. Heart failure and arrhythmias resulting from cardiac amyloidosis are a frequent cause of sudden death in centenarians.

Some structurally normal proteins cause amyloidosis when they are overproduced. The most common situation is the chronic overproduction of immunoglobulin light chains by an abnormal plasma cell clone. This is seen in many otherwise healthy old people (see Chapter 15). The amyloid can deposit in any organ system except the brain, with widely varying clinical consequences. A similar situation is observed for **serum amyloid A (SAA) protein,** which is normally associated with plasma lipoproteins. SAA is overproduced in inflammatory conditions, sometimes by as much as 100-fold. In chronic inflammatory diseases, SAA can form amyloid in the spleen and elsewhere. It also facilitates amyloid formation by other proteins because it binds tightly to the amyloid fibrils and thereby accelerates their formation or impairs their breakdown.

In advanced stages of type 2 diabetes mellitus, a small (37 amino acids) polypeptide known as **amylin or islet amyloid polypeptide (IAPP)** forms amyloid in the islets of Langerhans. Amylin is a hormone that is released by the pancreatic β-cells together with insulin. Possibly as a result of chronic oversecretion in the early stages of type 2 diabetes, amylin eventually deposits as amyloid in the islets of Langerhans. It is thought to contribute to the "burnout" of β-cells in the late stages of the disease.

Amyloidosis can be caused by a structurally abnormal protein. For example, normal transthyretin forms

Table 2.2 Some Forms of Amyloidosis

Type	Offending Protein	Sites of Deposition	Cause
Transthyretin amyloidosis	Transthyretin	Heart, kidneys, respiratory tract	Old age
AL amyloidosis	Immunoglobulin light chains	Systemic (excluding brain), sometimes local foci	Plasma cell dyscrasias (see Chapter 15)
AA amyloidosis	Serum amyloid A protein	Systemic (excluding brain)	Chronic inflammation
Dialysis-associated amyloidosis	β₂-microglobulin	Bones, joints	Hemodialysis
Type 2 diabetes mellitus	Islet amyloid polypeptide	Pancreatic islets	Oversecretion?
Alzheimer disease	β-amyloid precursor protein	Brain	Age-related, inherited mutation, Down syndrome

amyloid only late in life. However, some people are born with a point mutation that leads to a structurally abnormal transthyretin having a single amino acid substitution. More than 80 such mutations have been described, and most of them are amyloidogenic. Carriers of such mutations develop amyloidosis that leads to death in the second to sixth decade of life.

Hemodialysis is yet another setting in which amyloidosis can develop. In this case the culprit is β_2-microglobulin, a small cell surface protein that is involved in immune responses. To some extent, β_2-microglobulin detaches from the cells and appears in the blood plasma. Being small and water soluble, it is cleared mainly by the kidneys.

However, its removal by hemodialysis is inefficient, and its level can rise 50-fold in patients undergoing long-term hemodialysis. Under these conditions, β_2-microglobulin deposits as amyloid in bones and joints, causing painful arthritis.

NEURODEGENERATIVE DISEASES ARE CAUSED BY PROTEIN AGGREGATES

Most forms of amyloidosis spare the central nervous system because the offending proteins are rejected by the blood-brain barrier. However, aggregates of misfolded proteins can form in the brain itself, eventually

CLINICAL EXAMPLE 2.2: Alzheimer Disease

Alzheimer disease is the leading cause of senile dementia, affecting about 25% of people older than 75 years. Autopsy findings include **senile plaques** consisting of **β-amyloid (Aβ)** in the extracellular spaces and degenerating axons known as **neurofibrillary tangles** that are filled with aggregates of excessively phosphorylated tau protein.

Aβ is formed by the proteolytic cleavage of β-amyloid precursor protein (APP), a membrane protein that traverses the lipid bilayer of the plasma membrane by means of an α-helix. After an initial cleavage that is catalyzed by the protease **β-secretase,** another protease called **γ-secretase** cleaves the remaining polypeptide within the lipid bilayer of the plasma membrane, creating an intracellular fragment and the extracellular Aβ (**Fig. 2.16**). γ-Secretase cleavage is imprecise, and extracellular polypeptides of 40 and 42 amino acids can be formed. Less than 10% of the product is Aβ-42, but this form is far more amyloidogenic than Aβ-40. It folds into a form that contains a parallel β-pleated sheet with two stretches of 10 to 12 amino acids each.

This structure polymerizes into amyloid fibrils, forming the senile plaques.

Small aggregates of Aβ can interfere with membranes and therefore are toxic for the neurons. Through unknown mechanisms, Aβ appears to cause the abnormal phosphorylation and aggregation of tau protein in the axons.

Neurofibrillary tangles rather than senile plaques are most closely related to the severity of the disease, but Aβ seems to initiate the disease process. APP is encoded by a gene on chromosome 21, which is present in three instead of the normal two copies in patients with Down syndrome. Many patients with Down syndrome develop Alzheimer disease before the age of 50 years, probably because of overproduction of APP. Early-onset Alzheimer disease can be inherited as an autosomal dominant trait, caused by point mutations either in APP or in subunits of the γ-secretase complex. In many cases these mutations lead to overproduction of Aβ-42. The development of drugs that inhibit β-secretase or shift the cleavage specificity of γ-secretase away from the formation of Aβ-42 has not yet been successful, and Alzheimer disease still is incurable.

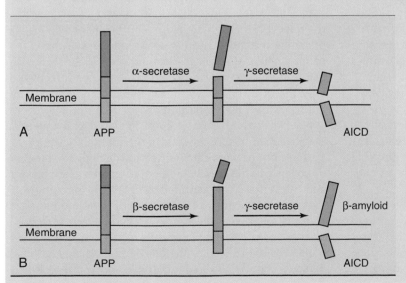

Figure 2.16 Degradation of β-amyloid precursor protein (APP). **A,** Cleavage by α-secretase followed by γ-secretase produces only innocuous products. **B,** Cleavage by β-secretase followed by γ-secretase produces β-amyloid. In Alzheimer disease, β-amyloid polymerizes into aggregates and eventually forms insoluble fibrils. *AICD,* β-Amyloid precursor protein intracellular domain.

killing the neurons. Because the brain has little extracellular space, most of these protein deposits are intracellular, and they do not always have the classic amyloid structure.

One example is **tau protein,** which stabilizes the microtubules in the axons of neurons. Its affinity for microtubules is regulated by reversible phosphorylation and dephosphorylation of serine and threonine side chains. In several neurodegenerative diseases, including **Alzheimer disease** and **frontotemporal dementia,** excessively phosphorylated ("hyperphosphorylated") tau protein forms filamentous aggregates in the axons, causing their eventual demise. Some people are born with a structurally abnormal tau protein that is more prone to abnormal phosphorylation, detaches more easily from the microtubules, or is more prone to aggregation after it has been phosphorylated and has detached from the microtubules. Most of these patients develop an inherited form of frontotemporal dementia with parkinsonism.

Another problem protein is **α-synuclein,** a small (140 amino acids), unstably folded, membrane-associated intracellular protein that can aggregate into cytoplasmic granules called **Lewy bodies.** Most patients with **Parkinson disease** have Lewy bodies in their ailing dopamine neurons. Parkinson disease is a motor disorder manifested as tremor, rigor, and akinesia. It is the second most common neurodegenerative disease after Alzheimer disease, affecting 1% to 3% of people older than 65 years. People who are born with structurally abnormal variants of α-synuclein or who overproduce structurally normal α-synuclein as a result of gene duplication or triplication can develop early-onset forms of Parkinson disease.

PROTEIN MISFOLDING CAN BE CONTAGIOUS

An unusual type of neurodegeneration is caused by aggregates of the **prion protein (PrP).** The normal cellular prion protein **(PrP^C)** is an abundant protein in the nervous system, where it is tethered to the outer surface of the plasma membrane by a glycosylphosphatidylinositol anchor (see Chapter 12). Smaller amounts are present in other organs and in blood and cerebrospinal fluid. Little is known about its normal function, although knockout mice lacking PrP have mild to moderate neurological abnormalities.

Creutzfeldt-Jacob disease (CJD) is a rare disease (incidence one per million per year) of middle-aged and old people in whom mental deterioration progresses to death within weeks or months. At autopsy the brain is found to be riddled with holes; therefore, this type of disease is characterized as a **spongiform encephalopathy.**

CJD develops when the normal PrP^C refolds itself into the abnormal PrP^{Sc} (Sc stands for "scrapie"), which forms aggregates in the brain. Most cases are sporadic, but some are inherited as an autosomal dominant trait. The offending point mutations increase the likelihood that PrP refolds itself into the aggregation-prone form.

What sets prion diseases apart from other protein misfolding diseases is their potentially infectious nature. Not only does PrP^{Sc} join hands with other molecules of

---

CLINICAL EXAMPLE 2.3: Kuru

During the 1950s, health officers in a remote part of Papua New Guinea became aware of a deadly disease that afflicted women and teenage girls of the local Fore tribe. The disease was known as *kuru*, after the local word for "trembling." The victims developed tremors, became unable to walk, sometimes laughed compulsively, and died within 1 year after the onset of symptoms. The similarity of the brain pathology with that of the sheep disease scrapie was soon noted, but the origin of the disease remained a mystery. Finally, its transmissibility to nonhuman primates could be shown. Unlike a virus, the infectious agent contained no nucleic acid. Therefore the term "prion" (*p*roteinaceous *i*nfectious *on*ly) was coined for this novel pathogen.

The Fore had adopted the custom of mortuary cannibalism in the early years of the twentieth century: They honored their dead by eating them. Through this practice, kuru was transmitted. Actually, the main route of infection was not through the gastrointestinal tract.

Like other proteins, prions are destroyed by enzymes in the stomach and intestine, and intact proteins are not readily absorbed. Most likely women and girls acquired the infection through small cuts in the skin while preparing the meals. Kuru was rare in parts of the country where the bodies were stewed on hot stones before they were carved up. Prions lose their infectivity after thorough heating because, like other proteins, they are subject to heat denaturation.

Most likely the kuru epidemic originated with a person who had died of spontaneous or inherited CJD. This person's prions were transmitted to the body's eaters, or more likely to the cooks, and then to the next set of cooks and eaters. Kuru was acquired by cannibals the same way that vCJD was acquired by Britons who were too intimate with the meat of cattle that were afflicted by mad cow disease. In both cases the disease is triggered when a few molecules of PrP^{Sc} enter the body and then induce the person's own PrP^C to fold into the disease-causing PrP^{Sc}.

PrP^{Sc} to form insoluble aggregates, it also induces neighboring molecules of PrP^C to refold into PrP^{Sc}, leading to a chain reaction. CJD is not normally transmitted among humans, but the sheep equivalent of CJD, known as scrapie, can be naturally transmitted among sheep. During the 1980s, when cattle in Britain were fed insufficiently heated meat-and-bone meal prepared from sheep carcasses, many cattle developed the bovine equivalent of CJD and scrapie, known as *bovine spongiform encephalopathy* or "mad cow disease." Some humans developed **variant Creutzfeldt-Jacob disease (vCJD)** after consuming the meat of infected cattle. Kuru is a transmissible spongiform encephalopathy in humans.

SUMMARY

Proteins consist of 20 different amino acids held together by peptide bonds. The covalent structure of the protein, defined by the amino acid sequence, disulfide bonds, and other covalent bonds, is called its *primary structure*. Higher-order structures are formed by noncovalent interactions.

Regular, repetitive folding patterns are called *secondary structures*. The most important secondary structures are the α-helix and β-pleated sheet, both stabilized by hydrogen bonds between the peptide bonds. The tertiary structure, which is prominent in globular proteins, is the overall folding pattern of the polypeptide. It is stabilized mainly by hydrophobic interactions between amino acid side chains. Some proteins consist of two or more polypeptides (subunits). Their subunit composition and interactions define the protein's quaternary structure.

Disulfide bonds between cysteine side chains can be formed within the polypeptide (intra-chain) or between polypeptides (inter-chain). Nonpolypeptide components, known as prosthetic groups, also are present in many proteins.

The noncovalent higher-order structure of proteins can be destroyed by heating, detergents, nonpolar organic solvents, heavy metals, and extreme pH. This process of denaturation destroys the protein's biological properties. Many laboratory methods for the separation of proteins from biological samples are available.

Some proteins are prone to misfolding, thus forming structures with a high content of β-pleated sheets that aggregate into insoluble fibrils. Extracellular protein deposits of this kind, known as amyloid, accumulate in old age and in many diseases. When formed in the brain, either within or outside the cells, misfolded proteins can lead to neurodegenerative diseases including Alzheimer and Parkinson disease. Prion protein, once in a misfolded state, can even bend other prion protein molecules into the pathogenic conformation.

Further Reading

Aguzzi A, Baumann F, Brem J: The prion's elusive reason for being, *Annu Rev Neurosci* 31:439–477, 2008.

Ballatore C, Lee VM-Y, Trojanowski Q: Tau-mediated neurodegeneration in Alzheimer's disease and related disorders, *Nat Rev Neurosci* 8:663–670, 2007.

Blaber ML, Zhang X-J, Matthews BW: Structural basis of amino acid α-helix propensity, *Science* 260:1637–1640, 1993.

Branden C, Tooze J: *Introduction to protein structure*, New York, 1998, Garland Science Publishing.

Caughey B, Baron GS, Chesebro B, Jeffrey M: Getting a grip on prions: oligomers, amyloids, and pathological membrane interactions, *Annu Rev Biochem* 78:177–204, 2009.

Cole SL, Vassar R: The role of amyloid precursor protein processing by BACE1, the β-secretase, in Alzheimer disease pathophysiology, *J Biol Chem* 283:29621–29625, 2008.

Franks F, editor: *Characterization of proteins*, Totowa, NJ, 1988, Humana Press.

Fukuchi S, Homma K, Minezaki Y, Gojobori T, Nishikawa K: Development of an accurate classification system of proteins into structured and unstructured regions that uncovers novel structural domains: its application to human transcription factors, *BMC Struct Biol* 9:26, 2009.

Goedert M, Spillantini M: A century of Alzheimer's disease, *Science* 314:777–781, 2006.

Kamoun PP: Denaturation of globular proteins by urea: breakdown of hydrogen or hydrophobic bonds? *Trends Biochem Sci* 13:424–425, 1988.

Pepys MB: Amyloidosis, *Annu Rev Med* 57:223–241, 2006.

Thinakaran G, Koo EH: Amyloid precursor protein trafficking, processing, and function, *J Biol Chem* 283:29615–29619, 2008.

Thomas PJ, Qu B-H, Pedersen PL: Defective protein folding as a basis of human disease, *Trends Biochem Sci* 20:456–459, 1995.

Wolfe MS: Tau mutations in neurodegenerative diseases, *J Biol Chem* 284:6021–6025, 2008.

1. The component of a water-soluble globular protein that is most likely to be present in the center of the molecule rather than on its surface is

   A. A glutamate side chain
   B. A histidine side chain
   C. A phenylalanine side chain
   D. A phosphate group covalently linked to a serine side chain
   E. An oligosaccharide covalently linked to an asparagine side chain

2. The following structure is an oligopeptide that is acetylated at its amino end and amidated at its carboxyl end, making the terminal groups nonionizable. This oligopeptide has a p*I* close to

   Acetyl-Ala-Glu-Ser-Lys-Gly-amide

   A. 4.3
   B. 5.1
   C. 6.0
   D. 7.5
   E. 10.8

3. Human blood plasma contains about 7% protein. These plasma proteins have p*K* values close to 4 or 5. In the test tube, these proteins will form an insoluble precipitate after all of the following treatments *except*

   A. Boiling the serum for 5 minutes
   B. Adding sodium chloride to a concentration of 35%
   C. Adjusting the pH to 4.5
   D. Boiling the serum with 6*N* hydrochloric acid for 10 hours
   E. Mixing one volume of plasma with two volumes of pure alcohol

4. A genetic engineer wants to produce athletes with increased hemoglobin concentration in the erythrocytes, to improve oxygen supply to the muscles. To do so, the water solubility of the hemoglobin molecule must be increased. Which of the following amino acid changes on the surface of the hemoglobin molecule is most likely to increase its water solubility?

   A. Arg → Lys
   B. Leu → Phe
   C. Gln → Ser
   D. Ala → Asn
   E. Ser → Ala

5. Your grandmother has become increasingly forgetful during the past 2 years. Last week she actually got lost on the way back from the grocery store a few blocks down the road. One treatment that could perhaps help her would be a drug that

   A. Reduces the synthesis of transthyretin
   B. Reduces the formation of immunoglobulins
   C. Inhibits the activity of β-secretase
   D. Reduces the formation of α-synuclein
   E. Adds phosphate groups to tau protein

6. While attending your great-grandfather's 100th birthday, he tells you that his doctor warned him that his heart is getting weak. The most likely cause of this is an abnormally folded form of

   A. Serum amyloid A protein
   B. β2-microglobulin
   C. β-amyloid
   D. Prion protein
   E. Transthyretin

Chapter 3
OXYGEN TRANSPORTERS: HEMOGLOBIN AND MYOGLOBIN

The human body consumes about 500 g of molecular oxygen per day. This amount of oxygen cannot be transported physically dissolved in blood plasma. At the oxygen partial pressure of 90 torr that prevails in the lung capillaries, 1 L of plasma can dissolve only 2.8 ml (4.1 mg) of O_2. Without oxygen-binding proteins, the 8000 L of blood that the heart pumps to the tissues every day would be able to supply only about 30 g of oxygen, which is 6% of the total requirement. Fortunately, human blood contains 150 g of the oxygen-binding protein **hemoglobin** per liter, locked up in the erythrocytes. Thanks to hemoglobin, 1 L of blood can dissolve 280 mg of oxygen, about 70 times more than hemoglobin-free blood plasma. The binding of oxygen to hemoglobin, known technically as **oxygenation,** is reversible:

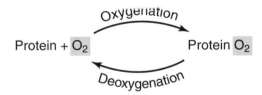

Therefore oxygen binds to oxygen-binding proteins when oxygen is plentiful, and is released when it is scarce.

THE HEME GROUP IS THE OXYGEN-BINDING SITE OF HEMOGLOBIN AND MYOGLOBIN

None of the functional groups in the common amino acids can bind molecular oxygen. Therefore oxygen binding to hemoglobin and its close relative myoglobin requires the prosthetic group **heme.**

Heme consists of a porphyrin, called **protoporphyrin IX,** with a ferrous iron chelated in its center (*Fig. 3.1*). Protoporphyrin IX contains four five-member, nitrogen-containing **pyrrole rings,** held together by methine (—CH=) bridges and decorated with methyl (—CH$_3$), vinyl (—CH=CH$_2$), and propionate (—CH$_2$—CH$_2$—COO$^-$) side chains. The most important part of the

heme group is its iron. Like other heavy metals, ionized iron can form coordination bonds with the free electron pairs of oxygen and nitrogen atoms. The iron in heme is bound to the nitrogen atoms of the four pyrrole rings. In hemoglobin and myoglobin, the iron forms a fifth bond with a nitrogen atom in a histidine side chain of the apoprotein. This histidine is called the **proximal histidine.** An optional sixth bond can be formed with molecular oxygen:

His

Iron can exist in a ferrous (Fe^{2+}) and a ferric (Fe^{3+}) state. Ferric iron is the more oxidized form because it can be formed from ferrous iron by the removal of an electron:

Fe^{2+} Fe^{3+}

Ferrous iron
(reduced form)

Ferric iron
(oxidized form)

By definition, the removal of an electron qualifies as oxidation. *The heme iron in hemoglobin and myoglobin is always in the ferrous state.* Even during oxygen binding it is not oxidized to the ferric form. It becomes oxygenated but not oxidized.

CLINICAL EXAMPLE 3.1: Cyanosis

The porphyrin ring system contains conjugated double bonds (double bonds alternating with single bonds), which absorb visible light. *These double bonds are responsible for the color of human blood.* The color of oxygenated hemoglobin is red, and the color of deoxyhemoglobin is blue. Conditions in which hemoglobin becomes deoxygenated to an abnormal extent lead to blue discoloration of the lips and other mucous membranes. Pulmonary and circulatory failure lead to cyanosis, as does severe anemia. A less serious situation is cold exposure, which leads to peripheral vasoconstriction, slows the flow of blood through the capillaries, and thereby leads to more complete deoxygenation.

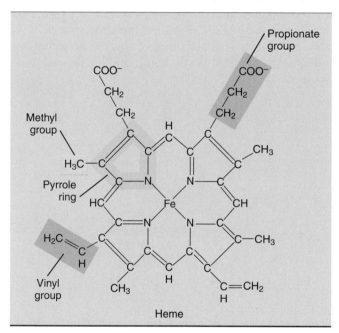

Figure 3.1 Structure of the heme group in hemoglobin and myoglobin. Note that the upper part of the group is hydrophilic because of the charged propionate side chains, whereas the lower part is hydrophobic. The conjugated double bonds in the ring system are responsible for its color. Oxyhemoglobin is red, and deoxyhemoglobin blue.

MYOGLOBIN IS A TIGHTLY PACKED GLOBULAR PROTEIN

Myoglobin is a relative of hemoglobin but occurs only in muscle tissue, where its function is short-term storage of oxygen for muscle contraction. It consists of a single polypeptide with 153 amino acids and a tightly bound heme group (molecular weight 17,000 D [17 kDa]). *About 75% of the amino acid residues participate in α-helical structures.* Eight α-helices with lengths between 7 and 23 amino acids are connected by nonhelical segments (*Fig. 3.2*). Starting from the amino terminus, the helixes are designated by capital letters A through H. The positions of the amino acid residues are specified by the helix letter and their position in the helix. For example, the proximal histidine, which is in position 93 of the polypeptide counting from the amino end, is designated His F8 because it is the eighth amino acid in the F helix.

Many of the α-helices are **amphipathic,** with hydrophobic amino acid residues clustered on one edge and hydrophilic residues on the other. The hydrophilic edge contacts the surrounding water, and the hydrophobic edge faces inward to the center of the molecule. *The interior of myoglobin is filled with tightly packed nonpolar side chains, and hydrophobic interactions are the major stabilizing force in its tertiary structure.*

The heme group is tucked between the E and F helices, properly positioned by hydrophobic interactions with amino acid side chains and the bond between the iron and the proximal histidine. On the side opposite the proximal histidine, the heme iron faces the **distal histidine** (His E7) without binding it. The cavity between the distal histidine and the heme iron is just large enough to accommodate an oxygen molecule.

Like most cytoplasmic proteins, *myoglobin contains no disulfide bonds.* Its tertiary structure is maintained only by noncovalent forces.

THE RED BLOOD CELLS ARE SPECIALIZED FOR OXYGEN TRANSPORT

Hemoglobin is found only in erythrocytes, or red blood cells (RBCs). Erythrocytes are released from the bone marrow and then circulate for about 120 days before they are scavenged by phagocytic cells in the spleen and other tissues. *Erythrocytes have no nucleus* and therefore are no longer able to divide and to synthesize proteins; they are dead. Their hemoglobin is inherited from their nucleated precursors in the bone marrow. They also lack mitochondria and therefore do not consume any of the oxygen they transport. They cover their modest energy needs by the anaerobic metabolism of glucose to lactic acid. In essence, erythrocytes are bags filled with hemoglobin at a concentration of 33%, physically dissolved in the cytoplasm.

THE HEMOGLOBINS ARE TETRAMERIC PROTEINS

Whereas myoglobin consists of a single polypeptide with its heme group, *hemoglobin has four polypeptides, each with its own heme.* Humans have several types of hemoglobin (*Table 3.1*). **Hemoglobin A (HbA),** which contains two α-chains and two β-chains, is the major adult hemoglobin. The **minor adult hemoglobin (HbA$_2$)** and **fetal hemoglobin (HbF)** also have two α-chains, but instead of the β-chains, HbA$_2$ has δ-chains and HbF has γ-chains.

The α-chains have 141 amino acids, and the β-, γ-, and δ-chains have 146 amino acids. *All of these chains*

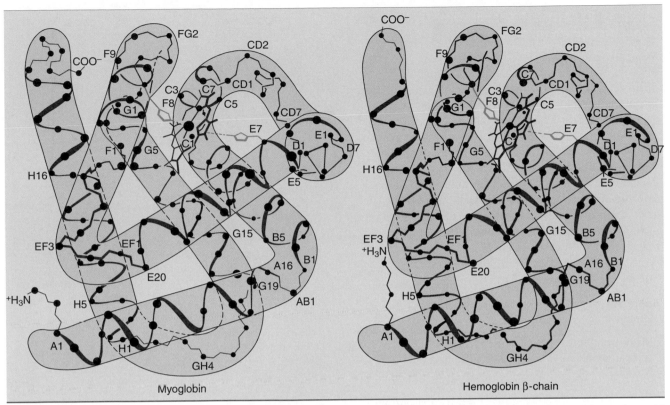

Figure 3.2   Tertiary structures of myoglobin and the β-chain of hemoglobin. Only the α-carbons are shown. The amino acid residues are designated by their position in one of the eight helices (A through H, starting from the amino terminus) or nonhelical links. For example, the proximal histidine F8, is the eighth amino acid in the F helix, counting from the amino end.

Table 3.1   Most Important Human Hemoglobins*

Type	Subunit Structure	Importance
Major adult (HbA)	$\alpha_2\beta_2$	97% of adult hemoglobin
Minor adult (HbA$_2$)	$\alpha_2\delta_2$	2%–3% of adult hemoglobin
Fetal (HbF)	$\alpha_2\gamma_2$	Major hemoglobin in second and third trimesters of pregnancy

*See also Chapter 9.

are structurally related. The α- and β-chains are identical in 64 of their amino acids. The β- and γ-chains differ in 39 their 146 amino acids, and the β- and δ-chains differ in 10.

Although hemoglobin chains are distant relatives of myoglobin, only 28 amino acids are identical in α-chains, β-chains, and myoglobin. These conserved amino acids include the proximal and distal histidines and some of the other amino acids contacting the heme group. Many of the nonconserved amino acid positions are "conservative" substitutions. This means that corresponding amino acids have similar physical properties.

Each hemoglobin subunit folds itself into a shape that strikingly resembles the tertiary structure of myoglobin (see *Fig. 3.2*). Therefore *hemoglobin looks like four myoglobin molecules glued together.* Like myoglobin, each hemoglobin subunit has a hydrophobic core and a hydrophilic surface. The subunits interact mainly through hydrogen bonds and salt bonds, without any disulfide bonds.

OXYGENATED AND DEOXYGENATED HEMOGLOBIN HAVE DIFFERENT QUATERNARY STRUCTURES

The subunits of deoxyhemoglobin are held together by eight salt bonds between the polypeptides as well as by hydrogen bonds and other noncovalent interactions. Upon oxygenation, the salt bonds break and a new set of hydrogen bonds forms. Subunit interactions are weaker in oxyhemoglobin than in deoxyhemoglobin. Therefore the conformation of deoxyhemoglobin is called the **T** (tense, or taut) **conformation,** and that of oxyhemoglobin is called the **R** (relaxed) **conformation** (*Fig. 3.3*).

The conformation of hemoglobin changes with oxygenation because the bond distances between the heme iron and the five nitrogen atoms with which it is complexed shorten when oxygen binds. This distorts the shape of the heme group and pulls on the F helix to which the proximal histidine (F8) belongs. The interactions with the other subunits are destabilized, and the shape of the whole molecule is shifted toward the R conformation.

CLINICAL EXAMPLE 3.2: Microcytic Hypochromic Anemia

Between 38% and 53% of the blood volume consists of RBCs (or erythrocytes). This percentage can be determined by centrifuging the blood for some minutes. Because of their high protein content, RBCs have a higher density than plasma and settle to the bottom. The percentage of the total volume occupied by this cellular sediment of red cells is called the **hematocrit** (*Table 3.2*).

Patients whose blood hemoglobin falls below the normal range of 12% to 17% are said to have **anemia.** They usually have a reduced hematocrit as well. Chronic anemia can have many causes, including hemolysis (destruction of RBCs), bone marrow failure (aplastic anemia), and impaired DNA synthesis and cell division in RBC precursors (megaloblastic anemia).

Table 3.2 Characteristics of Red Blood Cells and Hemoglobin

Diameter of RBCs	7.3 μm
Lifespan of RBCs	120 days
No. of RBCs	4.2–5.4 million/mm^3 (female)
	4.6–6.2 million/mm^3 (male)
Intracorpuscular hemoglobin concentration	33%
Hematocrit*	38%–46% (female)
	42%–53% (male)
Hemoglobin in whole blood	12%–15% (female)
	14%–17% (male)

RBC, Red blood cell.

*Hematocrit = percentage of blood volume occupied by blood cells; measured by centrifugation of whole blood.

Conditions that impair hemoglobin synthesis lead to microcytic hypochromic anemia. Causes include the inability to synthesize enough α-chains or β-chains, inability to synthesize the porphyrin portion of heme, or iron deficiency. The most common cause is iron deficiency due to poor nutrition and/or chronic blood loss (see Chapter 29). Other conditions (e.g., vitamin B$_6$ deficiency) impair the synthesis of the porphyrin. In the group of genetic diseases called the thalassemias, the synthesis of hemoglobin α-chains or β-chains is impaired (see Chapter 9). Because RBCs are little more than bags filled with hemoglobin, reduced hemoglobin synthesis leads to cells that both are too small (microcytosis) and have a reduced hemoglobin concentration (hypochromia).

The most important biological difference between the two conformations is their oxygen-binding affinity. *The R conformation binds oxygen 150 to 300 times more tightly than does the T conformation.*

Proteins that can assume alternative higher-order structures are called **allosteric proteins.** The alternative conformations of an allosteric protein interconvert

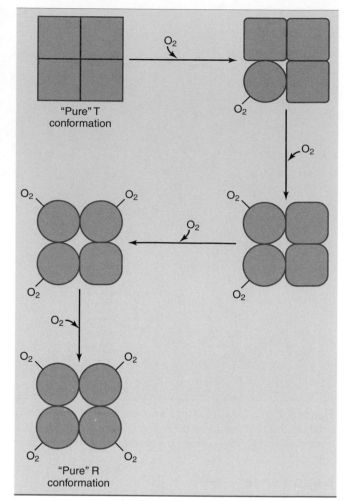

Figure 3.3 Simplified model of the transition from T to R conformation during successive oxygenations of hemoglobin. Partially oxygenated hemoglobin spends most of its time in intermediate conformational states. In actuality, different conformations ranging from "pure" T to "pure" R exist in equilibrium in each oxygenation state.

spontaneously, and their equilibrium is affected by ligand binding. A **ligand** (from Latin *ligare* meaning "to bind") is any small molecule that binds reversibly to a protein.

Erythrocytes contain the enzyme methemoglobin reductase, which uses the coenzyme NADH (the reduced form of nicotinamide adenine dinucleotide) to reduce methemoglobin back to hemoglobin. Inherited deficiency of this enzyme is another rare cause of congenital methemoglobinemia.

OXYGEN BINDING TO HEMOGLOBIN IS COOPERATIVE

The **oxygen-binding curve** describes the fractional saturation of the heme groups at varying oxygen partial pressures. The oxygen partial pressure (pO$_2$) is about 100 torr in the lung alveoli, 90 torr in the lung capillaries, and between 30 and 60 torr in the capillaries of most tissues. In contracting muscles, pO$_2$ can fall to 20 torr.

Only ferrous iron (Fe^{2+}) binds molecular oxygen. Ferric iron (Fe^{3+}) does not. Oxidation of the heme iron in hemoglobin to the ferric state produces methemoglobin, which is useless for oxygen transport. Methemoglobin is responsible for the brown color of dried blood. Normally less than 1% of the circulating hemoglobin is in the form of methemoglobin, but aniline dyes, aromatic nitro compounds, inorganic and organic nitrites, and other oxidizing chemicals can cause excessive methemoglobin formation. Methemoglobinemia is treated with reducing agents (e.g., methylene blue), which reduce the ferric iron back to the ferrous state.

The heme iron is somewhat protected from oxidant attack by its binding to the apoprotein, which leaves only one side of the iron accessible for oxygen and other oxidizing agents. Structural abnormalities of hemoglobin that lead to "loose" binding of the heme group cause congenital methemoglobinemia. This happens, for example, when the proximal histidine is replaced by a tyrosine residue.

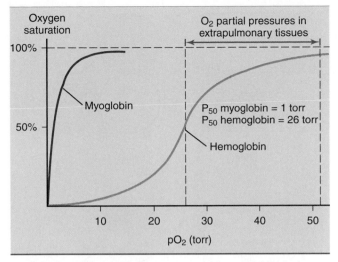

Figure 3.4 Oxygen-binding curves of hemoglobin and myoglobin. P_{50} is defined as the oxygen partial pressure at which half of the heme groups are oxygenated.

Figure 3.4 shows that *myoglobin binds oxygen far tighter than does hemoglobin.* Myoglobin is half-saturated with oxygen at 1 torr, whereas hemoglobin requires 26 torr. This difference in oxygen affinity facilitates the transfer of oxygen from the blood to the tissue.

The shapes of the oxygen-binding curves differ as well. The myoglobin curve is hyperbolic, which is expected for a simple equilibrium reaction of the following type:

$$Mb + O_2 \rightleftharpoons Mb \bullet O_2$$

The binding curve of hemoglobin is sigmoidal. Why? Completely deoxygenated hemoglobin is mainly in the T conformation, which has a very low oxygen affinity. This accounts for the flat part of the curve below about 10 torr. However, with increasing oxygen partial pressure, the first heme nevertheless becomes oxygenated. Oxygenation of the first heme destabilizes the T conformation and shifts the structure toward the R conformation. This repeats itself after binding of the second and third oxygen molecules. *Oxygen binding to a heme group in hemoglobin increases the oxygen affinities of the remaining heme groups.* This is called **positive cooperativity.**

Cooperativity improves hemoglobin's efficiency as an oxygen transporter. Without cooperativity, an 81-fold increase of pO_2 would be required to raise the oxygen saturation from 10% to 90%. For hemoglobin, however, a 4.8-fold increase is sufficient to do the same. Due to positive cooperativity, hemoglobin is about 96% saturated in the lung capillaries ($pO_2 = 90$ torr) but only 33% saturated in the capillaries of working muscle ($pO_2 = 20$ torr). Less oxygen is extracted in other tissues so that the mixed venous blood is still 60% to 70% oxygenated. Although this oxygen is useless under ordinary conditions, it can keep a person alive for a few minutes after acute respiratory arrest.

2,3-BISPHOSPHOGLYCERATE IS A NEGATIVE ALLOSTERIC EFFECTOR OF OXYGEN BINDING TO HEMOGLOBIN

2,3-Bisphosphoglycerate (BPG) is a small organic molecule that is present in RBCs at a concentration of about 5 mmol, roughly equimolar with hemoglobin:

Most of it is noncovalently bound to hemoglobin. One molecule of BPG is positioned in a central cavity between the subunits, forming salt bonds with positively charged amino acid residues in the two β-chains. *BPG binds to the T conformation but not the R conformation of hemoglobin.* Therefore it stabilizes only the T conformation, favoring it over the R conformation (*Fig. 3.5*). Because the T conformation has the lower oxygen affinity, *BPG decreases the oxygen-binding affinity.*

BPG is a physiologically important regulator of oxygen binding to hemoglobin. The BPG concentration in RBCs increases in hypoxic conditions, including lung diseases, severe anemia, and adaptation to high altitude. This barely affects oxygenation in the lung capillaries, but *it enhances the unloading of oxygen in the tissues whose oxygen partial pressures are in the steep part of the oxygen-binding curve* (*Fig. 3.6*).

BPG is described as a **negative allosteric effector** with regard to oxygen binding to hemoglobin because it lowers the oxygen affinity. A **positive allosteric effector** increases the oxygen affinity.

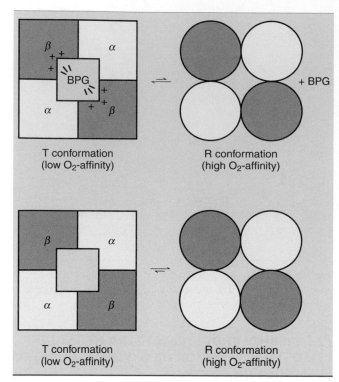

Figure 3.5 Effect of 2,3-bisphosphoglycerate (BPG) on the equilibrium between the T and R conformations of hemoglobin. The salt bonds between BPG and the β-chains stabilize the T conformation.

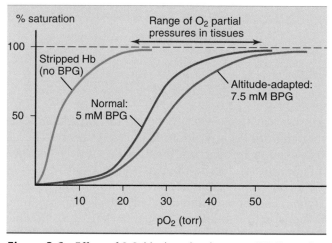

Figure 3.6 Effect of 2,3-bisphosphoglycerate (BPG) on the oxygen-binding affinity of hemoglobin (Hb).

Hemoglobin is not the only allosteric protein. Allosteric enzymes are regulated by positive and negative allosteric effectors that enhance or inhibit enzymatic catalysis, respectively (see Chapter 4). These effectors bind to regulatory sites on the enzyme that are outside of the catalytic sites. *Most allosteric proteins consist of more than one subunit, and the subunit interactions are affected by ligand binding.*

FETAL HEMOGLOBIN HAS A HIGHER OXYGEN-BINDING AFFINITY THAN DOES ADULT HEMOGLOBIN

In HbA, BPG forms salt bonds with the amino termini of the β-chains and with the side chains of Lys EF6 and His H21 in the β-chains. In the γ-chains of HbF, His H21 is replaced by an uncharged serine residue. Therefore *BPG binds less tightly to HbF than to HbA*, and it reduces the oxygen affinity of HbF less than that of HbA. Thus HbF has a higher oxygen affinity than does HbA. It is half-saturated at 20 torr compared to 26 torr for HbA. *This facilitates the transfer of oxygen from the maternal blood to the fetal blood in the capillaries of the placenta.*

CLINICAL EXAMPLE 3.4: Carbon Monoxide Poisoning

Carbon monoxide (CO) is a product of incomplete combustion, and a small amount is even formed in the human body (see Chapter 27). *CO binds to the ferrous iron in hemoglobin and myoglobin with 200 times higher affinity than O_2.* This kind of interaction is called **competitive antagonism** because CO and O_2 compete for the same binding site. In addition to keeping O_2 off the heme iron, bound CO greatly increases the oxygen-binding affinities of the remaining heme groups. This further impairs oxygen transport.

Despite its high affinity, *CO binding is reversible.* In a normally breathing patient with CO poisoning, O_2 gradually displaces the CO from the heme iron. The CO is exhaled through the lungs, and the patient recovers slowly in the course of several hours. Carbon monoxide poisoning can be treated with hyperbaric oxygen, which accelerates this process.

Acute CO poisoning is seen after attempted suicide by inhaling car exhaust gas and in people trapped in burning buildings. Throbbing headache, confusion, and fainting on exertion occur when 30% to 50% of the heme groups are occupied by CO, and a CO saturation of 80% is rapidly fatal. *Patients with CO poisoning are not cyanotic* because CO hemoglobin has a bright cherry-red color. Smokers have 4% to 8% of their hemoglobin in the CO form. Therefore smoking is not a good habit for patients who suffer from poor tissue oxygenation, such as those with angina pectoris (myocardial ischemia).

THE BOHR EFFECT FACILITATES OXYGEN DELIVERY

Metabolic activity can acidify the environment by two mechanisms. One is the formation of carbon dioxide (CO_2), which reacts with water to form carbonic acid:

$$CO_2 + H_2O \rightleftharpoons H_2CO_3 \rightleftharpoons HCO_3^- + H^+$$

The other mechanism is the formation of lactic acid from glucose or glycogen, which is the only way cells can make at least some ATP (adenosine triphosphate) without consuming oxygen. Lactic acid is formed in exercising muscles and under oxygen-deficient conditions (see Chapter 21).

An acidic environment reduces the oxygen affinity of hemoglobin, resulting in the release of bound oxygen. This is called the **Bohr effect.** It occurs because protons (H^+) are released from hemoglobin when oxygen binds:

$$\text{Hemoglobin} + O_2 \rightleftharpoons \text{Hemoglobin} \cdot O_2 + nH^+$$

In the backward reaction, oxygen is released when protons bind to hemoglobin. About 0.7 protons bind when one oxygen molecule leaves. An increased proton concentration pushes the reaction to the left, releasing oxygen from hemoglobin.

In addition to its acidifying action, CO_2 reduces the oxygen affinity of hemoglobin by covalent binding to the terminal amino groups of the α- and β-chains. This reaction forms **carbamino hemoglobin:**

$$\text{Hemoglobin} \longrightarrow NH_2 + CO_2$$

$$\text{Hemoglobin} \longrightarrow NH \longrightarrow \overset{\overset{\displaystyle O}{\|}}{C} \longrightarrow O^- + H^+$$

This reversible reaction proceeds spontaneously, without the need for an enzyme. Carbamino hemoglobin has a lower oxygen affinity than does unmodified hemoglobin. Like the pH effect, the CO_2 effect ensures that *oxygen is most easily released in actively metabolizing tissues where it is most needed.*

CLINICAL EXAMPLE 3.5: 2,3-BPG and Blood Banking

Blood for transfusion can be stored at 2°C to 6°C for about 4 weeks. Whole blood is used for patients who have suffered from severe blood loss after accidents or surgery. Anemic patients are best treated with packed RBCs.

Among the adverse changes that occur in erythrocytes during storage is the loss of 2,3-BPG. As much as 90% of BPG is lost after storage for 3 weeks, resulting in an abnormally high oxygen affinity of hemoglobin. After transfusion it takes up to 24 hours to restore BPG to a normal level.

Simply adding 2,3-BPG to the stored blood is ineffective because BPG, like other phosphorylated compounds, does not cross the erythrocyte membrane. BPG synthesis requires glycolytic intermediates and ATP. To prevent ATP depletion, blood is stored in the presence of glucose, which is the only fuel for erythrocytes. Adenine also is added in most cases. Phosphate and glycolytic intermediates, such as dihydroxyacetone or pyruvate, can be added to the blood to minimize the depletion of BPG.

MOST CARBON DIOXIDE IS TRANSPORTED AS BICARBONATE

CO_2 has a higher water solubility compared to O_2; therefore, some of it is transported physically dissolved in plasma. Another portion is transported as the carbamino group by hemoglobin and by plasma proteins.

However, 80% of the CO_2 is transported from the peripheral tissues to the lungs as inorganic bicarbonate (*Fig. 3.7*). CO_2 diffuses into the erythrocyte, where the enzyme **carbonic anhydrase** rapidly establishes equilibrium among CO_2, H_2O, and carbonic acid. Most of the carbonic acid dissociates into a proton and the bicarbonate anion. Although the proton binds to hemoglobin as part of the Bohr effect, the bicarbonate leaves the cell in exchange for a chloride ion. This exchange requires an anion channel in the membrane. The bicarbonate is now transported to the lungs, physically dissolved in the plasma. In the lung capillaries, all of these processes run in reverse while the CO_2 is exhaled.

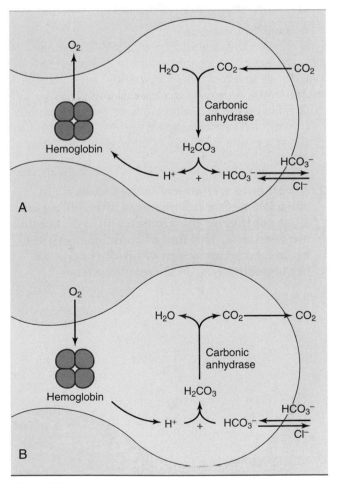

Figure 3.7 Major mechanism of carbon dioxide transport. Note that all processes are reversible. Their direction is determined by the concentrations of the involved substances in the extrapulmonary tissues (**A**) and in the lung capillaries (**B**).

SUMMARY

Oxygen-binding proteins are required because molecular oxygen is poorly soluble in body fluids. Hemoglobin in RBCs and myoglobin in the muscles are structurally related proteins that use heme as a prosthetic group. Myoglobin consists of a single polypeptide with a single heme group. Hemoglobin has four polypeptides, each with its own heme. Adult hemoglobin (HbA) has two α-chains and two β-chains, and fetal hemoglobin (HbF) has two α-chains and two γ-chains. Myoglobin has a far higher oxygen-binding affinity compared to the hemoglobins, and HbF has a slightly higher oxygen affinity than does HbA.

Hemoglobin (but not myoglobin) has allosteric properties. Positive cooperativity between the heme groups leads to a sigmoidal oxygen-binding curve. BPG and protons are negative allosteric effectors that decrease the oxygen-binding affinity. Hemoglobin deficiency, clinically known as anemia, occurs in many clinical conditions. Hemoglobin can also be poisoned by substances that oxidize the ferrous heme iron to the ferric state and by the competitive antagonist CO, which blocks the oxygen-binding site on the heme iron.

QUESTIONS

1. **A pharmaceutical company is trying to develop a drug that improves tissue oxygenation by increasing the percentage of oxygen that is released from hemoglobin during its passage through the capillaries of extrapulmonary tissues. It is hoped this drug will become a popular doping agent for athletes. The company should try a drug that**

   A. Binds to the heme iron
   B. Inhibits the degradation of 2,3-BPG, thereby increasing its concentration in erythrocytes
   C. Binds to ion channels in the RBC membrane, thereby increasing the intracellular pH
   D. Binds to the R conformation of hemoglobin but not the T conformation
   E. Induces the synthesis of hemoglobin γ-chains in adults

2. **A worker in a chemical factory loses consciousness a few minutes after falling into a vat containing the aromatic nitro compound nitrobenzene. This loss of consciousness may be caused by an action of nitrobenzene on hemoglobin, most likely resulting from**

   A. Competitive inhibition of oxygen binding
   B. Oxidation of the heme iron to the ferric state
   C. Reductive cleavage of disulfide bonds between the hemoglobin subunits
   D. Hydrolysis of peptide bonds in hemoglobin α- and β-chains
   E. Inhibition of hemoglobin synthesis

3. **The oxygen-binding curve of hemoglobin is sigmoidal *because***

   A. The binding of oxygen to a heme group increases the oxygen affinities of the other heme groups
   B. The heme groups of the α-chains have a higher oxygen affinity than do the heme groups of the β-chains
   C. The distal histidine allows the hemoglobin molecule to change its conformation in response to an elevated carbon dioxide concentration
   D. The subunits are held in place by interchain disulfide bonds
   E. The solubility of the hemoglobin molecule changes with its oxidation state

Chapter 4
ENZYMATIC REACTIONS

The living cell is a cauldron in which thousands of chemical reactions proceed at the same time. Hardly any of these reactions would proceed at any noticeable rate if their starting materials, or **substrates,** were simply mixed in a test tube by an overoptimistic chemist. The chemist could possibly force the reactions by increasing the temperature or by using a nonselective catalyst, such as a strong acid or a strong base. But the human body is not in this lucky position because body temperature and pH must be kept within narrow limits.

Therefore living things depend on highly selective catalysts called **enzymes.** By definition, *a catalyst is a substance that accelerates a chemical reaction without being consumed in the process.* Because it is regenerated at the end of each catalytic cycle (*Fig. 4.1*), a single molecule of the catalyst can convert many substrate molecules into product. Only a tiny amount of the catalyst is needed.

The **thermodynamic properties** of a reaction are related to energy balance and equilibrium, whereas **kinetic properties** are related to the speed (velocity, or rate) of the reaction. Enzymes do not change the equilibrium of a reaction or its energy balance; they only make the reaction go faster. *Enzymes change the kinetic but not the thermodynamic characteristics of the reaction.*

THE EQUILIBRIUM CONSTANT DESCRIBES THE EQUILIBRIUM OF THE REACTION

In theory, all chemical reactions are reversible. The reaction equilibrium can be determined experimentally by mixing substrates (or products) with a suitable catalyst and allowing the reaction to proceed to completion. At this point, the concentrations of substrates and products can be measured to determine the **equilibrium constant** K_{equ}, which is defined as *the ratio of product concentration to substrate concentration at equilibrium.* For a simple reaction

$$A \rightleftharpoons B$$

the equilibrium constant is

$$K_{equ} = \frac{[B]}{[A]}$$

[B] and [A] are the molar concentrations of product B and substrate A *at equilibrium.*

When more than one substrate or product participate, their concentrations have to be multiplied. For the reaction

$$A + B \rightleftharpoons C + D$$

the equilibrium constant is

$$K_{equ} = \frac{[C] \times [D]}{[A] \times [B]}$$

The alcohol dehydrogenase (ADH) reaction provides an example:

(1) $\quad H_3C-CH_2OH + NAD^+$
$\qquad$ Ethanol

$\qquad \rightleftharpoons H_3C-CHO + NADH + H^+$
$\qquad\qquad$ Acetaldehyde

NAD^+ (nicotinamide adenine dinucleotide) is a coenzyme that accepts hydrogen in this reaction (see Chapter 5). The equilibrium constant of the reaction is

(2) $\quad K_{equ} = \dfrac{[Acetaldehyde] \times [NADH] \times [H^+]}{[Ethanol] \times [NAD^+]}$

$\qquad = 10^{-11} M$

From *Equation (2)* we can calculate the relative concentrations of acetaldehyde and ethanol at equilibrium when $[NADH] = [NAD^+]$ and pH = 7.0:

(3) $\quad \dfrac{[Acetaldehyde]}{[Ethanol]} = 10^{-11} M \times \dfrac{[NAD^+]}{[NADH]} \times \dfrac{1}{[H^+]}$

$\qquad\qquad = 10^{-11} M \times 1 \times 10^7$

$\qquad\qquad = 10^{-4}$

There is 10,000 times more ethanol than acetaldehyde at equilibrium!

Under aerobic conditions, however, NAD^+ is far more abundant than NADH in the cell. When $[NAD^+]$ is 1000

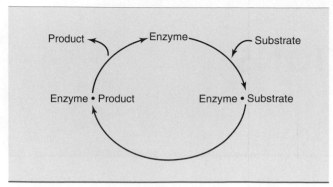

Figure 4.1 The catalytic cycle. The substrate has to bind to the enzyme to form a noncovalent enzyme-substrate complex (*Enzyme•Substrate*). The actual reaction takes place while the substrate is bound to the enzyme. Note that the enzyme is regenerated at the end of the catalytic cycle.

times higher than [NADH], *Equation (3)* assumes the numerical values of

$$\frac{[\text{Acetaldehyde}]}{[\text{Ethanol}]} = 10^{-11} \times 1000 \times 10^7$$
$$= 10^{-1}$$
$$= \frac{1}{10}$$

The pH also is important. At pH of 8.0 and $[\text{NAD}^+]/[\text{NADH}]$ ratio of 1000, for example, *Equation (3)* yields

$$\frac{[\text{Acetaldehyde}]}{[\text{Ethanol}]} = 10^{-11} \times 1000 \times 10^8$$
$$= 10^0$$
$$= 1$$

This example shows that a reaction can be driven toward product formation by raising the concentration of a substrate or lowering the concentration of a product.

To adapt the equilibrium constant to physiological conditions, a "biological equilibrium constant," K'_{equ}, is used. In the definition of K'_{equ}, a value of 1.0 is assigned to the water concentration if water participates in the reaction, and a value of 1.0 to a proton concentration of 10^{-7} mol/L (pH = 7.0) if protons participate in the reaction. The K'_{equ} of the alcohol dehydrogenase reaction, for example, is not 10^{-11} mol/L but 10^{-4} mol/L. At a pH of 8.0 in the preceding example, the proton concentration would be given a numerical value of 10^{-1}.

THE FREE ENERGY CHANGE IS THE DRIVING FORCE FOR CHEMICAL REACTIONS

During chemical reactions, energy is either released or absorbed. This is described as the **enthalpy change ΔH**:

(4) $\quad \Delta H = \Delta E + P \times \Delta V$

ΔE is the heat that is released or absorbed. It is measured in either kilocalories per mole (kcal/mol) or kilojoules per mole (kJ/mol, where 1 kcal = 4.184 kJ). By convention, *a negative sign of ΔE means that heat is released; a positive sign indicates that heat is absorbed.* P is the pressure, and ΔV is the volume change. $P \times \Delta V$ is the work done by the system. It can be substantial in a car motor when the volume in the cylinder expands against the pressure of the piston, but volume changes are negligible in the human body. Therefore $\Delta H \approx \Delta E$. *The enthalpy change describes the difference in the total chemical bond energies between the substrates and products.*

Reactions are driven not only by ΔH but by the **entropy change (ΔS)** as well. *Entropy is a measure of the randomness or disorderliness of the system.* A cluttered desk is often cited as an example of a high-entropy system. A positive ΔS means that the system becomes more disordered during the reaction. Entropy change and enthalpy change are combined in the **free energy change ΔG**:

(5) $\quad \Delta G = \Delta H - T \times \Delta S$

where T = absolute temperature measured in Kelvin.

ΔG *is the driving force of the reaction.* Like ΔE and ΔH in *Equation (4)*, it is measured in kilocalories per mole (kcal/mol) or kilojoules per mole (kJ/mol). A negative sign of ΔG defines an **exergonic reaction.** It can proceed only in the forward direction. A positive sign of ΔG signifies an **endergonic reaction.** It can proceed only in the backward direction. *At equilibrium, ΔG equals zero.*

Equation (5) shows that a reaction can be driven by either a decrease in the chemical bond energies of the reactants (negative ΔH) or an increase in their randomness (positive $T \times \Delta S$). Low energy content and high randomness are the preferred states. Like most students, Nature tends to slip from energized order into energy-depleted chaos.

Entropy changes are small in most biochemical reactions, but *diffusion is an entropy-driven process* (*Fig. 4.2, A*). There is no making and breaking of chemical bonds during diffusion. Therefore the enthalpy change ΔH is zero. This leaves the $T \times \Delta S$ part of *Equation (5)* as the only driving force. Thus diffusion can produce only a random distribution of the dissolved molecules.

The human body is a very orderly system. To maintain this improbable and therefore thermodynamically disfavored state of affairs, *biochemical reactions must antagonize the spontaneous increase in entropy. Equation (5)* shows that a reaction can reduce entropy (negative $T \times \Delta S$) only when it consumes chemical bond energy (negative ΔH). In other words, *the human body must consume chemical bond energy to maintain its low-entropy state.*

In the example of *Figure 4.2, B and C,* the cell maintains a sodium gradient across the membrane by pumping

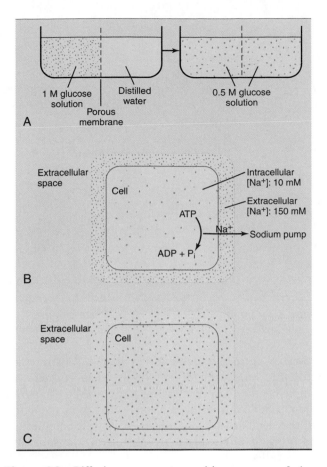

Figure 4.2 Diffusion as an entropy-driven process. **A,** In a hypothetical two-compartment system, molecules diffuse until their concentrations are equal. This is the state of maximal entropy. **B,** The living cell maintains a gradient of sodium ions across its plasma membrane. The cell can maintain this gradient, which represents a low-entropy state, only by "pumping" sodium out of the cell. The pump is fueled by the chemical bond energy in adenosine triphosphate *(ATP). ADP,* Adenosine diphosphate; P_i, inorganic phosphate. **C,** The dead cell lacks ATP; therefore, it cannot maintain its sodium gradient. A high-entropy state develops spontaneously, with intracellular $[Na^+]$ = extracellular $[Na^+]$.

sodium out of the cell (negative $T \times \Delta S$). Sodium pumping is driven by the hydrolysis of adenosine triphosphate (ATP) to adenosine diphosphate (ADP) and inorganic phosphate (P_i) (negative ΔH). Without ATP the gradient dissipates, the entropy of the system increases, and the cell dies. That is what death and dying are all about: a sharp rise in the entropy of the body.

THE STANDARD FREE ENERGY CHANGE DETERMINES THE EQUILIBRIUM

The free energy change ΔG is affected by the relative reactant concentrations. It is not a property of the reaction as such. To describe the energy balance of a reaction, the **standard free energy change,** $\Delta G^{0\prime}$, must be defined: $\Delta G^{0\prime}$ *is the free energy change under standard*

conditions. Standard conditions are defined by a concentration of 1 mol/L for all reactants (except protons and water) at a pH of 7.0. As in the definition of $K^\prime_{equ}$, values of 1 are assigned both to the water concentration and to the proton concentration at pH 7.

For the reaction

$$A + B \rightarrow C + D$$

the standard free energy change $\Delta G^{0\prime}$ is related to the real free energy change ΔG by *Equation (6)*:

$$(6) \quad \Delta G = \Delta G^{0\prime} + R \times T \times \log_e \frac{[C] \times [D]}{[A] \times [B]}$$

$$= \Delta G^{0\prime} + R \times T \times 2.303 \times \log \frac{[C] \times [D]}{[A] \times [B]}$$

where R = gas constant, and T = absolute temperature measured in Kelvin. The numerical value of R is 1.987 $\times 10^{-3}$ kcal $\times$ mol^{-1} $\times$ K^{-1}. At a "standard temperature" of 25°C (298K), *Equation (6)* assumes the form of

$$(7) \quad \Delta G = \Delta G^{0\prime} + 1.364 \times \log \frac{[C] \times [D]}{[A] \times [B]}$$

At equilibrium, $\Delta G = 0$, and *Equation (7)* therefore yields

$$(8) \quad \Delta G^{0\prime} = -1.364 \times \log \frac{[C] \times [D]}{[A] \times [B]}$$

The reactant concentrations under the logarithm are now the equilibrium concentrations. Their ratio defines the biological equilibrium constant $K^\prime_{equ}$

$$(9) \quad \frac{[C] \times [D]}{[A] \times [B]} = K^\prime_{equ}$$

Substituting *Equation (9)* into *Equation (8)* yields

$$(10) \quad \Delta G^{0\prime} = -1.364 \times \log K^\prime_{equ}$$

There is a negative logarithmic relationship between $\Delta G^{0\prime}$ and the equilibrium constant $K^\prime_{equ}$ (Table 4.1). When $\Delta G^{0\prime}$ is negative, product concentrations are higher than substrate concentrations at equilibrium; when it is positive, substrate concentrations are higher.

ENZYMES ARE BOTH POWERFUL AND SELECTIVE

There is no compelling reason why only proteins should catalyze reactions, and catalytic ribonucleic acids (RNAs) are known to exist. By and large, however, *almost all enzymes are globular proteins.*

Enzymes can accelerate a chemical reaction enormously. Many reactions that proceed within minutes in the presence of an enzyme would require thousands of years to reach their equilibrium in the absence of a catalyst. The **turnover number** describes the catalytic power of the enzyme. It is defined as the *maximal*

Table 4.1 Relationship between the Equilibrium Constant K'_{equ} and the Standard Free Energy Change $\Delta G^{0'}$

K'_{equ}	$\Delta G^{0'}$ (kcal/mol)
10^{-5}	6.82
10^{-4}	5.46
10^{-3}	4.09
10^{-2}	2.73
10^{-1}	1.36
1	0
10	−1.36
10^{2}	−2.73
10^{3}	−4.09
10^{4}	−5.46
10^{5}	−6.82

Table 4.2 Approximate Turnover Numbers of Some Enzymes

Enzyme	Turnover Number (s^{-1})*
Carbonic anhydrase	600,000
Catalase	80,000
Acetylcholinesterase	25,000
Triose phosphate isomerase	4,400
α-Amylase	300
Lactate dehydrogenase (muscle)	200
Chymotrypsin	100
Aldolase	11
Lysozyme	0.5
Fructose 2,6-bisphosphatase	0.1

*Turnover numbers are measured at saturating substrate concentrations. They depend on the assay conditions, including temperature and pH.

number of substrate molecules converted to product by one enzyme molecule per second. ***Table 4.2*** lists the turnover numbers of some enzymes.

Another key property of enzymes is their **substrate specificity.** Typically, each reaction requires its own enzyme. For example, when an enzyme is inhibited by a drug or is deficient because of a genetic defect, only one reaction is blocked.

THE SUBSTRATE MUST BIND TO ITS ENZYME BEFORE THE REACTION CAN PROCEED

Enzymatic catalysis, like sex, requires intimate physical contact. It starts with the formation of an **enzyme-substrate complex:**

$$E + S \rightleftharpoons E{\cdot}S$$

where E = free enzyme, S = free substrate, and $E{\cdot}S$ = enzyme-substrate complex.

In the enzyme-substrate complex, the substrate is bound noncovalently to the **active site** on the surface of the enzyme protein. The active site contains the functional groups for substrate binding and catalysis. If a prosthetic group participates in the reaction as a coenzyme, it is present in the active site.

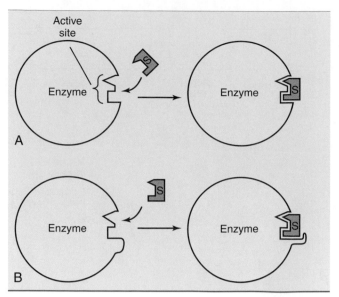

Figure 4.3 Two models of enzyme-substrate binding. **A,** Lock-and-key model. **B,** Induced-fit model. *S,* Substrate.

According to the **lock-and-key model,** substrate and active site bind each other because their surfaces are complementary. In many cases, however, substrate binding induces a conformational change in the active site that leads to further enzyme-substrate interactions and brings catalytically active groups to the substrate. This is called **induced fit** (***Fig. 4.3***).

The enzyme's substrate specificity is determined by the geometry of enzyme-substrate binding. If the substrate is optically active, generally only one of the isomers is admitted. This is to be expected because the enzyme, being formed from optically active amino acids, is optically active itself. A three-point attachment (shown schematically in ***Fig. 4.4***) is the minimal requirement for stereoselectivity.

RATE CONSTANTS ARE USEFUL FOR DESCRIBING REACTION RATES

The rate (velocity) of a chemical reaction can be described by a rate constant k:

$$A \xrightarrow{\; k \;} B$$

In this one-substrate reaction, the reaction rate is defined by

(11) $V = k \times [A]$

The rate constant has the dimension s^{-1} (per second), and the velocity V is the change in substrate concentration per second.

For a reversible reaction, the forward and backward reactions must be considered separately:

(12) $A \underset{k_{-1}}{\overset{k_1}{\rightleftharpoons}} B$

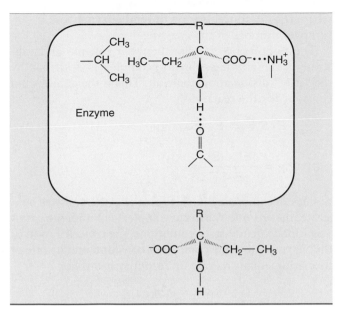

Figure 4.4 Three-point attachment is the minimal requirement for stereoselectivity. In this hypothetical example, the enzyme-substrate complex is formed by a salt bond, a hydrogen bond, and a hydrophobic interaction. The substrate binds, whereas its enantiomer *(bottom)*, is not able to form an enzyme-substrate complex.

$$(13) \quad \begin{aligned} V_{\text{forward}} &= k_1 \times [A] \\ V_{\text{backward}} &= k_{-1} \times [B] \end{aligned}$$

At equilibrium, $V_{\text{forward}} = V_{\text{backward}}$. Therefore the net reaction is zero:

$$(14) \quad k_1 \times [A] = k_{-1} \times [B]$$

$$(15) \quad \frac{[B]}{[A]} = \frac{k_1}{k_{-1}} = K_{\text{equ}}$$

Equation (15) shows that the equilibrium constant K_{equ}, previously defined as [B]/[A] at equilibrium, is also the ratio of the two rate constants.

The forward reaction in *Equation (12)* is a **first-order reaction**. In a first-order reaction, *the reaction rate is directly proportional to the substrate concentration*. When the substrate concentration [A] is doubled, the reaction rate V is doubled as well. Uncatalyzed one-substrate reactions follow first-order kinetics. A classic example is the decay of a radioactive isotope.

When two substrates participate, the reaction rate is likely to depend on the concentrations of both substrates. This is called a **second-order reaction**. For

$$A + B \xrightarrow{\;k\;} C + D$$

the following is obtained:

$$(16) \quad V = k \times [A] \times [B]$$

Doubling the concentration of one substrate doubles the reaction rate; doubling the concentrations of both raises it fourfold.

A **zero-order reaction** is independent of the substrate concentration. No matter how many substrate molecules are present in the test tube, only a fixed number is converted to product per second:

$$(17) \quad V = k$$

Zero-order kinetics are observed only in catalyzed reactions when the substrate concentration is high, and the amount and turnover number of the catalyst, rather than the substrate availability, is the limiting factor.

ENZYMES DECREASE THE FREE ENERGY OF ACTIVATION

Reactions with a negative ΔG *can* occur. In reality, however, many of these reactions do *not* occur at a perceptible rate. The reason is that in both catalyzed and uncatalyzed reactions, *the substrate must pass through a transition state before the product is formed*. The structure of the transition state is intermediate between substrate and product, but its free energy content is higher. Therefore it is unstable and decomposes almost instantly to form either substrate or product. *The formation of the transition state is the rate-limiting step in the overall reaction.*

The overall reaction shown in *Figure 4.5* is exergonic because the product has lower free energy content than the substrate, but the formation of the transition state from the substrate is endergonic. *The free energy difference between substrate and transition state is called the free energy of activation* ($\Delta G'_{\text{act}}$). It is an energy barrier that must be overcome by the kinetic

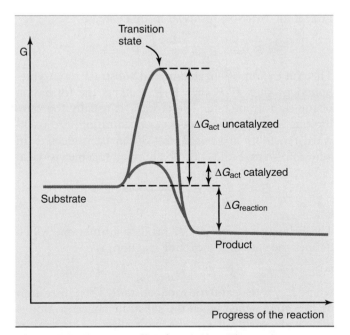

Figure 4.5 Energy profile of a reaction. The enzyme facilitates the reaction by decreasing the free energy content of the transition state. ——, Uncatalyzed reaction; ——, catalyzed reaction. ΔG_{act}, free energy of activation.

energy of the reacting molecules as they collide with each other.

Most chemical systems are **meta-stable,** that is, they are thermodynamically unstable but kinetically stable. The human body is meta-stable in an oxygen-containing atmosphere. CO_2 and H_2O have lower free energy than do molecular oxygen and the organic molecules in the human body, but humans do not self-combust spontaneously because the free energy of activation is too high.

Enzymes stabilize the transition state and decrease its free energy content. As a result, *the enzyme increases the reaction rate by decreasing the free energy of activation.* Forward and backward reactions are accelerated in proportion; therefore, *the equilibrium of the reaction remains unchanged.*

MANY ENZYMATIC REACTIONS CAN BE DESCRIBED BY MICHAELIS-MENTEN KINETICS

In Michaelis-Menten kinetics, a few simple (or simplistic) assumptions are made about enzymatic catalysis:

1. The reaction has only one substrate.
2. The substrate is present at much higher molar concentration than the enzyme.
3. Only the initial reaction rate is considered, at a time when product is virtually absent and the backward reaction negligible.
4. The course of the reaction is observed for only a very short time period; the changes in substrate and product concentrations that take place as the reaction proceeds are neglected.

Enzymatic reactions proceed in three steps:

$$E + S \underset{}{\overset{①}{\rightleftharpoons}} E \cdot S \overset{②}{\rightleftharpoons} E \cdot P \overset{③}{\rightleftharpoons} E + P$$

The conversion of enzyme-bound substrate to enzyme-bound product $E \cdot S \rightleftharpoons E \cdot P$ requires the formation of the transition state. Therefore it is usually the rate-limiting step. At low product concentration, the backward reactions in steps 2 and 3 can be neglected. In addition, steps 2 and 3 can be lumped together to yield

$$E + S \underset{k_{-1}}{\overset{k_1}{\rightleftharpoons}} E \cdot S \overset{k_{cat}}{\longrightarrow} E + P$$

The velocity or rate (V) of product formation, which defines the rate of the overall reaction, is

(18) $\quad V = k_{cat} \times [E \cdot S]$

where k_{cat} is the **catalytic rate constant.** The upper limit of V is approached when the substrate concentration is high and nearly all enzyme molecules are present as enzyme-substrate complex. Therefore the maximal reaction rate (V_{max}) is

(19) $\quad V_{max} = k_{cat} \times [E_T]$

where $[E_T]$ = concentration of total enzyme, and k_{cat} = turnover number of the enzyme.

The tightness of binding between enzyme and substrate in the enzyme-substrate complex is described by the **"true" dissociation constant.** This is the equilibrium constant for the reaction

$$E \cdot S \rightleftharpoons E + S:$$

(20) $\quad K_D = \dfrac{[E] \times [S]}{[E \cdot S]} = \dfrac{k_{-1}}{k_1}$

Besides decomposing back to free enzyme and free substrate, the enzyme-substrate complex can undergo catalysis. Under steady-state conditions, the concentration of the enzyme-substrate complex is constant, and its rate of formation equals its rate of decomposition. For

$$E + S \underset{k_{-1}}{\overset{k_1}{\rightleftharpoons}} E \cdot S \overset{k_{cat}}{\longrightarrow} E + P$$

the following is obtained:

(21) $\quad \underbrace{k_1 \times [E] \times [S]}_{\substack{\text{Rate of formation} \\ \text{of } E \cdot S}} = \underbrace{k_{-1} \times [E \cdot S]}_{\substack{\text{Rate of dissociation} \\ \text{of } E \cdot S \text{ to } E + S}} + \underbrace{k_{cat} \times [E \cdot S]}_{\substack{\text{Rate of product} \\ \text{formation}}}$

which yields

(22) $\quad k_1 \times [E] \times [S] = (k_{-1} + k_{cat}) \times [E \cdot S]$

and

(23) $\quad \dfrac{[E] \times [S]}{[E \cdot S]} = \dfrac{k_{-1} + k_{cat}}{k_1} = K_m$

This is the definition of the **Michaelis constant, K_m.** Because k_{cat} usually is far smaller than k_{-1}, K_m is numerically similar to the true dissociation constant of the enzyme-substrate complex [*Equation (20)*].

The meaning of K_m becomes clear when *Equation (23)* is remodeled to yield

(24) $\quad \dfrac{[E]}{[E \cdot S]} = \dfrac{K_m}{[S]}$

or

(25) $\quad [E \cdot S] = [E] \times \dfrac{[S]}{K_m}$

These equations show that when the substrate concentration $[S] = K_m$, the concentration of the enzyme-substrate complex $E \cdot S$ equals that of the free enzyme E: K_m *is the substrate concentration at which the enzyme is half-saturated with its substrate.* Because the reaction rate is proportionate to the concentration of the enzyme-substrate complex [*Equation (18)*], K_m *is also the substrate concentration at which the reaction rate is half-maximal.*

The total enzyme (E_T) is present as free enzyme and enzyme-substrate complex:

$$(26) \quad [E] + [E \cdot S] = [E_T]$$

or

$$(27) \quad [E] = [E_T] + [E \cdot S]$$

To obtain the Michaelis-Menten equation, *Equations (24)* and *(27)* are first combined:

$$(28) \quad \frac{[E_T] - [E \cdot S]}{[E \cdot S]} = \frac{K_m}{[S]}$$

This becomes

$$(29) \quad \frac{[E_T]}{[E \cdot S]} - 1 = \frac{K_m}{[S]}$$

and

$$(30) \quad \frac{[E_T]}{[E \cdot S]} = \frac{K_m}{[S]} + 1 = \frac{K_m}{[S]} + \frac{[S]}{[S]} = \frac{K_m + [S]}{[S]}$$

Combining *Equations (18)* and *(19)* yields

$$(31) \quad \frac{V_{max}}{V} = \frac{[E_T] \times k_{cat}}{[E \cdot S] \times k_{cat}} = \frac{[E_T]}{[E \cdot S]}$$

Equations (30) and *(31)* now can be combined to obtain the Michaelis-Menten equation:

$$(32) \quad \frac{V_{max}}{V} = \frac{K_m + [S]}{[S]}$$

or

$$(33) \quad V = V_{max} \times \frac{[S]}{K_m + [S]}$$

K_m AND V_{max} CAN BE DETERMINED GRAPHICALLY

The derivation of K_m and V_{max} is not merely a joyful intellectual exercise for the student. These kinetic properties can actually be used to predict reaction rates at varying substrate concentrations.

Figure 4.6 shows what happens when a fixed amount of enzyme is incubated with varying concentrations of substrate. At substrate concentrations far below K_m, the reaction rate is almost directly proportionate to the substrate concentration, and the reaction shows first-order kinetics. Eventually, however, the reaction rate approaches V_{max}. At substrate concentrations far higher than K_m, the reaction becomes nearly independent of the substrate concentration and shows zero-order kinetics. Almost all enzyme molecules are present as enzyme-substrate complex, and the reaction is limited no longer by substrate availability but by the amount and turnover number of the enzyme. K_m is the point on the x-axis that corresponds to ½V_{max} on the y-axis.

In a double-reciprocal plot, known as the **Lineweaver-Burk plot** (*Fig. 4.7*), the relationship between $1/V$ and

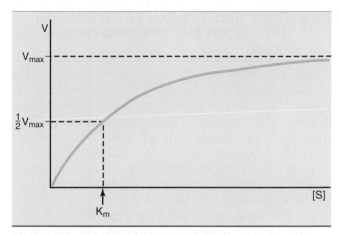

Figure 4.6   Relationship between reaction rate (V) and substrate concentration ($[S]$) in a typical enzymatic reaction. K_m, Michaelis constant; V_{max}, maximal reaction rate.

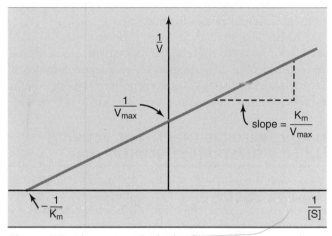

Figure 4.7   Lineweaver-Burk plot for a typical enzymatic reaction. It is derived from the equation $1/V = 1/V_{max} + K_m/V_{max} \times 1/[S]$. K_m, Michaelis constant; V, reaction rate; V_{max}, maximal reaction rate.

$1/[S]$ becomes a straight line. It corresponds to the equation

$$(34) \quad \frac{1}{V} = \frac{1}{V_{max}} + \frac{K_m}{V_{max}} \times \frac{1}{[S]}$$

which is obtained by turning the Michaelis-Menten equation [*Equation (33)*] upside down. The intersection of this line with the y-axis is $1/V_{max}$, and its intersection with the x-axis is $-1/K_m$.

The transition from first-order to zero-order kinetics with increasing substrate concentration can be compared to ticket sales in a bus terminal. When passengers are scarce, the number of tickets sold per minute depends directly on the number of passengers: Tickets are sold with first-order kinetics. However, during rush hour, when a line forms, the rate of ticket sales is no longer limited by passenger availability but by the turnover number of the ticket clerk. No matter how long the line, it progresses at a constant rate, V_{max}. Tickets are now sold with zero-order kinetics.

SUBSTRATE HALF-LIFE CAN BE DETERMINED FOR FIRST-ORDER BUT NOT ZERO-ORDER REACTIONS

Figure 4.8 shows how the substrate of an irreversible reaction gradually disappears by being converted to product. The slope of the curve is the reaction rate. The rate of a zero-order reaction remains constant over time; therefore, we get a straight line. The first-order reaction, in contrast, slows down as less and less substrate is left, and its rate approaches zero asymptotically.

The **half-life** is the time period during which one half of the substrate is consumed in a first-order reaction. Zero-order reactions do not have a half-life.

Many drugs are metabolized by enzymes in the liver. The drug concentration usually is so far below the K_m of the metabolizing enzyme that it is metabolized with first-order kinetics. Consequently, the drug's half-life can be determined by measuring its plasma concentrations at different points in time.

Alcohol metabolism is very different. The alcohol level is so high after a few drinks that the metabolizing enzyme, alcohol dehydrogenase, is almost completely saturated. Therefore a constant amount of about 10 g/hr is metabolized no matter how drunk a person is (*Fig. 4.9*).

K_{cat}/K_m PREDICTS THE ENZYME ACTIVITY AT LOW SUBSTRATE CONCENTRATION

V_{max} depends directly on the enzyme concentration [*Equation (19)*]: Doubling the enzyme concentration doubles the reaction rate. Therefore *the amount of an enzyme is most conveniently determined by measuring its activity at saturating substrate concentrations*. This is done in the clinical laboratory when serum enzymes are determined for diagnostic purposes (see Chapter 15). Enzyme activities can be expressed as **international units (IUs).** One IU is defined as *the amount of enzyme that converts one*

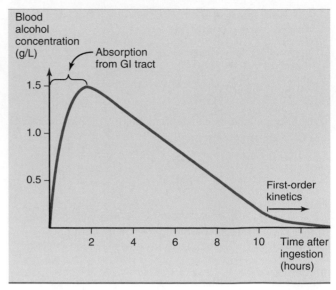

Figure 4.9 Blood alcohol concentration after the ingestion of 120 g of ethanol. The linear decrease of the alcohol level 2 to 10 hours after ingestion shows that a zero-order reaction limits the rate of alcohol metabolism. *GI,* Gastrointestinal.

micromole (μmol) of substrate to product per minute. Because V_{max} depends on temperature, pH, and other factors, the incubation conditions must be specified.

However, most enzymes in the living cell work with substrate concentrations far below their K_m. *At these low substrate concentrations, the k_{cat}/K_m ratio is the best predictor of the actual reaction rate.* This is apparent when *Equations (18)* and *(25)* are combined:

$$(35) \quad V = \frac{k_{cat}}{K_m} \times [E] \times [S]$$

When the substrate concentration is far below K_m, almost all the enzyme molecules are present as free enzyme rather than enzyme-substrate complex, and

$$[E] \approx [E_T]$$

Therefore *Equation (35)* yields

$$(36) \quad V \approx \frac{k_{cat}}{K_m} \times [E_T] \times [S]$$

It now is evident that at a very low substrate concentration, the reaction rate depends directly on enzyme concentration $[E_T]$, substrate concentration $[S]$, and k_{cat}/K_m. K_m is a measure of the affinity between enzyme and substrate, where a low K_m signifies high affinity, and k_{cat} is the turnover number of the enzyme.

ALLOSTERIC ENZYMES DO NOT CONFORM TO MICHAELIS-MENTEN KINETICS

Not all enzymes show simple Michaelis-Menten kinetics. For example, the sigmoidal relationship between substrate concentration and reaction rate (*Fig. 4.10*) is typical for an allosteric enzyme with more than one active site and positive cooperativity between the active

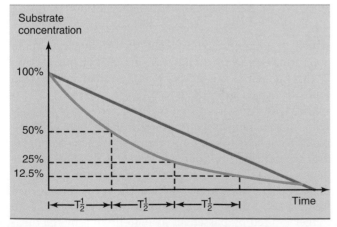

Figure 4.8 Disappearance of substrate is traced for a zero-order reaction (—) and a first-order reaction (—). The half-life ($T_{1/2}$) is defined as the time period during which half of the substrate is converted to product in the first-order reaction.

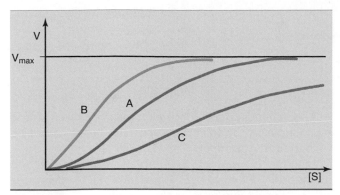

Figure 4.10 Plot of velocity (*V*) against substrate concentration ([*S*]) for an allosteric enzyme with positive cooperativity. *Line A,* Enzyme alone; *line B,* with positive allosteric effector; *line C,* with negative allosteric effector; V_{max}, maximal reaction rate.

sites. This curve would not yield a straight line in the Lineweaver-Burk plot.

More important are the responses of enzymes to **allosteric effectors.** Positive allosteric effectors activate the enzyme, and negative allosteric effectors inhibit it. *These regulatory molecules bind to sites other than the substrate-binding site.* Their binding is noncovalent and therefore reversible. Allosteric effectors can change both the enzyme's affinity for substrate (K_m) and its turnover number (k_{cat}).

Allosteric enzymes occupy strategic locations in metabolic pathways where they are regulated by substrates or products of the pathway.

ENZYME ACTIVITY DEPENDS ON TEMPERATURE AND pH

Chemical reactions are accelerated by increased temperature. The greater the activation energy ΔG_{act} of the reaction, the greater is its temperature dependence. The Q_{10} **value** is the factor by which the reaction is accelerated when the temperature rises by 10°C. Most uncatalyzed reactions have Q_{10} values between 2 and 5. Enzymatic reactions have lower activation energies, so their Q_{10} values are most commonly between 1.7 and 2.5. At very high temperatures, however, enzymes become irreversibly denatured. This produces the relationship shown in *Figure 4.11.*

The temperature dependence of enzymatic reactions contributes to the increased metabolic rate during fever. Presumably it also is responsible for the fact that humans cannot tolerate body temperatures higher than 42°C to 43°C. The most sensitive enzymes already start denaturing at temperatures above this limit. Protein denaturation is time dependent, and an enzyme that survives a temperature of 45°C for some minutes may well denature gradually during the course of several hours.

Hypothermia is far better tolerated than hyperthermia, and the temperature of the toes can fall close to 0°C on a cold winter day. This temperature blocks nerve conduction and muscle activity, but it does not

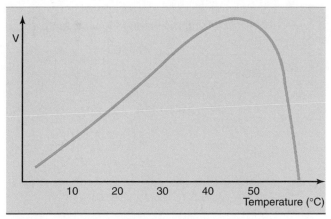

Figure 4.11 Temperature dependence of a typical enzymatic reaction. *V,* Reaction rate.

kill the cells. However, *the metabolic rate is depressed at low temperatures.* Therefore a slowdown in the vital functions of the brain and heart limits a person's tolerance of hypothermia. Also, a vicious cycle develops when decreased metabolism reduces heat production during hypothermia. *Hypothermia makes cells and tissues more resistant to hypoxia* because it decreases their oxygen consumption. Organs used for transplantation can be preserved in the cold for many hours.

Enzymes are also affected by pH (*Fig. 4.12*), mainly because *the protonation state of catalytically active groups in the enzyme depends on pH.* The pH values of tissues and body fluids are tightly regulated to satisfy the pH requirements of the enzymes. Deviations of more than 0.5 pH units from the normal blood pH of 7.4 are fatal. Inside the cells, typical pH values are 6.5 to 7.0 in the cytoplasm, 7.5 to 8.0 in the mitochondrial matrix, and 4.5 to 5.5 in the lysosomes.

DIFFERENT TYPES OF REVERSIBLE ENZYME INHIBITION CAN BE DISTINGUISHED KINETICALLY

Competitive inhibitors are structurally related to the normal substrate of the enzyme. They compete with the substrate by binding noncovalently to the active site of the

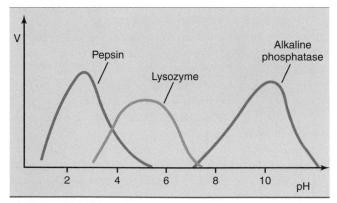

Figure 4.12 pH dependence of some enzymes. *V,* Reaction rate.

enzyme. For example, the mitochondrial enzyme succinate dehydrogenase (SDH) catalyzes the following reaction:

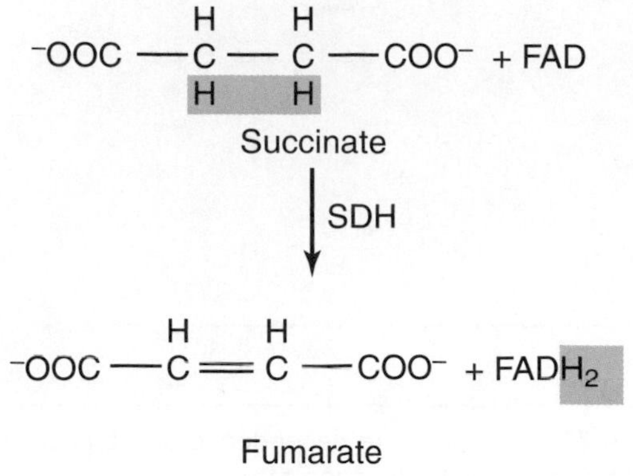

$$^-OOC \longrightarrow \underset{\underset{H}{|}}{\overset{\overset{H}{|}}{C}} \longrightarrow \underset{\underset{H}{|}}{\overset{\overset{H}{|}}{C}} \longrightarrow COO^- + FAD$$

Succinate

SDH

$$^-OOC \longrightarrow \overset{\overset{H}{|}}{C} = \overset{\overset{H}{|}}{C} \longrightarrow COO^- + FADH_2$$

Fumarate

CLINICAL EXAMPLE 4.1: Methanol Poisoning

Methanol is sometimes swallowed by people who read "methyl alcohol" on a label and mistake it for the real stuff. Methanol itself is not very obnoxious, but it is converted to the toxic metabolites formaldehyde and formic acid in the body (**Fig. 4.13**). Formaldehyde (otherwise used to preserve cadavers) is chemically reactive, and formic acid causes acidosis. Blindness and death can result from methanol poisoning.

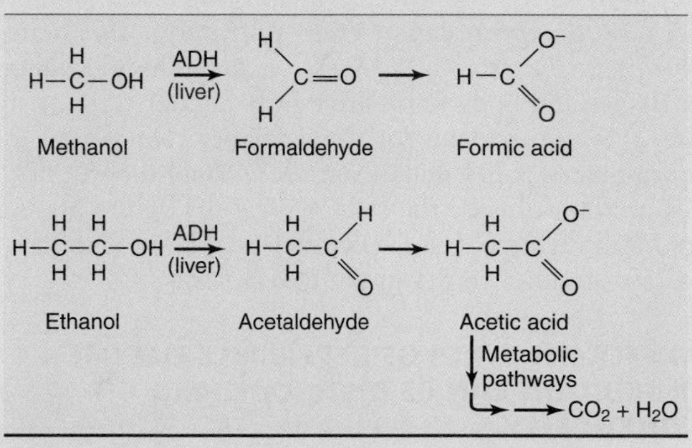

$$H\underset{\underset{H}{|}}{\overset{\overset{H}{|}}{C}}OH \xrightarrow[\text{(liver)}]{ADH} \underset{H}{\overset{H}{C}}=O \longrightarrow H\overset{}{C}\overset{O^-}{\underset{O}{\diagdown}}$$

Methanol   Formaldehyde   Formic acid

$$H\underset{\underset{H}{|}}{\overset{\overset{H}{|}}{C}}\underset{\underset{H}{|}}{\overset{\overset{H}{|}}{C}}OH \xrightarrow[\text{(liver)}]{ADH} H\underset{\underset{H}{|}}{\overset{\overset{H}{|}}{C}}\overset{H}{C}\overset{}{\underset{O}{\diagdown}} \longrightarrow H\underset{\underset{H}{|}}{\overset{\overset{H}{|}}{C}}\overset{}{C}\overset{O^-}{\underset{O}{\diagdown}}$$

Ethanol   Acetaldehyde   Acetic acid

Metabolic pathways
$\longrightarrow CO_2 + H_2O$

Figure 4.13 Role of alcohol dehydrogenase (ADH) in the metabolism of methanol and ethanol. The two substrates compete for the enzyme. Therefore ethanol inhibits the formation of toxic formaldehyde and formic acid from methanol.

The methanol-metabolizing enzyme alcohol dehydrogenase can metabolize ethanol as well. It actually has a higher affinity (lower K_m) for ethanol than for methanol. However, whereas methanol metabolites accumulate in the body, ethanol metabolites are channeled smoothly into the major metabolic pathways where they are rapidly oxidized to carbon dioxide and water. They do not accumulate to toxic levels. When ethanol is administered to a patient with methanol poisoning, the formation of the toxic methanol metabolites is delayed because ethanol competes with methanol for the enzyme. The patient remains drunk but alive.

This reaction is competitively inhibited by malonate:

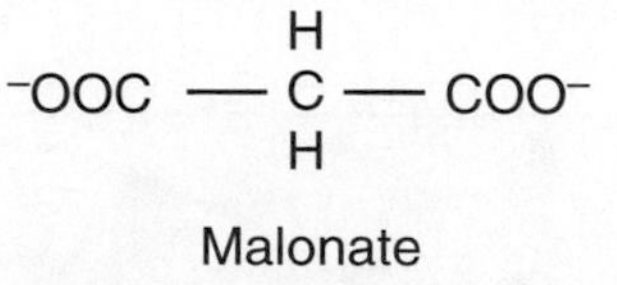

$$^-OOC \longrightarrow \underset{\underset{H}{|}}{\overset{\overset{H}{|}}{C}} \longrightarrow COO^-$$

Malonate

Malonate binds to the enzyme by the same electrostatic interactions as the substrate succinate, but it cannot be converted to a product.

In other cases, such as **Clinical Example 4.1**, the inhibitor is converted to a product: *Two alternative substrates can compete for the enzyme.*

Competitive inhibitors do not change V_{max} because inhibitor binding is reversible and can be overcome by high concentrations of the substrate. However, substrate binding to the enzyme is impaired, and the apparent binding affinity is decreased. Therefore *competitive inhibitors increase* K_m (**Fig. 4.14**).

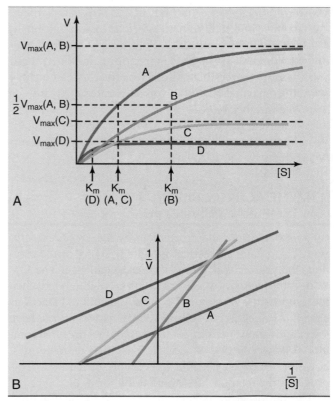

Figure 4.14 Effects of inhibitors on enzymatic reactions. *Line A,* Uninhibited enzyme; *line B,* competitive inhibitor; *line C,* noncompetitive inhibitor; *line D,* uncompetitive inhibitor. For noncompetitive inhibition, it is assumed that the inhibitor binds equally well to the free enzyme and the enzyme-substrate complex (see text for discussion). The kinetic effects of irreversible inhibitors resemble those shown for the noncompetitive inhibitor. **A,** Reaction rate (*V*) plotted against substrate concentration ([*S*]). **B,** In the Lineweaver-Burk plot, the effects of inhibitors on V_{max} (maximal reaction rate) and K_m (Michaelis constant) are reflected in changes of the intercepts with the *y*-axis and *x*-axis, respectively.

Noncompetitive inhibitors are structurally unrelated to the substrate and bind to the enzyme protein outside of the substrate-binding site. They do not necessarily prevent substrate binding, but they block enzymatic catalysis. *If the noncompetitive inhibitor binds equally well to the free enzyme and the enzyme-substrate complex, it reduces V_{max} without changing K_m.*

Uncompetitive inhibitors bind only to the enzyme-substrate complex but not to the free enzyme. *They thereby reduce both K_m and V_{max}.* Unlike competitive inhibitors, which are most effective at low substrate concentrations, *uncompetitive inhibitors work best when the substrate concentration is high.*

COVALENT MODIFICATION CAN INHIBIT ENZYMES IRREVERSIBLY

Competitive, noncompetitive, and uncompetitive inhibitors bind noncovalently to the enzyme. Therefore their actions are reversible. Enzyme activity is fully restored when the inhibitor is removed, for example, by extensive dialysis in the test tube, or by metabolic inactivation or renal excretion in the body. **Irreversible inhibitors**, however, form a covalent bond with the enzyme. The chemically modified enzyme is dead, and *this type of inhibition can be overcome only by the synthesis of new enzyme.*

ENZYMES ARE CLASSIFIED ACCORDING TO THEIR REACTION TYPE

Enzymes are most commonly named after their substrate and their reaction type, with the suffix *-ase* at the end. For example, monoamine oxidase is an enzyme that oxidizes monoamines, and catechol-O-methyltransferase transfers a methyl group to an oxygen in a catechol.

According to their reaction type, enzymes are grouped into the following six classes.

Oxidoreductases

Oxidoreductases catalyze oxidation-reduction reactions: electron transfers, hydrogen transfers, and reactions involving molecular oxygen.

Dehydrogenases transfer hydrogen between a substrate and a coenzyme, most commonly NAD (nicotinamide adenine dinucleotide), NADP (nicotinamide adenine dinucleotide phosphate), FAD (flavin adenine dinucleotide), or FMN (flavin mononucleotide). These enzymes are named after the substrate from which hydrogen is removed. For example,

CLINICAL EXAMPLE 4.2: Organophosphate Poisoning

Organophosphates are irreversible inhibitors of acetylcholinesterase, the enzyme that degrades the neurotransmitter acetylcholine at cholinergic synapses (see Chapter 16). The organophosphate inactivates acetylcholinesterase by forming a covalent bond with an essential serine residue in its active site:

Serine residue (in acetylcholinesterase)

Sarin

Without the free hydroxyl group of the serine side chain, the enzyme is completely inactive. Acetylcholine is no longer degraded and accumulates at cholinergic synapses in skeletal muscles, the autonomic nervous system, and the brain. Overstimulation of acetylcholine receptors leads to paralysis, autonomic dysfunction, and delirium.

Organophosphates have two uses. Those that are most potent on the acetylcholinesterase of insects are used as agricultural pesticides, and those that work best on the human enzyme are "nerve gases" that are of interest to terrorists and the military.

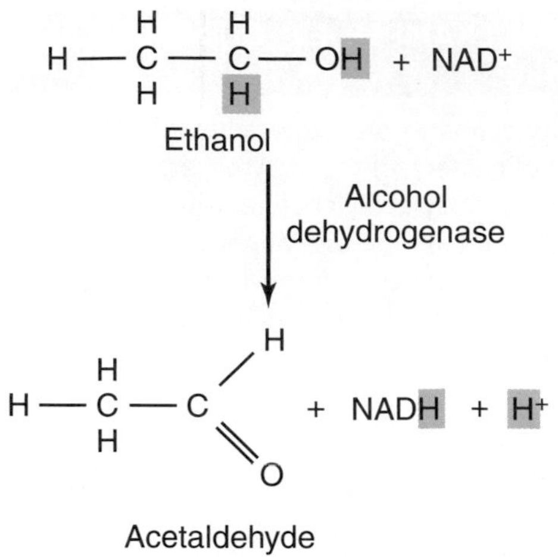

Ethanol

Alcohol
dehydrogenase

Acetaldehyde

Oxygenases use molecular oxygen as a substrate. **Dioxygenases** incorporate both oxygen atoms of O_2 into their substrate; **monooxygenases** incorporate only one. Most **hydroxylases** are monooxygenases:

$$\text{Substrate}-\text{H} + O_2 + \text{NADPH} + \text{H}^+$$
$$\downarrow$$
$$\text{Substrate}-\text{OH} + \text{NADP}^+ + H_2O$$

In this reaction, the second oxygen atom reacts with the reduced coenzyme NADPH to form water.

Peroxidases use hydrogen peroxide or an organic peroxide as one of their substrates. **Catalase** is technically a peroxidase. It degrades hydrogen peroxide to molecular oxygen and water:

$$H_2O_2 \longrightarrow H_2O + \frac{1}{2}O_2$$

Transferases

Transferases transfer a group from one molecule to another.

Kinases transfer phosphate from ATP to a second substrate. They are named according to the substrate to which the phosphate is transferred. For example,

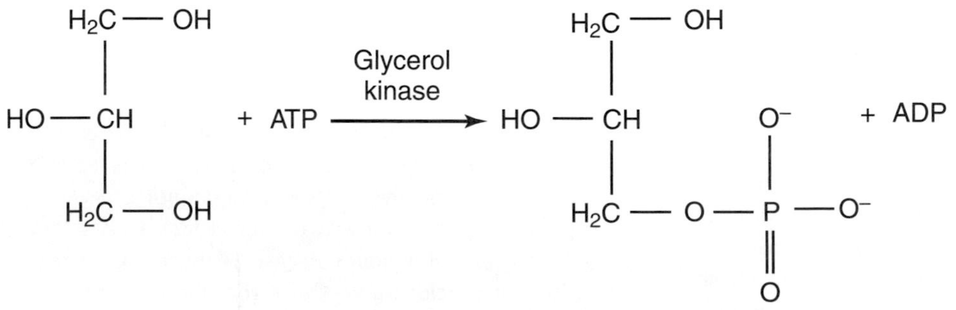

Glycerol

Glycerol
3-phosphate

Other examples of transferases include **phosphorylases**, which cleave bonds by the addition of inorganic phosphate; **glycosyl transferases**, which transfer a monosaccharide to an acceptor molecule; the **transaminases** (see Chapter 26); and the **peptidyl transferase** of the ribosome (see Chapter 6).

Hydrolases

Hydrolases cleave bonds by the addition of water. Digestive enzymes and lysosomal enzymes are hydrolases. Their names indicate the substrates or bonds on which they act. Examples include peptidases (proteases), esterases, lipases, and phosphatases. For example, acetylcholinesterase cleaves an ester bond in acetylcholine.

If the substrate is polymeric, the cleavage specificity of the enzyme is indicated by the prefixes *endo-* (from Greek meaning "inside") and *exo-* (from Greek meaning "outside"). For example, an exopeptidase cleaves amino acids from the end of a polypeptide, and an endopeptidase cleaves internal peptide bonds.

Lyases

Lyases remove a group nonhydrolytically, forming a double bond. Examples are the **dehydratases**:

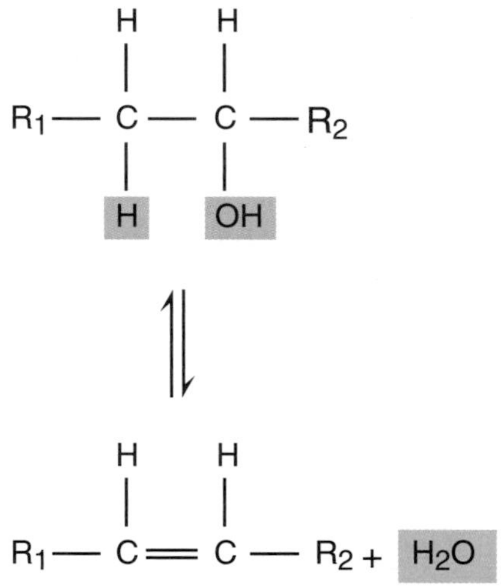

and decarboxylases:

$$R\!-\!C\!\!\underset{OH}{\overset{O}{<}} \longrightarrow R\!-\!H + O\!=\!C\!=\!O$$

Many lyase reactions proceed in the opposite direction, creating a new bond and obliterating a double bond in one of the substrates. These enzymes are called **synthases.**

Isomerases

Isomerases interconvert positional, geometric, or optical isomers.

Ligases

Ligases couple the hydrolysis of a phosphoanhydride bond to the formation of a bond. These enzymes are often called **synthetases.** For example, glutamine synthetase couples ATP hydrolysis to the formation of the amide bond in glutamine:

$$COO^-$$
$$|$$
$$(CH_2)_2$$
$$|$$
$$H_3^+N \!-\! CH \!-\! COO^- \qquad + NH_3 + ATP$$

Glutamate

↓ Glutamine synthetase

$$\overset{O}{\overset{\|}{C}} \!-\! NH_2$$
$$|$$
$$(CH_2)_2$$
$$|$$
$$H_3^+N \!-\! CH \!-\! COO^- \qquad + ADP + P_i$$

Glutamine

DNA ligase and **aminoacyl–tRNA synthetases** (see Chapter 6) are other examples. The biotin-dependent carboxylases (see Chapter 21) also are classified as ligases.

ENZYMES STABILIZE THE TRANSITION STATE

Enzymes can stabilize the transition state of the reaction by making its formation a more likely event, thereby increasing the entropy of the transition state, or by forming energetically favorable noncovalent interactions with the transition state, thereby reducing its enthalpy. Four mechanisms of enzymatic catalysis can be distinguished:

1. **Entropy effect:** The transition state can form only when the substrates of a two-substrate reaction collide in the correct geometric orientation and with sufficient energy to bring them to the transition state. The enzyme increases the likelihood of such an event by binding the two substrates to its active site in close proximity and in the correct geometric orientation.
2. **Stabilization of the transition state:** The enzyme forms favorable interactions with the transition state of the reaction, thereby reducing its free energy content and the free energy of activation.
3. **General acid-base catalysis:** Catalysis requires ionizable groups on the enzyme that accept or donate protons during the reaction. Enzymes can also provide electron pair donors and acceptors, which are known as Lewis bases and Lewis acids, respectively. Because the ionizable groups on the enzyme must be in the correct protonation state, *general acid-base catalysis is the most important reason for the pH dependence of enzymatic reactions.* For example, if the reaction requires a deprotonated glutamate side chain with a pK of 4.0 as a general base and a protonated histidine side chain with a pK of 6.0 as a general acid, only pH values between 4.0 and 6.0 will allow high reaction rates.
4. **Covalent catalysis:** The enzyme forms a transient covalent bond with the substrate. The serine proteases described in the following paragraph are the most prominent example.

CHYMOTRYPSIN FORMS A TRANSIENT COVALENT BOND DURING CATALYSIS

The serine proteases cleave peptide bonds with the help of a serine residue in their active site. The pancreatic enzyme **chymotrypsin** is a typical example. When chymotrypsin binds its polypeptide substrate, it forms a hydrophobic interaction with an amino acid side chain in the substrate. The peptide bond that is formed by the carboxyl group of this hydrophobic amino acid is targeted for cleavage. This peptide bond is placed right

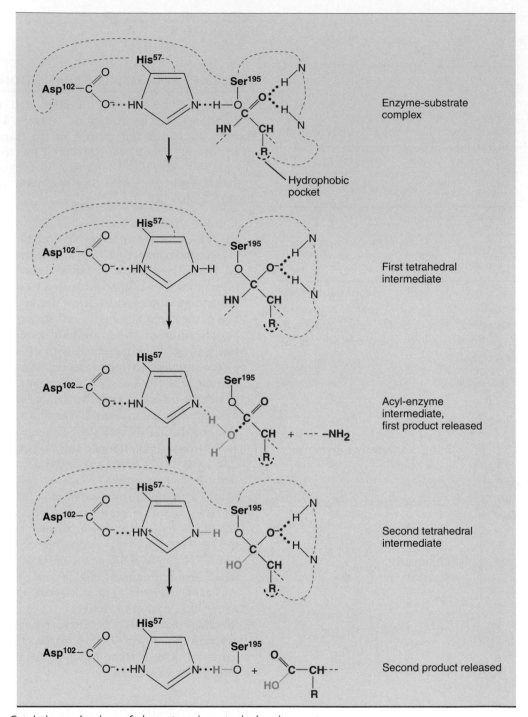

Figure 4.15 Catalytic mechanism of chymotrypsin, a typical serine protease.

on the hydroxyl group of the catalytic serine residue in the active site, Ser-195 (*Fig. 4.15*).

In addition to Ser-195, catalysis requires a deprotonated histidine residue, His-57, and a deprotonated aspartate residue, Asp-102. The numbers indicate the positions of the amino acids in the polypeptide, counting from the N-terminus. Although widely separated in the amino acid sequence of the protein, these three amino acids are hydrogen bonded to each other in the active site of the enzyme.

Chymotrypsin cleaves the bond in a sequence of two reactions. In the first reaction, the peptide bond in the substrate is cleaved, and one of the fragments binds covalently to the serine side chain to form an **acyl-enzyme intermediate**. In the second reaction, this intermediate is cleaved hydrolytically.

The acyl-enzyme intermediate does not qualify as a transition state because it occupies a valley in the free energy graph, rather than a peak (*Fig. 4.16*). The transition states in both reactions are negatively charged

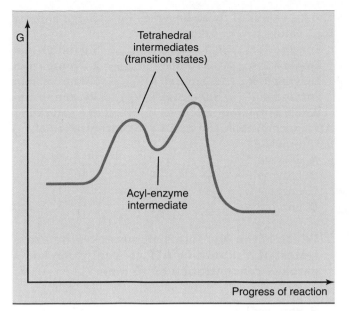

Figure 4.16 Energy profile for the reaction of a serine protease. *G*, Free energy.

tetrahedral intermediates that are stabilized by hydrogen bonds with two N-H groups in the main chain of the enzyme.

To form the negatively charged transition state, *a proton must be transferred from the hydroxyl group of Ser-195 to His-57*. Asp-102 remains negatively charged throughout the catalytic cycle. It forms a salt bond with the protonated but not the deprotonated form of His-57, thereby stabilizing the protonated form and increasing the proton affinity of the histidine.

The serine proteases are a large family of enzymes that includes the digestive enzymes trypsin, chymotrypsin, and elastase, and blood clotting factors including thrombin. They all use the same catalytic mechanism but have different substrate specificities. Chymotrypsin cleaves peptide bonds on the carboxyl side of large hydrophobic amino acids. Trypsin contains a negatively charged aspartate residue in its substrate-binding pocket and therefore prefers peptide bonds formed by positively charged amino acids. Elastase

cleaves bonds formed by glycine. Thrombin is highly selective for a small number of plasma proteins, including fibrinogen.

SUMMARY

Chemical reactions proceed to an equilibrium state at which the rates of the forward and backward reactions are equal, driven by the free energy change that accompanies the reaction. Enzymes cannot change the equilibrium of the reaction. They can only increase the reaction rate.

Enzymatic catalysis starts with the formation of a noncovalent enzyme-substrate complex. While bound to the enzyme, the substrate is converted to an unstable transition state that decomposes almost immediately to form either substrate or product. The enzyme accelerates the reaction by making the formation of the transition state more likely and by stabilizing the transition state energetically.

The Michaelis constant K_m is the substrate concentration at which the reaction rate is half-maximal. It is determined mainly by the binding affinity between enzyme and substrate. At substrate concentrations far lower than K_m, the reaction rate increases almost linearly with increasing substrate concentration. The reaction shows first-order kinetics. However, at substrate concentrations far higher than K_m, the reaction rate can hardly be increased by further increases of the substrate concentration because most of the enzyme is already present as enzyme-substrate complex. The reaction shows zero-order kinetics.

The rate of enzymatic reactions increases with increasing temperature, typically with a doubling of the reaction rate for a temperature increase of about 10°C. The pH also is important because most enzymes use ionizable groups for catalysis. These groups must be in the proper protonation state.

Many drugs and toxins act as specific enzyme inhibitors. Some bind to the enzyme reversibly, through noncovalent interactions. Others form a covalent bond with the enzyme, thereby destroying its catalytic activity permanently.

QUESTIONS

1. **During a drug screening program, you find a chemical that decreases the activity of the enzyme monoamine oxidase. A fixed dose of the chemical reduces the catalytic activity of the enzyme by the same percentage at all substrate concentrations, with a decrease in V_{max}. K_m is unaffected. This inhibitor is**

   A. Definitely a competitive inhibitor
   B. Definitely a noncompetitive inhibitor
   C. Definitely an irreversible inhibitor
   D. Either a competitive or an irreversible inhibitor
   E. Either a noncompetitive or an irreversible inhibitor

2. **The irreversible enzymatic reaction**

$$\text{Oxaloacetate} + \text{Acetyl} - \text{coenzyme A (CoA)} \rightarrow \text{Citrate} + \text{CoA} - \text{SH}$$

   is inhibited by high concentrations of its own product citrate. This product inhibition can be overcome, and a normal V_{max} can be restored, when the oxaloacetate

concentration is raised but not when the acetyl-CoA concentration is raised. This observation suggests that citrate is

A. An irreversible inhibitor reacting with the oxaloacetate binding site of the enzyme

B. A competitive inhibitor binding to the acetyl-CoA binding site of the enzyme

C. A competitive inhibitor binding to the oxaloacetate binding site of the enzyme

D. A noncompetitive inhibitor binding to the acetyl-CoA binding site of the enzyme

E. A noncompetitive inhibitor binding to the oxaloacetate binding site of the enzyme

3. An enzymatic reaction works best at pH values between 6 and 8. This is compatible with the assumption that the reaction mechanism requires two ionizable amino acid side chains in the active site of the enzyme, possibly

A. Protonated glutamate and deprotonated aspartate

B. Protonated histidine and deprotonated lysine

C. Protonated glutamate and deprotonated histidine

D. Protonated arginine and deprotonated lysine

E. Protonated cysteine and deprotonated histidine

4. A biotechnology company has cloned four different forms of the enzyme money synthetase, which catalyzes the reaction

Garbage + ATP → Money + ADP + Phosphate + H$^+$

The K_m values of these enzymes for garbage and the V_{max} values are as follows:

Enzyme 1: K_m = 0.1 mmol/L, V_{max} = 5.0 mmol/min

Enzyme 2: K_m = 0.3 mmol/L, V_{max} = 2.0 mmol/min

Enzyme 3: K_m = 1.0 mmol/L, V_{max} = 5.0 mmol/min

Enzyme 4: K_m = 3.0 mmol/L, V_{max} = 20 mmol/min

Which of the four enzymes is fastest at a saturating ATP concentration and a garbage concentration of 0.01 mmol/L?

A. Enzyme 1

B. Enzyme 2

C. Enzyme 3

D. Enzyme 4

5. Which of the four forms of money synthetase is fastest at a saturating ATP concentration and a garbage concentration of 10 mmol/L?

A. Enzyme 1

B. Enzyme 2

C. Enzyme 3

D. Enzyme 4

6. If the money synthetase reaction is freely reversible, which of the following manipulations would be best to favor money formation over garbage formation and to increase the [Money]/[Garbage] ratio at equilibrium?

A. Decreasing the pH value

B. Adding another enzyme that destroys ADP

C. Using a very low concentration of ATP

D. Increasing the temperature

E. Adding a noncompetitive inhibitor

Chapter 5
COENZYMES

Coenzymes are nonpolypeptide components that participate in enzymatic reactions. They are required because only a limited number of functional groups are available in polypeptides. For example, there are no groups that can easily transfer hydrogen or electrons and none that can bind molecular oxygen, and there are no energy-rich bonds. Whenever such structural features are required for enzymatic catalysis, a coenzyme is needed. Each coenzyme is concerned with a specific reaction type, such as hydrogen transfer, methylation, or carboxylation. Thus, test-savvy students can predict the coenzyme of a reaction from the reaction type.

There are two types of coenzymes. A **cosubstrate** is promiscuous, associating with the enzyme only for the purpose of the reaction. It becomes chemically modified in the reaction and then diffuses away for a next liaison with another enzyme. A true **prosthetic group,** in contrast, is monogamous. It is permanently bonded to the active site of the enzyme, either covalently or noncovalently, and stays with the enzyme after completion of the reaction.

Some coenzymes can be synthesized in the body de novo ("from scratch"), but others contain a vitamin or are vitamins themselves. Reactions that depend on such a coenzyme are blocked when the vitamin is deficient in the diet.

ADENOSINE TRIPHOSPHATE HAS TWO ENERGY-RICH BONDS

Metabolic energy is generated by the oxidation of carbohydrate, fat, protein, and alcohol. This energy must be harnessed to drive endergonic chemical reactions, membrane transport, and muscle contraction. Nature has solved this task with a simple trick: *Exergonic reactions are used for the synthesis of the energy-rich compound adenosine triphosphate (ATP), and the chemical bond energy of ATP drives the endergonic processes.* In this sense, ATP serves as the energetic currency of the cell (*Fig. 5.1*).

ATP is a ribonucleotide, one of the precursors for ribonucleic acid (RNA) synthesis. It does not contain a vitamin, and the whole molecule can be synthesized from simple precursors (see Chapter 28). Its most important part is a string of three phosphate residues, bound to carbon 5 of ribose and complexed with a magnesium ion (*Figs. 5.2* and *5.3*).

The first phosphate is linked to ribose by a phosphate ester bond, but *the two bonds between the phosphates are energy-rich phosphoanhydride bonds.* The free energy changes shown in *Figure 5.2* apply to standard conditions. The actual free energy change for the hydrolysis of ATP to ADP + inorganic phosphate (P_i) depends on pH, ionic strength, and the concentrations of ATP, ADP, phosphate, and magnesium. It is close to -11 or -12 kcal/mol under "real-cell" conditions. ATP can be hydrolyzed to ADP and phosphate:

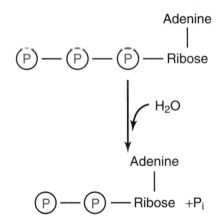

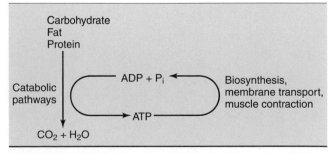

Figure 5.1 The function of adenosine triphosphate (*ATP*) as the "energetic currency" of the cell. *ADP,* Adenosine diphosphate; P_i, inorganic phosphate.

55

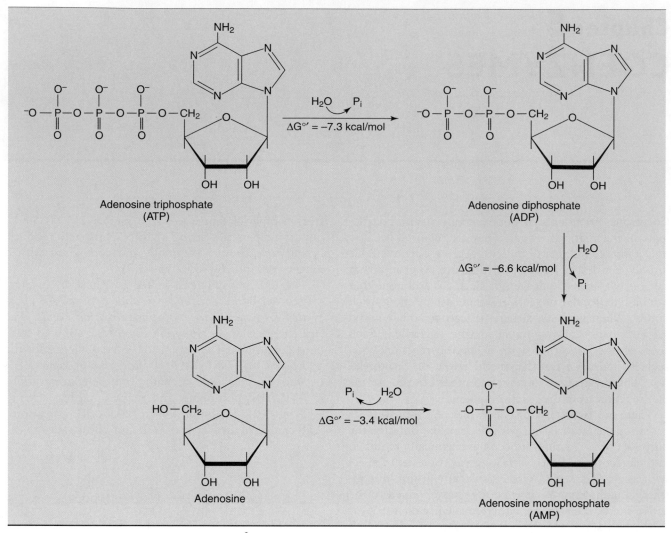

Figure 5.2 Sequential hydrolysis of ATP. $\Delta G^{0\prime}$, Standard free energy change; P_i, inorganic phosphate.

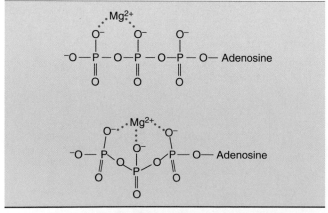

Figure 5.3 Magnesium complexes formed by adenosine triphosphate (ATP). Complexes are the actual substrates of ATP-dependent enzymes.

or to adenosine monophosphate (AMP) and inorganic pyrophosphate (PP_i):

The PP_i formed in the second reaction still contains an energy-rich phosphoanhydride bond:

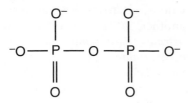

PP_i is rapidly hydrolyzed by pyrophosphatases in the cell. Because this removes PP_i from the reaction equilibrium, the cleavage of ATP to $AMP + PP_i$ releases far more energy than the cleavage to $ADP +$ phosphate.

ATP IS THE PHOSPHATE DONOR IN PHOSPHORYLATION REACTIONS

Table 5.1 lists the most important uses of ATP. Only phosphorylation reactions and the coupling to endergonic reactions are considered here.

Phosphorylation is the covalent attachment of a phosphate group to a substrate, most commonly by the formation of a phosphate ester bond. Assume that the cell is to convert glucose to glucose-6-phosphate, a simple phosphate ester:

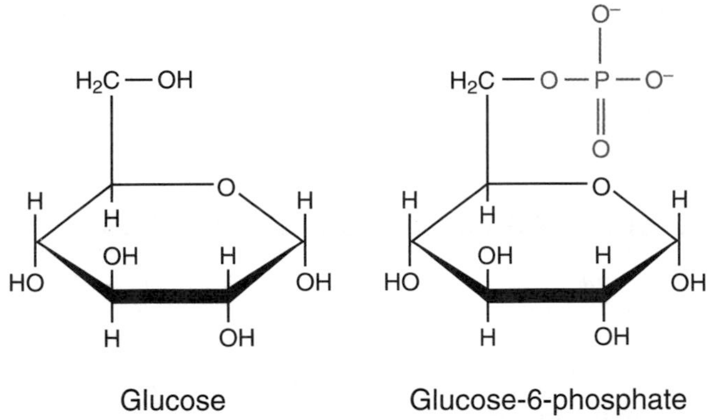

One possibility is to synthesize glucose-6-phosphate by reacting free glucose with P_i:

$$\text{Glucose} + P_i \xrightarrow{\text{Glucose 6-phosphatase}} \text{Glucose-6-phosphate} + H_2O$$

The enzyme glucose-6-phosphatase really exists, but the $\triangle G^{0\prime}$ of the reaction is $+3.3$ kcal/mol. This translates into an equilibrium constant (K_{equ}) of about 4×10^{-3} L/mol. At an intracellular phosphate concentration of 10 mmol/L, there would be 25,000 molecules of glucose for each molecule of glucose-6-phosphate! Things look better when ATP supplies the phosphate group:

$$\text{Glucose} + \text{ATP} \xrightarrow{\text{Hexokinase}} \text{Glucose-6-phosphate} + \text{ADP}$$

Table 5.1 Uses of ATP

Table 5.1 Uses of ATP

Process	Function
RNA synthesis	Precursor
Phosphorylation	Phosphate donor
Coupling to endergonic reactions	Energy source
Active membrane transport	Energy source
Muscle contraction	Energy source
Ciliary motion	Energy source

RNA, Ribonucleic acid.

The $\triangle G^{0\prime}$ of this reaction is -4.0 kcal/mol. The difference in the $\triangle G^{0\prime}$ values of the hexokinase and glucose-6-phosphatase reactions (7.3 kcal/mol) corresponds to the free energy content of the phosphoanhydride bond in ATP. Now the equilibrium constant is about 10^3. When the cellular ATP concentration is 10 times higher than the ADP concentration, there are 10,000 molecules of glucose-6-phosphate for each molecule of glucose at equilibrium!

ATP HYDROLYSIS DRIVES ENDERGONIC REACTIONS

Phosphorylations are not the only reactions driven in the desired direction by ATP. For example, the following reaction takes place in the mitochondria:

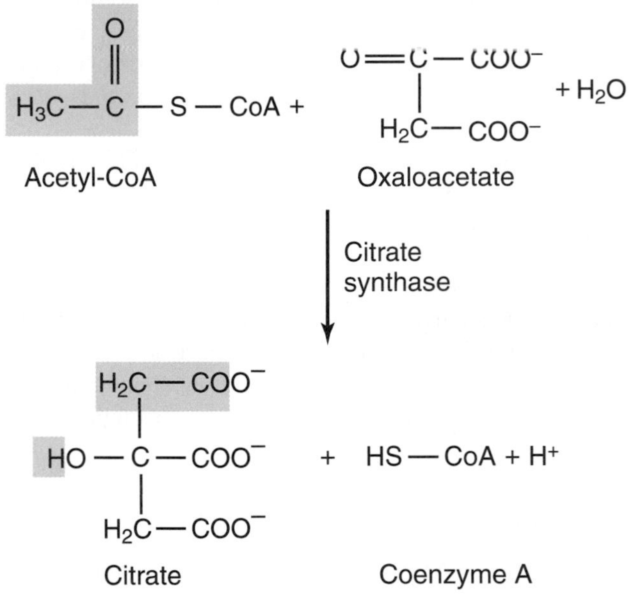

The $\triangle G^{0\prime}$ of this reaction is -8.5 kcal/mol. Therefore it is essentially irreversible in the direction of citrate formation. In the cytoplasm, however, the enzyme ATP-citrate lyase couples this reaction to ATP synthesis:

$$\text{Acetyl-CoA} + \text{Oxaloacetate} + \text{ADP} + P_i \rightarrow$$
$$\text{Citrate} + \text{Coenzyme A} + \text{ATP}$$

The $\triangle G^{0\prime}$ of this reaction is -1.2 kcal/mol, which is the sum of the free energy changes for citrate formation

(−8.5 kcal/mol) and ATP synthesis (+7.3 kcal/mol). The reaction now is reversible and can, under suitable conditions, make oxaloacetate from citrate.

CELLS ALWAYS TRY TO MAINTAIN A HIGH ENERGY CHARGE

ATP can reach a cellular concentration of 5 mmol/L (2.5 g/L, or 0.25%) in some tissues, but the life expectancy of an ATP molecule is only about 2 minutes. Although the total body content of ATP is only about 100 g, *60 to 70 kg is produced and consumed every day.*

In the cell, the enzyme adenylate kinase (adenylate = AMP) maintains the three adenine nucleotides in equilibrium:

$$\text{ATP} + \text{AMP} \xrightleftharpoons{\text{Adenylate kinase}} 2\ \text{ADP}$$

The energy status of the cell can be described either as the [ATP]/[ADP] ratio or as the **energy charge:**

$$\text{Energy charge} = \frac{[\text{ATP}] + \frac{1}{2}[\text{ADP}]}{[\text{ATP}] + [\text{ADP}] + [\text{AMP}]}$$

The energy charge can vary between 0 and 1. Healthy cells always maintain a high energy charge, with [ATP]/[ADP] ratios of 5 to 200 in different cell types. The energy charge drops when either ATP synthesis is impaired, as in hypoxia (oxygen deficiency), or ATP consumption is increased, as in contracting muscle. *When the energy charge approaches zero, the cell is dead.*

The nucleotides **guanosine triphosphate (GTP)**, **uridine triphosphate (UTP)**, and **cytidine triphosphate (CTP)** are present at lower concentrations than ATP. GTP rather than ATP is used as an energy source in some enzymatic reactions. UTP activates monosaccharides for the synthesis of complex carbohydrates (see Chapter 14), and CTP plays a similar role in phospholipid synthesis (see Chapter 24). The monophosphate, diphosphate, and triphosphate forms are in equilibrium through kinase reactions:

$$\left.\begin{array}{l}\text{GMP}\\\text{UMP}\\\text{CMP}\end{array}\right\} + \text{ATP} \xrightleftharpoons[]{\substack{\text{Nucleoside}\\\text{monophosphate}\\\text{kinases}}} \left.\begin{array}{l}\text{GDP}\\\text{UDP}\\\text{CDP}\end{array}\right\} + \text{ADP}$$

and

$$\left.\begin{array}{l}\text{GDP}\\\text{UDP}\\\text{CDP}\end{array}\right\} + \text{ATP} \xrightleftharpoons[]{\substack{\text{Nucleoside}\\\text{diphosphate}\\\text{kinase}}} \left.\begin{array}{l}\text{GTP}\\\text{UTP}\\\text{CTP}\end{array}\right\} + \text{ADP}$$

DEHYDROGENASE REACTIONS REQUIRE SPECIALIZED COENZYMES

In **redox reactions,** electrons are transferred from one substrate to another, either alone or along with protons.

The cosubstrates nicotinamide adenine dinucleotide (NAD) and nicotinamide adenine dinucleotide phosphate (NADP) accept and donate hydrogen (electron + proton) in dehydrogenase reactions. Nicotinamide, which is derived from the vitamin niacin (see Chapter 29), is the hydrogen-carrying part of these coenzymes (*Fig. 5.4*). The additional phosphate in NADP does not affect the hydrogen transfer potential, but it is a recognition site for enzymes. Most dehydrogenases use either NAD alone or NADP alone.

Both coenzymes acquire two electrons and a proton during catabolic reactions, but *NADH feeds its electrons into the respiratory chain of the mitochondria, and NADPH feeds them into biosynthetic pathways.* Therefore NADH is required for the synthesis of ATP, and NADPH is required for the synthesis of reduced products, such as fatty acids and cholesterol, from more oxidized precursors (*Fig. 5.5*).

Some dehydrogenases use flavin adenine dinucleotide (FAD) or flavin mononucleotide (FMN) instead of NAD or NADP (*Fig. 5.6*). Unlike NAD and NADP, *the flavin coenzymes are tightly bound to the apoprotein either noncovalently or by a covalent bond.* These proteins are called **flavoproteins** (from Latin *flavus* meaning "yellow") because the oxidized flavin coenzymes are yellow.

COENZYME A ACTIVATES ORGANIC ACIDS

Coenzyme A (CoA) is a soluble carrier of acyl groups (*Fig. 5.7*). The business end of the molecule is a sulfhydryl group, and its structure is abbreviated as CoA-SH. The sulfhydryl group forms energy-rich thioester bonds with many organic acids (e.g., acetic acid):

$$\begin{array}{c}\quad\quad\quad\overset{\displaystyle O}{\overset{\displaystyle \|}{}}\\ \text{CoA} - \text{S} - \text{C} - \text{CH}_3\end{array}$$

Acetyl-CoA

and fatty acids:

$$\begin{array}{c}\quad\quad\quad\overset{\displaystyle O}{\overset{\displaystyle \|}{}}\\ \text{CoA} - \text{S} - \text{C} - (\text{CH}_2)_{14} - \text{CH}_3\end{array}$$

Palmitoyl-CoA

The thioester bonds have free energy contents between 7 and 8 kcal/mol. *In biosynthetic reactions, the acid is transferred from CoA to an acceptor molecule.* For

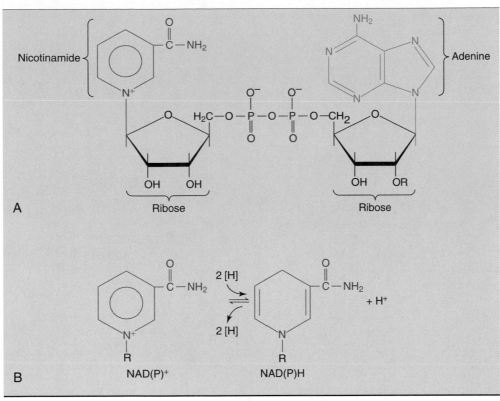

Figure 5.4 Structures of nicotinamide adenine dinucleotide (NAD$^+$) and nicotinamide adenine dinucleotide phosphate (NADP$^+$). **A,** Structures of the coenzymes. For NAD$^+$, R = —H; for NADP$^+$, R = —PO$_3^{2-}$. **B,** The reversible hydrogenation of the nicotinamide portion in NAD and NADP.

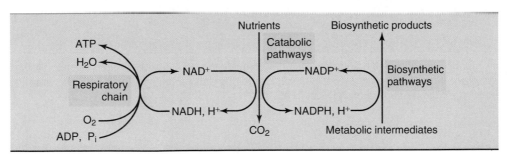

Figure 5.5 Metabolic functions of nicotinamide adenine dinucleotide *(NAD)* and nicotinamide adenine dinucleotide phosphate *(NADP)*.

example, this occurs during acetylation reactions (the "A" in "coenzyme A" stands for "acetylation") and in the synthesis of triglycerides (see Chapter 23).

S-ADENOSYL METHIONINE DONATES METHYL GROUPS

Methylation reactions transfer a methyl group (—CH$_3$) to an acceptor molecule. The donor of the methyl group is in most cases *S*-adenosyl methionine (SAM) (*Fig. 5.8*), which can be synthesized from ATP and the amino acid methionine. The methylation reaction converts SAM to *S*-adenosyl homocysteine (SAH), which can be converted

back to SAM in a sequence of reactions (see Chapter 26). Like CoA, SAM is a cosubstrate rather than a prosthetic group.

Several other coenzymes participate in enzymatic reactions. These coenzymes, summarized in *Table 5.2*, will be discussed in the context of the metabolic reactions in which they participate.

MANY ENZYMES REQUIRE A METAL ION

Some enzymes contain a transition metal such as iron, zinc, copper, or manganese in their active site. *These metals can easily switch between different oxidation states and therefore are suitable for electron transfer reactions:*

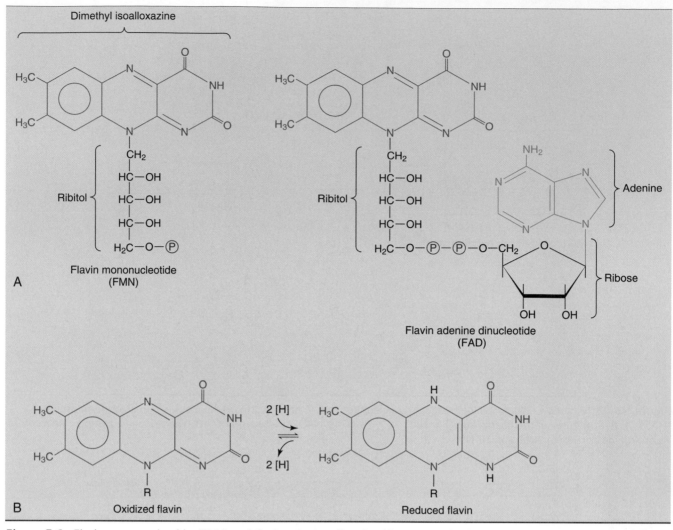

Figure 5.6 Flavin mononucleotide *(FMN)* and flavin adenine dinucleotide *(FAD)* as hydrogen carriers. **A,** Structures of the coenzymes. The structure formed from the dimethyl isoalloxazine ring and ribitol is called riboflavin (vitamin B$_2$). **B,** Hydrogen transfer by the dimethyl isoalloxazine ring of FMN and FAD.

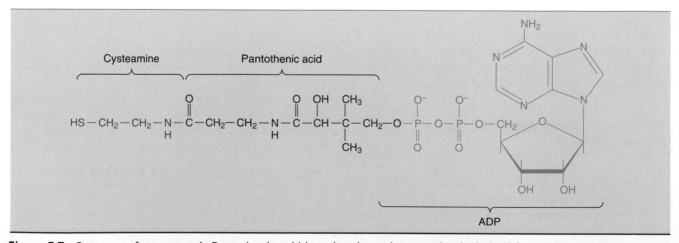

Figure 5.7 Structure of coenzyme A. Pantothenic acid is a vitamin, and cysteamine is derived from the amino acid cysteine.

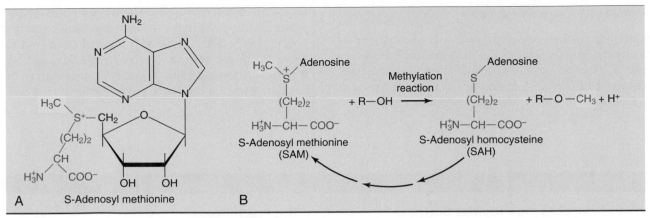

Figure 5.8   S-Adenosyl methionine (SAM) as a methyl group donor. **A**, Structure of the coenzyme. **B**, Formation of a methoxyl group in a SAM-dependent methylation.

Table 5.2   Summary of the Most Important Coenzymes

Coenzyme	Present as	Functions in	Vitamin*
Adenosine triphosphate (ATP)	Cosubstrate	Energy-dependent reactions	—
Guanosine triphosphate (GTP)	Cosubstrate	Energy-dependent reactions	—
Uridine triphosphate (UTP)	Cosubstrate	Activation of monosaccharides	—
Cytidine triphosphate (CTP)	Cosubstrate	Phospholipid synthesis	—
Nicotinamide adenine dinucleotide (NAD) and nicotinamide adenine dinucleotide phosphate (NADP)	Cosubstrate	Hydrogen transfers	Niacin
Flavin adenine dinucleotide (FAD) and flavin mononucleotide (FMN)	Prosthetic group	Hydrogen transfers	Riboflavin
Coenzyme A	Cosubstrate	Acylation reactions	Pantothenic acid
S-Adenosyl methionine (SAM)	Cosubstrate	Methylation reactions	—
Heme	Prosthetic group	Electron transfers	—
Biotin	Prosthetic group	Carboxylation reactions	Biotin
Tetrahydrofolate (THF)	Cosubstrate	One-carbon transfers	Folic acid
Pyridoxal phosphate (PLP)	Prosthetic group	Amino acid metabolism	B_6
Thiamin pyrophosphate (TPP)	Prosthetic group	Carbonyl transfers	Thiamin (B_1)
Lipoic acid	Prosthetic group	Oxidative decarboxylations	—

*The vitamins are discussed in Chapter 29.

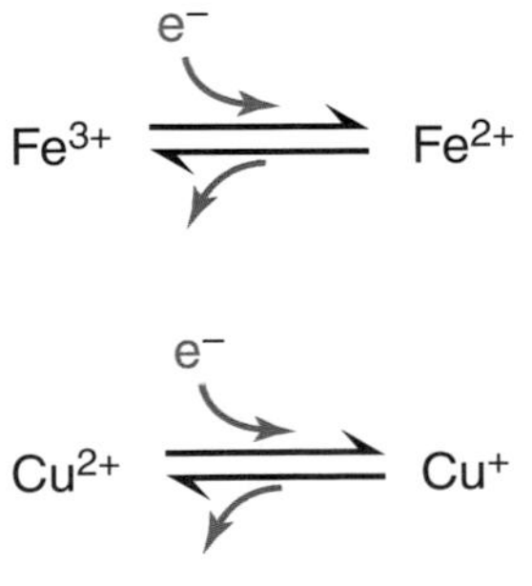

$$Fe^{3+} \;\xrightleftharpoons{e^-}\; Fe^{2+}$$

$$Cu^{2+} \;\xrightleftharpoons{e^-}\; Cu^+$$

In other cases the metal acts as a Lewis acid, or electron-pair acceptor. This occurs in many oxygenase reactions, when ferrous iron (Fe^{2+}) or monovalent copper (Cu^+) binds molecular oxygen. Another example is the carbonic anhydrase reaction shown in *Figure 5.9*.

In this case, the electron density on the oxygen of a water molecule is increased by binding to a zinc ion. This makes the water more reactive for a nucleophilic attack on the carbon of CO_2.

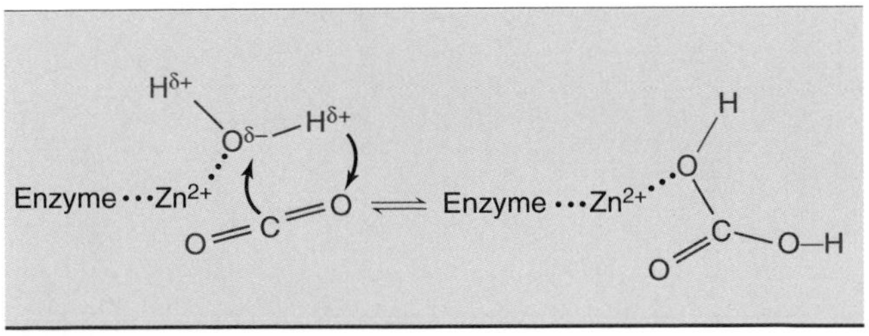

Figure 5.9   Catalytic mechanism of carbonic anhydrase. This enzyme catalyzes the reversible reaction $CO_2 + H_2O \rightleftharpoons H_2CO_3$.

SUMMARY

Some coenzymes are tightly bound to the enzyme as prosthetic groups, whereas others are soluble cosubstrates. They are required because they offer structural features and chemical reactivities that are not present in simple polypeptides. Many coenzymes are specialized for different reaction types. The more important coenzymes include ATP for energy-dependent reactions; NAD, NADP, FAD, and FMN for hydrogen transfers; coenzyme A for activation of organic acids; and SAM for methylation reactions. Some enzymes catalyze their reaction with the help of a heavy metal in their active site.

QUESTIONS

1. Protein kinases are enzymes that phosphorylate amino acid side chains of proteins in ATP-dependent reactions. A protein kinase can be classified as

   A. Oxidoreductase
   B. Hydrolase
   C. Isomerase
   D. Lyase
   E. Transferase

2. Cyanide is a potent inhibitor of cell respiration that prevents the oxidation of all nutrients. Therefore cyanide will definitely reduce the cellular concentration of

   A. Heme groups
   B. $FADH_2$
   C. CoA
   D. ATP
   E. SAM

3. The reaction

   Succinyl-CoA + GDP + P_i
   $\rightarrow$ Succinate + CoA-SH + GTP

   has a standard free energy change $\Delta G^{0\prime}$ of −0.8 kcal/mol. If the free energy content of a phosphoanhydride bond in GTP is 7.3 kcal/mol, what would be the standard free energy change of following reaction?

   Succinyl-CoA + H_2O $\rightarrow$ Succinate + CoA-SH

   A. −8.1 kcal/mol
   B. +6.5 kcal/mol
   C. +8.1 kcal/mol
   D. −6.5 kcal/mol
   E. +0.8 kcal/mol

Part TWO

GENETIC INFORMATION: DNA, RNA, AND PROTEIN SYNTHESIS

Chapter 6

DNA, RNA, AND PROTEIN SYNTHESIS

A typical human cell contains about 10,000 different proteins, which are synthesized according to instructions that are sent from the chromosome to the ribosome in the form of **messenger ribonucleic acid (mRNA)**. Therefore gene expression requires two steps (*Fig. 6.1*):

1. **Transcription** is the synthesis of an mRNA molecule in the nucleus. The mRNA is the carbon copy of a deoxyribonucleic acid (DNA) strand.
2. **Translation** is the synthesis of the polypeptide by the ribosome, guided by the base sequence of the mRNA.

A **gene** is a length of DNA that directs the synthesis of a messenger RNA and polypeptide, or of a functional RNA that is not translated into a polypeptide. It consists of a transcribed sequence and regulatory sites. A **chromosome** is a very long DNA molecule with hundreds or thousands of genes.

As it is expressed, the genetic message is amplified. A single gene can be transcribed into thousands of mRNA molecules, and each mRNA can be translated into thousands of polypeptides. For example, a red blood cell contains 5×10^8 copies of the hemoglobin β-chain, but the nucleated red blood cell precursors that make the hemoglobin have only two copies of the β-chain gene.

ALL LIVING ORGANISMS USE DNA AS THEIR GENETIC DATABANK

Living things are grouped into two major branches on the basis of their cell structure. The **prokaryotes** include bacteria, actinomycetes, blue-green algae, and archaea, and the **eukaryotes** include protozoa, plants, and animals. *Only eukaryotic cells are compartmentalized into organelles by intracellular membranes.* Structures that are present in eukaryotic but not prokaryotic cells include the following:

1. A **nucleus** surrounded by a twofold membrane.
2. **Mitochondria**, with a twofold membrane, are the powerhouses of the cell. They turn food and oxygen into adenosine triphosphate (ATP).
3. The **endoplasmic reticulum**, bounded by a single membrane, processes membrane proteins, membrane lipids, and secreted proteins.

4. The **Golgi apparatus** is a sorting station that sends secreted proteins, lysosomal enzymes, and membrane components to their proper destinations.
5. **Lysosomes** are vesicles filled with hydrolytic enzymes. They degrade many cellular macromolecules as well as substances that the cell engulfs by endocytosis.
6. **Peroxisomes** contain enzymes that generate and destroy toxic hydrogen peroxide.
7. **Cytoskeletal fibers** give structural support to the cell. They are also required for cell motility and intracellular transport.

Differences between prokaryotes and eukaryotes are summarized in *Figure 6.2* and *Table 6.1*. Despite these differences, all living cells have three features in common:

1. *All cells are surrounded by a plasma membrane,* which is a flimsy, fluid, flexible structure that forms a diffusion barrier between the cell and its environment.
2. *All cells generate metabolic energy,* which they use for biosynthesis, maintenance of cell structure, and cell motility.
3. *All cells store genetic information in the form of DNA,* which the cells use to reproduce themselves and to direct the synthesis of RNA and protein.

This chapter describes DNA replication and protein synthesis in prokaryotes. The corresponding processes in eukaryotes (see Chapter 7) are similar but are often more complex.

DNA CONTAINS FOUR BASES

DNA is a polymer of nucleoside monophosphates (also called nucleotides) (*Fig. 6.3, B*). Its structural backbone consists of alternating phosphate and 2-deoxyribose residues that are held together by phosphodiester bonds involving carbon-3 and carbon-5 of the sugar. Carbon-1 forms a β-N-glycosidic bond with one of the four bases shown in *Figure 6.4*.

One end of the DNA strand has a free hydroxyl group at C-5 of the last 2-deoxyribose. The other end has a free hydroxyl group at C-3. The carbons of 2-deoxyribose are numbered by a prime (′) to distinguish

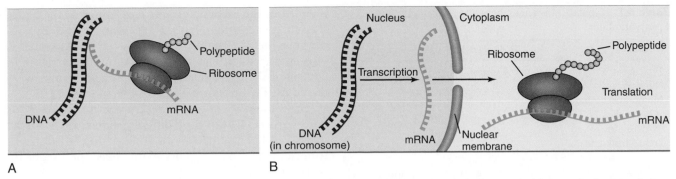

Figure 6.1 Expression of genetic information. In all organisms, the DNA of the gene is first copied into a single-stranded molecule of messenger RNA (mRNA). This process is called transcription. During ribosomal protein synthesis, the base sequence of the mRNA specifies the amino acid sequence of a polypeptide. This is called translation. **A,** In prokaryotic cells, translation starts before transcription is completed. **B,** Eukaryotic cells have a nuclear membrane. Therefore transcription and translation take place in different compartments: transcription in the nucleus and translation in the cytoplasm.

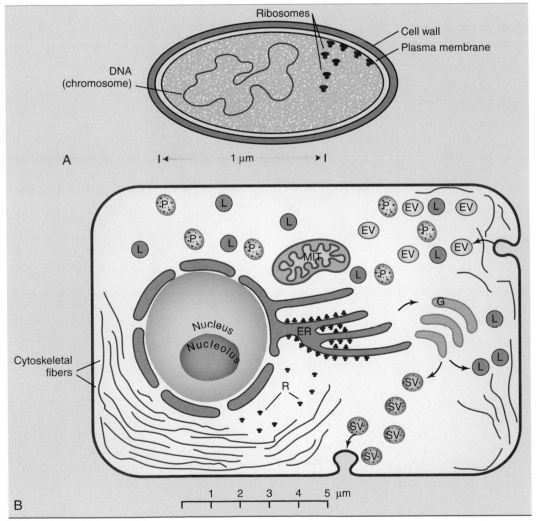

Figure 6.2 Typical elements of prokaryotic and eukaryotic cell structure. **A,** Typical bacterial (prokaryotic) cell. **B,** Typical human (eukaryotic) cell. *ER,* Endoplasmic reticulum; *EV,* endocytotic vesicle; *G,* Golgi apparatus; *L,* lysosome; *MIT,* mitochondrion; *P,* peroxisome; *R,* ribosome; *SV,* secretory vesicle.

Table 6.1 Typical Differences between Prokaryotic and Eukaryotic Cells

Property	Prokaryotes	Eukaryotes
Typical size	0.4–4 μm	5–50 μm
Nucleus	–	+
Membrane-bounded organelles	–	+
Cytoskeleton	–	+
Endocytosis and exocytosis	–	+
Cell wall	+ (some –)	+ (plants) – (animals)
No. of chromosomes	1 (+plasmids)	>1
Ploidy	Haploid	Haploid or diploid
Histones	–	+
Introns	–	+
Ribosomes	70S	80S

them from the carbon and nitrogen atoms of the bases; therefore, each strand has a 5′ end and a 3′ end. By convention, the 5′ terminus of a DNA (or RNA) strand is written at the left end and the 3′ terminus at the right end. Thus the tetranucleotide in *Figure 6.4* can be written as ACTG but not GTCA.

The variability of DNA structure is produced by its base sequence. With four different bases, there are 4^2 (or 16) different dinucleotides and 4^3 (or 64) different trinucleotides, and 4^{100} possibilities exist for a sequence of 100 nucleotides.

DNA FORMS A DOUBLE HELIX

Cellular DNA is double stranded, and almost all of it is present as a **double helix,** as first described by James Watson and Francis Crick in 1953. The most prominent features of the Watson-Crick double helix (*Figs. 6.5 to 6.7*) are as follows:

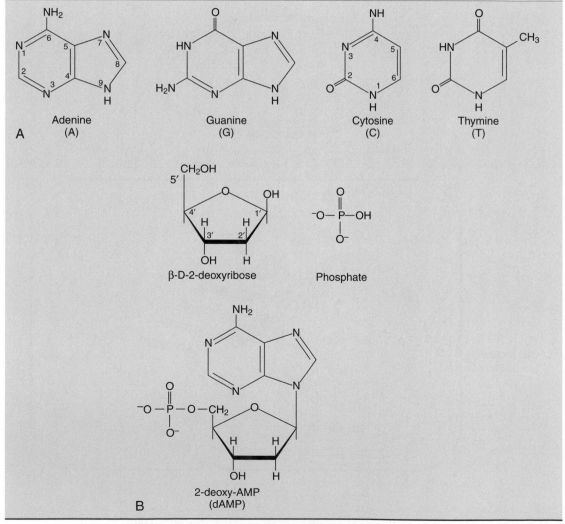

Figure 6.3 The building blocks of DNA. **A,** Structures of the four bases, 2-deoxyribose, and phosphate. The bases A and G are purines, and C and T are pyrimidines. **B,** Structure of 2-deoxy-adenosine monophosphate (dAMP), one of the four 2-deoxyribonucleoside monophosphates (also called 2-deoxynucleotides) in the repeat structure of DNA. Note that a nitrogen atom of the base is bound by a β-*N*-glycosidic bond to C-1 of 2-deoxyribose, whereas C-5 forms a phosphate ester bond.

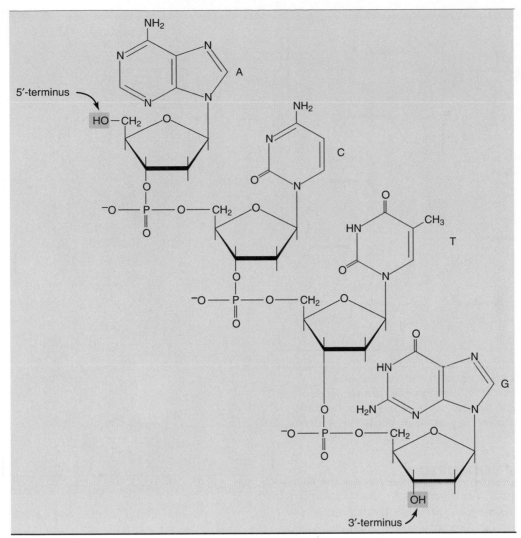

Figure 6.4 Structure of the (2-deoxy-)tetranucleotide ACTG. The DNA strands in chromosomes are far larger, with lengths of many million nucleotide units. *A*, Adenine; *C*, cytosine; *G*, guanine; *T*, thymine.

1. *The two strands of the double helix have opposite polarity, meaning they run in opposite directions.* Base pairing is always antiparallel, not only in the DNA double helix but also in other base-paired structures formed by DNA or RNA.

2. *The 2-deoxyribose/phosphate backbones of the two strands form two ridges on the surface of the molecule.* The phosphate groups are negatively charged.

3. *The bases face inward to the helix axis, but their edges are exposed.* They form the lining of two grooves that are framed by the ridges of the sugar-phosphate backbone. Because the *N*-glycosidic bonds are not exactly opposite each other (see *Fig. 6.7*), the two grooves are of unequal size. They are called the **major groove** and the **minor groove.**

4. *In each of the two strands, successive bases lie flat, one on top of the other,* like a stack of pancakes. The flat surfaces of the bases are hydrophobic, and successive bases in a strand form numerous van der Waals interactions.

5. *Bases in opposite strands interact by hydrogen bonds.* Adenine (A) always pairs with thymine (T) in the opposite strand, and guanine (G) with cytosine (C). Therefore the molar amount of adenine in the double-stranded DNA always equals that of thymine, and the amount of guanine equals that of cytosine. A-T base pairs are held together by two hydrogen bonds, and G-C base pairs by three. Most important, *the base sequence of one strand predicts exactly the base sequence of the opposite strand*. This is essential for DNA replication and DNA repair.

6. *The double strand is wound into a right-handed helix.* Each turn of the helix has about 10.4 base pairs and advances about 3.4 nm along the helix axis. The double helix is rather stiff, but it can be bent and twisted by DNA-binding proteins.

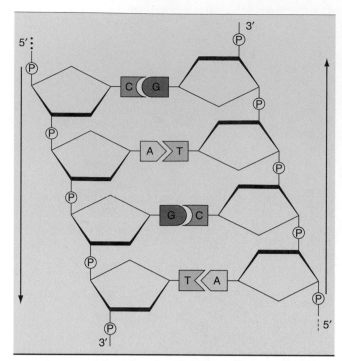

Figure 6.5 Schematic view of the DNA double strand. Note that the strands are antiparallel and that only A-T and G-C base pairs are permitted. Therefore the base sequence of one strand predicts the base sequence of the opposite strand. *A*, Adenine; *C*, cytosine; *G*, guanine; *P*, phosphate; *T*, thymine.

DNA CAN BE DENATURED

Like other noncovalent structures, *the Watson-Crick double helix disintegrates at high temperatures.* Heat denaturation of DNA is also called **melting.** Because A-T base pairs are held together by two hydrogen bonds and G-C base pairs by three, *A-T–rich sections of the DNA unravel more easily than G-C–rich regions when the temperature is raised* (***Figs. 6.8*** and ***6.9***). At physiological pH and ionic strength, this typically happens between 85°C and 95°C.

Heat denaturation decreases the viscosity of DNA solutions because the single strands are more flexible than the stiff, resilient double helix. It also increases the ultraviolet light absorbance at 260 nm, which is caused by the bases, because base pairing and base stacking are disrupted.

Other ways to denature DNA include decreased salt concentration, extreme pH, and chemicals that disrupt hydrogen bonding or base stacking.

When cooled slowly, denatured DNA "renatures" spontaneously. This process is called **annealing.** Whereas small DNA molecules anneal almost instantaneously, large molecules require seconds to minutes.

DNA IS SUPERCOILED

Many naturally occurring DNA molecules are circular. When a linear duplex is partially unwound by one or several turns before it is linked into a circle, the

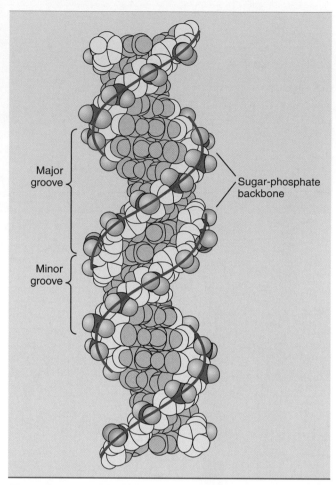

Figure 6.6 Space-filling model of the Watson-Crick double helix (B-DNA).

number of base pairs per turn of the helix is greater than the usual 10.4. The torsional strain in this molecule leads to supercoiling of the duplex around its own axis, much as a telephone cord twists around itself. This is called a **negative supertwist.** The opposite situation, in which the helix is overwound, is called a **positive supertwist.**

Most cellular DNAs are negatively supertwisted, with 5% to 7% fewer right-handed turns than expected from the number of their base pairs. *This underwound condition favors the unwinding of the double helix during DNA replication and transcription.*

The supertwisting of DNA is regulated by two types of **topoisomerase.** Type I topoisomerases cleave one strand of the double helix, creating a molecular swivel that relaxes supertwists passively. Type II topoisomerases are more complex. They cleave both strands and allow an intact helix to pass through this transient double-strand break, before resealing the break. Type II topoisomerases hydrolyze ATP to pump negative supertwists into the DNA (***Fig. 6.10***).

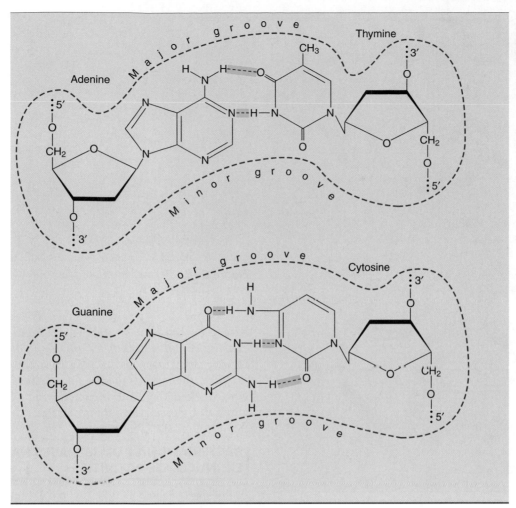

Figure 6.7 Cross-sections through an adenine-thymine (A-T) and a guanine-cytosine (G-C) base pair in the DNA duplex. The A-T base pair is held together by two hydrogen bonds [---] and the G-C base pair by three.

DNA REPLICATION IS SEMICONSERVATIVE

DNA makes identical copies of itself, which are transmitted to the daughter cells during mitosis and even to the next generation through the gametes. In this sense, DNA is the only immortal molecule in the body. The organism is best understood as an artificial environment, created by genes for the benefit of their own continued existence.

DNA is replicated in two steps (**Fig. 6.11**):

1. *The double helix unwinds to produce two single strands.* This requires ATP-dependent enzymes to break the hydrogen bonds between bases. DNA unwinding creates the **replication fork.** This is the place where the new DNA strands are synthesized.
2. *A new complementary strand is synthesized for each of the two old strands.* This is possible because the base sequence of each strand predicts the base sequence of the complementary strand.

DNA replication is called **semiconservative** because one strand in the daughter molecule is always old and the other strand is newly synthesized.

DNA IS SYNTHESIZED BY DNA POLYMERASES

The steps in DNA replication are best known in *Escherichia coli,* an intestinal bacterium that has enjoyed the unfaltering affection of generations of molecular biologists.

The key enzymes of DNA replication in *E. coli,* as in all other cells, are the **DNA polymerases.** *DNA polymerases synthesize the new DNA strand stepwise, nucleotide by nucleotide, in the 5'→3' direction.* The precursors are the deoxyribonucleoside triphosphates: deoxy-adenosine triphosphate (dATP), deoxy-guanosine triphosphate (dGTP), deoxy-cytosine triphosphate (dCTP), and deoxy-thymidine triphosphate (dTTP). DNA polymerase elongates DNA strands by linking the proximal phosphate of an incoming nucleotide to the 3'-hydroxyl group at the end of the growing strand (**Fig. 6.12**). The pyrophosphate formed in this reaction is rapidly cleaved to inorganic phosphate by cellular pyrophosphatases.

Prior unwinding of the double helix is required because the DNA polymerases require a single-stranded DNA as a **template.** While synthesizing the new strand

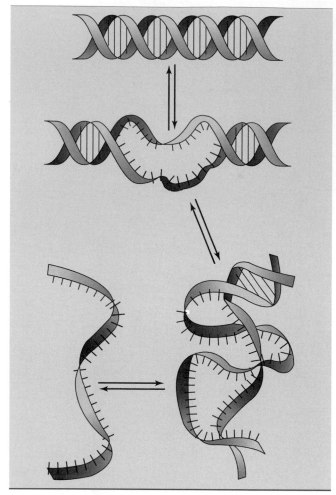

Figure 6.8 Melting of DNA.

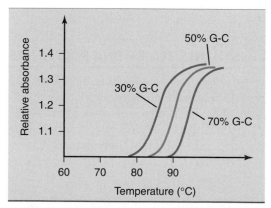

Figure 6.9 Melting of DNA, monitored by the increase of ultraviolet light absorbance at 260 nm. The melting temperature increases with increased guanine-cytosine (G-C) content of the DNA. It is also affected by ionic strength and pH. The melting temperature is the temperature at which the increase in ultraviolet absorbance is half-maximal.

in the $5' \rightarrow 3'$ direction, the enzyme moves along the template strand in the $3' \rightarrow 5'$ direction.

DNA polymerases are literate enzymes. They read the base sequence of their template and make sure that each base that they add to the new strand pairs with the

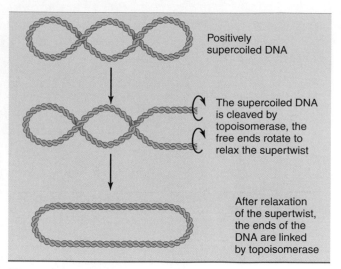

Figure 6.10 Relaxation of positive supertwists in DNA by a type II topoisomerase.

base in the template strand. Therefore *the new strand is exactly complementary to the template strand.* The DNA polymerases are lacking in creative spirit. They are like the scribe monks in medieval monasteries, who worked day and night copying old manuscripts without understanding their content.

BACTERIAL DNA POLYMERASES HAVE EXONUCLEASE ACTIVITIES

A **nuclease** is an enzyme that cleaves phosphodiester bonds in a nucleic acid. Deoxyribonucleases (DNases) cleave DNA, and ribonucleases (RNases) cleave RNA. Nucleases that cleave internal phosphodiester bonds are called **endonucleases,** and those that cleave bonds at the 5′ end or the 3′ end are called **exonucleases.**

Nobody is perfect, and even DNA polymerase sometimes incorporates a wrong nucleotide in the new strand. This can create a lasting **mutation,** which can be deadly if it leads to the synthesis of a faulty protein. To minimize such mishaps, the bacterial DNA polymerases are equipped with a **3′-exonuclease activity** that they use for proofreading. When the nucleotide that has been added to the 3′ end of a growing chain fails to pair with the base in the template strand, it is removed by the 3′-exonuclease activity (***Fig. 6.13***). *This proofreading mechanism reduces the error rate from 1 in 10^4 or 1 in 10^5 to less than 1 in 10^7.*

Most bacterial DNA polymerases also have a **5′-exonuclease activity** (see ***Fig. 6.13***). This activity is not used for proofreading, but it cleaves damaged DNA strands during DNA repair and erases the RNA primer during DNA replication.

Escherichia coli has three DNA polymerases. They differ in their affinity for the DNA template and consequently in their **processivity,** the number of nucleotides they polymerize before dissociating from the template:

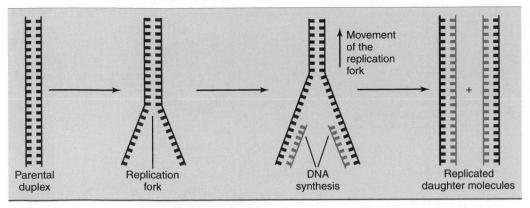

Figure 6.11 Semiconservative mechanism of DNA replication.

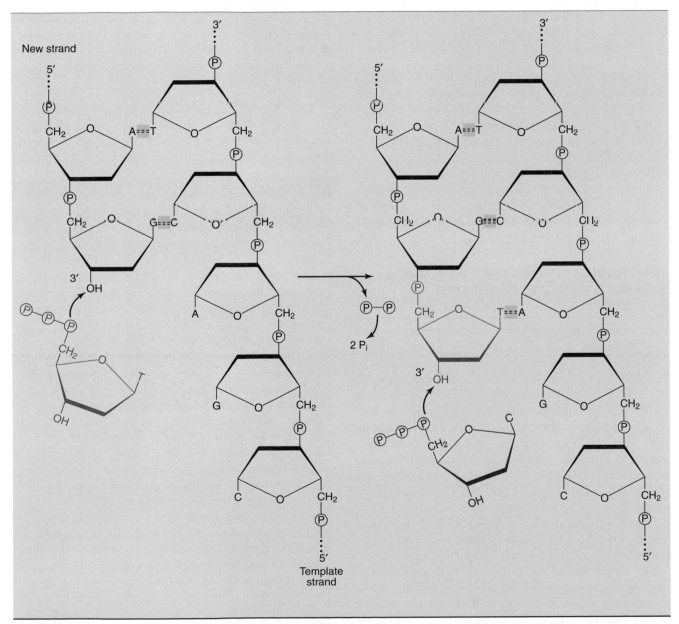

Figure 6.12 Template-directed synthesis of DNA by DNA polymerases. *A*, Adenine; *C*, cytosine; *G*, guanine; *P*, phosphate; *T*, thymine.

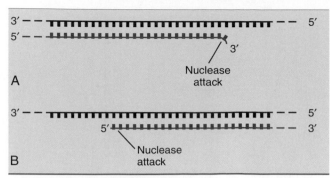

Figure 6.13 Exonuclease activities of bacterial DNA polymerases. The products of these cleavages are nucleoside 5'-monophosphates. **A,** 3'-Exonuclease activity. Only mismatched bases are removed from the 3' end of the newly synthesized DNA strand. This activity is required for proofreading. **B,** 5'-Exonuclease activity. Base-paired nucleotides are removed from the 5' end. This activity is required to erase the RNA primer during DNA replication and to remove damaged portions of DNA during DNA repair.

- **Poly I** has low processivity and falls off its template after polymerizing only a few dozen nucleotides. This enzyme is used for DNA repair (see Chapter 9) and plays only an accessory role in DNA replication.
- **Poly II** has a somewhat higher processivity. It is involved with DNA repair as well.
- **Poly III** is the major enzyme of DNA replication. With the help of a specialized clamp protein, it binds tightly to its template and polymerizes hundreds of thousands of nucleotides in one sitting, at a rate of about 800 nucleotides per second.

UNWINDING PROTEINS PRESENT A SINGLE-STRANDED TEMPLATE TO THE DNA POLYMERASES

Escherichia coli has a single circular chromosome with 4.6 million base pairs and a length of 1.3 mm. This is 1000 times the diameter of the cell. The replication of this chromosome starts at a single site, known as **oriC.** The 245 base-pair sequence of oriC binds multiple copies of an initiator protein that triggers the unwinding of the double helix. This creates two replication forks that move in opposite directions. *Unwinding and DNA synthesis proceed bidirectionally from oriC until the two replication forks meet at the opposite side of the chromosome* (**Fig. 6.14**). The replication of the whole chromosome takes 30 to 40 minutes.

Strand separation is achieved by an ATP-dependent **helicase** enzyme. The *E. coli* helicase that is in charge of DNA replication is known as the **dnaB protein.**

The unwinding of the DNA causes overwinding of the double helix ahead of the moving replication fork. To prevent a standstill, positive supertwisting is relieved by **DNA gyrase,** a type II topoisomerase. *DNA gyrase relaxes positive supertwists passively and induces negative supertwists by an ATP-dependent mechanism.*

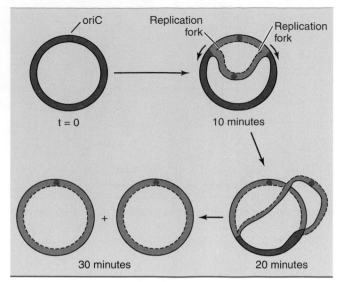

Figure 6.14 Replication of the circular chromosome of *Escherichia coli.* Replication proceeds bidirectionally from a single replication origin (*oriC*). *Dashed lines* indicate new strands.

Once the strands have been separated in the replication fork, they associate with a single-stranded DNA binding protein (**SSB protein**). This keeps them in the single-stranded state.

CLINICAL EXAMPLE 6.1: Gyrase Inhibitors

Chemotherapeutic agents are weapons of mass destruction that doctors use to exterminate undesirable life forms, such as bacteria, fungi, parasites, and cancer cells. To be used effectively in the patient, chemotherapeutic agents must perform their mission without collateral damage to normal cells. As a rule, bacteria are more easily killed in the human body than are fungi and parasites because they are more different from human cells than are the eukaryotic pathogens. Cancer cells are most difficult to eradicate because they are too similar to the normal cells from which they evolved.

DNA replication is an attractive target because it is essential for the continued existence of all cells. Several chemotherapeutic agents are inhibitors of topoisomerases. **Ciprofloxacin** and **nalidixic acid** are important antibiotics. They inhibit bacterial type II topoisomerases, including gyrase. Human topoisomerases are sufficiently different from the bacterial enzymes to be unaffected.

Drugs that inhibit human type II topoisomerases, including **etoposide** and **doxorubicin,** are used for cancer treatment. They have some selectivity for cancer cells because cancer cells divide more rapidly than normal cells and have more replication-associated topoisomerase action. The commonly used drugs do not prevent the initial DNA double-strand cleavage by the topoisomerase, but they delay or prevent the reconnection of the broken ends.

ONE OF THE NEW DNA STRANDS IS SYNTHESIZED DISCONTINUOUSLY

None of the known DNA polymerases can assemble the first nucleotides of a new chain. This task is left to **primase** (dnaG protein), a specialized RNA polymerase that is tightly associated with the dnaB helicase in the replication fork. Primase synthesizes a small piece of RNA, only about 10 nucleotides long. *This small RNA, base paired with the DNA template strand, is the primer for poly III (**Fig. 6.15, A**).*

DNA polymerases synthesize only in the $5' \rightarrow 3'$ direction, reading their template $3' \rightarrow 5'$. Because the parental double strand is antiparallel, only one of the new DNA chains, the **leading strand,** can be synthesized by a poly III molecule that simply travels with the replication fork. The other strand, called the **lagging strand,** has to be synthesized piecemeal.

This requires the repeated action of the primase, followed by poly III. Together they produce DNA strands of about 1000 nucleotides, each with a tiny piece of RNA at the $5'$ end. The pieces are called **Okazaki fragments.** The RNA primer is soon removed by the $5'$-exonuclease activity of poly I, and the gaps are filled by its polymerase activity.

Poly I cannot connect the loose ends of two Okazaki fragments. This is the task of a **DNA ligase,** which links the phosphorylated $5'$ terminus of one fragment with the free $3'$ terminus of another. The hydrolysis of a phosphoanhydride bond in NADH (in bacteria) or ATP (in humans) is required for this reaction (**Fig. 6.16**).

Figure 6.15, B, shows that the enzymes of DNA replication are aggregated in large complexes. The helicase is associated with the primase to ensure that strand separation is followed almost immediately by synthesis of the new strand. DNA is synthesized by **DNA polymerase III holoenzyme,** a large complex with two copies of the catalytically active core enzyme (subunit structure $\alpha\epsilon\theta$) held together by two τ subunits. One copy of the core enzyme synthesizes the leading strand, and the other synthesizes the lagging strand. This dimeric core enzyme associates with other polypeptides and finally with the clamp protein β to form the holoenzyme with a subunit structure of $(\alpha\epsilon\theta)_2\tau_2\gamma_2\delta\delta'\chi\psi\beta_2$ and a molecular weight of 900,000.

RNA PLAYS KEY ROLES IN GENE EXPRESSION

There are only two strictly chemical differences between DNA and RNA: RNA contains ribose instead of 2-deoxyribose, and it contains uracil instead of thymine. Thymine and uracil are distinguished only by a methyl group. Because this methyl group does not participate in base pairing, *both uracil and thymine pair with adenine (**Table 6.2**).*

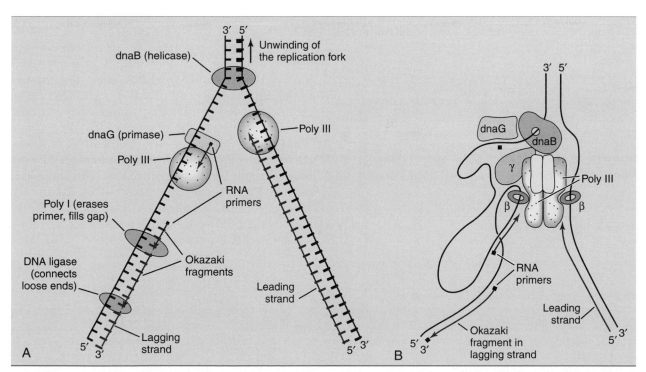

Figure 6.15 Replication fork of *Escherichia coli.* **A,** Because new DNA can be synthesized only in the $5' \rightarrow 3'$ direction, one of the two new strands (the "lagging strand") is synthesized piecemeal. The primer has to be removed from the lagging strand by DNA polymerase I (*Poly I*), and the Okazaki fragments have to be connected by DNA ligase. **B,** Model for the actual assembly of proteins in the bacterial replication fork. Note that the DNA template for the lagging strand has to spool through the β clamp backward to account for the direction of DNA synthesis. β, Clamp protein; γ, clamp loader; *dnaB,* helicase; *dnaG,* primase; *Poly III,* DNA polymerase III.

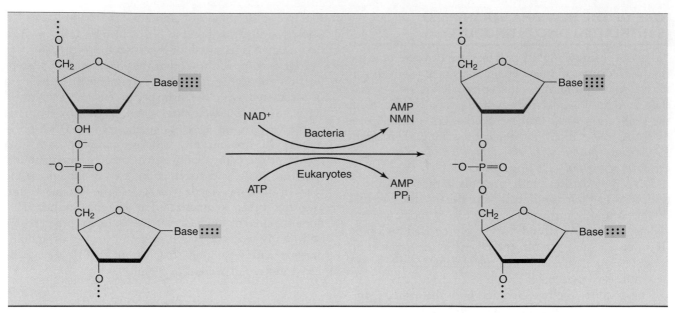

Figure 6.16 Reaction of DNA ligase. The two DNA strands have to be base paired with a complementary strand in a DNA duplex. *AMP*, Adenosine monophosphate; *ATP*, adenosine triphosphate; *NAD*⁺, nicotinamide adenine dinucleotide; *NMN*, nicotinamide mononucleotide (contains nicotinamide + ribose + phosphate); *PPᵢ*, inorganic pyrophosphate.

RNA can form a double helix with dimensions similar to those of DNA but is present in single-stranded form in cells. RNA strands can nevertheless fold back on themselves to form short antiparallel double-helical segments between complementary sequences. Most RNA molecules contain both unpaired and base-paired portions. RNA can also base pair with DNA to form a DNA-RNA hybrid. Hybridization is the base pairing (or annealing) of different kinds of nucleic acid (e.g., messenger RNA with genomic DNA) or of nucleic acids from different origins (e.g., human DNA with chimpanzee DNA).

Most RNAs play roles in gene expression and protein synthesis, but only **mRNA** is translated into protein. **Ribosomal RNA (rRNA)** is a major constituent of the ribosome, and **transfer RNAs (tRNAs)** are small cytoplasmic RNAs that bind amino acids covalently and deliver them to the ribosome for protein synthesis (*Table 6.3*). More than 80% of all RNA in *E. coli* is rRNA and only 3% is mRNA, although about one third of the RNA synthesized in this organism is mRNA. This is because bacterial mRNA has an average lifespan of only 3 minutes. Most human mRNAs, on the other hand, live for 1 to 10 hours before they succumb to cellular nucleases.

Table 6.2 Differences between DNA and RNA

Property	DNA	RNA
Sugar	2-Deoxyribose	Ribose
Bases	A, G, C, T	A, G, C, U
Strandedness in vivo	Double strand	Single strand
Typical size	Often >10^6 base pairs	60–20,000 bases
Function	Genetic information	Gene expression

A, Adenine; *C*, cytosine; *DNA*, deoxyribonucleic acid; *G*, guanine; *RNA*, ribonucleic acid; *T*, thymine; *U*, uracil.

Table 6.3 Properties of rRNA, tRNA, and mRNA

Property	rRNA	tRNA	mRNA
Relative abundance	Most abundant	Less abundant	Least abundant
Molecular weight (in *Escherichia coli*)	1.2×10^6 0.55×10^6 3.6×10^4	$2\text{–}3 \times 10^4$	Heterogeneous
Location (in eukaryotes)	Ribosomes, nucleolus	Cytoplasm	Nucleus, cytoplasm
Function	Structure of ribosomal subunits, peptidyl transferase activity	Brings amino acids to the ribosome	Transmits information for protein synthesis

mRNA, Messenger ribonucleic acid; *rRNA*, ribosomal ribonucleic acid; *tRNA*, transfer ribonucleic acid.

THE σ SUBUNIT RECOGNIZES PROMOTERS

RNA is synthesized by **RNA polymerase** (*Table 6.4*). Bacterial RNA polymerase consists of a core enzyme with the subunit structure $\alpha_2\beta\beta'\omega$ and a σ (sigma) subunit that is only loosely bound to the core enzyme. *The σ subunit recognizes transcriptional start sites, and the core enzyme synthesizes RNA.*

Before starting transcription, RNA polymerase has to bind to a **promoter,** a sequence of about 60 base pairs at the start of the gene. The promoter is recognized by the σ subunit, which binds to the promoter and positions the core enzyme over the transcriptional start site.

The RNA polymerase then separates the DNA double helix over a length of about 18 base pairs, starting at a conserved A-T–rich sequence about 10 base pairs upstream of the transcriptional start site. Strand separation is essential because *transcription, like DNA replication, requires a single-stranded template.*

The σ subunit separates from the core enzyme after the formation of the first 5 to 15 phosphodiester bonds. This marks the transition from the initiation phase to the elongation phase of transcription. The core enzyme now moves along the template strand of the gene while synthesizing the RNA transcript at a rate of about 50 nucleotides per second.

The promoters of different genes look quite different. Only two short segments, located about 10 base pairs and 35 base pairs upstream of the transcriptional start site, are similar in all promoters. Even these sequences are variable, but we can define a **consensus sequence** of the most commonly encountered bases (*Fig. 6.17*).

This diversity is required because genes must be transcribed at different rates. Some are transcribed up to 10 times per minute, whereas others are transcribed only once every 10 to 20 minutes. The rate of transcriptional initiation depends on the base sequence of the promoter. In general, *the more the promoter resembles the consensus sequence, the higher is the rate of transcription.*

DNA IS FAITHFULLY COPIED INTO RNA

RNA synthesis resembles DNA synthesis in most respects (*Fig. 6.18*). ATP, GTP, CTP, and uridine triphosphate (UTP) are the precursors, and RNA is synthesized in the $5'{\rightarrow}3'$ direction (*Fig. 6.19*). However, unlike the DNA polymerases, RNA polymerase can do without a primer. It starts a new chain simply by placing a nucleotide in the first position.

Table 6.4 Comparison of Bacterial DNA Polymerases and RNA Polymerase

Property	DNA Polymerase I	DNA Polymerase III	RNA Polymerase
Subunit structure	Single polypeptide	8 Subunits	$\alpha\alpha_2\,\beta\beta'\omega\sigma$
Molecular weight	$\approx$103,000	$\approx$170,000*	$\approx$450,000
Substrates	dATP, dGTP, dCTP, dTTP	dATP, dGTP, dCTP, dTTP	ATP, GTP, CTP, UTP
Direction of synthesis	$5'{\rightarrow}3'$	$5'{\rightarrow}3'$	$5'{\rightarrow}3'$
Template required	DNA	DNA	DNA
Primer required	Yes	Yes	No
Speed (bases/s)	10–20	600–1000	$\approx$50
3'-Exonuclease activity	Yes	Yes	No
5'-Exonuclease activity	Yes	No	No

ATP, Adenosine triphosphate, *CTP*, cytosine triphosphate; *dATP*, deoxy-adenosine triphosphate, *dCTP*, deoxy-cytosine triphosphate; *dGTP*, deoxy-guanosine triphosphate; *DNA*, deoxyribonucleic acid; *dTTP*, deoxy-thymidine triphosphate; *GTP*, guanosine triphosphate; *RNA*, ribonucleic acid; UTP, uridine triphosphate.

*Core enzyme ($\alpha + \varepsilon + \theta$ subunits) only. Several other polypeptides are associated with this core enzyme in vivo.

P_R	CGGCATGATATTGACTTATTGAATAAAATTGGG	TAAATTTGACTCAACG
T7AI	AAAAGAGTTGACTTAAAGTCTAACCTATAG	GATACTTACAGCCAT
lac	ACCCCAGGCTTTACACTTTATGCTTCCGGCTCG	TATGTTGTGTGGAATT
araC	GCCGTGATTATAGACACTTTTGTTACGCGTTTT	TGTCATGGCTTTGGTC
trp	AAATGAGCTGTTGACAATTAATCATCGAACTAG	TTAACTAGTACGCAAG
bioB	CATAATCGACTTGTAAACCAAATTGAAAAGATT	TAGGTTTACAAGTCTA
tRNA_{tyr}	CAACGTAACACTTTACAGCGGCGCGTCATTTGA	TATGATGCGCCCCGCT
Str	TGTATATTTCTTGACACCTTTTCGGCATCGCCC	TAAAATTCGGCGTCCT
Tet	ATTCTCATGTTTGACAGCTTATCATCGATAAGC	TTTAATGCGGTAGTTT
Consensus sequence	TTGACA	TATAAT

Figure 6.17 Consensus sequence for promoters in *Escherichia coli.* All of these promoters are recognized by the major σ subunit of E. coli. Some belong to E. coli genes, and others belong to bacteriophages infecting E. coli. Only the base sequence of the coding strand (nontemplate strand) is shown. Colored bases to the right of the TATAAT consensus indicate start of transcription.

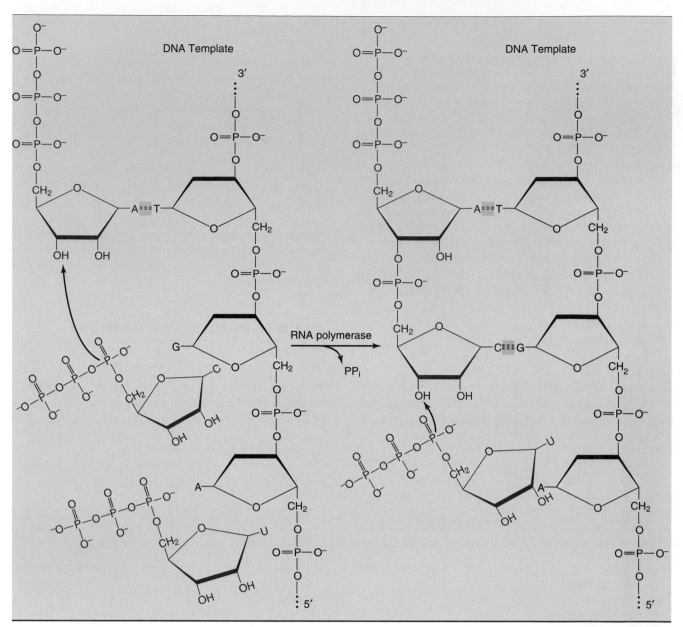

Figure 6.18 Formation of the first phosphodiester bond during transcription. The nucleotide at the 5′ terminus of the RNA remains in the 5′-triphosphate form. Compare this with the mechanism of DNA synthesis shown in *Figure 6.12*. *A*, Adenine; *C*, cytosine; *G*, guanine; *PP*$_i$, inorganic pyrophosphate; *T*, thymine.

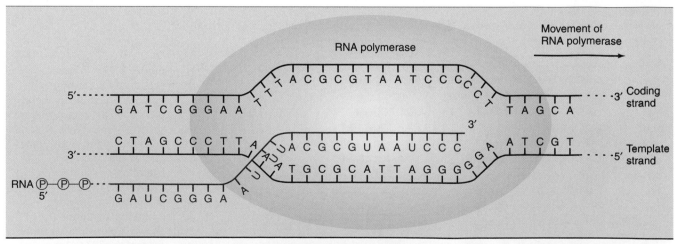

Figure 6.19 Elongation phase of transcription. RNA polymerase separates the double helix on a length of about 18 base pairs to form a "transcription bubble." Only one of the two DNA strands is used as a template. *A*, Adenine; *C*, cytosine; *G*, guanine; *P*, phosphate; *T*, thymine; *U*, uracil.

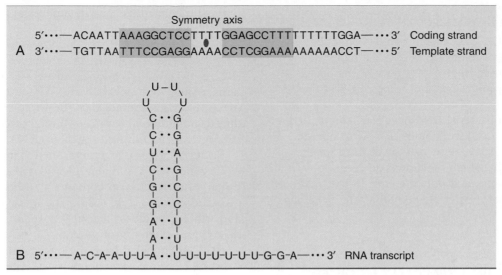

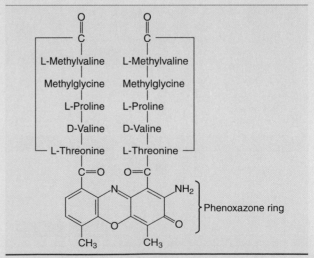

Figure 6.20   Termination sequence of a viral gene that is transcribed by the bacterial RNA polymerase. **A**, Sequence of DNA double strand. **B**, RNA transcript forms a hairpin loop. *A*, Adenine; *C*, cytosine; *G*, guanine; *T*, thymine; *U*, uracil.

The **template strand** of the DNA is antiparallel and complementary to the RNA. The opposite DNA strand, which has the same polarity and base sequence as the RNA transcript (T replacing U), is called the **coding strand** (see *Fig. 6.19*). RNA polymerase has no proofreading nuclease activity, and thus *it has an error rate of about 1 per 10,000*, which is 1000 times higher than the error rate of poly III. This can be tolerated because the damage caused by a single faulty RNA molecule is not nearly as great as the damage caused by a faulty DNA.

Transcription continues until the RNA polymerase runs into a **terminator** sequence at the end of the gene. Most terminators contain a **palindrome,** which is a type of symmetrical sequence in which the base sequence of one DNA strand traced in one direction from the symmetry axis is the same as the sequence of the opposite strand traced in the opposite direction. A palindrome is a word or sentence that reads the same in both directions, as in "Madam, I'm Adam."

When a palindrome is transcribed, the RNA transcript forms a **hairpin loop** by internal base pairing (*Fig. 6.20*), causing the RNA polymerase to dissociate from the DNA template and release the RNA.

CLINICAL EXAMPLE 6.2: Rifampicin

Rifampicin inhibits transcription by tight binding to the β subunit of bacterial RNA polymerase. This does not kill the bacteria, but it prevents their growth: The effect is bacteriostatic, not bactericidal. Rifampicin causes no collateral damage because eukaryotic RNA polymerases are not affected.

Rifampicin can be used for the treatment of bacterial infections, including tuberculosis. Its main limitation is the rapid development of drug resistance, because a point mutation that changes the rifampicin binding site on the β subunit can make the bacteria resistant.

Drug resistance mutations are not induced by the drug. They pop up randomly in bacterial populations but remain at very low frequency because they offer no advantage (or even a slight disadvantage) in the absence of the drug. However, when the bacteria are exposed to the drug and the susceptible cells are killed, the few drug-resistant mutants survive and take over the ecosystem. This is evolution in action, with organisms changing rapidly through mutation and selection. It makes the drug treatment of infectious diseases an arms race between pharmaceutical chemists designing new drugs and bacteria evolving resistance to the drugs.

CLINICAL EXAMPLE 6.3: Actinomycin D

Transcription can be inhibited by the microbial toxin **actinomycin D**. A planar phenoxazone ring in the molecule (*Fig. 6.21*) becomes intercalated (sandwiched)

Figure 6.21   Structure of actinomycin D.

Continued

between two G-C base pairs in double-stranded DNA, and two oligopeptide tails in the molecule clamp the drug to the minor groove of the double helix. RNA polymerase cannot transcribe past the bound drug.

Human and bacterial DNA have the same structure. Therefore actinomycin D binds equally to human and bacterial DNA, and it cannot be used for the treatment of bacterial infections. However, for unknown reasons, it is very effective in the treatment of Wilms tumor (nephroblastoma), a rare childhood cancer.

SOME RNAs ARE CHEMICALLY MODIFIED AFTER TRANSCRIPTION

The chemical modification of RNA after its synthesis by RNA polymerase is called **posttranscriptional processing.** Of the three major RNA types, **mRNA** is rarely processed in prokaryotes. It is translated as soon as it is synthesized, leaving no time for posttranscriptional modifications. In fact, *ribosomes attach to the 5′ end of bacterial mRNA and start translation long before the synthesis of the mRNA has been completed.* In eukaryotes, however, mRNA is processed extensively (see Chapter 7).

Ribosomal RNA is modified posttranscriptionally in both prokaryotes and eukaryotes. Each bacterial ribosome contains three molecules of rRNA: 5S, 16S, and 23S RNA. The "S" refers to the behavior of the molecule in the ultracentrifuge, and its numerical value is roughly related to its size.

These ribosomal RNAs are derived from a single long precursor RNA, which is cleaved into the three rRNAs by specific endonucleases. The ribosome contains a single copy of each rRNA, and this mechanism of synthesis guarantees that the three rRNAs are produced in equimolar amounts. Eukaryotes use a similar strategy for the synthesis of their rRNA (*Fig. 6.22*).

Bacterial rRNA contains methylated bases, and eukaryotic rRNA contains methylated ribose residues. Eukaryotic rRNA also contains a rather large amount of pseudouridine (*Fig. 6.23*). The methylation of bases and ribose residues requires *S*-adenosyl methionine (SAM) as a methyl group donor.

tRNA is modeled from the original transcript by the concerted action of endonucleases and exonucleases, and chemically modified bases are formed by the action of enzymes on the tRNA or tRNA precursors, both in prokaryotes and in eukaryotes (see *Fig. 6.23*).

THE GENETIC CODE DEFINES THE RELATIONSHIP BETWEEN BASE SEQUENCE OF mRNA AND AMINO ACID SEQUENCE OF POLYPEPTIDE

mRNA has only four bases, but polypeptides contain 20 amino acids. Therefore a single base in the mRNA cannot specify an amino acid in a polypeptide. A sequence of two bases can specify 4^2 (16) amino acids, and a sequence of three bases can specify 4^3 (64) amino acids.

In fact, *a sequence of three bases on the mRNA codes for an amino acid.* The ribosome reads these base triplets, or **codons,** in the $5′ \rightarrow 3′$ direction, the same

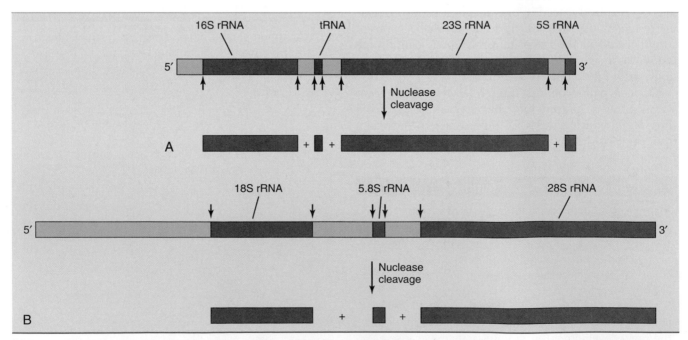

Figure 6.22 Processing of ribosomal RNA (rRNA) precursors in prokaryotes and eukaryotes. **A,** In *Escherichia coli.* **B,** In *Homo sapiens. tRNA,* Transfer RNA.

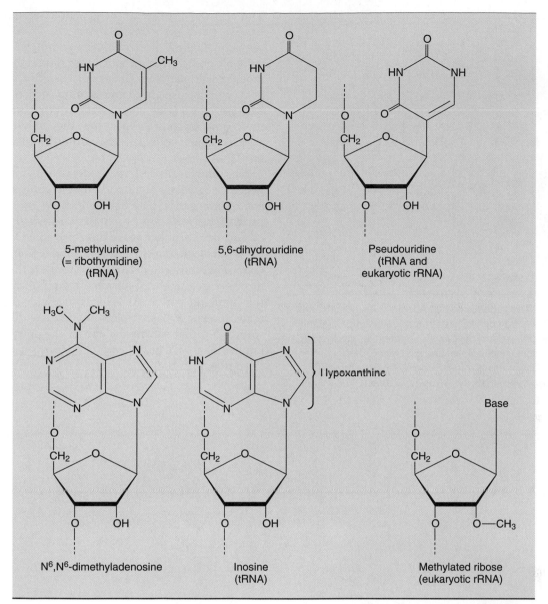

Figure 6.23 Some posttranscriptional modifications in transfer RNA (tRNA) and ribosomal RNA (rRNA). Hypoxanthine is introduced into tRNA by replacement of adenine. The other unusual bases shown here are produced by the enzymatic modification of existing bases.

direction in which the mRNA is synthesized by RNA polymerase. *As the ribosome moves along the mRNA in the 5'→3' direction, it synthesizes the polypeptide in the amino→carboxyl terminal direction.*

The important properties of the genetic code (*Fig. 6.24*) are as follows:

1. *It is colinear.* The sequence of amino acids in the polypeptide, from amino end to carboxyl end, corresponds exactly to the sequence of their codons in the mRNA, read from 5' to 3'.
2. *It is nonoverlapping and "commaless."* The codons are aligned without overlap and without empty spaces in between. Each base belongs to one and only one codon.

3. *It contains 61 amino acid coding codons and the three stop codons UAA, UAG, and UGA.* One of the amino acid coding codons, AUG, is also used as a start codon.
4. *It is unambiguous.* Each codon specifies one and only one amino acid.
5. *It is degenerate.* More than one codon can code for an amino acid.
6. *It is universal.* With the minor exception of the start codon AUG, which determines *N*-formyl methionine in prokaryotes and methionine in eukaryotes, the code is identical in prokaryotes and eukaryotes. Other minor variations occur in the small genomes of mitochondria and chloroplasts and in some single-celled eukaryotes.

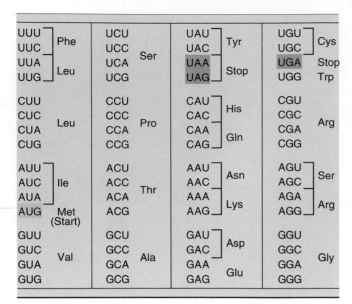

UUU ⎤ Phe UUC ⎦ UUA ⎤ Leu UUG ⎦	UCU UCC UCA ⎦ Ser UCG	UAU ⎤ Tyr UAC ⎦ UAA ⎤ Stop UAG ⎦	UGU ⎤ Cys UGC ⎦ UGA Stop UGG Trp
CUU CUC CUA ⎦ Leu CUG	CCU CCC CCA ⎦ Pro CCG	CAU ⎤ His CAC ⎦ CAA ⎤ Gln CAG ⎦	CGU CGC CGA ⎦ Arg CGG
AUU ⎤ AUC ⎥ Ile AUA ⎦ AUG Met (Start)	ACU ACC ACA ⎦ Thr ACG	AAU ⎤ Asn AAC ⎦ AAA ⎤ Lys AAG ⎦	AGU ⎤ Ser AGC ⎦ AGA ⎤ Arg AGG ⎦
GUU GUC GUA ⎦ Val GUG	GCU GCC GCA ⎦ Ala GCG	GAU ⎤ Asp GAC ⎦ GAA ⎤ Glu GAG ⎦	GGU GGC GGA ⎦ Gly GGG

Figure 6.24 The genetic code. *A,* Adenine; *Ala,* alanine; *Arg,* arginine; *Asn,* asparagine; *Asp,* aspartate; *C,* cytosine; *G,* guanine; *Cys,* cysteine; *Gln,* glutamine; *Glu,* glutamate; *Gly,* glycine; *His,* histidine; *Ile,* isoleucine; *Leu,* leucine; *Lys,* lysine; *Met,* methionine; *Phe,* phenylalanine; *Pro,* proline; *Ser,* serine; *Thr,* threonine; *Trp,* tryptophan; *Tyr,* tyrosine; *U,* uracil; *Val,* valine.

The near universality of the genetic code shows that *all surviving life on earth is descended from a common ancestor.* There is no way that a complex and arbitrary system such as the genetic code could have evolved independently in two lineages. Aliens from other planets would also need replicating genetic molecules because inheritance is an essential attribute of life, but there is no reason to expect that they would use the terrestrial genetic code. It is even doubtful that they would use DNA.

The universality of the code is also interesting for genetic engineers. It implies that *coding sequences of eukaryotic genes that are artificially introduced into prokaryotic cells can be expressed correctly.*

One final problem is the three possible **reading frames** for a colinear, nonoverlapping, and commaless triplet code. The ribosome decides among these three possibilities by searching the 5′-terminal region of the mRNA for the initiation codon AUG. Starting with AUG, it then reads successive base triplets as codons until it reaches a stop codon that signals the end of the polypeptide. This implies that *the 5′ and 3′ ends of the mRNA are not translated* (**Fig. 6.25**).

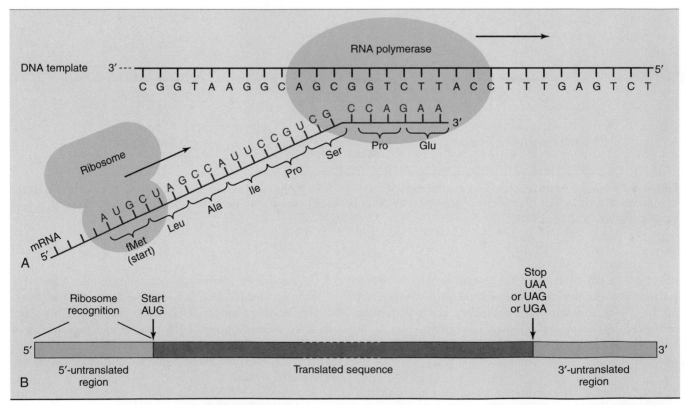

Figure 6.25 Reading frame of messenger RNA (mRNA) and importance of the start and stop codons. **A,** Determination of the reading frame. The ribosome identifies the start codon AUG, then reads successive base triplets as codons. The cotranscriptional initiation of translation depicted here is specific for prokaryotes. **B,** Overall structure of mRNA. mRNAs have a 5′-untranslated sequence upstream of the start codon and a 3′-untranslated sequence downstream of the stop codon. The 5′-untranslated region is required for initial binding of the mRNA to the ribosome during the initiation of translation. *A,* Adenine; *C,* cytosine; *G,* guanine; *T,* thymine; *U,* uracil.

TRANSFER RNA IS THE ADAPTER MOLECULE IN PROTEIN SYNTHESIS

The tRNAs are small RNAs, about 80 nucleotides long, that present amino acids to the ribosome for protein synthesis. Some of their common structural and functional features (**Fig. 6.26**) are as follows:

1. *The molecule is folded into a cloverleaf structure,* with three base-paired stem portions and three loops whose bases are unpaired.
2. *The 3′ terminus is the attachment site for an amino acid.* It ends with the sequence CCA, and the amino acid is bound to the ribose of the last nucleotide.
3. *One of the three loops of the cloverleaf contains the* **anticodon.** The three bases of the anticodon pair with the codon on the mRNA during protein synthesis.

The unique feature of tRNA is that it possesses both an anticodon to recognize the codon on the mRNA and a covalently bound amino acid. Thus *the tRNA matches the amino acid to the appropriate codon on the mRNA.*

AMINO ACIDS ARE ACTIVATED BY AN ESTER BOND WITH THE 3′ TERMINUS OF THE tRNA

A cytoplasmic **aminoacyl-tRNA synthetase** attaches an amino acid to the 3′ end of the tRNA, thereby converting it into an **aminoacyl-tRNA** (*Fig. 6.27*). The balance of the reaction is

$$\text{Amino acid} + \text{tRNA} + \text{ATP}$$

$$\downarrow$$

$$\text{Aminoacyl-tRNA} + \text{AMP} + \text{PP}_i$$

where AMP = adenosine monophosphate, and PP_i = inorganic pyrophosphate. The ester bond between amino acid and tRNA is almost as energy rich as a phosphoanhydride bond in ATP, but the reaction is nevertheless irreversible because the pyrophosphate is quickly hydrolyzed in the cell.

Aminoacyl-tRNA synthetases must be highly accurate because attachment of the wrong amino acid to a tRNA leads to the incorporation of a wrong amino acid

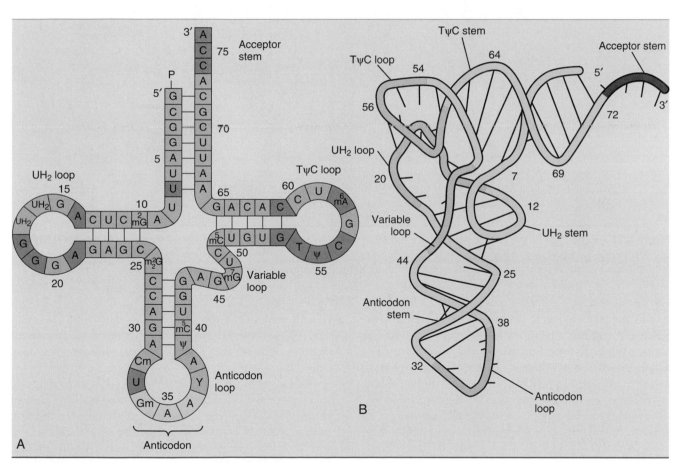

Figure 6.26   Structure of a typical transfer ribonucleic acid (tRNA), yeast tRNAPhe. Note the wide separation between the amino acid binding site ("acceptor stem") and the anticodon. **A,** "Cloverleaf" structure. Conserved bases are indicated by dark color. **B,** Tertiary structure. The three stem-loop structures of the cloverleaf are shown in *orange*. A, Adenine; C, cytosine; G, guanine; T, thymine; U, uracil. Modified nucleosides: ψ2, Pseudouridine; Cm, 2′-O-methyl cytidine; Gm, 2′-O-methylguanosine; m^2G, 2-methylguanosine; m_2^2G, 2,2-dimethylguanosine; m^5C, 5-methylcytidine; m^6A, 6-methyladenosine; m^7G, 7-methylguanosine; UH_2, dihydrouridine; Y, "hypermodified" purine.

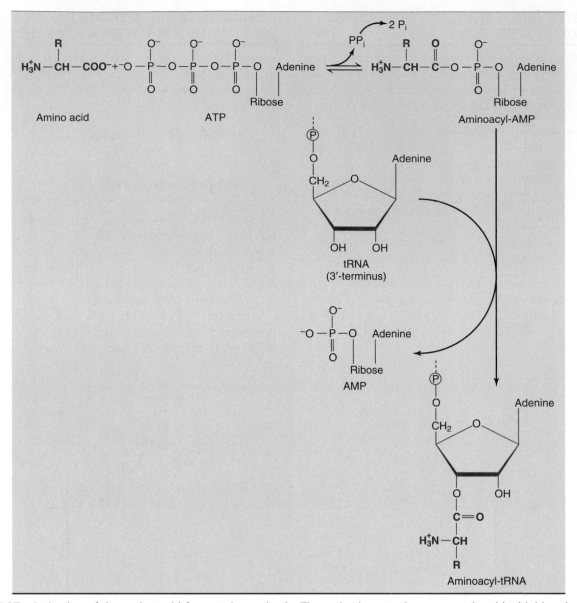

Figure 6.27 Activation of the amino acid for protein synthesis. The activation reactions are catalyzed by highly selective aminoacyl-tRNA synthetases in the cytoplasm. The aminoacyl-tRNA is the immediate substrate for ribosomal protein synthesis. *AMP*, Adenosine monophosphate; *ATP*, adenosine triphosphate; P_i, inorganic phosphate; PP_i, inorganic pyrophosphate.

in the protein. In fact, aminoacyl-tRNA synthetases make only about one mistake in every 40,000 couplings. When a mutation alters the specificity of an aminoacyl-tRNA synthetase, causing it to attach the wrong amino acid to a tRNA, the result will be a change in the genetic code. A mutation in the anticodon of a tRNA changes the genetic code as well, but such mutations are rarely observed because they are rapidly fatal.

MANY TRANSFER RNAs RECOGNIZE MORE THAN ONE CODON

During protein synthesis, *the codon of the mRNA base pairs with the anticodon of the tRNA in an antiparallel orientation*. With strict Watson-Crick base pairing, at least 61 different tRNAs would be needed for the 61 amino acid coding codons. However, most bacteria have fewer than 61 different tRNAs, and human mitochondria have only 22.

This is possible because the rules of base pairing are relaxed for the third codon base. Uracil at the 5′ end of the anticodon can pair not only with adenine (A) but also with guanine (G) at the 3′ end of the codon, and a G in this position can pair with cytosine (C) or uracil (U). Some tRNAs have hypoxanthine as their first anticodon base (the corresponding nucleoside is called inosine). Hypoxanthine can pair with A, U, or C. This freedom of base pairing is called **wobble.**

Wobble contributes to the degeneracy of the genetic code. As shown in *Figure 6.24*, codons specifying the same amino acid usually differ in the third codon base. This is the "wobble position," and in many cases the alternative codons are indeed read by the same tRNA.

RIBOSOMES ARE THE WORKBENCHES FOR PROTEIN SYNTHESIS

Although they enjoy the prestigious status of organelles, ribosomes are not surrounded by a membrane and do not form a separate cellular compartment. They are merely large, catalytically active ribonucleoprotein particles. In bacteria, they are either free floating in the cytoplasm or attached to the plasma membrane. In eukaryotes they are either free floating in the cytoplasm or attached to the membrane of the endoplasmic reticulum. *Escherichia coli* contains about 16,000 ribosomes, whereas a typical eukaryotic cell has more than one million.

Ribosomes consist of a large subunit and a small subunit. According to their sedimentation rate in the ultracentrifuge, bacterial ribosomes are described as 70S ribosomes, with 30S and 50S subunits. The ribosomes in the cytoplasm and on the endoplasmic reticulum of eukaryotes are a bit larger: 80S, with 40S and 60S subunits.

The composition of bacterial and eukaryotic ribosomes is summarized in *Table 6.5*. Each ribosomal RNA molecule and, with one exception, each ribosomal protein is present in only one copy per ribosome. The components are held together noncovalently, and ribosomal subunits can be assembled in the test tube by mixing ribosomal proteins and RNAs. In the cell,

ribosomes are assembled in the cytoplasm (prokaryotes) or the nucleolus (eukaryotes).

Some features of ribosomal protein synthesis are as follows:

1. To start protein synthesis, the ribosome binds to a site near the 5′ terminus of the mRNA.
2. mRNA is read in the 5′→3′ direction while the polypeptide is synthesized in the amino→carboxyl terminal direction.
3. The ribosome has a binding site for the tRNA that carries the growing polypeptide chain (**P site**) and another binding site for the incoming aminoacyl-tRNA (**A site**).
4. The ribosome forms the peptide bond, while peptidyl-tRNA and aminoacyl-tRNA are bound to these sites.
5. Energy-dependent steps in ribosomal protein synthesis require GTP, not ATP.
6. Some steps in protein synthesis require soluble cytoplasmic proteins known as initiation factors, elongation factors, and termination factors.
7. Each ribosome synthesizes only one polypeptide at a time, but an mRNA molecule is read simultaneously by many ribosomes.

THE INITIATION COMPLEX BRINGS TOGETHER RIBOSOME, MESSENGER RNA, AND INITIATOR tRNA

Positioning the mRNA correctly on the ribosome requires the conserved **Shine-Dalgarno sequence** in the 5′-untranslated region of the mRNA (consensus: AGGAGGU), about 10 nucleotides upstream of the AUG start codon. It base pairs with a complementary sequence on the 16S RNA in the small ribosomal subunit. Now the initiator tRNA can bind to the small ribosomal subunit while pairing its anticodon with the AUG start codon of the mRNA (*Fig. 6.28*). The initiator tRNA carries the modified amino acid N-formylmethionine (fMet), and therefore *all bacterial proteins are synthesized with fMet at the amino terminus.*

This **30S initiation complex** also contains three initiation factors. **IF-1** and **IF-3** prevent the ribosomal subunits from associating into a complete 70S ribosome. **IF-2**, which contains a bound GTP molecule, is required for binding of fMet-tRNA to the 30S initiation complex.

The **70S initiation complex** is formed when the 50S ribosomal subunit binds to the 30S initiation complex. The initiation factors are released while the bound GTP is hydrolyzed to GDP and inorganic phosphate.

The binding site for the initiator tRNA on the ribosome is called the **P site** because it is occupied by a peptidyl-tRNA during the elongation phase. A second tRNA binding site, the **A site** (A = aminoacyl-tRNA, or acceptor) is still empty. It receives incoming aminoacyl-tRNA molecules during the elongation phase.

Table 6.5 Features of Prokaryotic and Eukaryotic Ribosomes

Property	Escherichia coli	Homo sapiens (Cytoplasmic)*
Diameter (nm)	20	25
Mass (kD)	2700	4200
Sedimentation coefficient†		
Complete ribosome	70S	80S
Small subunit	30S	40S
Large subunit	50S	60S
RNA content	65%	50%
Protein content	35%	50%
rRNA, small subunit	16S	18S
rRNA, large subunit	5S, 23S	5S, 5.8S, 28S
No. of proteins		
Small subunit	21	34
Large subunit	34	50

RNA, Ribonucleic acid; rRNA, ribosomal ribonucleic acid.
*For mitochondrial ribosomes, see Chapter 7.
†S, Svedberg unit, describes the behavior of particles in the ultracentrifuge. Higher S values are associated with heavier particles, but they are not additive.

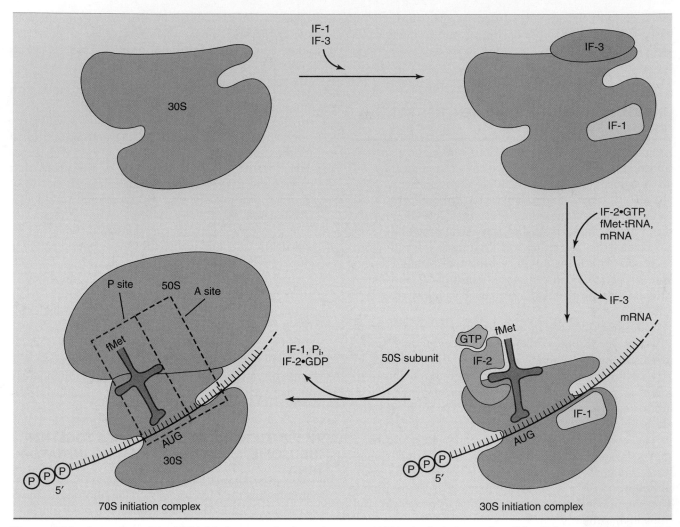

Figure 6.28   Formation of the 70S initiation complex in prokaryotes. *AUG* is the intiation codon. *fMet*, *N*-formylmethionine; *IF-1*, *IF-2*, and *IF-3*, initiation factors 1, 2, and 3, respectively; *mRNA*, messenger RNA; *P$_i$*, inorganic phosphate; *tRNA*, transfer RNA.

POLYPEPTIDES GROW STEPWISE FROM THE AMINO TERMINUS TO THE CARBOXYL TERMINUS

To start the elongation cycle of protein synthesis (*Fig. 6.29*), an aminoacyl-tRNA is placed in the A site of the ribosome along with the GTP-binding elongation factor Tu (**EF-Tu**). If (and only if) codon and anticodon match, the bound GTP is hydrolyzed to GDP, and EF-Tu with its bound GDP vacates the ribosome. The aminoacyl-tRNA remains in the A site, ready for peptide bond formation.

The first peptide bond is formed when fMet is transferred from the initiator tRNA to the amino acid residue on the aminoacyl-tRNA in the A site (*Fig. 6.30*). This reaction requires no external energy source because the free energy content of the ester bond in the fMet-tRNA ($\approx$7 kcal/mol) exceeds that of the peptide bond ($\approx$1 kcal/mol). The **peptidyl transferase** of the large ribosomal subunit that catalyzes peptide bond formation is not a ribosomal protein, but *it is an enzymatic activity*

of the 23S RNA in the large ribosomal subunit. Therefore the ribosome is an RNA enzyme, or **ribozyme.**

Peptide bond formation leaves a free tRNA in the P site and a peptidyl-tRNA in the A site. The free tRNA moves from the P site to an E site (E = exit) on the large ribosomal subunit before leaving the ribosome altogether, and the peptidyl-tRNA moves from the A site into the P site. Codon-anticodon pairing remains intact. Therefore *the ribosome moves along the mRNA by three bases*. This step is called **translocation.** It requires the GTP-binding elongation factor **EF-G** and is accompanied by the hydrolysis of the bound GTP (see *Fig. 6.29*). The speed of ribosomal protein synthesis is about 20 amino acids per second, and the error rate is about 1 for every 10,000 amino acids.

The stop codons UAA, UAG, and UGA have no matching tRNAs. Instead they are recognized by proteins called **termination factors** or **release factors,** which induce cleavage of the bond between polypeptide and tRNA. GTP hydrolysis takes place during translational termination.

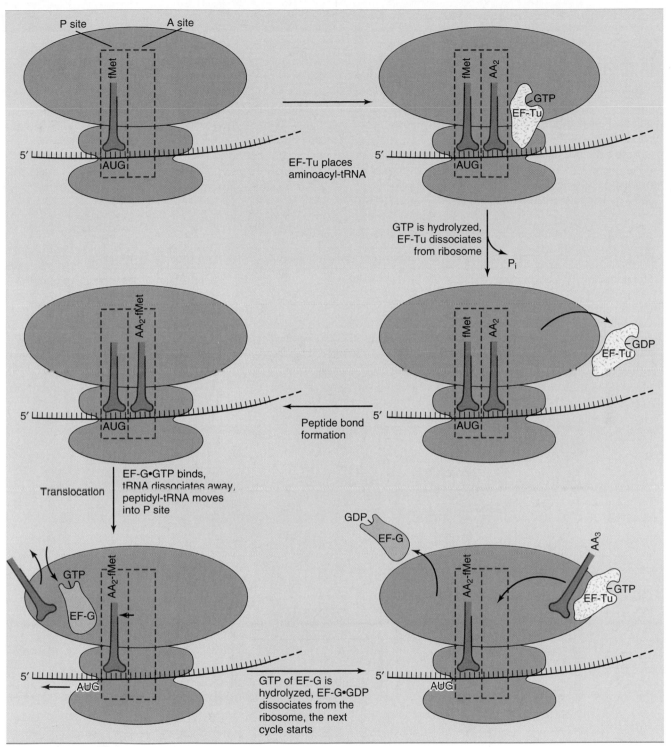

Figure 6.29   First elongation cycle of ribosomal protein synthesis, which introduces the second amino acid (*AA₂*). *EF-G*, Elongation factor *G*; *EF-Tu*, elongation factor Tu; *fMet*, *N*-formylmethionine; *GDP*, guanosine diphosphate; *GTP*, guanosine triphosphate; *tRNA*, transfer ribonucleic acid.

CLINICAL EXAMPLE 6.4: Streptomycin Resistance

Cells stop growing immediately when their protein synthesis is inhibited, and they die slowly when worn-out cellular proteins can no longer be replaced by new ones. Therefore it is not surprising that many of the antibiotics that microorganisms have invented for chemical warfare against their competitors are inhibitors of ribosomal protein synthesis.

These antibiotics bind to various sites on the ribosome and interfere with individual steps in protein synthesis (*Table 6.6*). Most are very selective, inhibiting protein synthesis in either prokaryotes or eukaryotes but not in both.

Bacteria can become resistant to ribosomally acting antibiotics by mutations that change the target of drug action. For example, streptomycin resistance can be produced by mutations in the gene for S12, a protein of the small ribosomal subunit to which this antibiotic binds. Even streptomycin-dependent bacterial mutants can be selected in the laboratory. In other cases of ribosomally acting antibiotics, mutations that alter the sequence of one or another ribosomal RNA can make the bacterium drug resistant.

Table 6.6 Some Antibiotic Inhibitors of Ribosomal Protein Synthesis

Drug	Target Organisms	Ribosomal Subunit Bound	Effect on Protein Synthesis
Streptomycin	Prokaryotes	30S	Inhibits initiation, causes misreading of mRNA
Tetracycline	Prokaryotes	30S	Inhibits aminoacyl-tRNA binding
Chloramphenicol	Prokaryotes	50S	Inhibits peptidyl transferase
Cycloheximide	Eukaryotes	60S	Inhibits peptidyl transferase
Erythromycin	Prokaryotes	50S	Inhibits translocation
Puromycin	Prokaryotes, eukaryotes	50S, 60S	Terminates elongation

mRNA, Messenger ribonucleic acid; *tRNA*, transfer messenger ribonucleic acid.

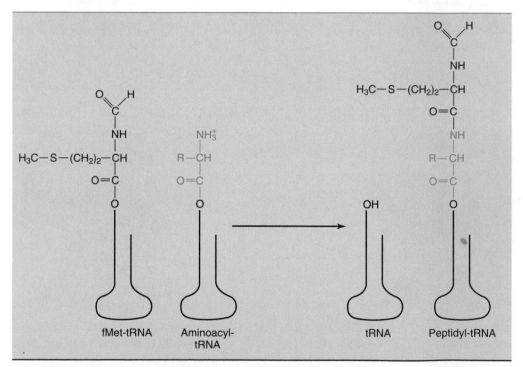

Figure 6.30 Formation of the first peptide bond in the peptidyl transferase reaction. *fMet*, N-Formylmethionine; *tRNA*, transfer ribonucleic acid.

PROTEIN SYNTHESIS IS ENERGETICALLY EXPENSIVE

GTP hydrolysis during initiation and termination are one-time expenses, but each elongation cycle requires the recurrent expense of two GTP bonds: one for placement, and the other for translocation. This adds to the two high-energy phosphate bonds in ATP that are expended for the synthesis of each aminoacyl-tRNA.

Therefore *at least four high-energy bonds are consumed for the synthesis of each peptide bond*. Rapidly growing bacteria devote 30% to 50% of their metabolic energy to protein synthesis, but the human body spends only about 5% of its energy for this purpose.

GENE EXPRESSION IS TIGHTLY REGULATED

Some proteins are needed at all times, so the genes that encode them are transcribed at a fairly constant rate at all times. These proteins are called **constitutive proteins,** and their genes are called **housekeeping genes** because they have to work continuously. **Inducible proteins,** in contrast, are synthesized only when they are needed. Their genes are transcribed only in response to external stimuli that signal a requirement for the encoded protein.

Bacteria have to adjust their metabolic activities to the nutrient supply. When a bacterium falls into a glass of milk, in which lactose is the major carbohydrate, the bacterium needs enzymes for lactose metabolism. In a glass of lemonade, in which sucrose is abundant, the bacterium needs enzymes of sucrose metabolism. In a glass of beer, the bacterium needs enzymes for alcohol oxidation. In short, having the enzymes for a catabolic, energy-generating pathway makes sense only when the substrate of the pathway is available.

The enzymes of a biosynthetic pathway, on the other hand, are required only when the end product is not available from external sources. For example, the enzymes of tryptophan synthesis are required only when the cell has to grow on a tryptophan-free medium.

Humans have to adjust their metabolism not only to nutrient supply and need for biosynthetic products, but also according to cell type. *All cells of the body have the same genes, but different cells make different proteins.*

For example, hemoglobin is synthesized by erythroid precursor cells in the bone marrow but not by neurons in the cerebral cortex. *Such differences are the result of cell-specific gene expression.*

A REPRESSOR PROTEIN REGULATES TRANSCRIPTION OF THE *LAC* OPERON IN *E. COLI*

Escherichia coli can use the disaccharide lactose (milk sugar) as a source of metabolic energy. Lactose is first transported across the plasma membrane by the membrane carrier **lactose permease,** then it is cleaved to free glucose and galactose by the enzyme **β-galactosidase** (*Fig. 6.31*). A third protein, **β-galactoside transacetylase,** is not required for lactose catabolism, but it acetylates several other β-galactosides. It probably is involved in the removal of nonmetabolizable β-galactosides from the cell.

As an intestinal bacterium, *E. coli* needs these three proteins only when its host drinks milk. In the absence of lactose, the cell contains only about 10 molecules of β-galactosidase, but several thousand molecules are present when lactose is the only carbon source. The levels of the permease and the transacetylase parallel exactly those of β-galactosidase.

The genes for these three proteins are lined up head to tail in the bacterial chromosome. They are regulated in concert because *they are transcribed from a single promoter.* The product of transcription is a *polycistronic mRNA* (from *cistron* meaning "gene"). The ribosome can synthesize three different polypeptides from this large mRNA because the stop codons of the first two genes are followed by a Shine-Dalgarno sequence and a start codon at which the synthesis of the next polypeptide is initiated.

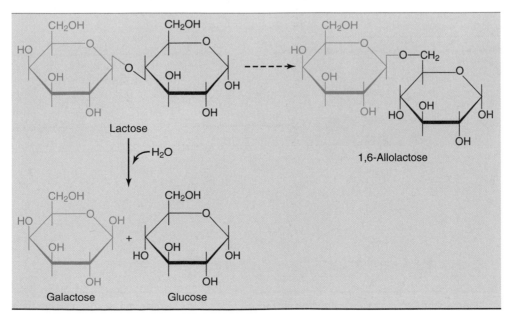

Figure 6.31 β-Galactosidase reaction. A small percentage of the substrate is not hydrolyzed but rather is isomerized to 1,6-allolactose in a minor side reaction.

The array of protein-coding genes, shared promoter, and associated regulatory sites is called an **operon,** and the protein-coding genes of the operon are called **structural genes.**

Wedged between the three structural genes and their shared promoter is an **operator** (*Fig. 6.32*), a short regulatory DNA sequence that binds the *lac* **repressor.** The repressor binding site (operator) overlaps with the binding site for RNA polymerase (promoter). Therefore *the RNA polymerase cannot bind to the promoter when the* lac *repressor is bound to the operator.*

The *lac* repressor is a tetrameric (from Greek τετρα meaning "four" and μεροσ meaning "part") protein with four identical subunits, encoded by a regulatory gene that is constitutively transcribed at a low rate. This gene is located immediately upstream of the *lac* operon.

In the absence of lactose, the *lac* repressor binds tightly to the operator and prevents transcription of the structural genes. In the presence of lactose, however, a small amount of 1,6-allolactose is formed. This minor side product of the β-galactosidase reaction (see *Fig. 6.31*) binds tightly to the *lac* repressor, changing its conformation by an allosteric mechanism. The repressor-allolactose complex no longer binds to the operator, and the structural genes can be transcribed. Thus 1,6-allolactose functions as an **inducer** of the *lac* operon.

ANABOLIC OPERONS ARE REPRESSED BY THE END PRODUCT OF THE PATHWAY

The tryptophan (*trp*) operon of *E. coli* codes for a set of five enzymes that are required for the synthesis of tryptophan. Thus the bacteria can synthesize their own tryptophan, but *this energetically expensive biosynthetic pathway is required only when external tryptophan is not available.*

The repressor of the *trp* operon is a dimeric protein that binds to an operator site about 20 to 30 nucleotides upstream of the transcriptional start site, in the middle of the promoter. It thereby prevents the binding of RNA polymerase (*Fig. 6.33*).

Unlike the *lac* repressor, the *trp* repressor cannot bind its operator without outside help. *It is an allosteric protein that becomes an active repressor only when it binds tryptophan.* Therefore the *trp* operon is repressed when tryptophan is abundant. In this system, the repressor protein is called an **aporepressor,** and tryptophan

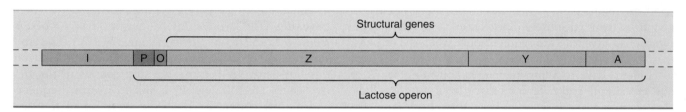

Figure 6.32 Structure of the lactose (*lac*) operon of *Escherichia coli*. Promoter (*P*), operator (*O*), and structural genes are contiguous in all bacterial operons. The regulatory gene that encodes the *lac* repressor (*I*) may or may not be located next to the operon. *A*, Gene for β-galactoside transacetylase; *Y*, gene for lactose permease; *Z*, gene for β-galactosidase.

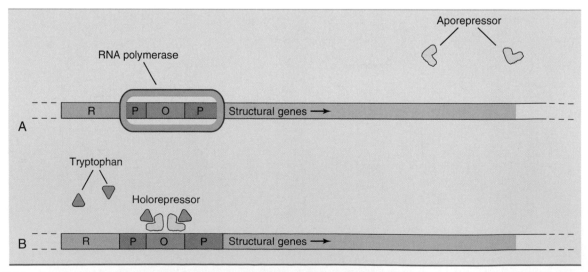

Figure 6.33 Regulation of the tryptophan (*trp*) operon of *Escherichia coli*. **A,** Tryptophan is absent. The aporepressor does not bind to the operator, and the structural genes are transcribed. **B,** Tryptophan is abundant. The "holorepressor" (aporepressor + tryptophan) binds to the operator. The binding of RNA polymerase is prevented, and the structural genes are not transcribed. *O*, Operator; *P*, promoter; *R*, regulatory gene.

is called a **corepressor**. This regulatory strategy is typical for biosynthetic operons.

GLUCOSE REGULATES THE TRANSCRIPTION OF MANY CATABOLIC OPERONS

When given the choice between glucose and lactose, *E. coli* metabolizes glucose first. The levels of β-galactosidase and the other products of the *lac* operon are very low as long as both sugars are present in the medium, and *the enzymes of lactose metabolism are induced only when glucose is depleted* (**Fig. 6.34**).

Glucose is the favored tasty treat of bacteria because it is more easily metabolized than lactose. The thrifty (or lazy) bacterium saves the expense for the synthesis of lactose-metabolizing enzymes by metabolizing glucose first. Not only the *lac* operon but also many other catabolic operons are repressed in the presence of glucose. This is called **catabolite repression**.

Catabolite repression is mediated by **cyclic adenosine monophosphate (cAMP)**. This small molecule serves as a second messenger of hormone action in humans (see Chapter 17), but in bacteria it is regulated by glucose. *The intracellular cAMP level is low when glucose is plentiful and high when it is scarce.*

When glucose is depleted and cAMP is abundant, cAMP binds to the dimeric **catabolite activator protein**

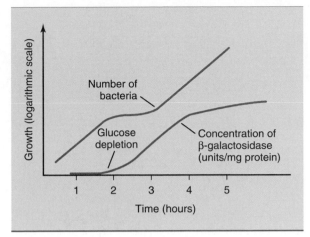

Figure 6.34 Growth of *Escherichia coli* bacteria on a mixture of glucose and lactose.

(CAP). CAP alone does not bind to DNA, but *the CAP-cAMP complex binds at the promoters of many catabolic operons*, including the *lac* operon (**Figs. 6.35 and 6.36, A**). The DNA-bound CAP-cAMP complex provides additional sites of interaction for RNA polymerase, thereby facilitating its binding to the promoter and the initiation of transcription.

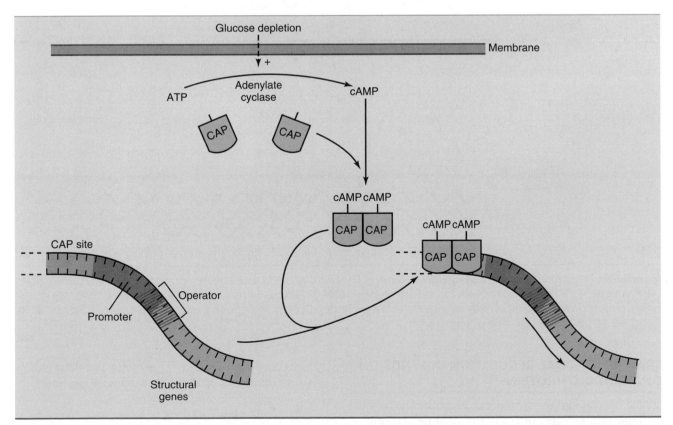

Figure 6.35 Mechanism of catabolite repression. The promoter of the *lac* operon is intrinsically weak and permits a high rate of transcription only when the complex of catabolite activator protein (*CAP*) and cyclic adenosine monophosphate (*cAMP*) is bound to the DNA of the promoter. The cAMP level is low in the presence of glucose but rises in the absence of glucose when the cAMP-forming enzyme adenylate cyclase is activated. The CAP binds the promoter only when it is complexed with cAMP.

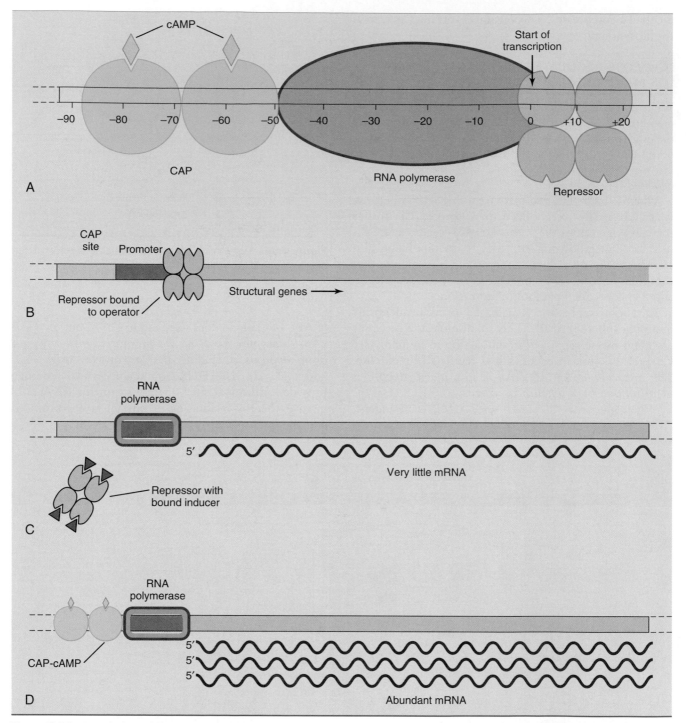

Figure 6.36 Regulation of the lactose operon. **A,** Binding sites for RNA polymerase, repressor, and catabolite activator protein (*CAP*)-cyclic AMP (*cAMP*). **B,** Lactose absent, glucose present. RNA polymerase cannot start transcription. **C,** Lactose present, glucose present. Weak binding of RNA polymerase to the promoter. **D,** Lactose present, glucose absent. Strong binding of RNA polymerase to promoter; high rate of transcription.

TRANSCRIPTIONAL REGULATION DEPENDS ON DNA-BINDING PROTEINS

The *lac* operon and the *trp* operon illustrate the following important features of transcriptional regulation:

1. *Gene expression is most commonly regulated at the level of transcription.* Regulation of mRNA processing and translation also occur, especially in eukaryotes, but transcriptional regulation is of prime importance.

2. *Prokaryotes coordinate the transcription of functionally related genes by arranging them in operons.* Eukaryotes, however, do not use this strategy. They work with monocistronic mRNAs, and functionally related genes need not be close together in the genome.

3. *Transcription is controlled by proteins that bind to regulatory DNA sequences in the vicinity of the transcriptional start site.* The proteins can recognize these sites because the edges of the DNA bases are exposed in the major and minor grooves of the double helix.

4. *Many transcriptional activators and repressors are allosterically controlled by small molecules such as 1,6-allolactose, cAMP, and tryptophan.* However, other control mechanisms are possible. These include interactions with other regulatory proteins and covalent modification by protein phosphorylation.

5. *DNA-binding gene regulator proteins act as either activators or repressors.* This action is called **positive control** or **negative control** of transcription, respectively. The stimulation of transcription by CAP-cAMP is an example of positive control, and the actions of the *lac* repressor and the *trp* repressor are examples of negative control.

6. *Many transcriptional regulators are either dimers (CAP,* trp *repressor) or larger oligomers (lac* repressor) *with identical or slightly different subunits.* Therefore their structures are symmetrical. The symmetry of the proteins is reflected in the DNA sequences to which they bind, which in many cases are palindromic (*Fig. 6.37*). The oligomeric nature of the gene regulators facilitates allosteric changes in their conformation, and their responses to effector molecules can be accentuated by positive cooperativity.

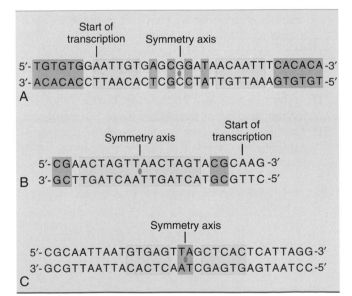

Figure 6.37 Incomplete palindromic sequences in the binding sites of transcriptional regulator proteins. Most transcriptional regulators bind their cognate DNA sites in a dimeric form, each subunit interacting with one leg of the palindrome left and right of the symmetry axis. **A,** The *lac* operator. **B,** The *trp* operator. **C,** The catabolite activator protein-cAMP binding site of the *lac* operon. *A,* Adenine; *C,* cytosine; *G,* guanine; *T,* thymine.

SUMMARY

DNA as it occurs in cells is a large double-stranded molecule with a length of several million nucleotides. It contains the four bases adenine (A), guanine (G), cytosine (C), and thymine (T), bound to a backbone of 2-deoxyribose and phosphate. Bases in opposite strands interact, forming A-T base pairs and G-C base pairs. Therefore the base sequence of one strand predicts the base sequence of the opposite strand.

For replication, the parental DNA double helix is unwound and new complementary strands are synthesized; one of the old strands is always used as a template. The new strands are synthesized by DNA polymerases, with deoxyribonucleoside triphosphates as precursors.

For gene expression, DNA is copied into RNA by RNA polymerase. This process is called transcription. The gene is defined as the length of DNA that codes for a polypeptide or for a functional RNA in cases in which the RNA is not translated into protein (e.g., rRNA and tRNA). The RNA transcript of a protein-coding gene is called a messenger ribonucleic acid (mRNA).

The most important principle discussed so far is that *all nucleic acid synthesis requires a DNA template.* DNA is the sovereign master of the organism because it alone controls the synthesis of DNA, RNA, and proteins.

The correspondence between the base sequence of the mRNA and the amino acid sequence of the encoded polypeptide is called the genetic code. The amino acids are specified by base triplets called codons. There are 61 amino acid coding codons and three stop codons. The amino acid coding codons are recognized by tRNAs during protein synthesis, and each tRNA presents the appropriate amino acid to the ribosome. During protein synthesis, the ribosome moves along the mRNA in the $5'\rightarrow3'$ direction while polymerizing the polypeptide in the amino$\rightarrow$carboxyl terminal direction.

Genes contain regulatory DNA sequences near the transcriptional start site that bind regulatory proteins. The enhancement of transcription by a DNA-binding protein is called positive control, and the inhibition of transcription is called negative control.

Further Reading

Benkovic SJ, Valentine AM, Salinas F: Replisome-mediated DNA replication, *Annu Rev Biochem* 70:181–208, 2001.

Froelich-Ammon SJ, Osheroff N: Topoisomerase poisons: harnessing the dark side of enzyme mechanism, *J Biol Chem* 270:21429–21432, 1995.

Gilmour DS, Fan R: Derailing the locomotive: transcription termination, *J Biol Chem* 283:661–664, 2008.

Kisselev LL, Buckingham RH: Translational termination comes of age, *Trends Biochem Sci* 25:561–566, 2000.

Kunkel TA: DNA replication fidelity, *J Biol Chem* 279: 16895–16898, 2004.

Vassylyev DG: Elongation by RNA polymerase: a race through roadblocks, *Curr Opin Struct Biol* 19:691–700, 2009.

Wilson DN: The A-Z of bacterial translation inhibitors, *Crit Rev Biochem Mol Biol* 44:393–433, 2009.

QUESTIONS

1. **The base triplet 5′-GAT-3′ on the template strand of DNA is transcribed into mRNA. The anticodon that recognizes this sequence during translation is**

   A. 5′-GAT-3′
   B. 5′-GAU-3′
   C. 5′-UAG-3′
   D. 5′-AUC-3′
   E. 5′-ATC-3′

2. **The high fidelity of DNA replication in *E. coli* would not be possible without**

   A. The high processivity of DNA polymerase III
   B. The S subunit of DNA polymerase I
   C. The 5′-exonuclease activity of DNA polymerase I
   D. The 3′-exonuclease activity of DNA polymerase III
   E. The extremely high accuracy of the aminoacyl-tRNA synthetases

3. **Stop codons are present on**

   A. The coding strand of DNA, where they signal the end of transcription
   B. The template strand of DNA, where they signal the end of transcription
   C. The mRNA, where they signal the end of translation
   D. The tRNA, where they signal the end of translation
   E. Termination factors, where they signal the end of translation

4. **As a result of a mutation, an *E. coli* cell produces an aberrant aminoacyl-tRNA synthetase that attaches not leucine but isoleucine to one of the leucine tRNAs. This kind of mutation would lead to**

   A. A disruption of codon-anticodon pairing during protein synthesis
   B. Premature chain termination during ribosomal protein synthesis
   C. Impaired initiation of ribosomal protein synthesis
   D. Inability of the aminoacyl-tRNA to bind to the ribosome
   E. A change in the genetic code

5. **Like lactose, the pentose sugar arabinose can be used as a source of metabolic energy by *E. coli*. The most reasonable prediction for the regulation of the arabinose-catabolizing enzymes would be that**

   A. Enzymes of arabinose catabolism are induced when glucose is plentiful
   B. A repressor protein prevents the synthesis of arabinose-catabolizing enzymes in the absence of arabinose
   C. The catabolite activator protein prevents the synthesis of arabinose-catabolizing enzymes in the absence of arabinose
   D. Arabinose acts as a corepressor that is required for the binding of the repressor to the operator
   E. Arabinose stimulates the synthesis of arabinose-catabolizing enzymes by raising the cellular cAMP level

Chapter 7
THE HUMAN GENOME

Although the clockwork of life is similar in prokaryotes and eukaryotes, eukaryotes are more complex. Prokaryotes must be mean and lean to ensure fast reproduction. Therefore they keep their genomes small and regulate gene expression in simple yet efficient ways. Eukaryotes, however, require genetic complexity to control their complex cellular and organismal structures and sophisticated lifecycles.

Humans, for example, have 700 times more DNA than *Escherichia coli,* but they have only six times more genes (*Table 7.1*). This disparity comes from the fact that 90% of *E. coli* DNA, but only 1.3% of human DNA, codes for proteins.

Gene regulation is more important than gene number. Multicellular eukaryotes have (almost) the same genes in every cell of the body, but different genes are expressed in different cell types and at different stages during the development of the organism. This requires control mechanisms of extraordinary complexity.

CHROMATIN CONSISTS OF DNA AND HISTONES

The prokaryotic chromosome is a naked circular DNA double helix with a length of about 1 mm. Eukaryotic chromosomes consists of a single linear DNA double helix with a length of several centimeters, which is tightly packaged with a set of **histone** proteins.

The histones are small basic proteins, with numerous positive charges on the side chains of lysine and arginine residues. These positive charges bind to the negatively charged phosphate groups of the DNA, and they neutralize at least 60% of the negative charges on DNA.

Eukaryotic cells have five major types of histones (*Table 7.2*). With the exception of histone H1, whose structure varies in different species and even in different tissues of the same organism, the histones are well conserved throughout the phylogenetic tree. For example, histones H3 and H4 from pea seedlings and calf thymus differ in only four and two amino acid positions, respectively. Presumably, the histones were invented by the very first eukaryotes, perhaps as early as 2 billion

years ago, and have served the same essential functions ever since.

Chromatin, named for its affinity for basic dyes such as hematoxylin and fuchsin, contains roughly equal amounts of DNA and histones. **Euchromatin** has a loose structure, whereas **heterochromatin** is more tightly condensed and deeper staining. *Genes are actively transcribed in euchromatin but are repressed in heterochromatin.*

THE NUCLEOSOME IS THE STRUCTURAL UNIT OF CHROMATIN

Under the electron microscope, euchromatin looks like beads on a string. The "string" is the DNA double helix, and the "beads" are **nucleosomes,** which are little disks formed from two copies each of histones H2A, H2B, H3, and H4. One hundred forty-six base pairs of DNA are wound around the histone core in a left-handed orientation. The DNA between the nucleosomes, typically 50 to 60 base pairs in length, can associate with a molecule of histone H1 (*Fig. 7.1*). This happens especially during the formation of higher-order chromatin structures.

Beads on a string are typical for euchromatin, but transcriptionally silent heterochromatin is present mainly in the form of the **30-nm fiber** (*Fig. 7.1, B*). The 30-nm fiber is about 40 times more compact than the stretched-out DNA double helix. Further compaction occurs during the formation of mitotic and meiotic chromosomes, when the 30-nm fiber attaches to chromosomal **scaffold proteins,** forming long loops (*Fig. 7.1, C*). Metaphase chromosomes are about 200 times more compact than the 30-nm fiber.

COVALENT HISTONE MODIFICATIONS REGULATE DNA REPLICATION AND TRANSCRIPTION

Transcription can take place only when the 30-nm fiber has disintegrated into the loose structure of euchromatin, and histones have been displaced from the DNA. *Whereas prokaryotic genes are transcribed unless transcription is prevented by a repressor, eukaryotic*

Table 7.1 Genomes of Various Organisms

Species	Type of Organism	Genome Size (Mega Base Pairs)	Gene Number
Prokaryotes			
Escherichia coli	Intestinal bacterium	4.639	4289
Mycoplasma genitalium	Genitourinary pathogen	0.58	468
Mycobacterium tuberculosis	Tubercle bacillus	4.447	4402
Rickettsia prowazekii	Typhus bacillus	1.111	834
Treponema pallidum	Syphilis spirochete	1.138	1041
Helicobacter pylori	Stomach ulcer bacterium	1.667	1590
Eukaryotes			
Saccharomyces cerevisiae	Baker's yeast	12.069	6300
Caenorhabditis elegans	Roundworm	97	19000
Drosophila melanogaster	Fruit fly	137	14000
Homo sapiens	Pride of creation	3000	25000

Table 7.2 Five Types of Histones

Type	Size (Amino Acids)	Location
H1	215	Linker
H2A	129	Nucleosome core
H2B	125	Nucleosome core
H3	135	Nucleosome core
H4	102	Nucleosome core

genes are silent unless the histones are removed from the DNA. The association between histones and DNA is regulated by covalent modifications of the histones:

1. *Acetylation of lysine side chains in histones destabilizes chromatin structures and favors transcription.* Acetylation eliminates the positive charges on the lysine side chains, thereby weakening the binding of the histones to DNA.
2. *Methylation of some lysine side chains in histones favors the formation of tightly condensed heterochromatin and reduces transcription, whereas methylations on other lysine and arginine side chains have the opposite effect.* These effects probably are mediated by nonhistone proteins that bind to the methylated histone.
3. *Phosphorylation of a threonine side chain in histone H2A is characteristic of mitosis and meiosis,* although its role in these processes is not well understood.
4. ATP-dependent **chromatin remodeling complexes** can loosen the nucleosome structure temporarily to facilitate transcription. Little is known about the constituents, regulation, and biological functions of these complexes.

These histone modifications are controlled by sequence-specific DNA binding proteins that regulate transcription ("transcription factors") and by DNA methylation.

DNA METHYLATION SILENCES GENES

About 3% of the cytosine in human DNA is methylated:

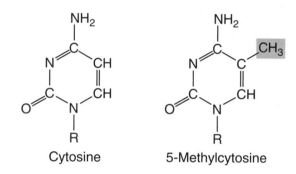

Cytosine   5-Methylcytosine

Methylcytosine is found in palindromic 5'-CG-3' sequences, which carry the methyl mark on the cytosines of both strands. *5-Methylcytosine causes chromatin condensation and gene silencing,* most likely by recruiting histone deacetylases. The methyl groups are introduced by two types of DNA methyltransferase: **de novo DNA methyltransferases,** which attach methyl groups to previously unmethylated CG sequences; and **maintenance DNA methyltransferases,** which methylate the new strand after DNA replication to complement a methyl mark on the old strand. Because of the maintenance DNA methyltransferases, *DNA methylation is heritable through the cell generations.* The term **epigenetic inheritance** is used to describe the transmission of DNA methylation patterns and histone modifications.

DNA methylation has several functions:

1. *Gene regulation:* About 60% of human genes possess **CG islands** near their promoters, whose methylation state is different in different tissues. The poor health of many cloned animals is attributed to the incomplete erasure of epigenetic marks when a somatic cell nucleus is introduced into an oocyte.

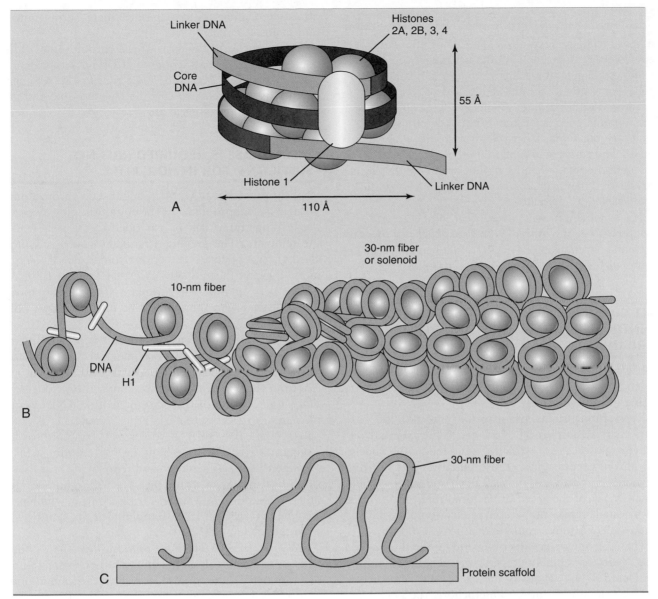

Figure 7.1 Structure of chromatin. **A,** The nucleosome. **B,** Formation of the 30-nm fiber. **C,** Attachment of the 30-nm fiber to the central protein scaffold of the chromosome. Each loop of the 30-nm fiber from one scaffold attachment to the next measures approximately 0.4 to 0.8 μm and contains 45,000 to 90,000 base pairs.

2. *Suppression of mobile elements*: CG sequences near mobile elements are kept in the methylated state in order to prevent transcription of the mobile elements.
3. *X inactivation*: The inactive second X chromosome of females ("Barr body") is kept in the condensed, heterochromatic state by widespread DNA methylation.
4. *Imprinting*: A few dozen human genes become methylated selectively in the male or female germ line. The embryo and fetus express these genes only from the maternally or paternally inherited chromosome, respectively. Because of imprinting, creation of a viable human being by fusing two oocytes in a test tube is not possible, which is bad news for lesbian couples.

CLINICAL EXAMPLE 7.1: Rett Syndrome

Rett syndrome is a severe neurological disease of females. Affected girls develop normally for the first 1 to 2 years after birth. After this age they lose the motor and cognitive skills they had already acquired and develop mental deficiency, seizures, autism, repetitive hand movements, and/or autonomic dysfunction. Death occurs between the ages of 12 and 40 years.

Rett syndrome is caused by a mutation of the gene encoding MeCP2 (methyl-cytosine binding protein-2), one of several proteins that repress transcription after binding to methylcytosine in DNA. However, MeCP2 has

Continued

other unrelated effects as well, including stimulatory effects on the transcription of many genes. The neurological aberrations are attributed to deranged gene expression in neurons and glial cells.

Classic Rett syndrome is limited to females because the mutated gene is located on the X chromosome. Heterozygous females have Rett syndrome, whereas males who carry the mutation on their single X chromosome die before birth. Rett syndrome usually is caused by a new mutation because affected females are too disabled to reproduce.

Milder MeCP2 mutations do occur in males, with symptoms ranging from mild mental deficiency to fatal neonatal encephalopathy. Such mutations have been found in 1.5% of mentally retarded males.

ALL EUKARYOTIC CHROMOSOMES HAVE A CENTROMERE, TELOMERES, AND REPLICATION ORIGINS

Chromosomes need specialized structures to ensure their structural integrity, replication, and transmission during mitosis (*Fig. 7.2*).

Replication origins are spaced about 100,000 base pairs apart. Multiple origins are needed because eukaryotic chromosomes are 10 to 100 times longer than bacterial chromosomes and because eukaryotic replication forks move at a rate of only 50 nucleotides per second, which is 6% of the speed of bacterial replication forks. With a single replication origin, replication of the largest human chromosome would take at least 1 month.

The **centromere** consists of several hundred thousand base pairs of highly repetitive, gene-free, tightly condensed DNA. Proteins attach to the centromeric heterochromatin to form a **kinetochore**, the immediate attachment point for the spindle fibers during mitosis and meiosis.

Telomeres form the ends of the chromosomes. They consist of the repeat sequence TTAGGG repeated in tandem between 500 and 5000 times. The telomeric repeats bind proteins to cap the chromosome end and protect it from enzymatic attack.

TELOMERASE IS REQUIRED (BUT NOT SUFFICIENT) FOR IMMORTALITY

Replication of linear DNA in eukaryotic chromosomes poses a special problem. At the end of the chromosome, the leading strand can be extended to the very end of the template. The lagging strand, however, is synthesized in the opposite direction from small RNA primers. Even in the unlikely case that the last primer is at the very end of the template strand, its removal would leave a gap that cannot be filled by DNA polymerase (*Fig. 7.3, A*).

The enzyme **telomerase** solves this problem by adding the telomeric TTAGGG sequence to the overhanging 3′ end. No DNA template is available for this reaction; therefore, *telomerase contains an RNA template*. One section of this 150-nucleotide RNA is complementary to the telomeric repeat sequence. By base pairing with the DNA, it serves as a template for the elongation of the overhanging 3′ terminus. This extended 3′ end is then used as a template for the extension of the opposite strand (see *Fig. 7.3, B* and *C*). Telomerase qualifies as a **reverse transcriptase**, which is an enzyme that uses an RNA template for the synthesis of a complementary DNA.

Telomerase is required for immortality. The Olympic gods were immortal, so presumably they expressed telomerase in all their cells. However, in the human body, only the cells of the germ line are immortal. They have

Figure 7.2 Maintenance structures of eukaryotic chromosomes.

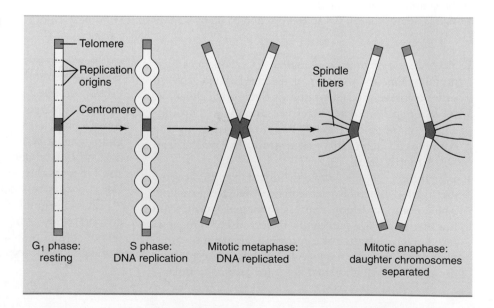

G₁ phase: resting — S phase: DNA replication — Mitotic metaphase: DNA replicated — Mitotic anaphase: daughter chromosomes separated

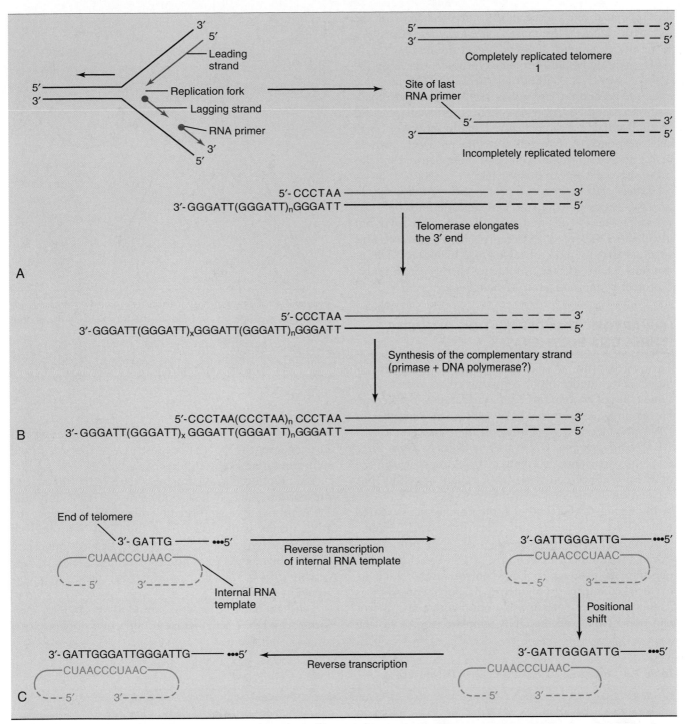

Figure 7.3 Terminal replication problem of telomeric DNA in eukaryotic chromosomes. **A,** The problem: One of the daughter chromosomes is incompletely replicated because DNA replication proceeds only in the 5′→3′ direction, and replication of the lagging strand ends at the site of the last RNA primer. **B,** The solution: Telomerase elongates the overhanging 3′ end of the incompletely replicated telomere. This is followed by synthesis of the complementary strand. Complementary strand synthesis most likely occurs by the regular mechanism of DNA replication. **C,** The hypothetical mechanism of telomere extension by telomerase.

telomerase; therefore, egg and sperm have long telomeres. The expression of telomerase tapers off during fetal development, and from that time on, the cells lose 50 to 100 base pairs of DNA from the telomeres with every round of DNA replication.

For example, fibroblasts can be grown in cell culture but eventually die after a few dozen mitotic divisions. Fibroblasts taken from an infant survive longer in cell culture than those taken from a senior citizen. However, the best predictor of fibroblast lifespan is not the chronological age of the donor but the length of the telomeric DNA. *Fibroblasts with long telomeres live long, and those with short telomeres die fast.*

The telomeres bind protective proteins that hide the ends of the DNA. Without telomeres, the chromosome ends are recognized as broken DNA in need of repair, and misguided DNA repair systems produce haphazard chromosomal rearrangements. Usually, however, aged cells respond to undersized telomeres with growth arrest and programmed cell death long before the telomeres have disappeared altogether.

Cancer cells express telomerase and are immortal. In order to become malignant, a somatic cell not only has to escape the controls that normally limit its growth but also has to find ways to derepress its telomerase. This suggests that the lack of telomerase in somatic cells is not only a curse that seals humans' earthly fate but also a protective mechanism to reduce the cancer risk.

EUKARYOTIC DNA REPLICATION REQUIRES THREE DNA POLYMERASES

The mechanism of eukaryotic DNA replication is incompletely understood. Although eukaryotes use the same types of protein as *E. coli*, the details are different. For example, eukaryotes have a far greater number of DNA polymerases. *The human genome encodes at least 14 DNA-dependent DNA polymerases.* At least three of them participate routinely in DNA replication. The others are concerned with DNA repair or with DNA replication across sites of DNA damage.

In lagging strand synthesis, the primase is associated with **DNA polymerase α.** This composite enzyme synthesizes about 10 nucleotides of RNA primer followed by about 20 nucleotides of DNA, before relinquishing its product to **DNA polymerase δ.** Like its bacterial counterpart polymerase III, polymerase δ owes its high processivity to its association with a clamp protein that holds it on the DNA template (*Fig. 7.4*). The

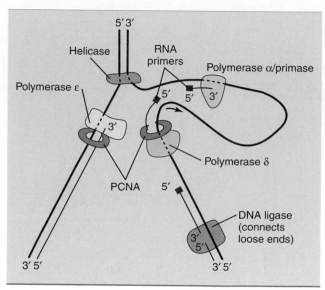

Figure 7.4 Eukaryotic replication fork. The two major DNA polymerases, δ and ε, are held on the template by the sliding clamp proliferating cell nuclear antigen (PCNA), the eukaryotic equivalent of the β-clamp in bacteria. The DNA template of the lagging strand spools backward through polymerase δ and PCNA (*arrow*) to create the loop on the right side.

eukaryotic clamp protein is known as **proliferating cell nuclear antigen (PCNA)** because it was first identified in proliferating but not quiescent cells.

Eukaryotic Okazaki fragments are only 100 to 200 nucleotides long. When polymerase δ runs into the RNA primer of the preceding Okazaki fragment, the RNA primer is displaced from the DNA and removed by a nuclease, most commonly the flap endonuclease **FEN1.** Polymerase α has no proofreading 3′-exonuclease activity (*Table 7.3*), and its errors are most likely corrected by polymerase δ.

Synthesis of the leading strand is most likely performed by **DNA polymerase ε,** although polymerase δ

Table 7.3 Properties of Eukaryotic DNA Polymerases

Polymerase	Location	MW	3′-Exonuclease Activity	Primase Activity	Processivity	Function
α	Nucleus	335,000*	−	+	Low	Initiates DNA replication
δ	Nucleus	170,000†	+	−	High	Replication of lagging strand, DNA repair
ε	Nucleus	256,000‡	+	−	High	Replication of leading strand, DNA repair
β	Nucleus	37,000	−	−	Low	DNA repair
γ	Mitochondria	160,000–300,000§	+	−	High	Replication and repair of mitochondrial DNA

DNA, Deoxyribonucleic acid; *MW,* molecular weight.
*With catalytic subunit of MW 165,000 D.
†With catalytic core of MW 125,000 D.
‡With catalytic core of MW 215,000 D.
§With catalytic subunit of MW 125,000 D.

can synthesize the leading strand and appears to be involved in leading strand synthesis in some situations.

MOST HUMAN DNA DOES NOT CODE FOR PROTEINS

Only 1.3% of the human genome codes for proteins. Genes are separated by vast expanses of noncoding DNA, including gene deserts extending over more than one million base pairs. Noncoding DNA is present even *within* the genes. Human genes are patchworks of **exons**, whose transcripts are processed to a mature mRNA, and **introns**. *Introns are transcribed along with the exons but are excised from the transcript before the messenger RNA (mRNA) leaves the nucleus.*

Human genes have between 1 and 178 exons, with an average of 8.8 exons and 7.8 introns. The average exon is about 145 base pairs long and codes for 48 amino acids, and the average polypeptide has a length of 440 amino acids. Introns are generally far longer than exons, and more than 90% of the DNA within genes belongs to introns (see *Fig. 7.12* for an example).

Why human genes have introns, why they have so many of them, and why the introns are so long are not known. Except for some intronic sequences that contribute to the regulation of gene expression by binding regulatory proteins, introns appear to be useless **junk DNA.**

However, the intron-exon structure of human genes is important for evolution. *Different structural and functional domains of a polypeptide are often encoded by separate exons.* For example, the immunoglobulin chains consist of several globular domains with similar amino acid sequence and tertiary structure, each encoded by its own exon (see Chapter 15). Immunoglobulin genes most likely arose by repeated **exon duplication** from a single-exon gene.

In other cases, exons from different genes appear to have combined to form a new functional gene. This is called **exon shuffling.** *The exons are the building blocks from which the multitude of eukaryotic genes has been assembled in the course of evolution.*

Figure 7.5 shows an overview of the composition of the human genome. One commentator wrote about the human genome: "In some ways it may resemble your garage/bedroom/refrigerator/life: highly individualistic, but unkempt; little evidence of organization; much accumulated clutter (referred to by the uninitiated as 'junk'); virtually nothing ever discarded; and the few patently valuable items indiscriminately, apparently carelessly, scattered throughout."

GENE FAMILIES ORIGINATE BY GENE DUPLICATION

Most protein-coding genes are present in only one copy in the haploid genome, but **duplicated genes,** with two identical or near-identical copies close together on the

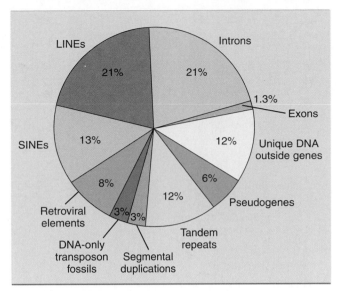

Figure 7.5 Approximate composition of the human genome. *LINEs,* Long interspersed elements; *SINEs,* short interspersed elements.

same chromosome, are seen occasionally. *Some genes that code for very abundant RNAs or proteins are present in multiple copies,* including the ribosomal RNA (rRNA) genes (≈200 copies), the 5S rRNA gene (≈2000 copies), the histone genes (≈20 copies), and most of the transfer RNA (tRNA) genes. In most cases, identical or near-identical copies of the gene are arranged in tandem, head to tail over long stretches of DNA, separated by untranscribed spacers.

Gene families consist of two or more similar but not identical genes that, in most cases, are positioned close together on the chromosome. They arise during evolution by repeated gene duplications, mostly during **crossing over** in prophase of meiosis I when homologous chromosomes align in parallel and exchange DNA by homologous recombination. Normal crossing over is a strictly reciprocal process in which the chromosome neither gains nor loses genes. However, *if the chromosomes are mispaired during crossing over, one chromosome acquires a deletion and the other a duplication* (*Fig. 7.6*). Through new mutations, a duplicated gene can acquire new biological properties and functions.

In many cases, however, one of the duplication products acquires crippling mutations that prevent its transcription or translation. The result is called a **pseudogene.** Pseudogenes still have the intron-exon structure of the functional gene from which they were derived, and they are located close to their functional counterpart on the chromosome.

THE GENOME CONTAINS MANY TANDEM REPEATS

Tandem repeats, also known as **simple-sequence DNA,** consist of a short DNA sequence of between two and a few dozen base pairs that is repeated head to tail many

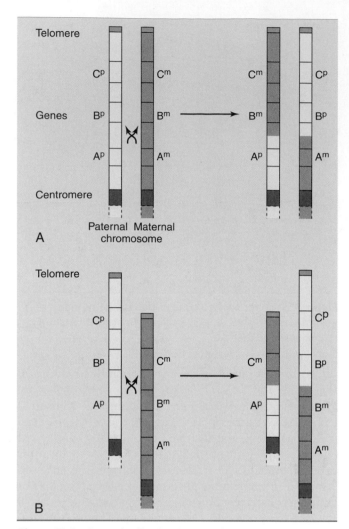

Figure 7.6 Gene duplication by crossing over between mispaired chromosomes in meiosis. **A,** Normal meiotic recombination. This is an example of homologous recombination, which requires similar or identical base sequence. It creates new combinations of the paternally derived and maternally derived genes. **B,** Recombination between mispaired chromosomes. One chromosome acquires a deletion and the other a duplication. Repeated gene duplications followed by divergent evolution of the duplicated genes create gene families.

times. The telomeric TTAGGG sequence is one example. *The centromeres have even more simple-sequence DNA than the telomeres, but the repeat sequences differ in different chromosomes.*

Microsatellites are interspersed tandem repeats outside the centromeres and telomeres. They usually have between two and five bases in the repeat unit that are repeated from a few times to more than 50 times in any one location. The same repeat can be present at multiple sites in the genome. Tandem repeats with longer repeat units are called **minisatellites.**

The length of tandem repeats is prone to change through mutation. Because most tandem repeats have no biological function (but see *Clinical Example 7.2*), the resulting length variations are innocuous and therefore are not removed by natural selection. They become part of normal genetic diversity and can be used for DNA fingerprinting and paternity testing.

SOME DNA SEQUENCES ARE COPIES OF FUNCTIONAL RNAs

As the degenerate offspring of duplicated genes, pseudogenes still have the intron-exon structure of the functional gene from which they were derived. **Processed pseudogenes** are a different type of gene derivative. *Processed pseudogenes consist only of exon sequences, with an oligo-A tract of 10 to 50 nucleotides at the 3′ end.* This structure is framed by direct repeats of between 9 and 14 base pairs (*Fig. 7.7*).

Processed pseudogenes arise during evolution by the reverse transcription of a cellular mRNA. The key enzyme in this process is **reverse transcriptase,** which transcribes the RNA into a complementary DNA (cDNA). The cDNA is then inserted into the genome by an **integrase** enzyme, which splices the cDNA into the genomic DNA. *Enzymes with reverse transcriptase and integrase activities are encoded by retrotransposons in the human genome.* These enzymes can also be introduced by infecting retroviruses (see Chapter 10).

Integration can occur virtually anywhere in the genome. Unlike pseudogenes, processed pseudogenes are not located near their functional counterparts. The direct repeats flanking the processed pseudogene are target site duplications that arise when an integrase enzyme inserts the cDNA into the chromosome. Having lost their promoter during retrotransposition, processed pseudogenes are rarely transcribed.

MANY REPETITIVE DNA SEQUENCES ARE (OR WERE) MOBILE

About 45% of the human genome consists of repetitive sequences with lengths of a few hundred to several thousand base pairs. They are not aligned in tandem but are scattered throughout the genome as **interspersed elements** (*Table 7.5*). These elements are repetitive because they can insert copies of themselves into new genomic locations. *These mobile elements can be understood as molecular parasites that infest the human genome.*

DNA transposons contain a gene for a transposase enzyme that is flanked by inverted repeats. The transposase catalyzes the duplication of the transposon and the insertion of a copy in a new genomic location (see Chapter 10). DNA transposons were active in the genomes of early primates, but in the human lineage they mutated into nonfunctionality approximately 30 million years ago. Only their molecular fossils can still be inspected.

CLINICAL EXAMPLE 7.2: Huntington Disease

Most microsatellites reside in nonessential "junk DNA," but some occur in the regulatory or coding sequences of genes. **Huntington disease** is caused by expansion of the trinucleotide repeat CAG in the coding sequence of a brain-expressed gene. In the normal gene, the CAG is repeated 6 to 34 times, coding for a polyglutamine tract in the protein huntingtin.

When the CAG sequence expands to a copy number in excess of 36, the result is a glutamine-expanded huntingtin protein that forms abnormal complexes with other proteins. These abnormal complexes kill cells in the basal ganglia of the brain and in the cerebral cortex, leading to an adult-onset disease with personality changes, a motor disorder, and progressive dementia.

The greater the trinucleotide expansion, the earlier is the onset of the disease. Because the trinucleotide repeat tends to expand further during father-to-child transmission, *the disease tends to become more severe in successive generations.* **Table 7.4** lists some other diseases that are caused by trinucleotide expansions.

Table 7.4 Diseases Caused by Expansion of a Trinucleotide Repeat Sequence in a Gene

Disease	Type of Disease	Inheritance	Amplified Repeat*	Repeat Number		Location in Gene
				Normal	Disease	
Huntington disease	Neural degeneration	AD	CAG	6-34	36-120	Coding sequence (Gln)
Myotonic dystrophy	Muscle loss, cardiac arrhythmia	AD	CTG	5-37	100-5000	3'-Untranslated region
Fragile X	Mental retardation	XR	CGG	6-52	200-3000	5'-Untranslated region
Friedreich ataxia	Loss of motor coordination	AR	GAA	7-22	200-1000	Intron

AD, Autosomal dominant; *AR*, autosomal recessive; *Gln*, glutamine; *XR*, X-linked recessive.
*A, Adenine; C, cytosine; G, guanine; T, thymine.

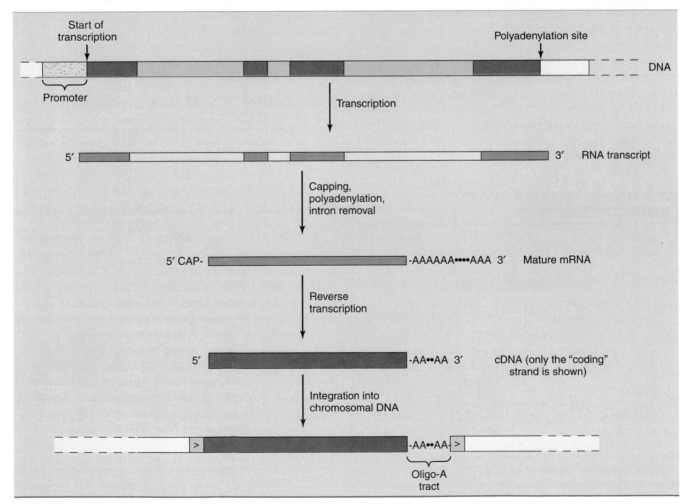

Figure 7.7 Origin of a processed pseudogene. ■, Exons; □, introns.

Table 7.5 Mobile Elements in Human Genome

Class	Length	Number in Genome	Encoded Proteins	Mode of Movement	Current Activity
DNA-only transposons	Variable, average 220 bp	400,000	Transposase (defunct)	Direct transposition	Fossils only
Retrovirus-like retrotransposons	Up to 10,000 bp, average 350 bp	700,000	Reverse transcriptase (usually defunct)	Retrotransposition	Few are still active
LINE-1 elements	Up to 6000 bp, most are truncated	900,000	Reverse transcriptase, RNA-binding protein	Retrotransposition	Still active
Alu sequences	Up to 300 bp, many are truncated	1,300,000	None	Retrotransposition	Still active

bp, Base pair; *DNA*, deoxyribonucleic acid; *LINE*, long interspersed element; *RNA*, ribonucleic acid.

The other mobile elements are **retrotransposons.** They are transcribed into RNA, then the RNA is copied into a cDNA by reverse transcriptase, and the cDNA is inserted into the genome.

Retroviral retrotransposons are descended from infecting retroviruses. This type of virus turns its RNA genome into a cDNA, which it inserts into the host cell genome (see Chapter 10). *Retroviral elements are integrated retroviruses that are no longer infectious because they have lost the ability to make the structural proteins of the virus particle.* However, they have multiplied *within* the genome because they retained, for some time at least, the ability to move into new genomic locations with the help of their reverse transcriptase and integrase. Like their retroviral ancestors, retroviral retrotransposons are flanked by long terminal repeat (LTR) sequences and therefore are also called **LTR retrotransposons.**

Almost all retroviral elements have lost the ability for retroposition. Only one family of these elements has been active in the human genome during the past six million years, since human ancestors separated from the ancestors of chimpanzees. *Most retroviral retrotransposons are the dead bodies of retroviruses, left to rot in the genomic soil.*

L1 ELEMENTS ENCODE A REVERSE TRANSCRIPTASE

L1 elements are the most abundant type of **long interspersed elements (LINEs).** A full-length L1 element has nearly 6000 base pairs and ends in a poly-A tract. It is framed by short direct repeats that originated during retrotransposition.

The human genome harbors about 900,000 L1 elements, but only about 5000 are full length. Most of the others are badly truncated at the 5′ end. Truncation is a common accident during retrotransposition. Different L1 elements in the human genome are identical in about 95% of their bases.

Full-length L1 elements contain two genes, but these genes are intact in only 60 to 100 of the 5000 full-length L1 elements. One of the two genes codes for an RNA-binding protein of unknown function, and the other for a protein with reverse transcriptase, nuclease, and integrase activities.

The element is transcribed by the cellular RNA polymerase II from an unusual promoter whose sequence becomes part of the 5′-untranslated region of the L1 messenger RNA. Reverse transcription and integration probably occur at the same time and are catalyzed by the same L1-encoded protein (*Fig. 7.8*). The short direct repeats flanking the element are target site duplications that arise during retrotransposition because the L1 endonuclease makes staggered cuts in the target DNA.

The L1 reverse transcriptase acts preferentially on the transcript of the L1 element. However, on occasion it produces a processed pseudogene by reverse transcribing and integrating a cellular mRNA (see *Fig. 7.7*).

ALU SEQUENCES SPREAD WITH THE HELP OF L1 REVERSE TRANSCRIPTASE

The most populous tribe of **short interspersed elements (SINEs)** is the **Alu sequences,** with 1.3 million copies in the haploid genome. A full-length Alu sequence measures 282 base pairs, contains an adenine-rich tract of between 7 and 50 base pairs at the 3′ end, and is flanked by direct repeats of 7 to 21 base pairs.

Alu sequences from different parts of the genome differ on average in about 20% of their bases. Some Alu sequences can be transcribed into RNA by RNA polymerase III, but they do not encode any proteins. However, *the RNA transcript of the Alu sequence can be reverse transcribed and integrated into the genome by the L1-encoded reverse transcriptase/integrase.*

L1 sequences might be the descendants of a virus, but Alu sequences are clearly of cellular origin. The Alu consensus sequence is more than 80% identical to the sequence of **7SL RNA,** a small cytoplasmic RNA that participates in the targeting of proteins to the endoplasmic reticulum (see Chapter 8).

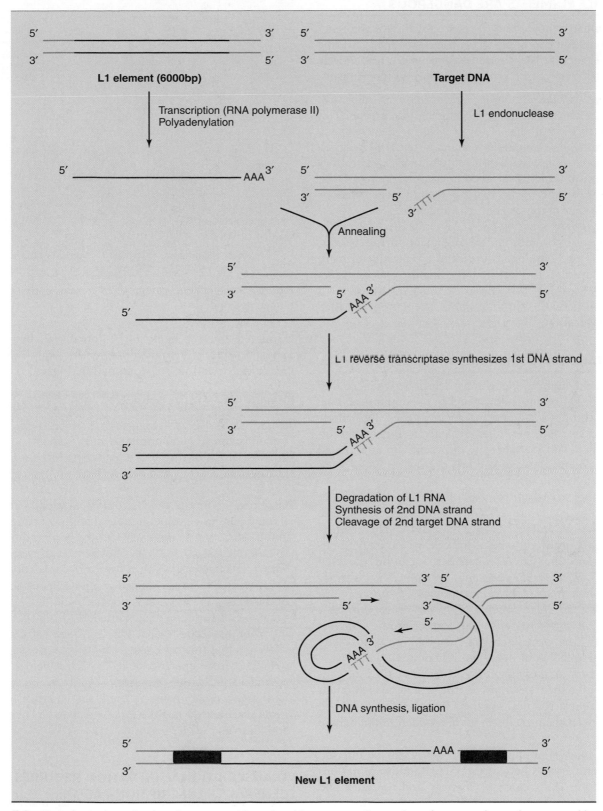

Figure 7.8 Hypothetical mechanism for retroposition of an L1 sequence. Formation of processed pseudogenes and insertions of Alu sequences use a similar mechanism.

MOBILE ELEMENTS ARE DANGEROUS

The human genome is a graveyard for the rotting relics of 4.3 million copies of largely useless, selfish, parasitic DNA elements. These mobile elements are not entirely harmless. They cause problems by several mechanisms:

1. *Gene disruption during retroposition:* Mobile elements can wreak havoc by jumping into a gene. This is a rare event that is responsible for a mere 0.3% of pathogenic mutations in humans (but 10% in mice).
2. *Chromosome breakage:* Even without successful retroposition, the L1-encoded nuclease can cause DNA double-strand breaks that can lead to large deletions and other chromosomal rearrangements.
3. *Illegitimate crossing-over:* Any repetitive sequence can cause chromosome misalignment during meiosis, when nonhomologous copies of a repetitive element pair up. This can lead to large duplications and deletions (see *Fig. 7.6, B*) as well as to transfers of DNA between chromosomes. The latter is called **translocation.**

HUMANS HAVE APPROXIMATELY 25,000 GENES

Most gene-hunting algorithms detect between 20,000 and 35,000 protein-coding genes in the human genome. These computer algorithms locate genes by telltale sequences such as promoter elements, a start codon followed by a substantial string of potentially amino acid coding codons, intron-exon junctions, stop codon, and polyadenylation signal.

Another approach consists of extracting RNA from cells, copying it into cDNA with the help of reverse transcriptase, and sequencing the cDNA. This method defines the **transcriptome** of the cell, which is the totality of transcribed DNA sequences that can be recovered as RNA. *Whereas the genome is the same in each cell of the human body, the transcriptomes of different cell types are different because different genes are transcribed in different cells.* The transcriptome contains not only the protein-coding mRNAs but also many noncoding RNAs of unknown function.

The sum total of expressed proteins is called the **proteome.** Like the transcriptome, the proteome is different in different cell types. *Figure 7.9* shows the presumed functions of the proteins that are encoded in the human genome.

The functional importance of DNA can be inferred from comparisons between species. Random mutations in the junk DNA cause no damage and therefore can survive. However, mutations in important coding and regulatory sequences are likely to disrupt gene function and to cause disease or functional impairments. Therefore they are removed by natural selection. As a result, *coding and regulatory sequences of genes show little variation among species, and the junk DNA shows much variation.* Some noncoding RNA transcripts are

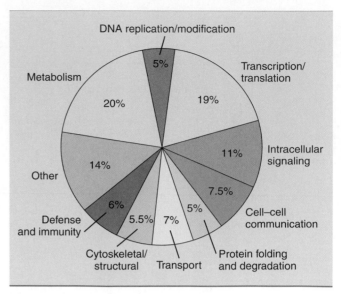

Figure 7.9 Functional categories of proteins encoded by the human genome.

conserved and are likely to be functional, but others appear to be unconstrained and most likely represent "leaky transcription" of nonfunctional DNA.

CLINICAL EXAMPLE 7.3: Heart-Breaking RNA

Acute myocardial infarction is not a genetic disease but a multifactorial condition that results from atherosclerosis of the coronary arteries. Risk factors include both lifestyle and genes. One case-control study investigated the association of acute myocardial infarction with more than 52,000 DNA variations throughout the genome in more than 3400 patients and 3700 controls. The study found a single-nucleotide variant, the less common allele of which was associated with a 35% increased risk of myocardial infarction. This polymorphism is included in a long RNA transcript of unknown function that is not translated into protein. This transcript was named MIAT (myocardial infarction-associated transcript). Only future studies can show whether this noncoding RNA is indeed associated with myocardial infarction and, if so, by which mechanism it confers disease susceptibility. Because MIAT is expressed mainly in the brain, its effects on cardiovascular risk might well be mediated by behavior and lifestyle.

TRANSCRIPTIONAL INITIATION REQUIRES GENERAL TRANSCRIPTION FACTORS

Eukaryotes use separate enzymes for the synthesis of rRNA, mRNA, and tRNA (*Table 7.6*).

RNA polymerase I synthesizes the common precursor of the 5.8S, 18S, and 28S rRNA in the nucleolus, where the ribosomal subunits are assembled. **RNA polymerase II** synthesizes the mRNA precursors, and

Table 7.6　Eukaryotic RNA Polymerases

Type	Location	Transcripts	Inhibition by α-Amanitin
I	Nucleolus	Pre-rRNA	−
II	Nucleus	Pre-mRNA	+++
III	Nucleus	tRNA, 5S rRNA	+
Mitochondrial	Mitochondria	Mitochondrial RNAs	−

mRNA, Messenger ribonucleic acid; *RNA*, ribonucleic acid; *rRNA*, ribosomal ribonucleic acid; *tRNA*, transfer ribonucleic acid.

RNA polymerase III synthesizes small RNAs including tRNAs and the 5S rRNA.

Transcription requires access of the RNA polymerase to the promoter at the 5′ end of the gene. To this effect, nucleosomes are excluded from the promoter by AT-rich sequences in the promoter and by transcription factors that bind to DNA sequences in the promoter.

Eukaryotic promoters are extremely variable. The **core promoter** includes 30 to 40 base pairs upstream of the transcriptional start site and serves as an assembly point for the **general transcription factors,** which are functionally equivalent to the bacterial σ subunit. They are named by the acronym TF, followed by the number of the RNA polymerase with which they work and an identifying letter. *The RNA polymerase must bind to the promoter-associated transcription factors before it can start transcription.*

One of the more frequently encountered promoter elements in protein-coding genes is the **TATA box** (consensus TATAAAA), located 25 to 30 base pairs upstream of the transcriptional start site. *Figure 7.10* shows how the general transcription factors are thought to assemble on TATA box-containing promoters. First the TATA-binding protein **TBP** binds to the TATA box. TBP is only one of about 14 subunits of transcription factor IID (**TFIID**). The other subunits, known as TBP-associated factors (**TAFs**), assemble on TBP while TBP is bound to the TATA box. Other transcription factors add to this complex, including **TFIIH,** which is unusual in being an ATP-dependent helicase and a protein kinase. It helps in strand separation during transcription, and it phosphorylates RNA polymerase II on multiple serine and threonine side chains.

Only about 10% of human genes possess a TATA box, and there are many alternative ways of assembling a preinitiation complex on core promoters. For example, some of the TAFs bind not only to TBP but also to promoter elements other than the TATA box.

GENES ARE SURROUNDED BY REGULATORY SITES

Within 200 or 300 base pairs upstream of the core promoter are binding sites for activator and repressor proteins that stabilize or destabilize the transcriptional initiation complex, respectively. Together with the "general" transcription factors on the core promoter, these sequence-specific activator and repressor proteins are loosely referred to as "transcription factors." They can affect transcriptional initiation in multiple ways:

1. They can physically interact with the general transcription factors or RNA polymerase to stabilize the transcriptional initiation complex.

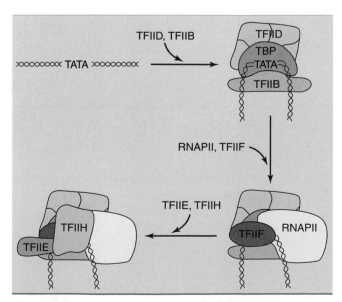

Figure 7.10　Formation of the transcriptional initiation complex by assembly of general transcription factors and RNA polymerase II (*RNAPII*). Transcription factor IID (*TFIID*) contains multiple subunits. One subunit, the TATA-binding protein (*TBP*), binds the TATA box. *TFIIB, TFIIE, TFIIF, TFIIH,* Transcription factor IIB, IIE, IIF, and IIH, respectively.

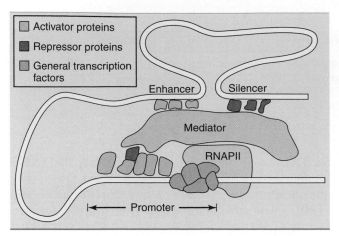

Figure 7.11 The mediator is a large protein complex that mediates the effects of activator and repressor proteins on transcriptional initiation. *RNAP II*, Ribonucleic acid polymerase II.

2. They can recruit histone-modifying enzymes or ATP-dependent chromatin remodeling complexes.
3. They can interact with the transcriptional initiation complex indirectly through a large protein complex with 20 to 30 subunits known as **mediator** (*Fig. 7.11*)

Binding sites for transcription factors are not restricted to the promoter but can be found thousands and sometimes up to one million base pairs away from the transcriptional start site in one of the gene's introns, in the junk DNA between the genes, or even in an intron of a neighboring gene. These binding sites tend to form clusters called **enhancers** or **silencers,** depending on whether they stimulate or depress transcription.

One gene can have multiple enhancers and silencers, and an enhancer or silencer can regulate a whole set of neighboring genes. Presumably, the transcription factors bound to these distant regulatory sites can affect transcription by looping of the DNA, which brings them in physical contact with the promoter-bound proteins or the mediator complex (see *Fig. 7.11*).

Typical enhancers look as if an overenthusiastic sorcerer's apprentice had stuffed as many binding sites for regulatory proteins as possible into as small a space as possible. *Figure 7.12* shows an example. Most binding sites are only 15 to 20 base pairs long. Many transcription factors respond to hormones, second messengers, or nutrients. Therefore their binding sites are called **response elements.**

GENE EXPRESSION IS REGULATED BY DNA-BINDING PROTEINS

About 6% of human genes code for proteins with DNA-binding domains and presumed functions in the regulation of gene expression, for a total of about 1500 candidate transcription factors. However, the DNA binding and regulatory functions have been verified for fewer than 100 of them.

Figure 7.12 Gene for the liver protein transthyretin (prealbumin), with its regulatory sites. The gene is drawn to scale to show its intron-exon structure and the multiple upstream binding sites for regulatory proteins. Note that the introns are far longer than the exons. Binding sites for regulatory proteins are clustered in the promoter and a distal enhancer. With the exception of AP1, which is present in all nucleated cells, the regulatory proteins are present in hepatocytes but not in most other cell types. ■, AP1; ○, C/EBP; ①, ③, and ④, hepatocyte nuclear factors 1, 3, and 4.

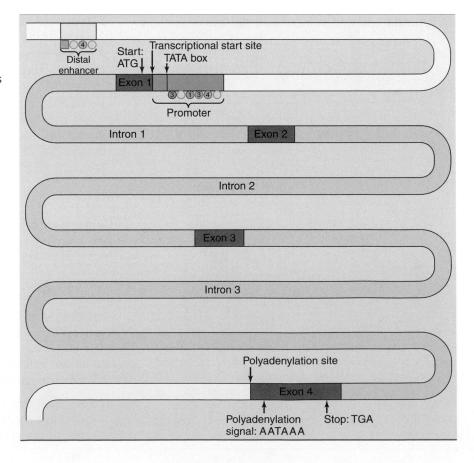

Most transcription factors bind to DNA in a dimeric form, either as homodimers of two identical subunits or as heterodimers of two slightly different subunits. The symmetry of the dimeric transcription factors is matched by their response elements, which tend to possess an incomplete dyad symmetry (see **Fig. 6.37**).

The dimeric transcription factors have a modular structure (**Table 7.7**, and **Figures 7.13** and **7.14**). A *DNA-binding module* recognizes the specific base sequence of the response element; a *dimerization module* forms the active dimeric state; and a *transcriptional activation (or inhibition) region* stimulates or inhibits transcription. Many transcription factors bind a **coactivator** or **corepressor** protein, which in turn interacts with the mediator or with RNA polymerase or recruits chromatin-modifying enzymes.

The **helix-turn-helix proteins, leucine zipper proteins,** and **helix-loop-helix proteins** (see *Table 7.7*) bind to DNA through an α helix, 20 to 40 amino acids long and with a high content of basic amino acid residues. This α helix fits into the major groove of the DNA double helix (see **Fig. 7.13, C**).

The **zinc finger proteins** contain between two and about a dozen zinc ions in their DNA-binding region, each complexed to four amino acid side chains: either four cysteines, or two cysteines and two histidines. The zinc finger is a loop of about 12 amino acid residues between two pairs of zinc-complexed amino acids (see **Fig. 7.14**).

The transcription factors dimerize through an amphipathic α helix that forms a two-stranded coiled coil in the dimeric protein (see **Fig. 7.13**). In the leucine zipper proteins, the hydrophobic edge of this amphipathic helix is formed by several leucine residues that are spaced exactly seven amino acids apart. Because the α helix has 3.6 amino acids per turn, these leucine residues all are on the same side of the helix, where they form hydrophobic interactions with the dimerization partner.

Transcription factors are regulated in several ways:

1. *Their own synthesis is regulated in a tissue-specific manner.* In essence, tissue-specific transcription factors regulate the synthesis of other tissue-specific transcription factors.

2. *Some are regulated by the reversible binding of a hormone.* The most prominent examples are the receptors for steroid hormones.

3. *Many are regulated by phosphorylation and dephosphorylation.* The protein kinases and protein phosphatases acting on the transcription factors are themselves responsive to growth factors, hormones, nutrients, and other external stimuli.

4. *Protein-protein interactions are important.* For example, the activation of transcription can be blocked by the binding of proteins to the transcriptional activator domain.

EUKARYOTIC MESSENGER RNA IS EXTENSIVELY PROCESSED IN THE NUCLEUS

The introns of human genes are transcribed along with the exons but are spliced out of the transcript in the nucleus. In addition, the two ends of the mRNA become modified.

1. *The 5′ end of the mRNA receives a cap.* The cap is a methylguanosine residue that is linked to the first nucleotide of the RNA through an unusual 5′-5′-triphosphate linkage (**Fig. 7.15**). The cap binds a set of proteins that protect the 5′ end of the mRNA from 5′-exonucleases, help guiding the mRNA through the nuclear pore complex into the cytosol, and are needed for the initial interaction between the mRNA and the ribosome.

2. *The 3′ end of the mRNA receives a poly-A tail of about 200 nucleotides.* Multiple copies of a **poly-A binding protein** (**PABP**) bind to the poly-A tail. This retards the action of 3′-exonucleases and allows the mRNA to survive for many hours or even a few days. Only the histone mRNAs have no poly-A tails, and consequently their half-lives are only a few minutes. Histones are synthesized only during S phase of the cell cycle when the DNA is replicated, and their synthesis must be switched off quickly once DNA replication is completed.

Only fully processed, mature mRNA translocates to the cytoplasm, where it is translated.

Table 7.7 Major Types of DNA-Binding Proteins in Eukaryotes

Structural Motif	Structural Features	Examples
Helix-turn-helix proteins	Two α helices separated by a β turn; "recognition helix" fitting in major groove of DNA	"Homeodomain" proteins (proteins regulating embryonic development); most prokaryotic repressors
Zinc finger proteins	Contain zinc bound to Cys and His side chains	Receptors for steroid and thyroid hormones
Leucine zipper proteins	Two α helices, one with basic residues for DNA binding, one with regularly spaced Leu for dimerization	C/EBP (gene activator in liver); c-Myc, c-Fos, c-Jun (growth regulators, proto-oncogene products)
Helix-loop-helix proteins	DNA-binding α helix and two dimerization helices separated by a nonhelical loop	Myo D-1, myogenin (proteins that induce muscle differentiation)

Cys, Cysteine; *DNA,* deoxyribonucleic acid; *His,* histidine.

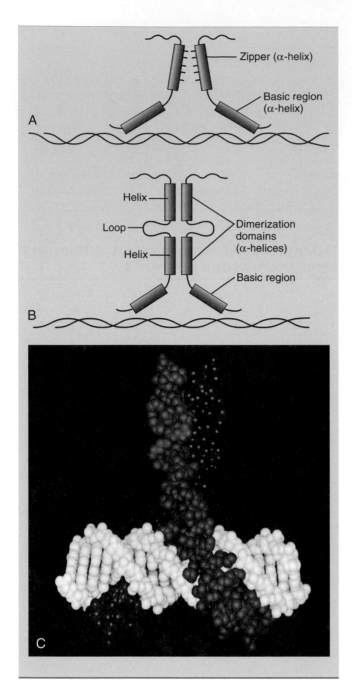

Figure 7.13 Binding of dimeric transcription factors to their response elements. The base sequences of the response elements show a dyad symmetry that matches the symmetry of the transcription factors. **A,** Schematic binding of a leucine zipper protein. The "zipper" is required for dimerization while the basic region binds to DNA. **B,** DNA binding by a helix-loop-helix protein. **C,** Computer graphic model of binding of the carboxyl-terminal portion ("basic region") of the leucine zipper protein C/EBF to its cognate binding site.

mRNA PROCESSING STARTS DURING TRANSCRIPTION

"Posttranscriptional" processing of mRNA actually is cotranscriptional. It occurs during transcription and is guided by proteins that are recruited by the RNA polymerase (*Fig. 7.16*).

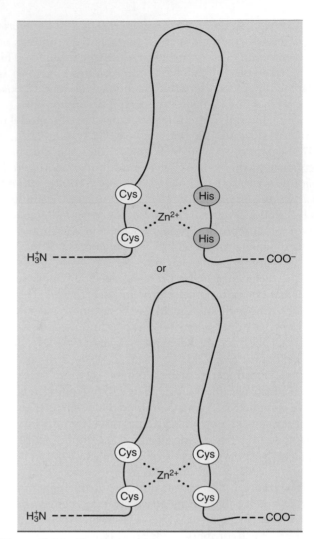

Figure 7.14 Zinc finger. This structural motif occurs in 2 to 12 copies in the DNA-binding region of the zinc finger proteins. The amino acid residues on each side of the zinc are separated by three or four amino acid residues, and the intervening loop contains approximately 12 residues. *Cys,* Cysteine; *His,* histidine.

The RNA is synthesized in the $5' \rightarrow 3'$ direction, and *5' capping is the first modification of the pre-mRNA.* It is done when about 25 nucleotides of the RNA have been polymerized.

Next, *the introns are removed by spliceosomes.* The spliceosome contains five small RNAs (U1, U2, U4, U5, and U6) with lengths between 106 and 185 nucleotides. These associate with proteins to form **small nuclear ribonucleoprotein particles (snRNPs ["snurps"]).** Overall, about 50 proteins are involved in splicing.

The intron-exon junctions of protein-coding nuclear genes are marked by more or less conserved consensus sequences. There is also a conserved "branch site" within the intron, about 30 nucleotides from the 3' end (*Fig. 7.17*). Splicing releases the intron as a cyclic lariat structure, with the 5' end bonded with the 2' hydroxyl group at the branch site.

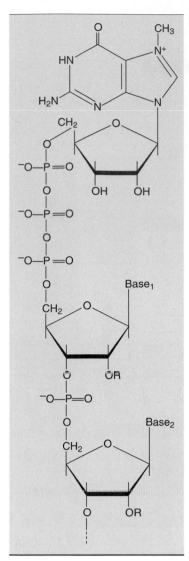

Figure 7.15 Structure of the cap at the 5′ end of eukaryotic messenger RNAs. Transfer and ribosomal RNAs do not have caps. *R,* H or CH_3.

only three initiation factors, eukaryotes have at least 12 initiation factors consisting of more than two dozen polypeptides. Only some of them are shown in *Figure 7.18. Eukaryotic mRNA does not have a ribosome-binding Shine-Dalgarno sequence in the 5′-untranslated region.* The initial binding between mRNA and ribosome is mediated by proteins instead.

Figure 7.18 shows that both ends of the mRNA are coated with proteins. The proteins at the 5′ end interact with the proteins on the poly-A tail, and they serve as translational initiation factors by interacting with proteins on the small (40S) ribosomal subunit.

With the help of these initiation factors, the ribosome scans the 5′-terminal region of the mRNA for the start codon AUG. Usually the first AUG is chosen, but in some mRNAs the second or third AUG is used. Once the initiator codon has been found, *methionine rather than N-formylmethionine is introduced as the first amino acid at the N-terminus of the polypeptide.*

The steps in the elongation cycle are analogous to those in bacterial protein synthesis, and the elongation factors are functionally equivalent (*Table 7.8*). However, *eukaryotes add only two amino acids per second to the growing polypeptide chain compared to 20 per second in bacteria.*

mRNA PROCESSING AND TRANSLATION ARE OFTEN REGULATED

Control of transcriptional initiation is the most efficient way to regulate gene expression because it avoids the energetically costly synthesis of unneeded mRNAs. Nevertheless, eukaryotes also use posttranscriptional controls, as follows.

Regulation of Messenger RNA Stability

Only about 5% of the RNA that is synthesized ever leaves the nucleus. mRNA must associate with proteins to guide it through the nuclear pore complexes. Improperly spliced mRNA that lacks the usual posttranscriptional modifications does not associate with these proteins. It is retained in the nucleus, where it is degraded by nucleases.

In the cytoplasm, the lifespan of mRNA is regulated by nucleases that degrade mRNA and by mRNA-binding proteins that protect mRNA from the nucleases. Thus *mutations that change the 3′ and 5′ untranslated regions of mRNA can disrupt protein synthesis by interfering with the binding of protective proteins.*

Tissue-Specific Initiation and Termination of Transcription

Some genes can be transcribed from alternative promoters, yielding transcripts with different 5′-terminal portions. Other genes have alternative polyadenylation

Finally, a **polyadenylation signal** (consensus AAUAAA) in the last exon recruits an endonuclease that cleaves the RNA about 20 nucleotides downstream. This cut marks the end of the last exon, and a poly-A tail is added enzymatically to the newly created 3′ end. Transcription can proceed for many hundred nucleotides beyond the polyadenylation site, but the cutoff tail of the transcript is discarded.

TRANSLATIONAL INITIATION REQUIRES MANY INITIATION FACTORS

Eukaryotic translation differs from the prokaryotic system (see Chapter 6) in the usual ways: It is more complex, and it is slower.

This is especially obvious in the initiation of translation. Whereas prokaryotic translation initiation requires

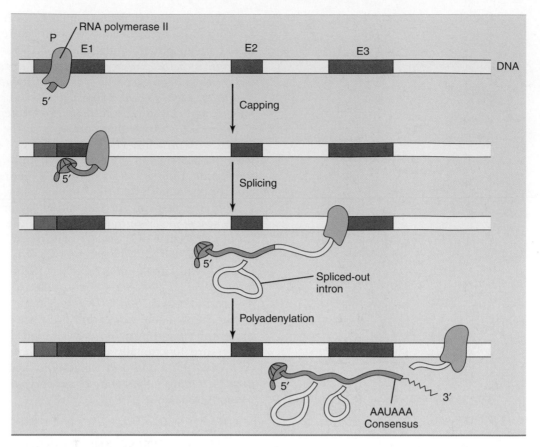

Figure 7.16 "Posttranscriptional" processing of mRNA actually takes place while RNA polymerase II is synthesizing the mRNA. *E1, E2, E3,* Exons; *P,* promoter.

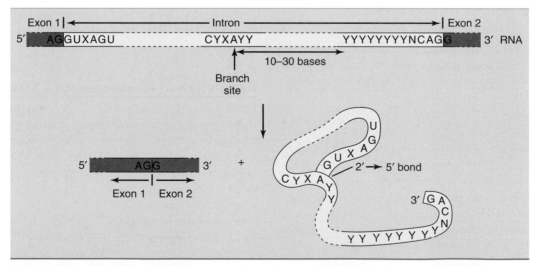

Figure 7.17 Splicing of introns from mRNA precursors. The consensus sequences base pair with RNA components of the spliceosomes. *A,* Adenine; *C,* cytosine; *G,* guanine; *N,* any base; *U,* uracil; *X,* purine; *Y,* pyrimidine.

sites and can produce transcripts with different 3′ ends. An example of the tissue-specific initiation of transcription is the use of alternative promoters in the gene for glucokinase (*Fig. 7.19*), an enzyme that is expressed only in the liver and the insulin-producing β-cells of the pancreas.

Tissue-Specific Splicing

Recognition of splice sites is regulated by tissue-specific proteins. Therefore an exon that is included in the mature mRNA in one cell type can be skipped in another. About 60% of human genes is thought to be subject to alternative splicing. Therefore the 20,000 to

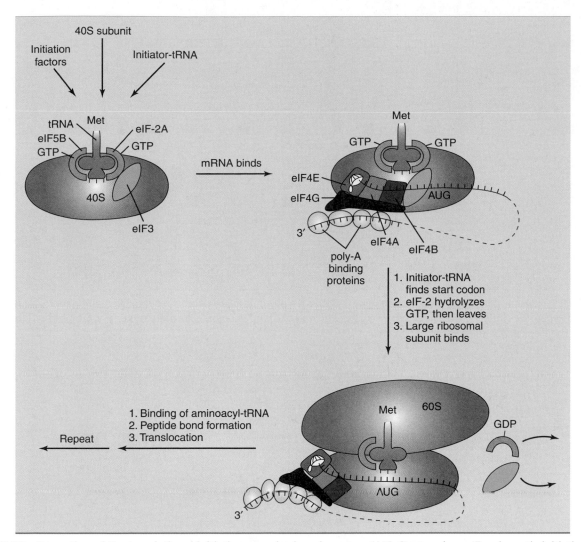

Figure 7.18 Formation of the translational initiation complex in eukaryotes. *AUG*, Start codon; *eIF*, eukaryotic initiation factor; *Met*, methionine.

Table 7.8 Initiation Factors and Elongation Factors of Eukaryotic Protein Synthesis

Eukaryotic Protein	Prokaryotic Equivalent	GTP Hydrolysis	Function
Initiation Factors			
eIF1	IF-3	−	Component of initiation complex eIF1A
	IF-1	−	Component of initiation complex
eIF2	EF-Tu subunit	+	Places initiator tRNA on 40S subunit
eIF-3 (10+ subunits)	—	−	Facilitates binding of initiator tRNA and mRNA
eIF4E	—	−	Cap-binding protein
eIF4A	—	−	RNA helicase
eIF4B	—	−	Facilitates scanning
eIF4G	—	−	Scaffold protein
eIF5	—	−	Activates GTPase activity of eIF2
eIF5B	IF-2	+	Stabilizes initiator tRNA binding to ribosome
Elongation Factors			
EF-1α	EF-Tu	+	Places aminoacyl-tRNA in A site of ribosome
EF-1βγ	EF-Ts	−	Regenerates GTP-bound form of EF-1α
EF-2	EF-G	+	Translocation

eIF, Eukaryotic initiation factor; *GTP*, guanosine triphosphate; *GTPase*, guanosine triphosphatase; *IF*, initiation factor; *mRNA*, messenger RNA; *tRNA*, transfer RNA.

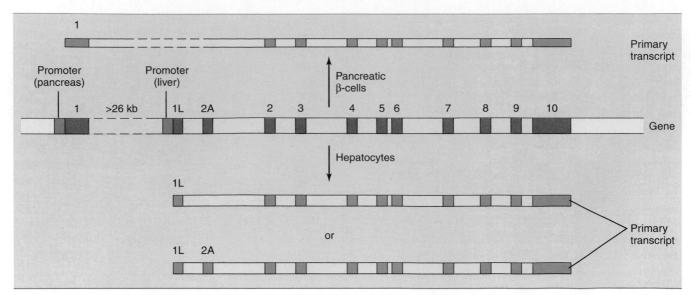

Figure 7.19 Transcription of the glucokinase gene. Alternative promoters are used in hepatocytes and pancreatic β-cells. The resulting polypeptides differ in the N-terminal region, which is encoded by exon 1 in the pancreas and by exon 1L or exons 1L and 2A in the liver. ■, Exon; □, intron.

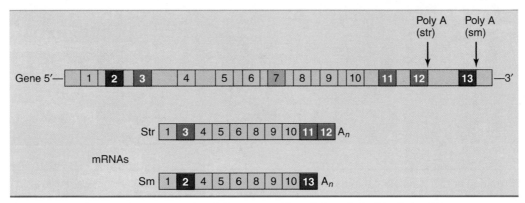

Figure 7.20 The tropomyosin gene is an example of tissue-specific splicing. Only 10 of the 13 exons are used in striated muscle, and nine are used in smooth muscle. Alternative polyadenylation signals are used in striated muscle and smooth muscle: *poly A (str)* and *poly A (sm)*.

30,000 human genes can make an estimated 50,000 different polypeptides. *Figure 7.20* shows an example.

Translational Repressors

Ribosomal protein synthesis can be regulated by mRNA-binding proteins. For example, the mRNA of the poly-A binding protein (PABP) has an oligo-A tract in its 5'-untranslated region. When PABP is abundant, it binds to this oligo-A tract to prevent its own continued synthesis.

Messenger RNA Editing

In mRNA editing, a base in the mRNA is altered enzymatically. If this creates or obliterates a stop codon, the length of the encoded polypeptide is altered. mRNA editing is rare in mammals, but when it occurs, it can produce alternative polypeptides from the same gene in different cell types.

CLINICAL EXAMPLE 7.5: Diphtheria

Diphtheria is a bacterial infection of the upper respiratory tract that leads to necrosis (death) of mucosal cells and airway obstruction. Prior to the introduction of antibiotics, diphtheria was a major cause of death in children. The offending bacterium, *Corynebacterium diphtheriae*, secretes a toxic protein that binds to a surface receptor on the mucosal cells and then is cleaved by a protease. One of the proteolytic fragments then enters the cell. *This active fragment is an enzyme that inactivates the elongation factor EF-2* (*Fig. 7.21*). A single toxin molecule is sufficient to inactivate thousands of EF-2 molecules. Strains of *Corynebacterium* that do not produce the toxin are peaceful members of the normal bacterial flora on skin and mucous membranes.

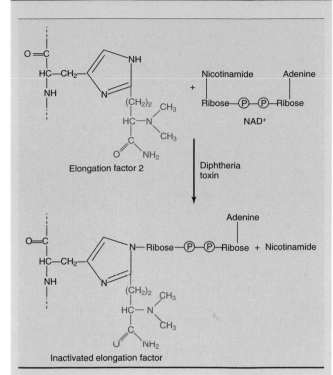

Figure 7.21 Covalent modification of the eukaryotic elongation factor 2 ("translocase") by diphtheria toxin. The amino acid side chain in the elongation factor is diphthamide, a posttranslationally modified histidine. *NAD*$^+$, Nicotinamide adenine dinucleotide.

SMALL RNA MOLECULES INHIBIT GENE EXPRESSION

Translation can be prevented by **RNA interference,** which is triggered by the appearance of a double-stranded RNA in the cell. The double-stranded RNA is processed by cellular RNases into small RNAs having lengths of about 22 nucleotides. The product is called **small interfering RNA (siRNA)** if it is derived from an external source and **micro-RNA (miRNA)** if it is derived from a cellular gene.

The siRNA or miRNA is targeted to a complementary sequence in an mRNA, whose translation it prevents selectively. *RNA interference serves two main functions: protection against RNA viruses and posttranscriptional regulation of gene expression.*

For defense against RNA viruses, the nuclease **dicer** cleaves long, double-stranded viral RNA into small pieces of about 22 nucleotides, which are transferred from dicer to an **RNA-induced silencing complex (RISC).** An RNA helicase in the RISC converts the RNA into single strands. This single-stranded siRNA binds to an **argonaute** protein, which forms the active core of the RISC.

The argonaute-bound siRNA guides the RISC to single-stranded viral mRNA with complementary base sequence. Base pairing of the argonaute-bound siRNA prevents the translation of the viral mRNA. In most cases this is followed by nuclease cleavage of the viral mRNA. One of the four argonaute proteins encoded by the human genome is an active RNase.

This general mechanism has been co-opted for the posttranscriptional regulation of gene expression. Endogenous miRNAs are derived either from noncoding transcripts or from introns of protein-coding genes. The miRNA precursors possess stem-loop structures with base-paired double-helical stems. The stem loops are processed by the RNases drosha and dicer, and the resulting miRNA is loaded on the RISC (*Fig. 7.22*). The argonaute-bound miRNA is complementary to a target sequence in a cellular mRNA, most commonly in its 3′-untranslated region.

Prevention of translation rather than mRNA cleavage is the most common outcome of miRNA binding to its target mRNA. This effect requires the pairing of only six bases in positions 2 to 7 of the miRNA to the mRNA.

Simple eukaryotes have about 100 miRNAs, but humans and other mammals have about 1000. Some miRNAs target only one or a few mRNAs, whereas others regulate hundreds. Between 30% and 80% of all human genes are believed to be regulated by at least one miRNA. Thus *a miRNA can coordinate gene expression by affecting all mRNAs containing a complementary sequence,* in the same way that a transcription factor can coordinate the expression of all genes that have binding sites for the transcription factor in their regulatory sites. The expression of most miRNA precursors is tissue specific or is restricted to distinct developmental stages.

miRNA appears to be capable of transcriptional silencing as well. In this case, a miRNA-loaded RISC recognizes targets on pre-mRNA while it is produced by RNA polymerase II. Upon target recognition the complex recruits histone-modifying enzymes that convert the gene into a heterochromatic state.

CLINICAL EXAMPLE 7.6: miRNAs in Alzheimer Disease

Alzheimer disease is caused by the aberrant processing of amyloid precursor protein (APP) to β-amyloid (see Chapter 2). When miRNA levels in postmortem brains of patients with Alzheimer disease were studied, one micro-RNA (miR-107) was present in reduced amount. Another study found reduced levels of three other miRNAs (miR-29a, miR-29b, and miR-9) in Alzheimer brains. These miRNAs target the mRNA for β-secretase, the enzyme that produces β-amyloid. We cannot be certain whether the reduced levels of these miRNAs are a cause or consequence of the disease, but it is conceivable that reduced levels of the miRNAs lead to enhanced expression of β-secretase and thereby to enhanced formation of β-amyloid.

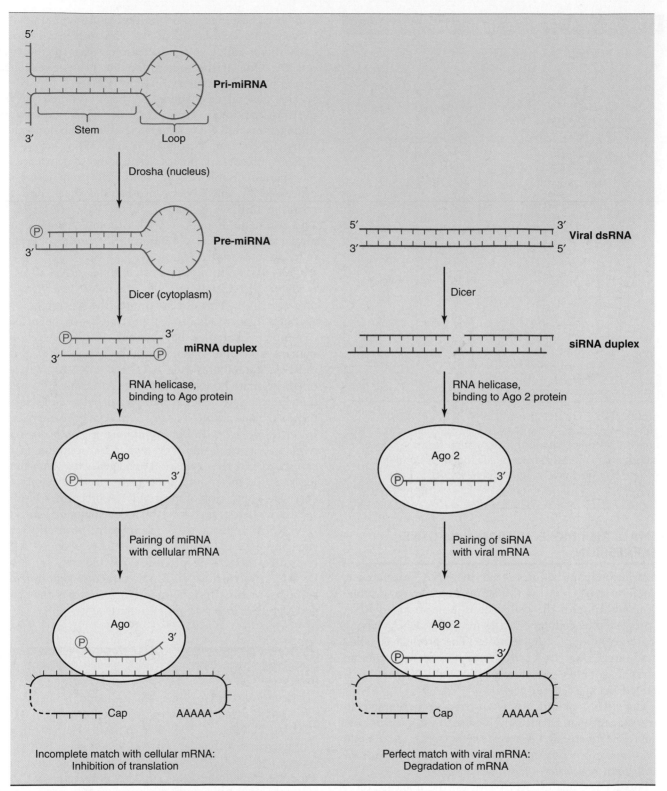

Figure 7.22 Formation of micro-RNA acid (*miRNA*) from a cellular transcript and small interfering RNA (*siRNA*) from double-stranded (*ds*) viral RNA. *Ago*, Argonaute protein.

MITOCHONDRIA HAVE THEIR OWN DNA

Human mitochondria contain 4 to 10 copies of a small circular chromosome with 16,569 base pairs of DNA. The genes for 13 polypeptides, 22 tRNAs, and 2 rRNAs (12S and 16S) are transcribed by a mitochondrial RNA polymerase, and the mRNA is translated by small mitochondrial ribosomes that are more similar to bacterial ribosomes than to human cytoplasmic ribosomes.

Table 7.9 Differences between the Genetic Code of Human Mitochondria and the Standard Code Used by Cytoplasmic Ribosomes

Codon	Standard Code	Mitochondrial Code
AUA	Ile	Met
AGA	Arg	Stop
AGG	Arg	Stop
UGA	Stop	Trp

This protein-synthesizing system exists because *mitochondria are the descendants of symbiotic bacteria.* More than 1.5 billion years ago, their already aerobic ancestors invaded a eukaryotic cell that had not yet learned the use of oxygen for ATP synthesis. What may have started as an attempt at parasitism soon turned into a peaceful coexistence, and in time the bacteria evolved (or degenerated) into the present-day mitochondria.

One after another, most of the original bacterial genes relocated into the nucleus, and for good reason. For a gene, the nucleus is a safer place than the mitochondrion because mitochondrial oxidation pollutes the environment with DNA-damaging superoxide and hydroxyl radicals. This means that *the human nuclear genome is of hybrid origin, being descended in part from a primordial eukaryote and in part from a symbiotic prokaryote.*

The reason for the continued existence of the mitochondrial genome is that once the mitochondrial genome was very small, it evolved small changes in the genetic code (*Table 7.9*). Because today the genetic code is different in the nucleus and the mitochondria, transfer of the remaining mitochondrial genes into the nucleus is no longer possible.

HUMAN GENOMES ARE VERY DIVERSE

When the genomes of two humans are compared, a difference is encountered about once every 1100 base pairs. For comparison, human DNA and chimpanzee DNA have about one difference every 80 base pairs. Most differences between humans are **single-nucleotide polymorphisms (SNPs)**, a replacement of a single base. The human genome contains 11 million SNPs with a minor allele frequency of more than 1%, and seven million of these have a minor allele frequency greater than 5%. The coding sequence of an average protein-coding gene has about four SNPs with a population frequency greater than 1% for the less common allele. Another common type of variation consists of small insertions and deletions of one or a few base pairs, collectively called **indels.**

Table 7.10 lists the density of these variations in different functional categories. Generally, *there is less variation in functional sequences than in presumed junk DNA.* For example, the frequencies of SNPs and

Table 7.10 Genetic Variations in the Genome of an Individual Human (Craig Venter) Compared to the Human Reference Genome

	Variations per 10,000 Base Pairs	
	SNPs	Indels
Total genome	7.8	0.9
Coding sequences	4.5	0.09
Coding sequences of disease genes	3.6	0.04
5'-Untranslated regions	5.5	0.3
3'-Untranslated regions	5.9	0.7
Splice sites	5.0	0.6
Promoter (1 kb upstream of start)	6.8	0.8
Introns	7.0	0.9
Conserved elements in introns	4.8	0.5
Conserved elements between genes	5.9	0.5
Alu sequences	9.0	2.6
L1 sequences	8.3	0.6
Tandem repeats	11.0	15

indel, Insertion or deletion; *SNP,* single-nucleotide polymorphism.

especially of insertions or deletions (indels) are lower in coding sequences of genes than in repetitive elements. The reason is that a new mutation in a coding sequence is likely to be disruptive and consequently is removed by natural selection. Similar mutations in functionless DNA, including the large majority of repetitive elements, can be carried through the generations because they are harmless. Even differences between humans and chimpanzees are greater in junk DNA than in functional sequences.

Indels in a coding sequence tend to be more disruptive than SNPs for protein structure and function and therefore are removed more efficiently. Even among the coding SNPs there is a bias in favor of **synonymous SNPs,** which do not change the amino acid sequence of the protein because they change a codon into a different codon that still codes for the same amino acid. Nearly 50% of the SNPs in coding sequences are synonymous.

Not all genes are equally important. *Only 7% of human genes is known to be associated with one or another genetic disease.* These "disease genes" are even less variable than protein-coding genes in general, presumably because they are more important. We know from studies in knockout mice that many genes can be lost entirely without leading to obvious abnormalities. Also many human genes are believed to be rather "unimportant" in the sense that the effects of mutations in these genes are too mild to be recognized as a genetic disease.

Some sequences outside protein-coding genes are well conserved between species and therefore are believed to be functional. Some are likely to code for functional RNAs, including miRNA precursors, whereas others are distal regulatory elements of protein-coding genes. *Table 7.10* shows that these conserved elements have little diversity within the human species as well.

HUMAN GENOMES HAVE MANY LOW-FREQUENCY COPY NUMBER VARIATIONS

Whereas SNPs and small indels originate as replication errors, most large deletions and duplications arise by crossing over between mispaired chromosomes (see *Fig. 7.6*).

These **copy number variations** have sizes between about 1000 and more than onemillion base pairs. Most individual copy number variants are rare, and only 30% to 40% of those that have been observed so far has a minor allele frequency greater than 1%. Between 5% and 10% of individuals have at least one copy number variant larger than 500,000 base pairs, and 1% to 2% of individuals have a variant of more than one million base pairs.

For any given individual, between 9 and 25 million base pairs of DNA are involved in structural variations. About three times more bases are involved in structural variations than in SNPs and small indels. In all, the structural variations that have been observed so far (often in a single individual or family) include up to 25% of the genome.

Copy number variants can affect a person's phenotype and possibly contribute to disease susceptibilities through **gene dosage effects**. However, if there are no impairments, a copy number variant can persist through the generations. It can even become a normal feature of the genome. Ancient duplications gave rise to gene families, and somewhat more recent ones are annotated as **segmental duplications** (see *Fig. 7.5*). Mutations that produce copy number variations are quite frequent. Even the genomes of identical twins sometimes differ in one or two of them. Most copy number changes seem to be at least slightly unfavorable, so they remain rare and tend to be selected out of the gene pool slowly while possibly contributing to disease on the way. This process is called **mutation-selection balance**.

SUMMARY

Eukaryotes package their DNA into chromatin with the help of small basic proteins called histones. The condensation state of the chromatin, and with it the accessibility of the genes for transcription, is regulated by covalent modifications of both histones and DNA.

Only 1.3% of human nuclear DNA codes for proteins. Human genes are interrupted by noncoding introns, and they are separated from neighboring genes by variable expanses of junk DNA. About 45% of the human genome is formed by the remnants of mobile DNA sequences that are best understood as "molecular parasites." These mobile elements can move into new genomic locations through an RNA intermediate in a process known as retro(trans)position.

Transcription is meticulously regulated by proteins that bind to promoters and other regulatory sites in and around the genes. The mRNA transcripts must be modified by capping, polyadenylation, and removal of introns before the mature mRNA is allowed to leave the nucleus for translation. Translation can be regulated as well, for example, by micro-RNAs that suppress translation by binding to specific mRNAs. A vast amount of variation in the human genome is responsible for individual differences in disease susceptibilities and other phenotypic traits.

Further Reading

Bandiera S, Hatem E, Lyonnet S, et al: microRNAs in diseases: from candidate to modifier genes, *Clin Genet* 77: 306–313, 2010.

Belancio VP, Hedges DJ, Deininger P: Mammalian non-LTR retrotransposons: for better or worse, in sickness and health, *Genome Res* 18:343–358, 2008.

Burgers PMJ: Polymerase dynamics at the eukaryotic DNA replication fork, *J Biol Chem* 284:4041–4045, 2009.

Carthew RW, Sontheimer EJ: Origins and mechanisms of miRNAs and siRNAs, *Cell* 136:642–655, 2009.

De Lange T: How telomeres solve the end-protection problem, *Science* 326:948–952, 2009.

Erson AE, Petty EM: MicroRNAs in development and disease, *Clin Genet* 74:296–306, 2008.

Frazer KA, Murray SS, Schork NJ, et al: Human genetic variation and its contribution to complex traits, *Nat Rev Genet* 10:241–251, 2009.

Friedman RC, Farh KK-H, Burge CB, et al: Most mammalian mRNAs are conserved targets of microRNAs, *Genome Res* 19:92–105, 2009.

Hernández G, Altmann M, Lasko P: Origins and evolution of the mechanisms regulating translation initiation in eukaryotes, *Trends Biochem Sci* 35:63–73, 2010.

Ho L, Crabtree GR: Chromatin remodeling during development, *Nature* 463:474–484, 2010.

International HapMap Consortium: A second generation human haplotype map of over 3.1 million SNPs, *Nature* 449:851–861, 2007.

Ishii N, Ozaki K, Sato H, et al: Identification of a novel noncoding RNA, MIAT, that confers risk of myocardial infarction, *J Hum Genet* 51:1087–1099, 2006.

Itsara A, Cooper GM, Baker C, et al: Population analysis of large copy number variants and hotspots of human genetic disease, *Am J Hum Genet* 84:148–161, 2009.

Kapp LD, Lorsch JR: The molecular mechanics of eukaryotic translation, *Annu Rev Biochem* 73:657–704, 2004.

Kapranov P, Willingham AT, Gingeras TR: Genome-wide transcription and the implications for genomic organization, *Nat Rev Genet* 8:413–423, 2007.

Khalil AM, Guttman M, Huarte M, et al: Many human large intergenic noncoding RNAs associate with chromatin-modifying complexes and affect gene expression, *Proc Natl Acad Sci U S A* 106:11667–11672, 2009.

Kim J-I, Ju YS, Park H, et al: A highly annotated whole-genome sequence of a Korean individual, *Nature* 460:1011–1015, 2009.

Loeb LA, Monnat RJ: DNA polymerases and human disease, *Nat Rev Genet* 9:594–604, 2008.

Müller F, Demény MA, Tora L: New problems in RNA polymerase II transcription initiation: matching the diversity of core promoters with a variety of promoter recognition factors, *J Biol Chem* 282:14685–14689, 2007.

Ng PC, Levy S, Huang J, et al: Genetic variation in an individual human exome, *PLoS Genet* 4:e1000160, 2008.

Pheasant M, Mattick JS: Raising the estimate of functional human sequences, *Genome Res* 17:1245–1253, 2007.

Ponting CP, Oliver PL, Reik W: Evolution and functions of long noncoding RNAs, *Cell* 136:629–641, 2009.

Pratt AJ, MacRae IJ: The RNA-induced silencing complex: a versatile gene-silencing machine, *J Biol Chem* 284: 17897–17901, 2009.

Sahin E, DePinho RA: Linking functional decline of telomeres, mitochondria and stem cells during ageing, *Nature* 464:520–528, 2010.

Sonenberg N, Hinnebusch AG: Regulation of translation initiation in eukaryotes: mechanisms and biological targets, *Cell* 136:731–745, 2009.

Vaquerizas JM, Kummerfeld SK, Teichmann SA, et al: A census of human transcription factors: function, expression and evolution, *Nat Rev Genet* 10:252–263, 2009.

Venters BJ, Pugh BF: How eukaryotic genes are transcribed, *Crit Rev Biochem Mol Biol* 44:117–141, 2009.

Villard L: MECP2 mutations in males, *J Med Genet* 44: 417–423, 2007.

Zoghbi HY: Rett syndrome: what do we know for sure? *Nat Neurosci* 12:239–240, 2009.

QUESTIONS

1. The reason why a fusion of two oocytes in the test tube cannot produce a viable child is

A. X inactivation would not be possible
B. Some imprinted genes would not be expressed
C. Transposons would become activated
D. Female-expressed genes would not be suppressed by male-derived miRNAs
E. Telomeres would shorten excessively, leading to early senility and death in utero

2. Some pharmaceutical companies are trying frantically to find inhibitors of telomerase. A telomerase inhibitor could, in theory, be used in an attempt to

A. Boost the synthesis of muscle proteins
B. Prevent viral infections
C. Cure cancer
D. Cure acquired immunodeficiency syndrome (AIDS)
E. Make people immortal

3. Alu sequences can cause diseases by jumping into new genomic locations. Their mobility depends on the following enzymatic activities:

A. Transposase and RNA polymerase
B. DNA polymerase and RNA replicase
C. Peptidyl transferase and transposase
D. Primase and integrase
E. RNA polymerase and reverse transcriptase

4. The report you have just received from the paternity testing laboratory states that analysis of polymorphic microsatellites was used. What exactly is a polymorphic microsatellite?

A. A sequence in the centromeric DNA
B. A piece of chromatin attached to the short arm of an acrocentric chromosome
C. A tandem repeat of variable length
D. A nonfunctional copy of a gene

E. A small RNA that regulates gene expression by targeting mRNAs

5. Eukaryotic enhancers are

A. Regulatory DNA sequences within the coding sequences of genes that affect the rate of transcriptional elongation
B. Binding sites for general transcription factors in the promoter
C. Proteins that bind to regulatory base sequences in DNA
D. DNA sequences outside the promoter region that contain multiple binding sites for regulatory proteins
E. Proteins that enhance the rate of translational initiation by binding to either the ribosome or the mRNA

6. In the year 2045, the Surgeon General determines that reverse transcriptase is hazardous to your health because it leads to insertional mutations. In order to eliminate reverse transcriptase from the human body, genetic engineers would have to excise all full-length, intact copies of

A. DNA transposons and Alu sequences
B. Retroviral retrotransposons and Alu sequences
C. L1 elements and Alu sequences
D. Pseudogenes and retroviral retrotransposons
E. L1 elements and retroviral retrotransposons

7. Deletion of a gene coding for a miRNA precursor is likely to result in

A. Increased translation of mRNAs
B. Misreading of the genetic code
C. Reduced stability of mRNAs
D. Acetylation of histones and enhanced transcription
E. Repression of retroposition by mobile elements

Chapter 8
PROTEIN TARGETING

Proteins have intricate higher-order structures that form through noncovalent interactions during and immediately after ribosomal protein synthesis. In addition, covalent structural modifications in most proteins must be introduced by specialized enzymes. These reactions are known collectively as **posttranslational processing,** which should not be confused with the post*transcriptional* processing of RNA.

The processed proteins must be sent to their proper destinations in the cell. This requires targeting signals and transport mechanisms. Finally, aged and partially denatured proteins must be destroyed in order to prevent toxic effects and protein aggregation. This chapter traces the fate of eukaryotic proteins from the cradle to the grave.

A SIGNAL SEQUENCE DIRECTS POLYPEPTIDES TO THE ENDOPLASMIC RETICULUM

Some ribosomes are free-floating in the cytoplasm, and others are attached to the membrane of the endoplasmic reticulum (ER). These ribosomes have the same structure but make different proteins. *Free cytoplasmic ribosomes synthesize the proteins of cytoplasm, nucleus, and mitochondria. ER-bound ribosomes synthesize secreted proteins, plasma membrane proteins, and the proteins of ER, Golgi apparatus, and lysosomes.*

Ribosomes attach to the ER membrane only when they synthesize a polypeptide containing a **signal sequence** of about 20 to 25 mainly hydrophobic amino acid residues at the amino end. As soon as it emerges from the ribosome, the signal sequence binds to a cytoplasmic **signal recognition particle (SRP),** which is formed from a small RNA molecule of about 300 nucleotides (the **7SL RNA**) and six protein subunits. *Binding of the SRP halts translation.* Translation is resumed only when the SRP-signal sequence-ribosome complex binds to an **SRP receptor** on the ER membrane (*Fig. 8.1*).

The SRP receptor brings the ribosome in contact with a **protein translocator,** which is a donut-shaped protein in the ER membrane. The tunnel on the large ribosomal subunit from which the growing polypeptide emerges is placed on the central hollow of the protein translocator while the SRP detaches. A pore opens in the translocator, through which the polypeptide passes into the lumen of the rough ER.

The signal sequence is no longer required beyond this stage. It is cleaved off by a **signal peptidase** on the inner surface of the ER membrane.

Soluble secreted proteins are ferried from the ER to the Golgi apparatus in transfer vesicles (*Fig. 8.2*). *The Golgi apparatus is a sorting station in which secreted proteins are packaged into secretory vesicles.* These vesicles are destined to fuse with the plasma membrane and release their contents by **exocytosis.** This system of organelles forms the **secretory pathway,** which is used by all protein-secreting cells in the body (*Table 8.1*).

Proteins of the plasma membrane are initially inserted in the ER membrane and then travel through the secretory pathway until they are deposited in the plasma membrane during exocytosis. Proteins of the ER membrane and the Golgi membrane are retained in their respective organelles.

GLYCOPROTEINS ARE PROCESSED IN THE SECRETORY PATHWAY

This road to the periphery is also an assembly line on which the proteins are modified covalently (*Table 8.2*). Disulfide bonds are formed with the help of a **protein disulfide isomerase** enzyme in the ER. However, the most important robots in this assembly line are **glycosyl transferases,** which build oligosaccharides on the side chains of serine, threonine, and asparagine in the protein. The precursors for these reactions are nucleotide-activated monosaccharides (*Figs. 8.3* and *8.4A,* and *Table 8.3*), whose synthesis is described in Chapter 22. *Most proteins that are processed through the secretory pathway are glycoproteins* (see *Fig. 8.3*).

O-linked oligosaccharides are bound to the oxygen in the side chains of serine and threonine. They are synthesized in the Golgi apparatus by the stepwise addition of monosaccharides.

N-linked oligosaccharides are bound to the nitrogen in the side chain of asparagine. N-*linked glycosylation*

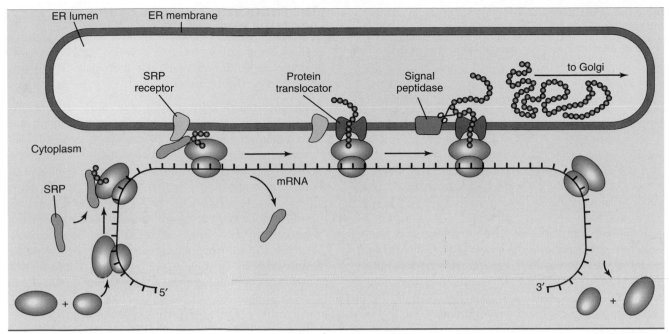

Figure 8.1 Synthesis of a secreted protein by ribosomes on the rough endoplasmic reticulum (*ER*). The ribosome forms a tight seal on the translocator during translocation, to prevent other molecules from diffusing in and out of the ER while the polypeptide is threaded through the pore. *mRNA*, Messenger RNA; *SRP*, signal recognition particle.

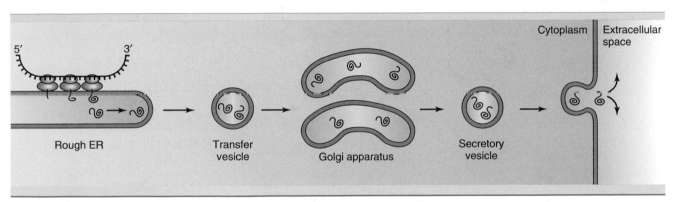

Figure 8.2 Secretory pathway. The proteins are transported to the cell periphery through the endoplasmic reticulum (*ER*), transfer vesicles, Golgi apparatus, and secretory vesicles. Release from the cell is by exocytosis (fusion of the secretory vesicle membrane with the plasma membrane).

Table 8.1 Use of the Secretory Pathway by Different Cell Types

Cell	Secreted Products	Reference Chapter
Pancreatic acinar cells	Zymogens (enzyme precursors)	19
Pancreatic β-cells	Insulin, C-peptide, amylin	16
Fibroblasts	Collagen, elastin, glycoproteins, proteoglycans	14
Goblet cells	Glycoproteins ("mucins"), proteoglycans	14
Intestinal mucosal cells	Chylomicrons	23
Hepatocytes	Serum albumin, other plasma proteins, very-low-density lipoprotein	15

starts with the construction of a mannose-rich oligosaccharide on **dolichol phosphate,** a lipid in the ER membrane. The whole oligosaccharide is then transferred to an asparagine side chain of a newly synthesized polypeptide (*Fig. 8.5*).

In the ER and Golgi apparatus, exoglycosidases remove the glucose residues and one or more of the mannose residues from the protein-bound oligosaccharide. The remaining core structure is again extended by glycosyl transferases in the Golgi apparatus.

Table 8.2 Posttranslational Processing in the Secretory Pathway

Type of Processing	Examples
Removal of signal sequence	All proteins of secretory pathway
Disulfide bond formation	Most proteins of secretory pathway
Glycosylation	Collagen, other glycoproteins, proteoglycans
Amino acid modifications	Collagen, elastin
Partial proteolytic cleavage	Insulin, other peptide and protein hormones

The oligosaccharides of glycoproteins range in size from two sugar residues in the simplest *O*-linked oligosaccharides to more than 15 in some of the more complex *N*-linked oligosaccharides. Most are branched, and in many cases the terminal positions are occupied by the acidic amino sugar **N-acetylneuraminic acid** (**NANA**) (see ***Fig. 8.3***).

The carbohydrate content of glycoproteins varies from less than 10% to greater than 50%. The oligosaccharides of glycoproteins affect their biological functions, including maintenance of their higher-order structure, water solubility, antigenicity, and regulation of the protein's metabolic fate.

THE ENDOCYTIC PATHWAY BRINGS PROTEINS INTO THE CELL

Besides being able to secrete proteins, cells can ingest proteins and other extracellular materials. Three processes can be distinguished.

1. **Phagocytosis** ("cell eating") (***Fig. 8.6***) is the uptake of solid particles into the cell. The particle first binds to components of the cell surface. The cytoplasm then flows around the particle by a mechanism that involves the polymerization and depolymerization of actin microfilaments, forming a phagocytic vacuole. The usual fate of the phagocytic vacuole is fusion with lysosomes and digestion of the engulfed particle by lysosomal enzymes. Unicellular eukaryotes (e.g., amoeba) use phagocytosis for their own nutrition. In the human body, however, the process is limited to macrophages, neutrophils, and dendritic cells. These professional phagocytes protect the body by eating aberrant cells and microbial invaders.
2. **Pinocytosis** ("cell drinking") is the nonselective uptake of fluid droplets into the cell. Pinocytic vesicles contain dissolved substances according to their concentrations in the extracellular medium. Secretory cells use pinocytosis to retrieve the membrane material that is added to the plasma membrane during exocytosis.

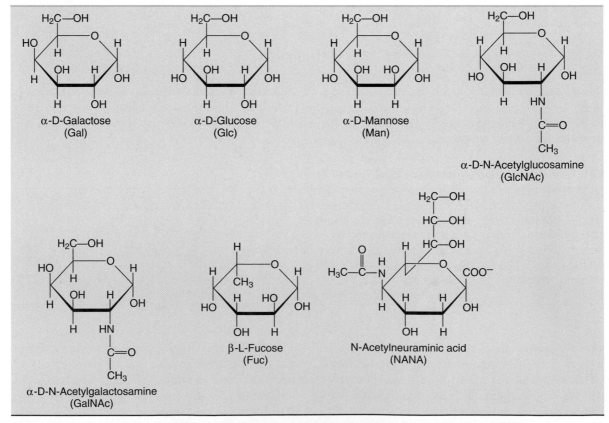

Figure 8.3 Structures of some monosaccharides in glycoproteins.

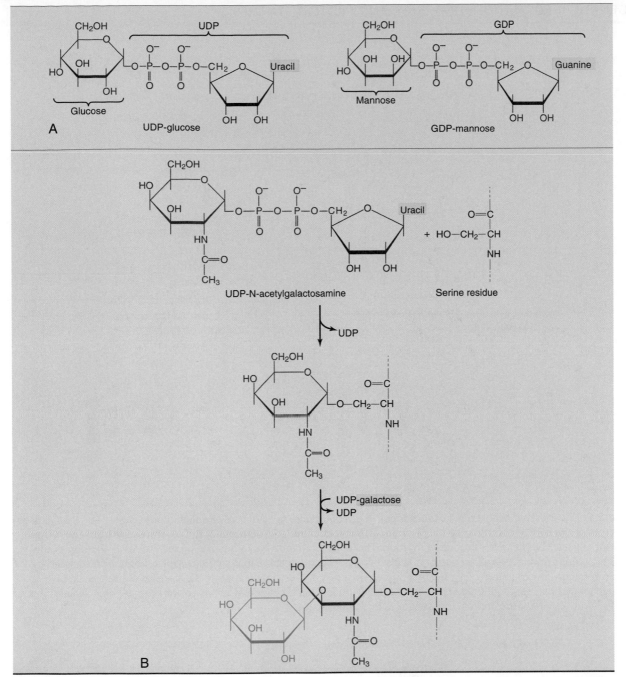

Figure 8.4 Synthesis of *O*-linked oligosaccharides in glycoproteins. **A,** Examples of activated monosaccharides used in the synthesis of oligosaccharides. The nucleotide is generally bound to the anomeric carbon (C-1 in the aldohexoses and their derivatives). **B,** Two steps in the synthesis of an *O*-linked oligosaccharide in a glycoprotein. Each reaction requires a specific glycosyltransferase in the Golgi apparatus. *GDP*, Guanosine diphosphate; *UDP*, uridine diphosphate.

Table 8.3 Monosaccharides Commonly Found in Glycoproteins

Monosaccharide	Type	Activated Form	Comments
Galactose (Gal)	Aldohexose	UDP-Gal	Common
Glucose (Glc)	Aldohexose	UDP-Glc	Rare in mature glycoproteins
Mannose (Man)	Aldohexose	GDP-Man	Very common in *N*-linked oligosaccharides
Fucose (Fuc)	6-Deoxyhexose	GDP-Fuc	Both in *O*- and *N*-linked oligosaccharides
N-Acetylglucosamine (GlcNAc)	Amino sugar	UDP-GlcNAc	Linked to asparagine in *N*-linked oligosaccharides
N-Acetylgalactosamine (GalNAc)	Amino sugar	UDP-GalNAc	Common
N-Acetylneuraminic acid (NANA)	A sialic acid (acidic sugar derivative)	CMP-NANA	In terminal positions of many *O*- and *N*-linked oligosaccharides

GDP, Guanosine diphosphate; *UDP,* uridine diphosphate; *CMP,* cytidine monophosphate.

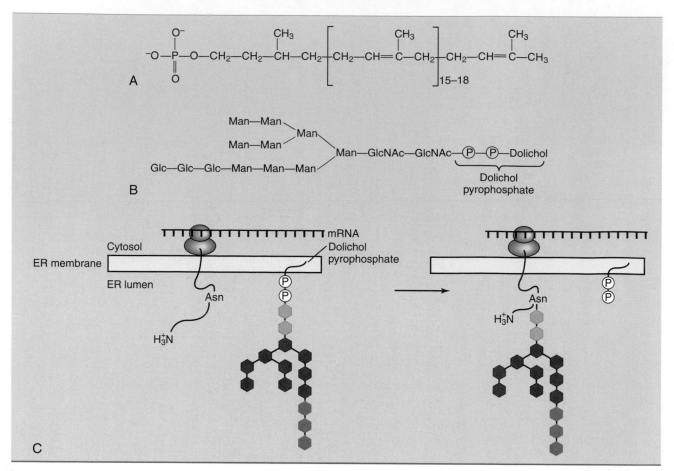

Figure 8.5 Synthesis of *N*-linked oligosaccharides in glycoproteins. **A,** Structure of dolichol phosphate. This lipid is used as a carrier of the core oligosaccharide in the endoplasmic reticulum (*ER*) membrane. **B,** Structure of the dolichol-bound precursor oligosaccharide in *N*-linked glycosylation. This oligosaccharide is synthesized by the stepwise addition of the monosaccharides from activated precursors. The second phosphate residue in dolichol pyrophosphate is introduced by UDP-α-D-*N*-acetylglucosamine (UDP-GlcNAc) during synthesis of the oligosaccharide. **C,** Transfer of the precursor oligosaccharide to an asparagine side chain of the polypeptide. This transfer reaction is cotranslational. *Asn,* Asparagine; *Glc,* α-D-Glucose; *Man,* α-D-mannose; *mRNA,* messenger RNA; *P,* phosphate.

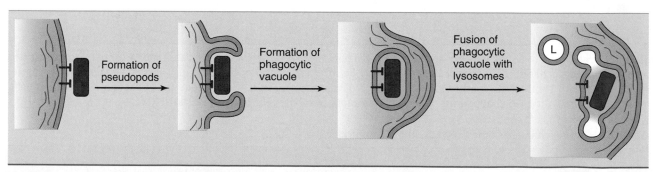

Figure 8.6 Phagocytosis is triggered by the binding of a solid particle to a protein in the plasma membrane that functions as a receptor (⊢). Pseudopods are formed that flow around the particle. This requires the reversible depolymerization and repolymerization of actin microfilaments (⌒) under the plasma membrane. The phagocytic vacuole fuses with lysosomes (*L*), and the particle is digested by lysosomal enzymes.

3. **Receptor-mediated endocytosis** (*Fig. 8.7*) is a mechanism for the selective uptake of soluble proteins and other high-molecular-weight materials. *Unlike pinocytosis, it requires a cell surface receptor to which the endocytosed product binds selectively.* Binding is followed by the clustering of receptor-ligand complexes on the cell surface and the formation of an endocytic vesicle.

Pinocytic and endocytic vesicles tend to fuse with each other and with intracellular vesicles to form larger

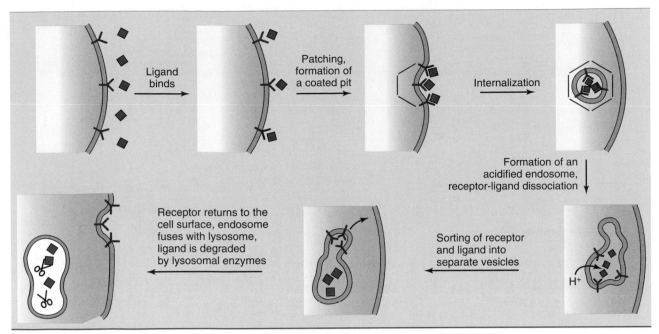

Figure 8.7 Receptor-mediated endocytosis is triggered by the binding of a ligand to a receptor in the plasma membrane. Fusion of the endocytic vesicle with intracellular vesicles creates an acidified endosome.

structures called **endosomes,** which become acidified to a pH of 5 to 6. Materials can be transferred from the endosome to the Golgi apparatus. More commonly, however, the endosome fuses with a lysosome to form a **secondary lysosome** in which the endocytosed material is digested by lysosomal enzymes. In most but not all cases, the receptor is recycled to the cell surface.

The most important uses of receptor-mediated endocytosis are as follows:

1. *Uptake of nutritive substances.* The uptake of low-density lipoprotein (see Chapter 25) and the iron-transferrin complex (see Chapter 29) are the most prominent examples.
2. *Waste disposal.* The uptake of "worn-out" plasma proteins and hemoglobin-haptoglobin complexes by hepatocytes or macrophages (see Chapter 15) is an example. The endocytosed products are digested by lysosomal enzymes.
3. *Mucosal transfer.* Single-layered epithelia can endocytose a protein on one side and exocytose it on the opposite side. This process is called transcytosis. The secretion of immunoglobulin A (IgA) across mucosal surfaces is an example (see Chapter 15).

Receptor-mediated endocytosis is initiated when the cytoplasmic protein **adaptin** is recruited to the plasma membrane by the ligand-bound receptor. The structural protein clathrin then binds to the adaptin, pulling the membrane into a **coated pit.** Within seconds, this structure is pinched off as a **coated vesicle** that is surrounded by a cagelike structure formed from clathrin (*Fig. 8.8*).

Other coat proteins and many different adaptor proteins are used for other types of vesicular transfer. They regulate the complex trafficking of vesicles and their contents in the intersecting secretory and endocytic pathways.

CLINICAL EXAMPLE 8.1: I-Cell Disease

I-cell disease is a rare, recessively inherited disease in which one of the enzymes for the attachment of mannose-6-phosphate to prospective lysosomal enzymes is deficient. As a result, *lysosomal enzymes are not sorted into the lysosomes but are secreted.* High levels of lysosomal enzymes circulate in the blood, and undegraded lipids and polysaccharides accumulate in the cells.

The accumulation of these products leads to mental deterioration, skeletal deformities, and death between 5 and 8 years of age. The disease is named after the inclusions of polysaccharides and glycolipids that are seen in the cells of these patients. Protein accumulation is not an important feature because proteins can be degraded by the proteasome as well as the lysosome.

LYSOSOMES ARE ORGANELLES OF INTRACELLULAR DIGESTION

Lysosomes are bags that are filled with hydrolytic enzymes, including glycosidases, proteases, phosphatases, and sulfatases. Their job description is the *breakdown of cellular macromolecules, especially of macromolecules that are taken up into the cell by phagocytosis, pinocytosis, and receptor-mediated endocytosis.* The lysosomal enzymes are synthesized at the rough ER and become glycosylated in the ER and Golgi apparatus. In the Golgi

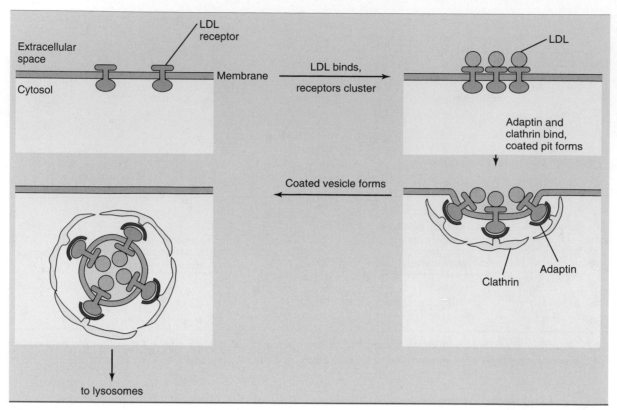

Figure 8.8 Receptor-mediated endocytosis of low-density lipoprotein (*LDL*). LDL is the most important source of cholesterol for most cells.

apparatus they finally acquire a **mannose-6-phosphate** residue on some of their N-linked oligosaccharides:

Mannose-6-phosphate is a molecular tag that acts like a postal address to route the enzymes to the lysosomes.

Inherited defects of lysosomal enzymes or lysosomal biogenesis result in **lysosomal storage diseases.** In most of these diseases, a single lysosomal enzyme is deficient. The substrate of the missing enzyme accumulates in the cell to a point where it impairs normal cellular function. In some diseases multiple lysosomal enzymes are affected (see *Clinical Example 8.1*).

CLINICAL EXAMPLE 8.2: Crohn Disease

Crohn disease is an inflammatory bowel disease that preferentially affects the terminal ileum. It is fairly common, with an incidence of about 5 per 100,000 person-years and prevalence between 100 and 150 per 100,000 in many populations. It is a seriously debilitating chronic condition that is treated with immune suppression or surgery. Crohn disease has long been attributed to an aberrant immune response to components of the normal bacterial flora in the intestine.

Variations in at least a dozen genes have been associated with risk of Crohn disease. One of the most consistent associations is with a single-nucleotide polymorphism (SNP) in the *ATG16L1* (autophagy-related 16-like 1) gene, one of more than 30 genes involved in autophagy. An A in the ancestral low-risk allele is replaced by a G in the high-risk allele, replacing the amino acid threonine with alanine.

Ordinarily, intestinal bacteria that have entered the cytoplasm of an intestinal mucosal cell are cleared by macroautophagy. A hypothesized consequence of the single amino acid substitution in the ATG16L1 protein is impaired sequestration of at least some kinds of bacteria in autophagosomes, which allows these bacteria to survive long enough to trigger an inflammatory response.

CELLULAR PROTEINS AND ORGANELLES ARE RECYCLED BY AUTOPHAGY

Lysosomes digest not only materials from outside the cell. They also dispose of worn-out cellular proteins and defective organelles in a process known as **autophagy** (literally, "self-eating").

The most important type is **macroautophagy.** It begins with the formation of a double membrane that encloses an organelle or a patch of the cytosol. The resulting structure, known as an **autophagosome,** fuses with a lysosome, and the contents are digested by lysosomal enzymes.

Macroautophagy is used for the disposal of organelles and protein aggregates that are too large to be handled by other mechanisms. It recycles peroxisomes and parts of the ER but is especially important for the removal of mitochondria. For example, the average lifespan of a liver mitochondrion is only 10 days. Macroautophagy is thought to contribute to quality control by removing defective organelles in preference to functional ones, but how the functional status of an organelle is assessed by the system is not known.

Another function of macroautophagy is the disposal of large protein aggregates. Finally, it is a mechanism for the elimination of bacteria and viruses that have invaded the cell (see *Clinical Example 8.2*).

POORLY FOLDED PROTEINS ARE EITHER REPAIRED OR DESTROYED

Formation of a protein's higher-order structure is no mean feat. Protein maturation can go awry, leading to misfolded proteins that are toxic to the cell or form obnoxious aggregates. According to one estimate, about one third of native proteins fail to fold properly and are degraded before they ever achieve a functional state.

Protein folding is assisted by helper proteins called **chaperones,** which bind to exposed hydrophobic patches on partly folded proteins. Repeated binding and dissociation of the chaperone, which is fueled by ATP hydrolysis, prevents aggregation and abnormal folding and gives the protein time to fold into its proper conformation.

Chaperones are abundant proteins in the cell, and their synthesis is further stimulated when the cell is exposed to elevated temperature. Therefore these chaperones are also called **heat shock proteins.** HSP70 (heat shock protein-70) is a type of chaperone that is concerned mainly with the education of young proteins that have just been synthesized or are still in the process of ribosomal synthesis. The **HSP60** chaperones are a different type that specializes in the reconditioning of aging proteins.

If the efforts of the chaperones are to no avail, the misfolded protein is marked for destruction by **ubiquitin,** a small protein with 76 amino acids that, as its name implies, is ubiquitous in all eukaryotic cells (*Fig. 8.9*). First, a **ubiquitin-conjugating enzyme (E1)** activates ubiquitin and transfers it to the E2 component of a **ubiquitin ligase (E2-E3 complex).**

The E3 component of the ubiquitin ligase recognizes the target protein and transfers the ubiquitin from E2 to the target protein. This process is repeated until a chain of four or more ubiquitins is attached to the target protein, which makes it eligible for degradation by the proteasome.

Humans have about 30 different E2 subunits and hundreds of E3 subunits. *Each ubiquitin ligase targets a different kind of structurally aberrant protein.* Some recognize the presence of oxidized amino acids in the protein, others recognize abnormal hydrophobic patches on the surface of partially denatured proteins, and still others recognize sequence motifs that are normally buried in the center of the protein but become exposed in misfolded proteins.

Some ubiquitin ligases recognize intact proteins that are naturally short lived in the cell, and some even respond to regulatory signals. This means that *the cell can regulate the lifespans of distinct classes of proteins.*

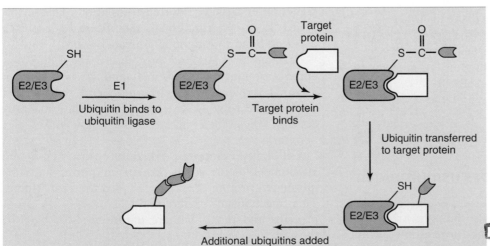

Figure 8.9 Ubiquitination of proteins. The multiubiquitin chain attached by ubiquitin ligase (E2/E3 complex) directs the target protein to the proteasome.

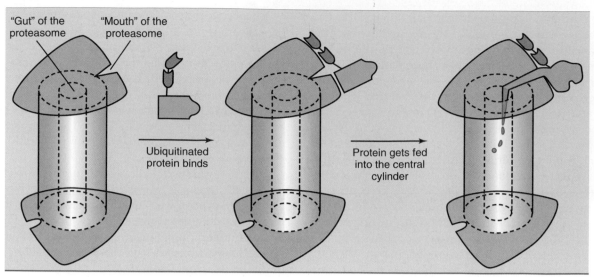

"Gut" of the proteasome "Mouth" of the proteasome

Ubiquitinated protein binds

Protein gets fed into the central cylinder

Figure 8.10 Proteasome. The cover on the hollow cylinder recognizes ubiquitinated proteins, denatures them, and feeds them into the central cavity, where they are degraded by proteases.

CLINICAL EXAMPLE 8.3: Proteasome Inhibitors as Anticancer Drugs

Drugs that inhibit the proteasome are highly toxic, but, like many other poisons, they can be useful in some situations. One such drug is **Bortezomib:**

Bortezomib

This boron-containing tripeptide analog inhibits the proteasome by binding with high affinity to its proteolytic sites. It was found to be effective in the treatment of multiple myeloma, an incurable malignancy of antibody-secreting plasma cells. The reason for its somewhat selective toxicity to cancer cells is not fully known. Its effectiveness is attributed to the accumulation of misfolded immunoglobulin chains in the cancer cells and to the accumulation of proteins that promote programmed cell death (apoptosis).

THE PROTEASOME DEGRADES UBIQUITINATED PROTEINS

Whereas the ubiquitin ligases are the judges that condemn a protein to death, the **proteasome** is the executioner. The proteasome is a hollow cylinder whose inner surface is lined with proteases, covered with a large cap on both sides (*Fig. 8.10*). The cap captures ubiquitinated proteins, denatures them with the help of ATP hydrolysis, and feeds them into the hollow cylinder for degradation.

Proteasomes are abundant in both the cytoplasm and the nucleus, and they constitute about 1% of the total cellular protein. The ER contains no proteasomes. However, misfolded and damaged proteins can be retrotranslocated from the ER lumen to the cytoplasm, where they are degraded by the ubiquitin-proteasome system.

SUMMARY

Peptide bond formation by the ribosome is only the first step in protein synthesis. The newly synthesized proteins have to fold themselves into their proper higher-order structure during translation. This is followed by posttranslational modifications such as disulfide bond formation and glycosylation.

Secreted proteins and proteins of the ER, Golgi apparatus, plasma membrane, and lysosomes have a signal sequence at their amino end that directs them to the rough ER. Their posttranslational processing takes place mainly in the ER and Golgi apparatus.

Cellular proteins are marked for destruction by the attachment of the small protein ubiquitin. The ubiquitinated proteins are then fed into the proteasome. This mechanism preferentially removes abnormal proteins and those that are naturally short lived in the cell.

Further Reading

Budarf ML, Labbe C, David G, et al: GWA studies: rewriting the story of IBD, *Trends Genet* 25:137–146, 2009.

Chang Y-Y, Juhasz G, Goraksha-Hicks P, et al: Nutrient-dependent regulation of autophagy through the target of rapamycin pathway, *Biochem Soc Trans* 37:232–236, 2009.

Collard F: The therapeutic potential of deubiquitinating enzyme inhibitors, *Biochem Soc Trans* 38:137–143, 2010.

Doherty GJ, McMahon HT: Mechanisms of endocytosis, *Annu Rev Biochem* 78:857–902, 2009.

Hatakeyama S, Nakayama KI: Ubiquitylation as a quality control system for intracellular proteins, *J Biochem* 134:1–8, 2003.

Mizushima N, Klionsky DJ: Protein turnover via autophagy: implications for metabolism, *Annu Rev Nutr* 27:19–40, 2007.

Navon A, Ciechanover A: The 26 S proteasome: from basic mechanisms to drug targeting, *J Biol Chem* 284:33713–33718, 2009.

Rapoport TA: Protein translocation across the eukaryotic endoplasmic reticulum and bacterial plasma membranes, *Nature* 450:663–669, 2007.

Rappoport JZ: Focusing on clathrin-mediated endocytosis, *Biochem J* 412:415–423, 2008.

Stipanuk MH: Macroautophagy and its role in nutrient homeostasis, *Nutr Rev* 67:677–689, 2009.

Turk B, Turk V: Lysosomes as "suicide bags" in cell death: myth or reality? *J Biol Chem* 284:21783–21787, 2009.

Van Wijk SJL, Timmers HTM: The family of ubiquitin-conjugating enzymes (E2s): deciding between life and death of proteins, *FASEB J* 24:981–993, 2010.

Wandinger SK, Richter K, Buchner J: The Hsp90 chaperone machinery, *J Biol Chem* 283:18473–18477, 2008.

QUESTIONS

1. A signal sequence has to be expected in the precursors of all the following proteins except

A. Ribosomal proteins

B. The sodium-potassium ATPase in the plasma membrane

C. Collagen in the extracellular matrix of connective tissues

D. Signal peptidase

E. Acid maltase, a lysosomal hydrolase

2. The deficiency of a ubiquitin ligase can potentially result in

A. Abnormal accumulation of ubiquitin in the cell

B. Failure to direct lysosomal proteins to the lysosomes

C. Excessive breakdown of some classes of proteins

D. Buildup of abnormal proteins in the cells

E. Increased mutation rate

Chapter 9

INTRODUCTION TO GENETIC DISEASES

In theory, one half of the genes in diploid somatic cells *should* be identical to genes in the father, the other half *should* be identical to genes in the mother, and the genes *should* be identical in all cells of the body. In reality, they are not—not quite. Maintaining a bloated genome of three billion base pairs is such a formidable task that replication errors and other molecular accidents are unavoidable. These errors are called **mutations,** and they are a major cause of disease and disability.

Somatic mutations can produce cells with reduced viability or impaired function. *They accumulate with age and contribute to normal aging.* The most dangerous somatic mutations are those that cause the cell to grow out of control. *Mutations of this type are the principal cause of cancer,* which is responsible for 20% of all deaths in the modern world. This implies that *all mutagenic agents are carcinogenic.*

Germline mutations arise in the gametes or their diploid ancestors in the gonads. They are transmitted to the offspring and can cause genetic diseases.

This chapter introduces the various types of mutation, their importance for disease, and the DNA repair systems that the body uses to protect itself against mutations. The chapter also presents the hemoglobinopathies as examples of genetic diseases with well-understood pathogenesis.

MUTATIONS ARE AN IMPORTANT CAUSE OF POOR HEALTH

According to one estimate, at least one new mutation can be expected to occur in each round of cell division, both in somatic cells and in the germ line. As a result, *the average child is born with an estimated 100 to 200 new mutations that were not present in the parents.* Most of them are single-base changes in nonfunctional DNA that cause no disease.

However, *an estimated one or two new mutations are "mildly detrimental."* This means they are not bad enough to cause a disease on their own, but they can impair physiological functions to some extent, and they can contribute to multifactorial diseases. Finally, *about 1 in 50 infants is born with a diagnosable genetic condition that can be attributed to a single major mutation.*

Children are, on average, a little sicker than their parents because they have new mutations on top of those inherited from the parents (see *Clinical Example 9.1*). This **mutational load** is kept in check by a form of natural selection called **purifying selection.** In most traditional societies, almost half of all children died before they had a chance to reproduce. We can only guess that those who died had, on average, more "mildly detrimental" mutations than those who survived. Therefore *the prevalence of disease-promoting mutations, and of the diseases themselves, is determined in large part by mutation-selection balance.*

FOUR TYPES OF GENETIC DISEASE

Four types of genetic disease are commonly distinguished.

1. **Aneuploidy** is an aberration in chromosome number, caused by faulty segregation of chromosomes during mitosis or meiosis. About 1 in 400 infants is born aneuploid. In **trisomy 21 (Down syndrome),** for example (*Fig. 9.1*), one of the smallest autosomes (non-sex chromosomes) is present in three rather than the usual two copies. Presumably the signs of Down syndrome are caused by overproduction of the proteins encoded by the 225 genes on chromosome 21. Most cases of aneuploidy originate in female meiosis I, and the risk rises with advanced maternal age.

2. **Chromosomal rearrangements** are caused by chromosome breakage or by recombination between mispaired chromosomes during meiosis. For example, in large **deletions,** part of a chromosome is lost. In **translocations,** part of a chromosome has been transferred to another chromosome. *Only chromosomal rearrangements that change the copy number of genes or that break up an important gene are likely to cause disease.* About 1 in 1000 infants is born with a symptomatic chromosomal rearrangement.

3. **Single-gene disorders,** also known as **mendelian disorders** because of their predictable inheritance patterns, are caused by mutations in a single gene. **Dominant diseases** are expressed in heterozygotes, who carry a single copy of the mutation. **Recessive diseases** are expressed only in homozygotes, who have the

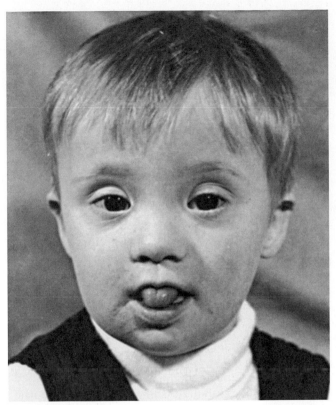

Figure 9.1 Physical appearance of a patient with Down syndrome. This disorder is characterized by moderately severe mental deficiency combined with physical stigmata.

mutation in both copies of the gene. Severe dominant diseases are often caused by a new mutation, whereas recessive mutations can be passed through many generations of unaffected carriers before they cause disease in a homozygote. *Figure 9.2* shows the types of protein that have been found mutated in genetic diseases.

4. **Multifactorial disorders,** also called **polygenic diseases** or **complex diseases,** are caused not by a single major mutation but by interacting genetic and environmental risk factors. *Most of the common diseases, from allergies to diabetes and coronary heart disease, are multifactorial.* Even susceptibility to infectious diseases is influenced by the patient's genetic constitution.

CLINICAL EXAMPLE 9.1: Paternal Age and Schizophrenia

About 1% of all people are diagnosed with schizophrenia at one or another time in their lives. This "multifactorial" disease manifests with delusions, hallucinations, and other thought disorders. The prevalence of schizophrenia is similar in all human populations, and its heritability is 60% to 80%. How can "schizophrenia genes" (actually, genetic variants that increase schizophrenia risk) be maintained at such high frequencies that they turn 1% of the population insane in each generation?

In most places, schizophrenics have fewer children than the average in the population. Unaffected relatives of schizophrenics, who are expected to carry some of the predisposing genes without expressing the disease, have no more children than everyone else. Therefore the offending genes should be eliminated by natural selection, but they are not.

The reason is shown by the observation that *the fathers of schizophrenics are, on average, a few years older than the fathers of unaffected people.* Maternal age has no independent effect. We know that new mutations leading to dominant diseases are more common in the children of older fathers because replication errors accumulate in the paternal germ line with advancing age. The spermatogonia of a 15-year-old boy have gone through an estimated 35 mitoses, but those of a 50-year-old man have gone through 800.

Molecular genetic studies are beginning to show that genetic liability to schizophrenia is caused by individually rare mutations in a fairly large number of genes. The effects of new mutations add to those of inherited mutations, raising the disease risk for the children of old fathers. The lesson for women is this: Take a young man rather than an old man as the father of your children!

SMALL MUTATIONS LEAD TO ABNORMAL PROTEINS

Base substitutions in the coding sequences of genes are responsible for about 60% of disease-causing mutations, and small insertions and deletions cause another 20% to 25%. Less than 1% of single-gene disorders are caused by a mutation in a regulatory site.

A **point mutation** is a change in a single base pair of the DNA. It is called **transition** if a purine is replaced by another purine or a pyrimidine by another pyrimidine, and it is called **transversion** if a purine is replaced by a pyrimidine or a pyrimidine by a purine.

In the coding sequence of a gene, the most common consequence of a point mutation is a single amino acid substitution in the polypeptide. For example:

-ACA-TTA-CGC- → -ACA-TCA-CGC-

-Thr-Leu-Arg- → -Thr-Ser-Arg-

This is called a **missense mutation.** Some missense mutations leave the biological functions of the protein intact, but others destroy them partially or completely. **Synonymous mutations,** also called **silent mutations,** are point mutations that do not change an amino acid because they create a new codon that still codes for the same amino acid. For example:

-ACA-TTA-CGC- → -ACA-CTA-CGC-

-Thr-Leu-Arg- → -Thr-Leu-Arg-

Figure 9.2 Functions of proteins that have been identified as targets of single-gene disorders in humans. In many cases, the functions are not known completely. Thus many proteins in the "ligand binding and protein-protein interactions" category in all likelihood are signal transducers, and many "DNA or RNA binding" proteins probably are transcriptional regulators.

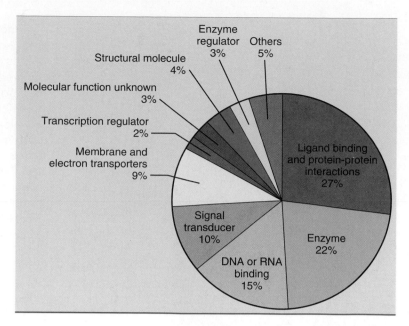

A **nonsense mutation** generates a premature stop codon. *It causes the premature termination of translation,* usually with the complete loss of function in the truncated protein. For example:

-ACA-TTA-CGC- → -ACA-TAA-CGC-

-Thr-Leu-Arg- → -Thr-Stop . . .

A **frameshift mutation** is caused by a small insertion or deletion. Although the amino terminal portion of the encoded protein is normal, the amino acid sequence is garbled beyond the site of the mutation because the messenger RNA (mRNA) is translated in the wrong reading frame. The protein product is most likely nonfunctional. For example:

-CTC-ATC-GGA-CTT- → -CTC-TCG-GAC-TT-

-Leu-Ile-Gly-Leu- → -Leu-Ser-Asp- . . .

However, the insertion or deletion of three base pairs, or any multiple of three, does not result in a frameshift.

Splice-site mutations change an intron-exon junction or the branch site within the intron. They cause the synthesis of an abnormally spliced protein.

Promoter mutations, as well as mutations in other regulatory sites, leave the structure of the polypeptide intact but change its rate of synthesis.

THE BASAL MUTATION RATE IS CAUSED MAINLY BY REPLICATION ERRORS

The **basal mutation rate,** which is observed in the absence of environmental mutagens, is caused mainly by errors during DNA replication. These replication errors have an important consequence. Because the number of mitotic divisions before formation of the gametes is far greater for spermatogonia than oogonia,

most base substitutions and small insertions and deletions originate in the paternal rather than the maternal germ line (see **Clinical Example 9.1**).

Spontaneous **tautomeric shifts** in the bases contribute to replication errors. For example, thymine normally is present in the keto form and pairs with adenine. Very rarely, however, it shifts spontaneously to the enol form, which pairs with guanine. If a thymine in the template strand happens to be in the rare enol form at the moment of DNA replication, G instead of A is incorporated in the new strand.

Similarly, adenine has a rare imino form that pairs with cytosine rather than thymine (**Fig. 9.3**). Fortunately, these bases spend very little time in their less stable forms; thus, mutations caused by tautomeric shifts are rare.

Mutations are also caused by short-lived, highly reactive free radicals that are formed during oxidative reactions in the cell, including superoxide and hydroxyl radicals. *Free radicals cause strand breaks and oxidation of bases in DNA.* They appear to be most important for mutagenesis in mitochondrial DNA.

MUTATIONS CAN BE INDUCED BY RADIATION AND CHEMICALS

Radiation is an avoidable cause of mutations. **Ionizing radiation,** including **x-rays** and **radioactive radiation,** is sufficiently energy rich to displace electrons from their orbitals. It damages DNA both directly, and indirectly through the formation of highly reactive hydroxyl radicals from water molecules. **DNA double-strand breaks** are the most important type of damage caused by ionizing radiation. *Ionizing radiation penetrates the whole body and therefore can cause both somatic and germline mutations.*

Ultraviolet radiation is a mutagenic component of sunlight. It cannot penetrate beyond the outer layers of the skin and therefore is unable to cause germline mutations. It only causes sunburn and skin cancer, mainly through the formation of **pyrimidine dimers** (*Fig. 9.4*).

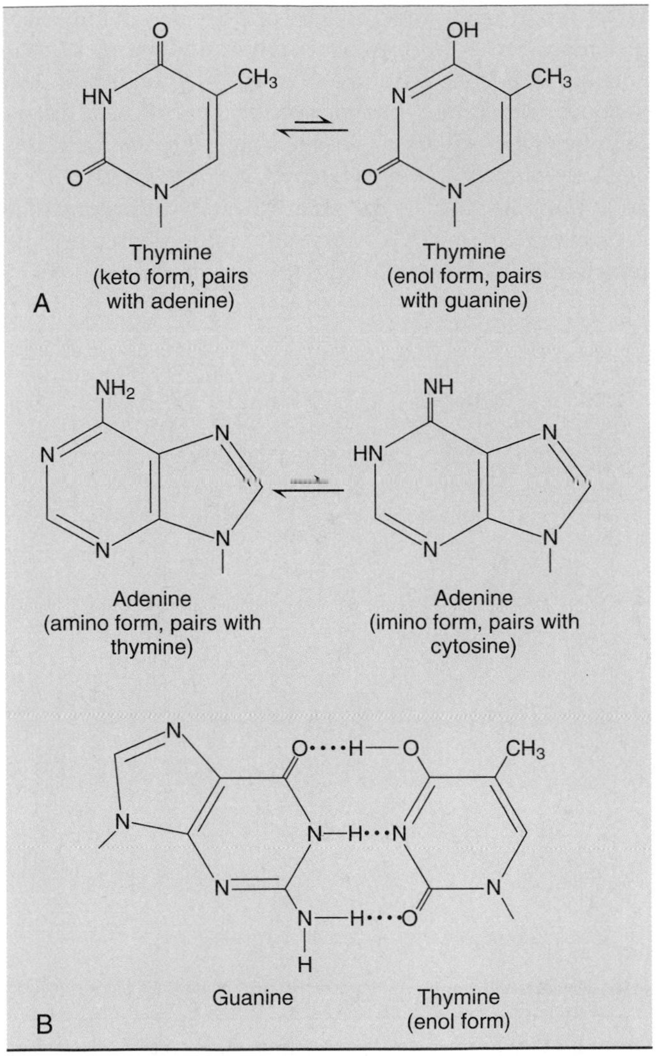

Many chemicals can act as mutagens.

1. **Base analogs** can cause mutations after their incorporation into DNA. **Bromouracil** is a structural analog of thymine:

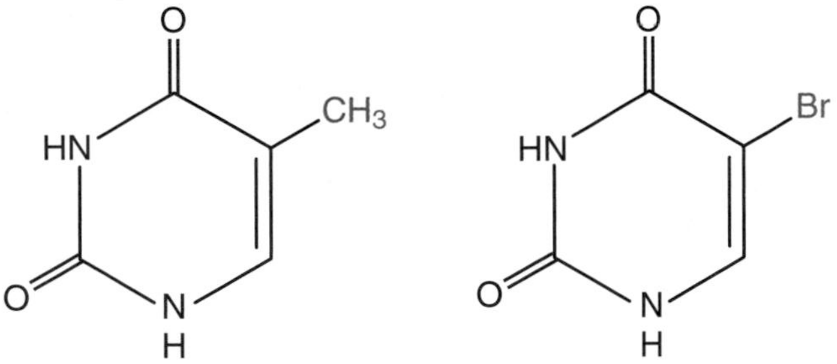

Thymine   5-Bromouracil

The enzymes of nucleotide synthesis and DNA synthesis treat bromouracil as thymine and incorporate it into the DNA, where it pairs with adenine. It is mutagenic because the enol form is more stable in bromouracil than in thymine, causing mutations through spontaneous tautomeric shifts.

2. **Alkylating agents** attach alkyl groups to nitrogen or oxygen atoms in the bases. Examples:

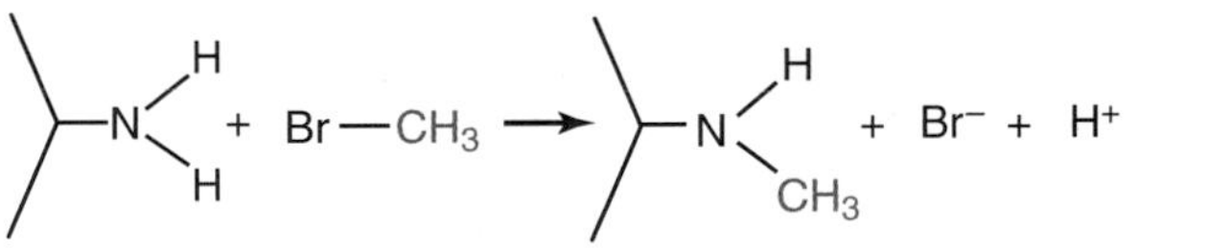

Methyl bromide

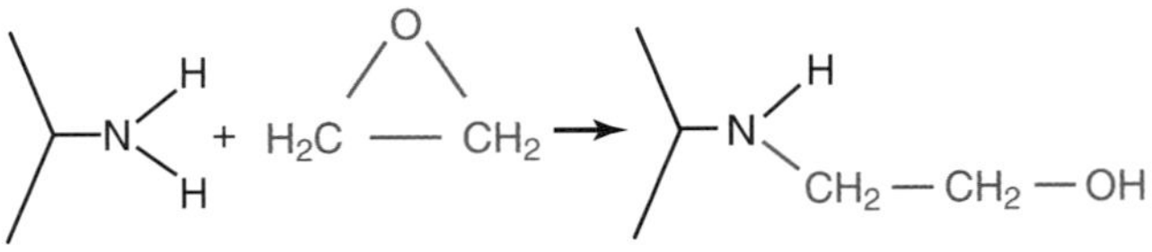

Ethylene oxide

Methyl bromide was used as a grain fumigant before it was banned for this use because of its carcinogenic properties. Ethylene oxide is used for the sterilization of surgical instruments. Nonenzymatic methylation

Figure 9.3 Spontaneous tautomeric shifts of DNA bases as a cause of point mutations. **A,** Alternative structures of thymine and adenine. **B,** Base pair between guanine and the enol form of thymine.

Thymine (keto form, pairs with adenine) / Thymine (enol form, pairs with guanine)

Adenine (amino form, pairs with thymine) / Adenine (imino form, pairs with cytosine)

Guanine / Thymine (enol form)

Figure 9.4 Formation of a thymine dimer by ultraviolet radiation. Note that the two thymine residues are in the same strand of the double helix.

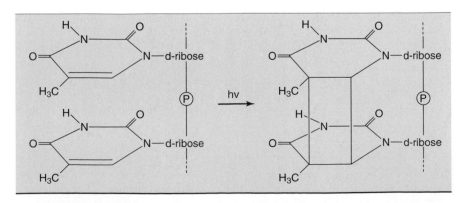

by *S*-adenosyl methionine (SAM, see Chapter 5) is an important endogenous source of methylated bases. About 4000 7-methylguanosine, 600 3-methyladenine, and 10 to 30 O^6-methylguanosine residues are formed by SAM in each cell per day.

3. **Deaminating agents** turn the bases adenine, guanine, and cytosine into hypoxanthine, xanthine, and uracil, respectively. These bases make aberrant base pairing and lead to errors during DNA replication (*Fig. 9.5*).

4. **Intercalating agents** are planar fused-ring structures that insert themselves between the stacked DNA bases, causing frameshift mutations during DNA replication (*Fig. 9.6*).

Mutagens are most mutagenic during the S phase of the cell cycle because mutagenesis during S phase leaves no time for repair of damaged DNA. This is the rationale

for radiation treatment of cancer. Cancer cells divide more frequently than normal cells and therefore more likely are in S phase when the radiation is applied.

MISMATCH REPAIR CORRECTS REPLICATION ERRORS

DNA repair is required as part of life's perennial struggle against the second law of thermodynamics (that entropy tends to rise over time). To maintain the genome, the repair enzymes have to proceed like a plumber who repairs a damaged pipe: *Locate the damage, remove the damaged part, and replace it with a good part.* Because of the great diversity of lesions that are generated in DNA every day, multiple repair systems with overlapping specificities are required.

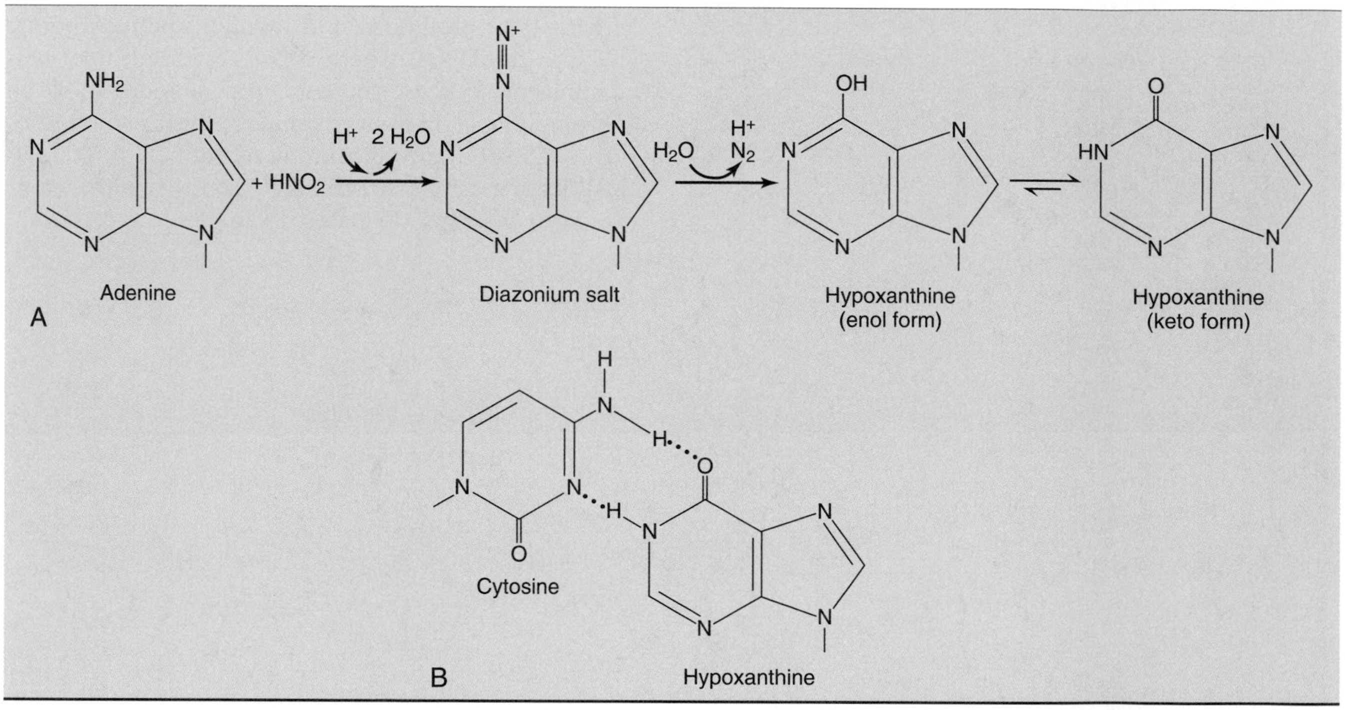

Figure 9.5 Action of a deaminating agent. HNO_2 can be formed from dietary nitrates in the intestine. **A,** Reaction of nitrous acid with adenine. **B,** Hypoxanthine pairs with cytosine instead of thymine.

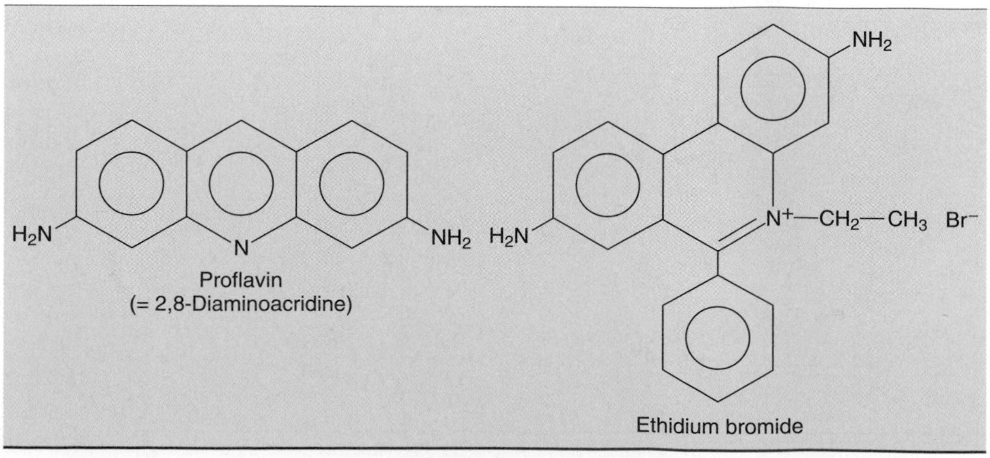

Figure 9.6 Structures of intercalating agents. These planar ring systems cause frameshift mutations by inserting themselves between the DNA bases.

Base mismatches that arise as replication errors pose a special problem for repair because the repair enzymes must distinguish between the intact old strand and the mutated new strand. Therefore **postreplication mismatch repair** requires at least two components: one to recognize the mismatch and the other to distinguish between the strands.

The new strand is distinguished from the old by the presence of frequent nicks. In the lagging strand, the nicks are present from the beginning until the Okazaki fragments are sealed by DNA ligase. However, even the leading strand is known to have occasional nicks.

The bound repair proteins recruit exonucleases to the nick, which then remove the DNA of the new strand between the nick and the mismatch, including the mismatch itself. This sets the stage for DNA polymerase δ and DNA ligase to fill the gap and connect the loose ends (***Fig. 9.7***). This system is most important for rapidly dividing cells (***Clinical Example 9.2***).

CLINICAL EXAMPLE 9.2: Colon Cancer

Like other cancers, colon cancer is caused by somatic mutations. However, some persons inherit a cancer-promoting mutation from a carrier parent or as a new mutation.

Hereditary nonpolyposis colon cancer (HNPCC, or Lynch syndrome) accounts for about 2% of all colon cancers. *These patients have inherited a heterozygous mutation in one of the four genes that are essential for mismatch repair.* Their cells still can repair mismatches because they have an intact backup copy of the gene.

However, when a cell loses this backup copy through a somatic mutation, it becomes a mutator that accumulates abundant mutations in each round of DNA replication. The effects are most dramatic for rapidly dividing cells, such as those in the colonic mucosa.

Most mutator cells slowly mutate to their death, but occasionally one of them mutates into a cancer cell.

Persons with this inherited cancer susceptibility have a greater than 50% risk of developing colon cancer by age 70 years. They also are at increased risk for other tumors. About 20% of spontaneous noninherited cancers, both of the colon and of other organs, are defective in mismatch repair as a result of either two successive somatic mutations or epigenetic silencing by promoter methylation.

MISSING BASES AND ABNORMAL BASES NEED TO BE REPLACED

The *N*-glycosidic bond between a purine base and 2-deoxyribose is the weakest covalent bond in the DNA. From 5000 to 10,000 purine bases hydrolyze spontaneously from DNA in each human cell every day.

The absence of a base is recognized by an **AP** (apurinic) **endonuclease** that cleaves the phosphodiester bond on the 5′ side of the abasic nucleotide. The 3′ phosphodiester bond is cleaved by DNA polymerase β, which also fills the resulting gap. Repair is completed by DNA ligase (***Fig. 9.8***).

Base excision repair removes abnormal bases. In this system, *a DNA glycosylase recognizes the abnormal base and cleaves its bond with 2-deoxyribose.* There are specialized DNA glycosylases for various deaminated, alkylated, and oxidized bases.

For example, 100 to 500 cytosines in the DNA are deaminated to uracil in each cell per day. Being recognized as an abnormal base, uracil is removed by a specialized uracil-DNA glycosylase. This reaction creates a baseless site that is recognized by AP endonuclease, and the remaining steps are identical to the repair of apurinic sites (see ***Fig. 9.8***).

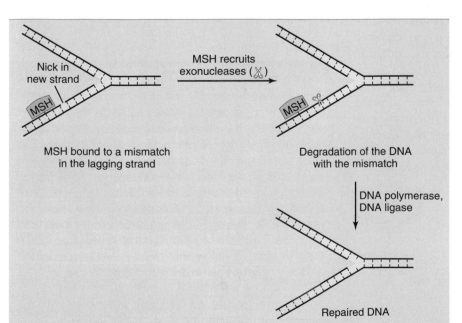

Figure 9.7 Postreplication mismatch repair. The damage is recognized by the MSH protein (MutS homolog, named after the corresponding protein in *Escherichia coli*). MSH binds to the mismatch and recruits exonucleases to degrade the portion of the new strand carrying the mismatch.

Nick in new strand

MSH recruits exonucleases (✂)

MSH

MSH bound to a mismatch in the lagging strand

Degradation of the DNA with the mismatch

DNA polymerase, DNA ligase

Repaired DNA

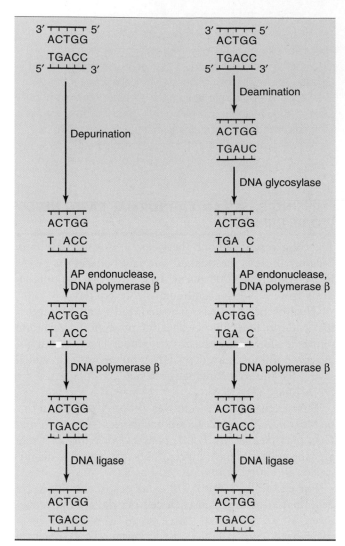

Figure 9.8 Repair of apurinic (*AP*) sites and of deaminated cytosine (uracil).

Cytosine deamination is a reason for having thymine rather than uracil in DNA. If DNA contained uracil, the deamination of cytosine could not be repaired because uracil would not be recognized and removed as an abnormal base. As a consequence, the mutation rate would be unpleasantly high.

The mutation rate is indeed unpleasantly high for 5-methylcytosine, which is important for gene silencing (see Chapter 7). The deamination of 5-methylcytosine produces thymine, which is a normal DNA base and therefore is less easily removed by base excision repair. Therefore *methylated CG sequences are mutational hot spots.*

5-Methylcytosine   Deamination →   Thymine

NUCLEOTIDE EXCISION REPAIR REMOVES BULKY LESIONS

Nucleotide excision repair can handle any lesion that is bulky enough to distort the geometry of the DNA double helix: pyrimidine dimers, adducts formed by covalent binding of large molecules to DNA, and some alkylated bases.

The components of the nucleotide excision repair system form a "repair crew" that scans the DNA, recognizes the lesion, and removes a piece of 25 to 30 nucleotides from the damaged strand. The resulting gap is filled by DNA polymerase δ or ε, followed by DNA ligase (*Fig. 9.9*).

One subsystem of nucleotide excision repair is specialized for the repair of transcribed genes. It is recruited when RNA polymerase encounters a lesion that makes transcription difficult. The importance of nucleotide excision repair is illustrated in *Clinical Examples 9.3* and *9.4.*

CLINICAL EXAMPLE 9.3: Xeroderma Pigmentosum

Patients with xeroderma pigmentosum (XP) present in infancy or early childhood with severe sunburn, numerous freckles, and ulcerative lesions on sun-exposed skin (*Fig. 9.10*). The lesions tend to progress to skin cancer, often before school age. Strict avoidance of sunlight is the mainstay of treatment, and malignant tumors must be removed as soon as they form. Some patients develop neurological degeneration as they grow older.

These patients have recessively inherited defects in genome-wide nucleotide excision repair, which make them unable to repair sunlight-induced DNA damage. There are about seven genetically distinct types, each caused by the deficiency of a different repair protein.

CLINICAL EXAMPLE 9.4: Cockayne Syndrome

Cockayne syndrome (CS) is a rare, recessively inherited disease. It is a progeroid syndrome that presents with growth retardation, neurological degeneration, and a wizened appearance. Patients die at about the age of 12 years with signs of early senility. Patients have only mild cutaneous photosensitivity and no cancer. CS is caused by defects in either one of two proteins that are required specifically for transcription-coupled nucleotide excision repair (NER). Some xeroderma pigmentosum mutations affect transcription-coupled NER and cause neurological degeneration similar to that of CS.

This pattern of abnormalities suggests that transcription-coupled NER is most important in terminally differentiated cells such as neurons, which can afford to concentrate their repair efforts on expressed genes. However, the CS proteins participate in basal transcription and some forms of base excision repair, as well as transcription-coupled NER. Therefore it is not known which function of these proteins is responsible for the clinical phenotype.

REPAIR OF DNA DOUBLE-STRAND BREAKS IS DIFFICULT

DNA single-strand breaks are common but can be repaired easily with the undamaged DNA strand serving as a template. DNA double-strand breaks are rare but are far more dangerous because they

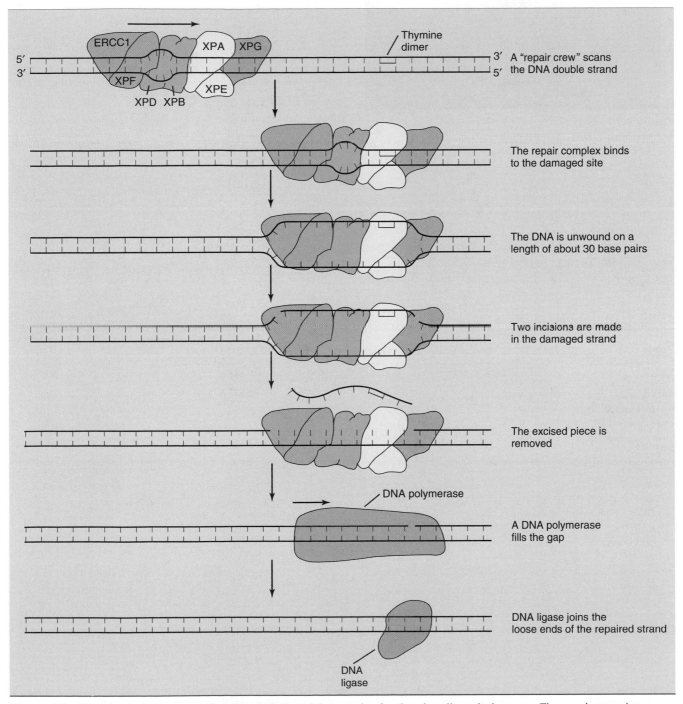

Figure 9.9 Hypothetical sequence of events during excision repair of a thymine dimer in humans. The repair complex may contain more than a dozen different polypeptides. Some of them (*XPB, XPD*) have helicase activity; others recognize the damage (*XPA, XPE*) or act as endonucleases (*XPG, ERCC1/XPF*). The "XP" in the names of many of the repair proteins stands for "xeroderma pigmentosum," a disease that is caused by defects of excision repair proteins. Each XP protein is related to a different subtype ("complementation group") of this disease.

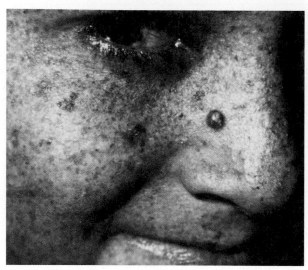

Figure 9.10 Cutaneous and ocular findings of xeroderma pigmentosum. Note the numerous hyperpigmented lesions on the skin and the conjunctivitis.

can lead to chromosome breakage and chromosomal rearrangements.

Nonhomologous end joining is the main repair pathway for double-strand breaks in quiescent cells. Proteins that act as "break sensors" bind to the broken ends of the DNA and recruit protein kinases, which activate repair enzymes and signal to the cell cycle machinery (**Table 9.1** and **Clinical Example 9.5**). Repair requires processing of the broken ends. *This is an error-prone type of "repair" that usually leads to the loss or addition of a few base pairs.*

Recombinational repair heals double-strand breaks without introducing a mutation but requires the presence of the homologous chromosome. *Therefore it is used mainly in late S phase and G2, when the DNA already has been replicated.* Recombinational repair uses the same mechanism as homologous recombination ("crossing-over") in prophase of meiosis I (**Fig. 9.11**). Indeed, *meiotic crossing-over is initiated by an enzymatically inflicted double-strand break in one of the chromosomes*

CLINICAL EXAMPLE 9.5: Ataxia-Telangiectasia

Patients with ataxia-telangiectasia, a recessively inherited disorder, suffer from immune dysfunction, sterility, cancer predisposition, extreme sensitivity to x-rays, and progressive cerebellar ataxia. Most are wheelchair-bound by the age of 14 years. The cause is a deficiency of the **ATM** (ataxia-telangiectasia mutated) **kinase**, which is recruited to sites of DNA

Table 9.1 Inherited Diseases Caused by a Defect in DNA Repair

Disease	Clinical Manifestation	Type of Protein Affected	Affected Function
Xeroderma pigmentosum	Cutaneous photosensitivity	Proteins of nucleotide excision repair	Genome-wide nucleotide excision repair
Cockayne syndrome	Poor growth, neurological degeneration, early senility	Proteins of nucleotide excision repair	Transcription-coupled nucleotide excision repair
Hereditary nonpolyposis colon cancer	Cancer susceptibility	Proteins of mismatch repair	Postreplication mismatch repair
Ataxia-telangiectasia	Motor incoordination, immune deficiency, chromosome breaks, lymphomas	Protein kinase activated by DNA double-strand breaks	Cell cycle arrest after DNA breakage
Seckel syndrome	Bird-headed dwarfism, microcephaly	Protein kinase activated by DNA damage	DNA repair signaling
Nijmegen breakage syndrome	Growth retardation, immunodeficiency, cancers	Activator of nuclear protein kinases	Signaling for double-strand break repair
Bloom syndrome	Poor growth, butterfly rash, immunodeficiency, cancer susceptibility, chromosome breaks	13 different proteins/genes	Recombinational repair?
Werner syndrome	Premature aging, short telomeres	DNA helicase and exonuclease	Unknown
Fanconi anemia	Anemia, leukemia, skeletal deformities, chromosome breakage	8 different proteins/genes	Repair of DNA cross-links?
Breast cancer susceptibility	Breast and ovarian cancer	BRCA1, BRCA2, interact with multiple repair proteins	Recombinational repair
Spinocerebellar ataxia	Motor incoordination	Several proteins/genes	Repair of DNA single-strand breaks

double-strand breaks where it becomes activated. ATM and two other protein kinases, **ATR** (ATM-related) **kinase** and **DNA-activated protein kinase**, phosphorylate more than 700 proteins in response to DNA double-strand breaks. The targets include signaling proteins that regulate cell cycle arrest and apoptosis. People carrying an ATM mutation in the heterozygous state do not have AT, but they do have a mildly increased risk of breast cancer.

HEMOGLOBIN GENES FORM TWO GENE CLUSTERS

Mutations that lead to abnormal hemoglobins illustrate the molecular mechanisms of genetic disease. These diseases, known as **hemoglobinopathies,** are the most common inherited diseases worldwide.

Figure 9.12 shows that hemoglobin genes are found in two clusters: α-like genes on chromosome 16 and β-like genes on chromosome 11. *Humans have two identical α-chain genes, both of which contribute about equally to the production of α-chains.* There are also two very similar γ-chain genes, $^A\gamma$ and $^G\gamma$, whose products differ only by the presence of either alanine or glycine in one of the amino acid positions.

Figure 9.13 shows the expression of hemoglobin genes during early development. The newborn has about 75% fetal hemoglobin (HbF) ($\alpha_2\gamma_2$) and 25% adult hemoglobin (HbA) ($\alpha_2\beta_2$). However, HbF becomes almost completely replaced by HbA within the first 4 months after birth.

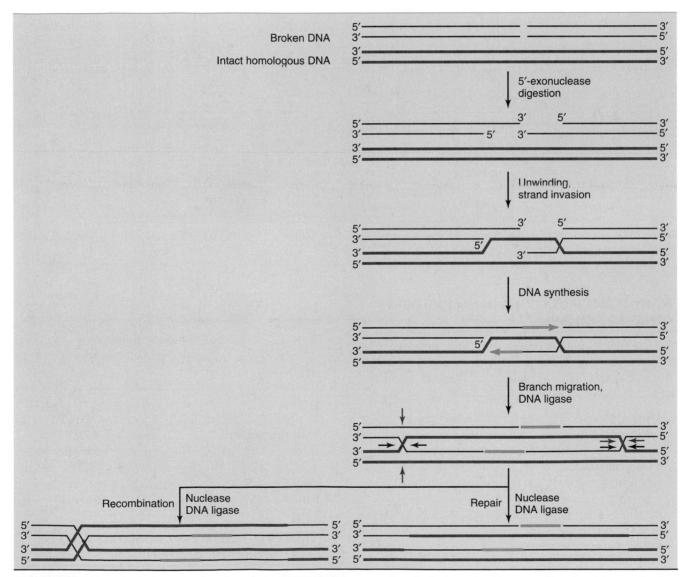

Figure 9.11 Hypothetical mechanism for repair of DNA double-strand breaks by homologous recombination. The mechanism is similar to meiotic recombination.

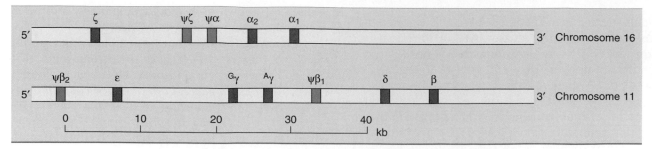

Figure 9.12 Structures of α- and β-like gene clusters. The two α-chain genes are identical, and the two γ-chain genes (^{G}γ and ^{A}γ) code for polypeptides with a single glycine or alanine substitution, respectively. ψ, Pseudogene.

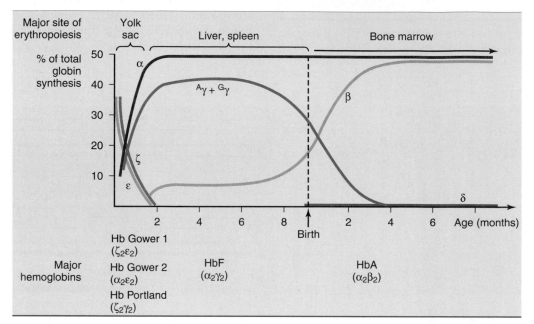

Figure 9.13 Synthesis of globin chains during different stages of development. *Hb*, Hemoglobin; *HbA*, adult hemoglobin; *HbF*, fetal hemoglobin.

MANY POINT MUTATIONS IN HEMOGLOBIN GENES ARE KNOWN

More than 900 hemoglobin variants are known. Most are single amino acid substitutions caused by a single base substitution in the gene, and most of them are harmless. However, some cause disease.

1. *Mutations affecting the heme-binding pocket cause methemoglobinemia.* Replacement of the proximal histidine by tyrosine, for example, makes the heme group inaccessible to methemoglobin reductase. Heterozygotes with this condition are cyanotic but otherwise in good health.
2. *Unstable hemoglobins cause hemolytic anemia.* Denatured hemoglobin forms insoluble protein aggregates in the erythrocytes that are known as **Heinz bodies.** The abnormal cells are removed by macrophages in the spleen, which results in anemia.
3. *Mutations affecting the interface between the subunits lead to abnormal oxygen binding affinity.*

Increased O_2 affinity leads to poor tissue oxygenation and a compensatory increase in erythropoiesis with polycythemia (increased number of red blood cells [RBCs]). Reduced O_2 affinity causes cyanosis (blue lips).

4. *Any mutation that prevents or grossly reduces the synthesis of α- or β-chains causes anemia, especially in the homozygous state.* Affected patients present with **thalassemia.**
5. *Hemoglobins with reduced water solubility cause sickling disorders.* Crystalline precipitates of the insoluble hemoglobin distort the shape of the cell, damage the membrane, and cause hemolysis.

SICKLE CELL DISEASE IS CAUSED BY A POINT MUTATION IN THE β-CHAIN GENE

Sickle cell disease is a severe hemolytic anemia that is most common in Africa but also occurs in India, Arabia, and the Mediterranean. *It is caused by the replacement of a glutamate residue in position 6 of the β-chain by valine:*

H_3^+N – Val–His– Leu – Thr – Pro – Glu – Glu ––·······

·······– CCT GAG GAG –·······

H_3^+N – Val–His– Leu – Thr – Pro – Val – Glu ––·······

·······– CCT GTG GAG –·······

Because the mutation changes the net charge of the molecule, the resulting **hemoglobin S** (**HbS,** subunit structure $\alpha_2\beta^S_2$) can be separated from HbA by electrophoresis (*Fig. 9.14*). HbS is synthesized at a normal rate, is stable, and has normal oxygen affinity. However, the replacement of a charged amino acid by a hydrophobic one reduces its water solubility. *Oxy-HbS is sufficiently soluble, but deoxy-HbS forms a fibrous precipitate in the cell.*

Only homozygotes (genotype SS) have sickle cell disease. Therefore the mode of inheritance is recessive. Until about 6 months after birth, infants are protected from the disease by the presence of fetal hemoglobin, which dilutes the HbS. After this age, HbS tends to precipitate in oxygen-depleted capillaries and veins, distorting the erythrocytes into bizarre, sicklelike shapes. Membrane damage can lead to rupture of the cell, or else the sickled cells are eliminated by splenic macrophages. This leads to anemia with hemoglobin levels anywhere between 6 and 12 g/dl.

The most ominous aspect of sickle cell disease is not the anemia but the tendency of the sickled cells to cause infarctions by blocking capillary beds. Painful bone and joint infarctions are common. Multiple renal infarctions can lead to kidney failure. Many patients develop poorly healing leg ulcers, and some are crippled by recurrent strokes.

Frequent attacks of severe pain in joints, bones, or abdomen, known as **painful crisis** or **sickling crisis,** impair the subjective well-being of the patients. Episodes of **aplastic crisis** (bone marrow failure) are far less common, and the sudden trapping of erythrocytes in

the enlarged spleen, known as **sequestration crisis,** can cause sudden death in children with the disease. These complications require blood transfusions. There is a high rate of mortality from infections, renal failure, and cerebrovascular accidents.

Patients with sickle cell disease should avoid anything that could lead to hypoxia, such as vigorous exercise, staying at high altitude, and drugs that depress respiration (e.g., heroin). Dehydration must be avoided because it leads to a temporary increase in the hemoglobin concentration. Indeed, *intravenous fluids are the standard treatment for sickling crisis.*

Anything that reduces the intracorpuscular concentration of hemoglobin or increases its oxygen affinity is beneficial. **Cyanate** increases the oxygen affinity of hemoglobin by covalent modification of the amino termini of the α- and β-chains:

Polypeptide — NH_2 + O = C = NH

cyanate

$$\downarrow$$

Polypeptide — NH — $\overset{\overset{\displaystyle O}{\|}}{C}$ — NH_2

Carbamoyl hemoglobin
(high O_2-affinity)

This reaction competes with the formation of carbamino hemoglobin, which has a reduced oxygen affinity (see Chapter 3):

Polypeptide — NH_2 + CO_2

$$\downarrow$$

Polypeptide — NH — $\overset{\overset{\displaystyle O}{\|}}{C}$ — O^- + H^+

Carbamino hemoglobin
(low O_2-affinity)

Because cyanate reacts not only with hemoglobin but also with the terminal amino groups of other proteins, it is too toxic for general use. Another possible treatment (although too dangerous for common use) is inhalation of low concentrations of carbon monoxide (CO). CO reduces sickling by converting some of the deoxy-HbS to the nonsickling CO-HbS.

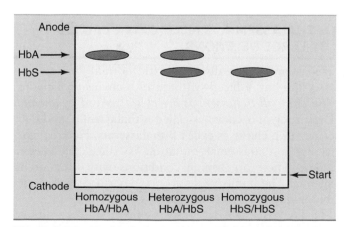

Figure 9.14 Electrophoresis of hemoglobin A (*HbA*) and hemoglobin S (*HbS*; sickle cell) at pH 8.6. Electrophoretic separation is possible because the sickle cell mutation removes a negative charge from the β-chain.

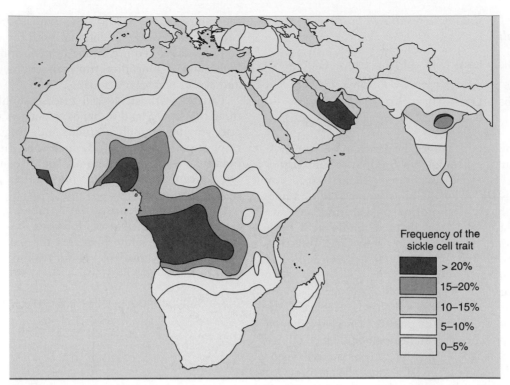

Figure 9.15 Prevalence of heterozygosity for hemoglobin S ("sickle cell trait") in the eastern hemisphere. In the United States, 8% of African Americans have the sickle cell trait, and approximately 1 in 600 has the disease.

SA HETEROZYGOTES ARE PROTECTED FROM TROPICAL MALARIA

HbS heterozygotes (genotype SA, or "sickle cell trait") have about 65% HbA and 35% HbS. Their RBCs do not sickle under ordinary conditions; therefore, *SA heterozygotes are healthy.*

Figure 9.15 shows the distribution of the sickle cell trait in the native populations of the Old World. The HbS allele is common in many tropical areas because *sickle cell heterozygotes have improved malaria resistance.* Natural selection favored the sickle cell allele in the heterozygous state, although homozygotes were likely to die before they had a chance to reproduce. This is a classic example of **heterozygote advantage.**

The connection between HbS and malaria is not surprising. The malaria parasite, *Plasmodium falciparum,* spends part of its lifecycle in erythrocytes, where it is protected from immune attack. The presence of HbS either reduces parasite growth or leads to early destruction of the parasitized cells in the spleen.

CLINICAL EXAMPLE 9.6: Hemoglobin SC Disease

Like HbS, hemoglobin C (HbC) has an amino acid substitution in position 6 of the β-chain. However, the original glutamate is replaced by lysine rather than valine. This hemoglobin variant originated between 2000 and 4000 years ago in an area of West Africa, where it was selected to high frequency because it improves malaria resistance of both homozygotes and heterozygotes.

Homozygosity for HbC leads to dehydration of RBCs and a mild hemolytic anemia. Because HbC and HbS both occur in African-descended populations, compound heterozygosity for the two mutant hemoglobins (SC disease) is not uncommon. SC disease presents as a milder variant of sickle cell disease, although some complications, such as retinal hemorrhages, are more common in patients with SC disease than in SS homozygotes.

α-THALASSEMIA IS MOST OFTEN CAUSED BY LARGE DELETIONS

Thalassemias are diseases with normal hemoglobin structure but reduced synthesis of α-chains or β-chains. Therefore *all thalassemias are characterized by anemia.* Deficiency of α-chains is called α-**thalassemia,** and deficiency of β-chains is called β-**thalassemia.** Heterozygosity for a thalassemia mutation is called **thalassemia minor.** These are benign conditions with little or no anemia. The homozygous forms, described as **thalassemia major,** are severe diseases.

α-Thalassemia is complex because the diploid genome contains four rather than two copies of the α-chain gene. Therefore *the severity of α-thalassemia depends on the number of α-chain genes that have been functionally lost (***Fig. 9.16***).* Deletions that remove

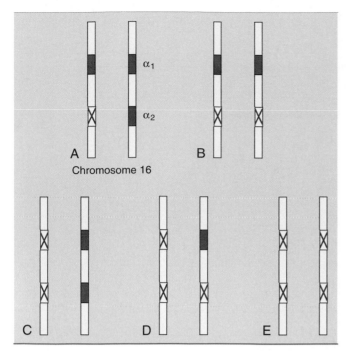

Figure 9.16 Deletion types in patients with α-thalassemia. **A,** One gene deleted ("silent carrier"): asymptomatic. **B,** Two genes deleted on different chromosomes: α-thalassemia minor, very mild anemia. **C,** Two genes deleted on the same chromosome: α-thalassemia minor, very mild anemia. **D,** Three genes deleted: hemoglobin H disease, moderately severe anemia. **E,** All four genes deleted: hemoglobin Bart disease, hydrops fetalis.

either one or both copies of the α-chain gene from the chromosome (α^+ and α^0 mutations, respectively) are the most common α-thalassemia mutations.

Because α-chains are present in fetal as well as adult hemoglobin, *a complete lack of α-chains is fatal before or at birth*. Fetuses with this defect produce an abnormal γ_4 tetramer (**hemoglobin Barts**), which has a 10-fold higher oxygen affinity than hemoglobin A and cannot function as an effective oxygen carrier. Infants who are born with only one intact α-chain gene can survive but have serious lifelong anemia. They form an unstable β_4 tetramer known as **hemoglobin H.**

Like the HbS mutation, thalassemia mutations appear to protect from malaria in the heterozygous state. Therefore *thalassemias are common only in tropical and subtropical areas*. α^+ Mutations occur in Africa, the Mediterranean basin, South Asia, and Southeast Asia. In some Indian and Melanesian populations, a majority of individuals either are silent carriers (one α-chain gene lost) or have α-thalassemia minor (two α-chain genes lost). α^0 Mutations are most common in Southeast Asia, where they are a frequent cause of stillbirth.

MANY DIFFERENT MUTATIONS CAN CAUSE β-THALASSEMIA

Some cases of β-thalassemia (and δβ thalassemia [*Fig. 9.17*]) are caused by large deletions, but most patients have single-base substitutions. In all, more than 200 β-thalassemia mutations have been identified. Splice-site mutations, promoter mutations, nonsense and frameshift mutations, and a mutation in the polyadenylation signal all have been observed in different patients. Three percent of the world population carries a β-thalassemia mutation, and 20 alleles account for 90% of the total. *Figure 9.18* shows an especially interesting type of β-thalassemia mutation.

Some β-thalassemia mutations only reduce β-chain synthesis (β^+-alleles), whereas others prevent β-chain synthesis altogether (β^0-alleles). Homozygous β^0-thalassemia is a severe disease with blood hemoglobin concentration less than 5% and HbF and HbA_2 as the only functional hemoglobins. Anemia does not develop until some months after birth, when HbF is phased out and β-chains become essential.

Because of the large number of mutations, most β-thalassemia "homozygotes" actually are **compound heterozygotes** who have two different mutations in their two β-chain genes. These patients show a wide range of residual β-chain production and clinical severity.

Most of the unpartnered α-chains that are present in β-thalassemia patients are degraded, but those that survive tend to form abnormal aggregates in the cells. Cells containing these aggregates are recognized as abnormal

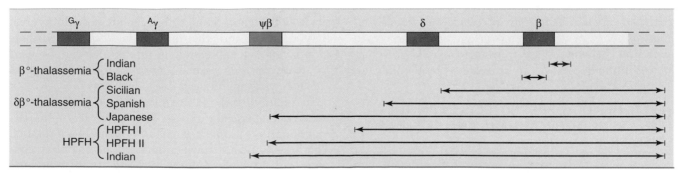

Figure 9.17 Deletions in the β-globin gene cluster. Deletions in the hereditary persistence of fetal hemoglobin (*HPFH*) group suggest that DNA sequences between the $^A\gamma$ and δ genes are important for the developmental switch-off of γ-chain synthesis.

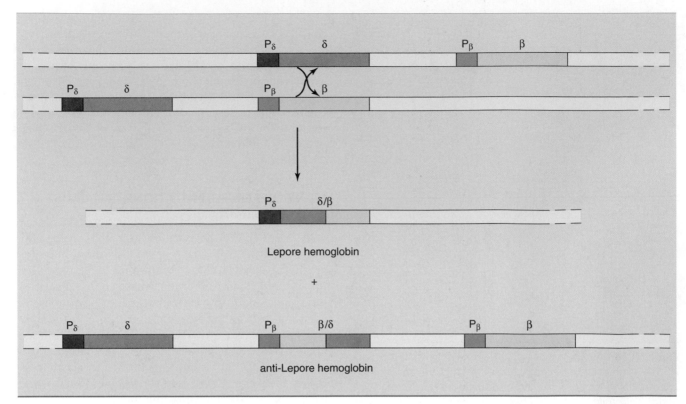

Figure 9.18 Creation of a Lepore hemoglobin. Crossing-over within a δ-chain gene that is misaligned with a β-chain gene during meiosis produces a fusion gene that starts as δ and continues as β. Because this fusion gene is transcribed from the weak δ-chain promoter, the resulting Lepore hemoglobin, which is a functional oxygen carrier, is produced at the rate of a normal δ-chain gene. Lepore hemoglobins are found in a minority of β-thalassemia patients.

by the macrophages in bone marrow and spleen and are consequently destroyed. Destruction of RBC precursors in the bone marrow and premature destruction of circulating RBCs in the spleen aggravate the anemia.

The bone marrow responds to the anemia by working overtime, and massive expansion of the red bone marrow leads to mild facial deformities ("chipmunk facies") and fragile bones. Eventually, extramedullary erythropoiesis develops in liver and spleen.

Untreated patients with homozygous β0-thalassemia are likely to die of severe anemia and intercurrent infections during infancy or childhood. Regular blood transfusions alone can keep them alive to an age of about 20 years, when they succumb to iron overload. *Severe anemia increases intestinal iron absorption, and repeated blood transfusions introduce additional iron that cannot be excreted.* Iron overload can be prevented with **iron chelators.** These drugs form soluble iron complexes in the body that can be excreted by the kidneys.

FETAL HEMOGLOBIN PROTECTS FROM THE EFFECTS OF β-THALASSEMIA AND SICKLE CELL DISEASE

Patients with β0-thalassemia can survive (although with difficulty) because they still possess small amounts of HbA$_2$ and HbF. HbF accounts for less than 2% of the hemoglobin in normal adults and occurs in only a fraction of RBCs. However, in homozygous β0-thalassemia, HbF is the major hemoglobin. *In these patients, the severity of the disease is inversely related to the HbF level.*

In certain patients, including those with some of the deletion types (see *Fig. 9.17*), the symptoms of β-thalassemia remain mild because of high levels of HbF expression. These conditions are called **hereditary persistence of fetal hemoglobin (HPFH).** Elevated levels of HbF are also seen in some nonthalassemic persons with near-normal levels of HbA. In some cases of nondeletion HPFH, the condition can be traced to a point mutation in the promoter region of one of the γ-chain genes.

Persistence of HbF in adults is protective in all β-chain abnormalities, including β-thalassemia and sickle cell disease. Some drugs, including hydroxyurea, butyric acid, and the antitumor drug azacytidine, induce γ-chain expression in adults and can be used for treatment of these diseases. Unfortunately, these agents have many undesirable side effects.

In addition to the HbF effect, there is an interaction between thalassemia and sickle cell disease. *Thalassemia mutations reduce the severity of sickle cell disease.* Thalassemic RBCs have a reduced hemoglobin concentration, which reduces sickling simply because the precipitation of insoluble HbS is concentration dependent.

SUMMARY

Mutations are changes in DNA structure that arise as spontaneous replication errors or as a consequence of DNA damage. Somatic mutations contribute to aging and are the principal cause of cancer, whereas germline mutations cause genetic diseases. Mutations can prevent the normal expression of a gene or cause the synthesis of a defective protein having impaired or abnormal biological properties.

Cells use a variety of DNA repair systems to keep the mutation rate at a tolerable level. Inherited defects of DNA repair are likely to increase the cancer risk or to cause signs of premature aging.

The hemoglobinopathies are classic examples of genetic diseases. In sickle cell disease, a Glu→Val substitution in the β-chain leads to a hemoglobin with abnormally low solubility in the deoxygenated state. The thalassemias are diseases in which structurally normal α-chains or β-chains are underproduced. The hemoglobinopathies are the most common genetic diseases in many parts of the world because heterozygous carriers of the offending mutations have improved malaria resistance.

Further Reading

Arnheim N, Calabrese P: Understanding what determines the frequency and pattern of human germline mutations, *Nat Rev Genet* 10:478–488, 2009.

Barrow E, Alduaij W, Robinson L, et al: Colorectal cancer in HNPCC: cumulative lifetime incidence, survival and tumour distribution. A report of 121 families with proven mutations, *Clin Genet* 74:233–242, 2008.

Bochukova EG, Huang N, Keogh J, et al: Large, rare chromosomal deletions associated with severe early-onset obesity, *Nature* 463:666–670, 2010.

Bodmer W, Bonilla C: Common and rare variants in multifactorial susceptibility to common diseases, *Nat Genet* 40:695–701, 2008.

Byrne M, Agerbo E, Ewald H, et al: Parental age and risk of schizophrenia: a case-control study, *Arch Gen Psychiatry* 60:673–678, 2003.

Caldecott KW: Single-strand break repair and genetic disease, *Nat Rev Genet* 9:619–631, 2008.

Claster S, Vichinsky EP: Managing sickle cell disease, *BMJ* 327:1151–1155, 2003.

Cleaver JE, Lam ET, Revet I: Disorders of nucleotide excision repair: the genetic and molecular basis of heterogeneity, *Nat Rev Genet* 10:756–768, 2009.

Crow JF: The origins, patterns and implications of human spontaneous mutation, *Nat Rev Genet* 1:40–47, 2000.

David SS, O'Shea VL, Kundu S: Base-excision repair of oxidative DNA damage, *Nature* 447:941–950, 2007.

Di Rienzo A: Population genetics models of common diseases, *Curr Opin Genet Dev* 16:630–636, 2006.

Dickson SP, Wang K, Krantz I, et al: Rare variants create synthetic genome-wide associations, *PLoS Biol* 8(1):e1000294, 2010.

Fanciulli M, Petretto E, Aitman TJ: Gene copy number variation and common human disease, *Clin Genet* 77:201–213, 2010.

Ferguson LR, Philpott M: Nutrition and mutagenesis, *Annu Rev Nutr* 28:313–329, 2008.

Fousteri M, Mullenders LHF: Transcription-coupled nucleotide excision repair in mammalian cells: molecular mechanisms and biological effects, *Cell Res* 18:73–84, 2008.

Giardine B, van Baal S, Kaimakis P, et al: HbVar database of human hemoglobin variants and thalassemia mutations: 2007 update, *Hum Mutat* Database 28:206, 2007.

Holloway JW, Yang IA, Holgate ST: Genetics of allergic disease, *J Allergy Clin Immunol* 125:S81–S94, 2010.

Knipscheer P, Räschle M, Smogorzewska A, et al: The Fanconi anemia pathway promotes replication-dependent DNA interstrand cross-link repair, *Science* 326:1698–1701, 2009.

Kulkarni A, Wilson DM: The involvement of DNA-damage and -repair defects in neurological dysfunction, *Am J Hum Genet* 82:539–566, 2008.

Kwiatkowski DP: How malaria has affected the human genome and what human genetics can teach us about malaria, *Am J Hum Genet* 77:171–192, 2005.

Li G-M: Mechanisms and functions of DNA mismatch repair, *Cell Res* 18:85–98, 2008.

Lieber MR: The mechanism of human nonhomologous DNA end joining, *J Biol Chem* 283:1–5, 2008.

Martinez SL, Kolodner RD: Functional analysis of human mismatch repair gene mutations identifies weak alleles and polymorphisms capable of polygenic interactions, *Proc Natl Acad Sci U S A* 107:5070–5075, 2010.

McKinnon PJ: DNA repair deficiency and neurological disease, *Nat Rev Neurosci* 10:100–112, 2009.

Mimitou EP, Symington LS: Nucleases and helicases take center stage in homologous recombination, *Trends Biochem Sci* 34:264–272, 2009.

Mitchell D: Revisiting the photochemistry of solar UVA in human skin, *Proc Natl Acad Sci U S A* 103:13567–13568, 2006.

Rund D, Rachmilewitz E: β-Thalassemia, *N Engl J Med* 353:1135–1146, 2005.

Sadelain M: Recent advances in globin gene transfer for the treatment of beta-thalassemia and sickle cell anemia, *Curr Opin Hematol* 13:142–148, 2006.

Somers CM, Cooper DN: Air pollution and mutations in the germline: are humans at risk? *Hum Genet* 125:119–130, 2009.

Svensson AC, Lichtenstein P, Sandin S, et al: Fertility of first-degree relatives of patients with schizophrenia: a three-generation perspective, *Schizophr Res* 91:238–245, 2007.

Wimmer K: Constitutional mismatch repair-deficiency syndrome: have we so far seen only the tip of the iceberg? *Hum Genet* 124:105–122, 2008.

QUESTIONS

1. You examine a 10-month-old infant who has numerous scaly and ulcerative skin lesions, premalignant changes, and areas of hyperpigmentation. These lesions are present only on sun-exposed skin. This is most likely caused by a defect in

   A. Postreplication mismatch repair
   B. Repair of DNA double-strand breaks
   C. Removal of deaminated bases
   D. Base excision repair
   E. Nucleotide excision repair

2. The most important type of DNA damage in the child described in Question 1 is

   A. DNA double-strand breaks
   B. Pyrimidine dimers
   C. Replication errors
   D. Insertions and deletions
   E. Base methylations

3. An 18-month-old girl of Middle Eastern ancestry, who initially was treated for recurrent lung infections, is found to have a blood hemoglobin concentration of 4.6%. The erythrocytes are smaller than normal and have a slightly irregular shape, and the mean intracorpuscular hemoglobin content is only 55% of normal. HbF and HbA$_2$ are elevated. This is most likely a case of

   A. Sickle cell disease
   B. A DNA repair defect
   C. α-Thalassemia major
   D. β-Thalassemia major
   E. β-Thalassemia minor

4. Some patients with sickle cell disease have relatively mild symptoms because they also have

   A. Bone marrow depression
   B. Elevated β-chain synthesis
   C. Reduced α-chain synthesis
   D. Reduced γ-chain synthesis
   E. Iron overload

5. In Europe and North America, the average age at reproduction has increased by several years during the past 50 years. What types of genetic mutations are likely to become more common as a result of increased maternal and paternal age?

   A. Aneuploidy in both advanced maternal and paternal age
   B. Maternal age: aneuploidy; paternal age: point mutations
   C. Maternal age: chromosomal rearrangements; paternal age: aneuploidy
   D. Maternal age: copy number changes; paternal age: aneuploidy
   E. Point mutations in both advanced maternal and paternal age

Chapter 10
VIRUSES

There are three essential attributes of life: a membrane that physically separates the living cell from its environment; the generation and utilization of metabolic energy; and reproduction.

Viruses have dispensed with cell structure and metabolism but are capable of reproduction. Being unable to generate the metabolic energy required for their reproduction, they depend on a living cell to replicate their nucleic acid and synthesize their proteins. Thus viruses are villains not by choice but by necessity.

All viruses are obligatory intracellular parasites. They do nothing useful for the organism that harbors them. They are encountered mainly as the causes of viral diseases. These diseases are difficult to treat because viruses are so simple that they offer few targets for drug development. This chapter introduces the life-cycles of the major types of viruses.

VIRUSES CAN REPLICATE ONLY IN A HOST CELL

The viral genome can be formed from any kind of nucleic acid: double-stranded DNA, single-stranded DNA, single-stranded RNA, or double-stranded RNA. Viruses are genetic paupers, with anywhere between 3 and 250 genes, in comparison with 4435 genes in *Escherichia coli* and 25,000 to 30,000 in *Homo sapiens*.

Outside the cell, the virus exists as a particle with viral nucleic acid wrapped into a protective protein coat, or **capsid**. Viral genomes are too small to encode large numbers of structural proteins. Therefore capsids are formed from a few proteins that polymerize into a regular, crystalline structure. The protein coat protects the nucleic acid from physical insults and enzymatic attack, and it is required to recognize and invade the host cell.

Many animal viruses are enclosed by an **envelope**, which is a piece of host cell membrane appropriated by the virus while it is budding out of its host cell. The envelope is studded with viral proteins, the **spike proteins** (*Fig. 10.1*).

The viral nucleic acid can be replicated only in the host cell, and *host cell ribosomes are required for the synthesis of the viral proteins.* Some viral proteins are enzymes for virus replication, and others form the capsid or appear as spike proteins in the viral envelope.

BACTERIOPHAGE T₄ DESTROYS ITS HOST CELL

Viruses that infect bacteria are called **bacteriophages** ("bacteria eaters") or simply "phages." Bacteriophage T_4 is a classic example. It is one of the most complex viruses known (*Fig. 10.2*), with a double-stranded DNA genome of about 150 genes tightly packed into the head portion of the virus particle. Attached to the head is a short neck followed by a cylindrical tail with two coaxial hollow tubes, a base plate, and six spidery tail fibers. This complex capsid consists of about 40 virus-encoded polypeptides, each present in many copies.

T_4 is constructed like a syringe that injects its DNA into the host cell. First, the tail fibers bind to a component of the bacterial cell wall that serves as a **virus receptor**. Next, the sheath of the tail contracts, its inner core penetrates the cell wall, and the viral DNA is injected into the cell. Only the DNA enters the host cell. The protein coat remains outside (*Fig. 10.3*).

Some viral genes are transcribed immediately by the bacterial RNA polymerase. One of these "immediate-early" genes encodes a DNase that degrades the host cell chromosome. The viral DNA is not attacked by this DNase because it contains hydroxymethyl cytosine instead of cytosine.

During later stages of the infection, viral proteins substitute for the σ subunit of bacterial RNA polymerase and direct the transcription of the "delayed-early" and "late" viral genes. The promoters of these genes are not recognized by the bacterial σ subunit.

The early viral proteins include enzymes for nucleotide synthesis, DNA replication, and DNA modification. The viral coat proteins are synthesized late in the infectious cycle, and *new virus particles are assembled from the replicated viral DNA and the newly synthesized coat proteins.* Finally, virus-encoded phospholipase and lysozyme destroy the bacterial plasma membrane and cell wall.

This mode of virus replication is called the **lytic pathway** because it ends with the lysis (destruction) of the

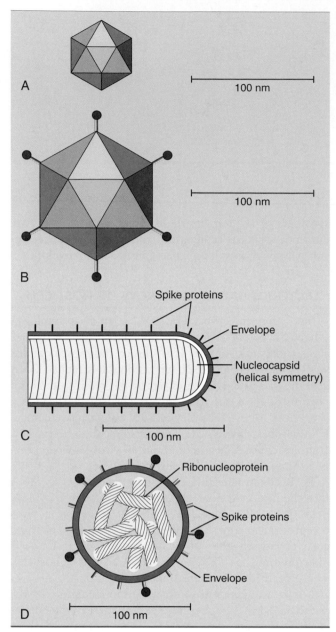

Figure 10.1 Sizes and structures of some typical viruses. **A,** Papilloma (wart) virus: a nonenveloped DNA virus of icosahedral shape (spherical symmetry). **B,** Adenovirus: another nonenveloped DNA virus. **C,** Rabies virus: an enveloped RNA virus. **D,** Influenza virus: an enveloped RNA virus containing eight segments of ribonucleoprotein with helical symmetry.

host cell. It takes approximately 20 minutes, and about 200 progeny viruses are released from the lysed host cell.

DNA VIRUSES SUBSTITUTE THEIR OWN DNA FOR THE HOST CELL DNA

Some but not all features of lytic infection by bacteriophage T4 are typical for viral infections in general:

1. *Infection begins with binding of the virus to the surface of its host cell.* A viral protein in the capsid or

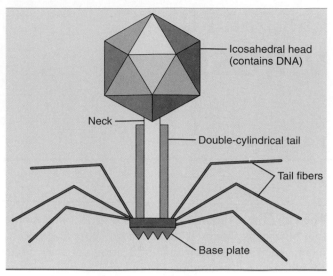

Figure 10.2 Structure of bacteriophage T4, one of the most complex DNA viruses known. Its capsid consists of approximately 40 different proteins.

the envelope binds selectively to a "virus receptor" on the host cell. Only cells that possess the virus receptor can be infected (***Clinical Example 10.1***). The human body can combat viral infections with antibodies that coat the viral surface proteins and thereby prevent them from binding to the virus receptor.

2. *Many bacteriophages inject their nucleic acid into the host cell.* Animal viruses use different strategies.

CLINICAL EXAMPLE 10.1: Genetic AIDS Resistance

The human immunodeficiency virus (HIV) is an enveloped virus that causes acquired immunodeficiency syndrome (AIDS) by infecting helper T cells and macrophages. HIV can invade these cells because they express a glycoprotein called CD4 on their cell surface. Entry of HIV into the cell is facilitated by coreceptors in the membrane, which interact with the CD4-bound virus. One of these coreceptors is CCR5, a cytokine receptor expressed primarily on macrophages.

This cytokine receptor seems to be nonessential for immune responses, as about 15% to 20% of Europeans are heterozygous for a 32–base-pair deletion in the *CCR5* gene (*CCR5-Δ32*), which prevents the synthesis of the receptor. Heterozygosity for this mutation delays the progression of HIV infection to clinical AIDS. Those lucky few who are homozygous for the mutation (up to 1 in 100 Europeans) are almost completely resistant to AIDS. The mutation is of recent origin. Whether it rose to its present frequency by chance or through darwinian selection by some infectious agent over the past one to five millennia is not known.

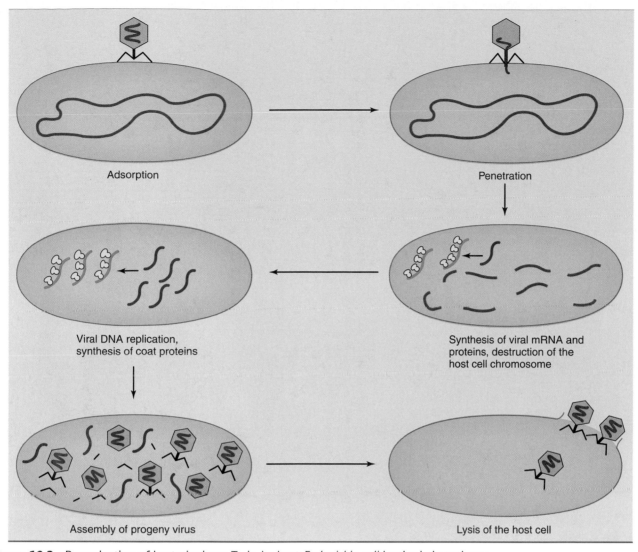

Figure 10.3   Reproduction of bacteriophage T$_4$ in its host *Escherichia coli* by the lytic pathway.

Some enveloped viruses fuse their envelope with the plasma membrane of the host cell, whereas others trigger their own endocytosis (*Fig. 10.4*).

3. *All viruses abuse the host cell ribosomes for the synthesis of their proteins.* DNA replication and transcription of the smaller viruses depend heavily on host cell enzymes, but larger viruses encode many of the required enzymes themselves.

4. *The viruses of eukaryotes replicate in either the nucleus or the cytoplasm.* Most DNA viruses replicate in the nucleus, where they can take advantage of the host's DNA and RNA polymerases, whereas most RNA viruses replicate in the cytoplasm.

5. *Many viruses inhibit vital processes of the host cell,* but T$_4$'s barbaric practice of cutting the host's DNA to pieces is not common among animal viruses.

6. *Bacteriophages kill their victims, but many virus-infected human cells survive.* In most cases, the infected human cells shed virus particles continuously.

λ PHAGE CAN INTEGRATE ITS DNA INTO THE HOST CELL CHROMOSOME

Like T$_4$ phage, λ phage is constructed as a syringe that injects its DNA into the host cell. Its genome, with about 50 genes, is a linear double-stranded DNA molecule of 48,502 base pairs with single-stranded ends of 12 nucleotides each. These single-stranded overhangs have complementary base sequences. They anneal (base pair) as soon as the viral DNA enters the host cell, and the viral genome is linked into a circle by bacterial DNA ligase (*Fig. 10.5*). Lytic infection can now proceed as described previously for T$_4$ phage.

Unlike T$_4$, however, λ phage can also pursue an alternative lifestyle. Rather than destroying its host cell by brute force, it can integrate itself into a specific site of the host cell chromosome, between the galactose and biotin operons. *The viral DNA is now part of the host cell chromosome* and is replicated during each

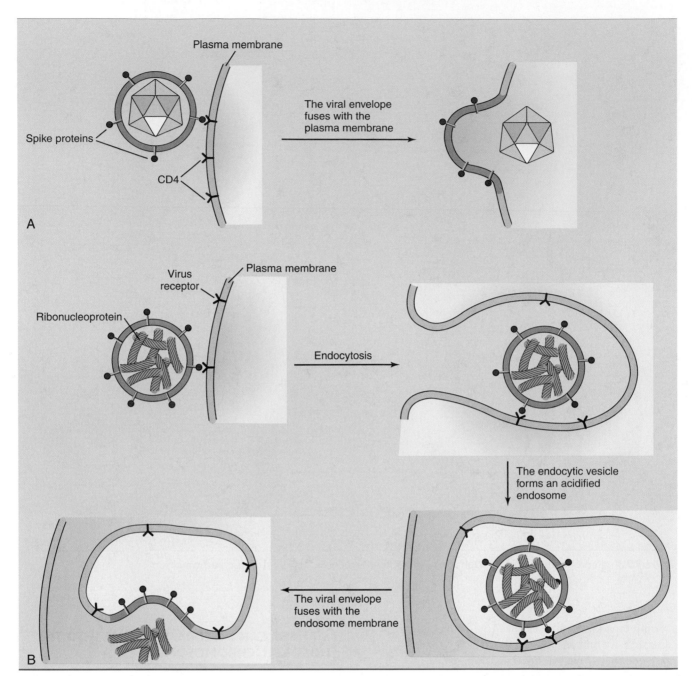

Figure 10.4 Two strategies for uptake of an enveloped virus into its host cell. An initial noncovalent binding between a viral spike protein and the host cell membrane is essential in both cases. **A,** Uptake of human immunodeficiency virus (a retrovirus) is triggered by binding to the membrane glycoprotein CD4. The uptake of the nucleocapsid into the cytoplasm does not depend on endocytosis but is effected by direct fusion of the viral envelope with the plasma membrane. Only CD4-positive cells can be infected by this virus. **B,** Uptake of influenza virus, an enveloped RNA virus. Endocytosis is triggered by binding of the virus to the cell surface. The fusion of the viral envelope with the membrane of the endosome is facilitated by the low pH (5.0–6.0) of this organelle.

cycle of cell division. This mode of virus replication is called the **lysogenic pathway** (*Fig. 10.6*). The integrated virus DNA is called a **prophage,** and the bacterium is characterized as **lysogenic.**

Integration of the viral DNA requires a virus-encoded **integrase.** Another viral gene, which becomes activated under the same conditions as the integrase gene, codes for the **λ repressor.** *The λ repressor maintains the*

lysogenic state by preventing the transcription of all viral genes except its own. It even makes the lysogenic bacterium resistant to reinfection by λ phage because the genes of any invading λ phage become repressed as well.

The lysogenic state can be maintained for many cell generations, but the viral genes can be reactivated. *Whenever the concentration of the λ repressor falls below a critical limit, the genes of the lytic pathway*

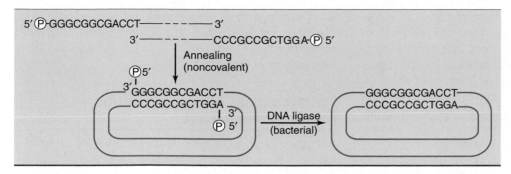

Figure 10.5 Circularization of λ phage DNA. This event takes place immediately after the entry of the viral DNA into the host cell and does not require virally encoded proteins. The circular DNA is then either replicated in the lytic pathway or integrated into the bacterial chromosome.

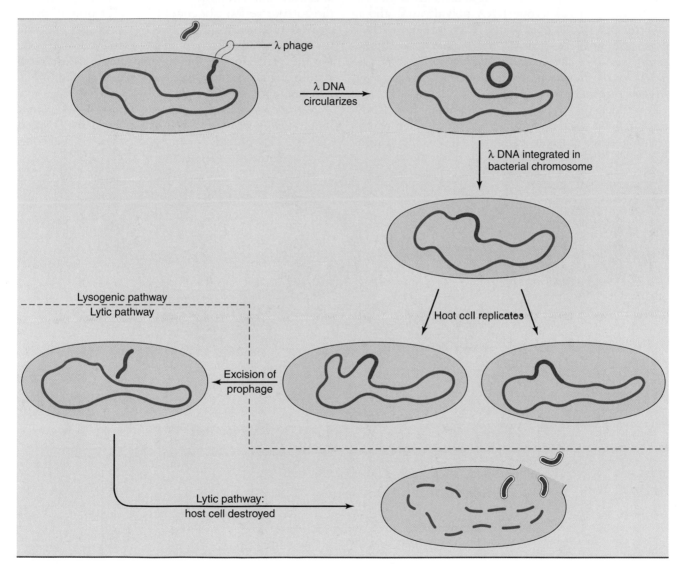

Figure 10.6 The lysogenic pathway of λ phage.

become derepressed. One of the derepressed genes codes for an enzyme that turns the prophage loose by cutting it out of the bacterial chromosome.

The lysogenic state is terminated when the bacterium suffers DNA damage from ultraviolet radiation or chemical mutagens. These conditions activate a bacterial protease that degrades the λ repressor. Like rats leaving a sinking ship, the virus leaves its troubled host.

RNA VIRUSES REQUIRE AN RNA-DEPENDENT RNA POLYMERASE

The lifecycles of RNA viruses tend to be simpler than those of DNA viruses because the viral RNA is translated directly by the host cell ribosomes, without the need for transcription. If the viral RNA is double stranded, only one of the strands, the + strand, serves as the viral messenger RNA (mRNA).

Replication of the viral genome requires an **RNA-dependent RNA polymerase,** also known as **RNA replicase** (*Fig. 10.7*). This enzyme is not present in healthy cells and therefore must be encoded by the virus. Single-stranded RNA viruses that have only the noncoding RNA strand in their genome must carry this enzyme in the virus particle. They require it to synthesize complementary + strands, which are then used as mRNA for the synthesis of the viral proteins.

Viral RNA replicases have no proofreading 3'-exonuclease activity, and their error rates are about as high as those of eukaryotic RNA polymerases, about one error per 10,000 nucleotides. Therefore most RNA viruses are small. In general, *the maximal functional genome size that can be maintained by an organism is limited by the fidelity of replication and the efficiency of repair mechanisms.*

Low fidelity of replication also implies that RNA viruses evolve fast and can elude host defenses by inventing new antigenic variants. This is the reason why there is no vaccine against the common cold. Rhinoviruses (cold viruses) are RNA viruses with high mutation rates. New strains arise all the time, making any vaccine obsolete very quickly.

RETROVIRUSES REPLICATE THROUGH A DNA INTERMEDIATE

Retroviruses contain two identical copies of a + RNA strand, about 10,000 nucleotides long, surrounded by a capsid and envelope. Their genome contains only three major genes: *gag* codes for a large protein that is cleaved into the capsid proteins by a protease, *pol* codes for reverse transcriptase and integrase, and *env* codes for the precursor of the spike proteins. Most retroviruses possess a few accessory genes in addition to *gag*, *pol*, and *env*.

Retroviruses copy their single-stranded RNA genome into a double-stranded DNA (complementary DNA, or cDNA). This process is catalyzed by the virus-encoded

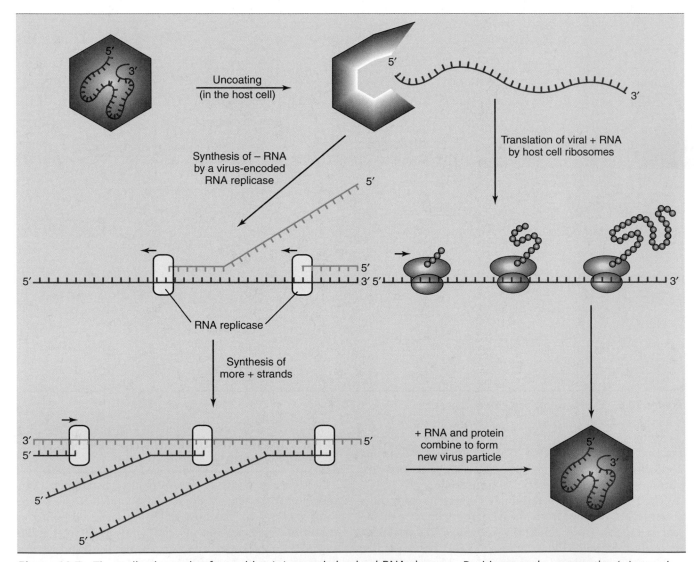

Figure 10.7 The replicative cycle of a positive (+)–stranded animal RNA virus. ⌐⌐, Positive strand; ⌐⌐, negative (−) strand.

enzyme **reverse transcriptase,** which is carried in the virus particle.

In the host cell, this imported reverse transcriptase catalyzes all steps in the synthesis of the viral cDNA (**Fig. 10.8**). In addition to several copies of the reverse transcriptase, the virus particle contains a transfer RNA (tRNA) from its previous host cell that is used as a primer for DNA synthesis.

The mechanism of reverse transcription shown in **Figure 10.8** implies that the cDNA ends in repeat sequences left and right that are known as **long terminal repeats (LTRs)** (**Fig. 10.9**). The LTRs are required for the integration of the retroviral cDNA into the host cell chromosome. The upstream LTR serves as a promoter for transcriptional initiation, and the downstream LTR contains a polyadenylation site for transcriptional termination.

Like the RNA replicases, reverse transcriptases do not proofread their product. Thus *retroviruses have high mutation rates.* This makes them fast-moving

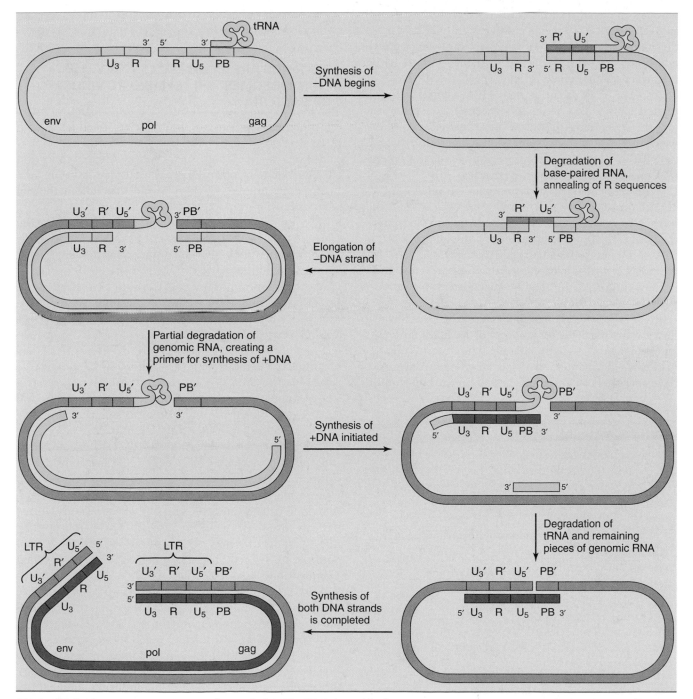

Figure 10.8 Reverse transcription of retroviral RNA. *PB,* Primer-binding sequence; *U₃, U₅, R,* noncoding sequences that become the long terminal repeats (LTR). ▫, RNA; ▪, negative (−) DNA strand; ■, positive (+) DNA strand.

Figure 10.9 Structure of integrated retroviral complementary DNA (cDNA). After integration into the host cell genome, all three genes are transcribed into a single mRNA. *gag*, *pol*, and *env* are the structural genes of the virus. LTR, long terminal repeat; ■, direct repeats (target site duplications).

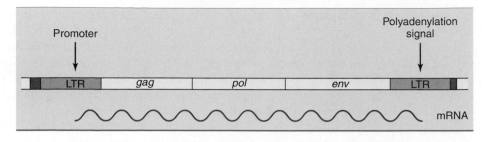

targets for the immune system and also for scientists who try to develop vaccines for retroviral diseases such as AIDS. An AIDS vaccine is still not in sight because of the high mutation rate of the retroviral *env* gene. In addition, drug treatment is difficult because drug-resistant strains emerge quickly (*Clinical Example 10.2*). The HIV that causes AIDS evolved from a related chimpanzee virus very recently, sometime during the twentieth century. This "instant evolution" was possible because of the short generation time of the virus, its high mutation rate, and the changed selection pressures in the new host species.

With the help of a virus-encoded **integrase**, *the cDNA produced by the reverse transcriptase becomes integrated into the host cell DNA.* After its integration, the viral cDNA is transcribed into a single long RNA by RNA polymerase II. This viral RNA has two uses. It is the mRNA for the synthesis of the viral proteins, and it is the genomic RNA that is packaged into new virus particles (*Fig. 10.10*).

In most retroviral infections the cell survives but produces virus particles for the rest of its lifetime. HIV is an exception. It actually kills the white blood cells that it infects. In Chapter 7 we saw that some retroviruses have managed to enter the human germ line millions

of years ago. By losing the ability to form infectious virus particles, these retroviruses evolved into the retroviral elements that litter the human genome today.

PLASMIDS ARE SMALL "ACCESSORY CHROMOSOMES" OR "SYMBIOTIC VIRUSES" OF BACTERIA

Plasmids are small circles of double-stranded DNA with between 2000 and 200,000 base pairs, found in prokaryotes and some lower eukaryotes. Their replication is controlled by plasmid genes that maintain an adequate copy number of the plasmid throughout the cell generations.

Most plasmids carry additional genes, but, unlike the chromosomal genes, *the plasmid genes are dispensable in most situations.* For example, plasmid genes can confer capabilities of toxin production, antibiotic resistance, degradation of unusual metabolic substrates, and genetic recombination. **R factor plasmids** (R for resistance) are especially important in medicine (*Fig. 10.11* and *Clinical Example 10.3*)

Some of the larger plasmids are infectious. A classic example is the **F factor** (F for fertility) of *E. coli*, a large plasmid with 94,500 base pairs. The F factor carries a set of about a dozen genes that control the formation of sex pili, which are hairlike processes that protrude from the cell surface in all directions.

Once an F factor–bearing cell (F$^+$ cell) encounters a cell without F factor (F$^-$ cell), a delicate bridge is formed between the cells by one of the sex pili. At the same time, one strand of the plasmid DNA is nicked, the double helix unravels, and one of the strands worms its way into the F$^-$ cell (*Fig. 10.12*). This is followed by the synthesis of a new cDNA strand in both the F$^+$ cell and the ex–F$^-$ cell. This type of DNA transfer is called **conjugation.**

The F factor behaves as an infectious agent that can spread in the bacterial population. Sometimes, the F factor acquires genes from the bacterial chromosome and transfers them into the F$^-$ cell along with its own genes. In rare cases, it even becomes integrated into the bacterial chromosome and pulls a complete copy of the chromosome into the F$^-$ cell during conjugation. Through these mechanisms, *the F factor enables the bacteria to exchange genetic information.*

CLINICAL EXAMPLE 10.2: Antiretroviral Drugs

Many antibiotics are available for the treatment of bacterial infections but few drugs for the treatment of viral infections. The reason is that viruses are too simple. They encode only a few proteins that can be targeted by drugs.

In the case of the human immunodeficiency virus (HIV), great effort has been expended for drug development. Most HIV drugs inhibit reverse transcriptase, integrase, or the viral protease that processes the precursors of the viral proteins. Other drugs inactivate two zinc fingers that are present in the precursor of the nucleocapsid proteins and that serve several functions during virus replication. Although the drugs can prolong the patient's life, cures are rarely achieved because effective doses of the drugs have serious side effects and because the virus tends to become resistant to the drugs.

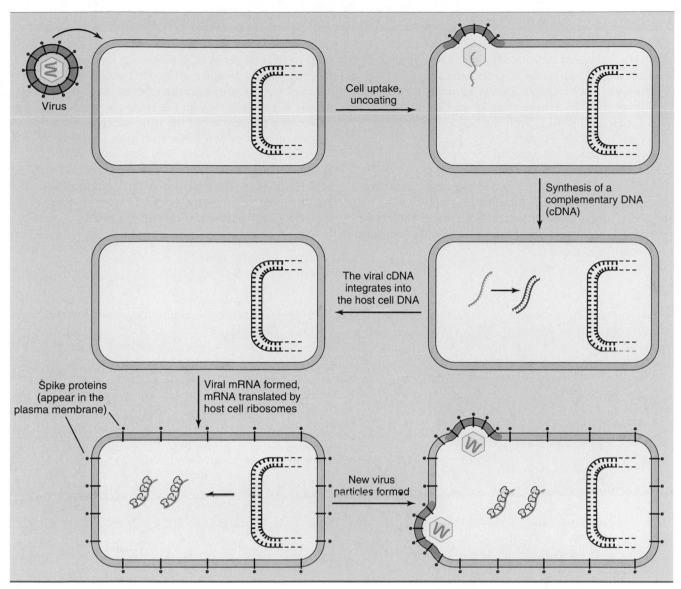

Figure 10.10   Lifecycle of a retrovirus. The viral reverse transcriptase converts the viral RNA (*green*) into a double-stranded DNA (*red*), which becomes integrated into the host cell genome.

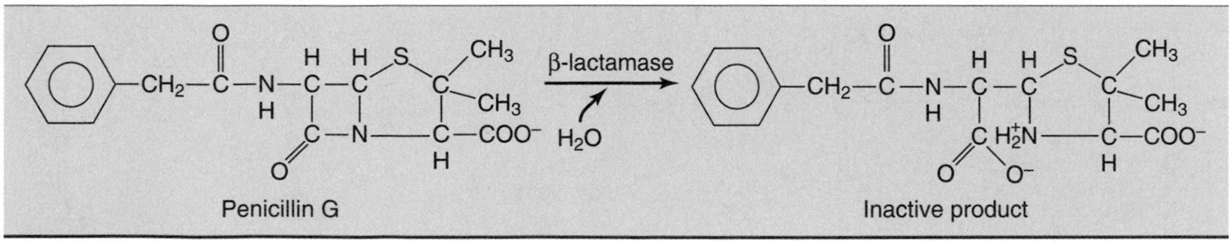

Figure 10.11   Action of β-lactamase ("penicillinase") on penicillin G. The gene for this enzyme is often found on R factor plasmids.

BACTERIA CAN EXCHANGE GENES BY TRANSFORMATION AND TRANSDUCTION

Bacteria can acquire new DNA by mechanisms other than conjugation (*Fig. 10.13*). In **transformation**, a piece of foreign DNA that has been taken up by the bacterium becomes integrated into the bacterial chromosome. Integration of the foreign DNA is possible by homologous recombination, which is the same mechanism that we encountered in Chapter 9 as a strategy for DNA repair and meiotic crossing-over. Some bacteria have specialized systems for the uptake of

CLINICAL EXAMPLE 10.3: Multidrug-Resistant *Staphylococcus aureus*

Staphylococcus aureus is one of the most common bacterial pathogens, causing skin infections, abscesses, and occasionally pneumonia, endocarditis, or osteomyelitis. When penicillin was introduced in the 1930s and 1940s, *S. aureus* was almost uniformly susceptible to this drug. With the passage of time, however, penicillin-resistant strains kept emerging. Today many strains are resistant not only to penicillin but to a broad range of antibiotics.

Many drug resistance genes encode drug-inactivating enzymes. For example, **β-lactamase** is a penicillin-degrading enzyme. In other cases, the resistance gene encodes a membrane transporter that actively transports drugs out of the cell. It turned out that, in many cases, drug-resistance genes in *S. aureus* are located on plasmids, some of which are self-transmissible. Many resistance genes are constituents of transposons that are mobile in the genome and therefore can be located either on a plasmid or on the bacterial chromosome.

Transmission of drug-resistance genes between bacterial "species" is sometimes observed. In one example, a strain of *S. aureus* that already was resistant to the antibiotic methicillin acquired a vancomycin-resistance gene from a vancomycin-resistant strain of the intestinal bacterium *Enterococcus fecalis*.

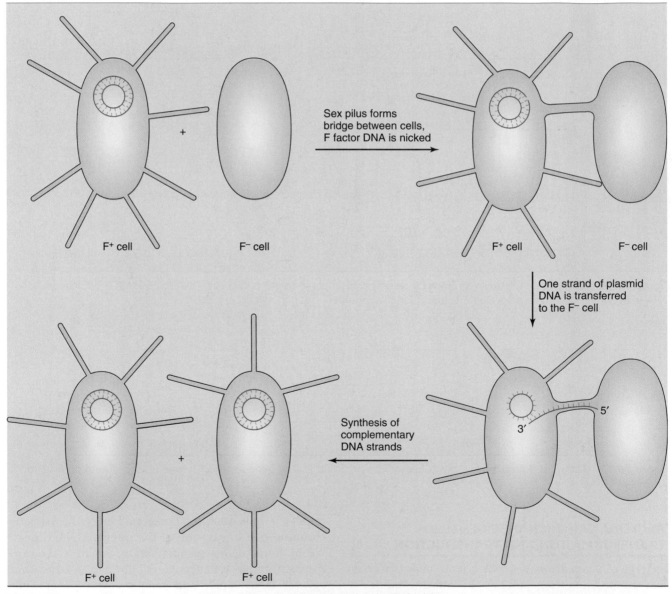

Figure 10.12 Cell-to-cell transfer of the F factor during conjugation in *Escherichia coli*.

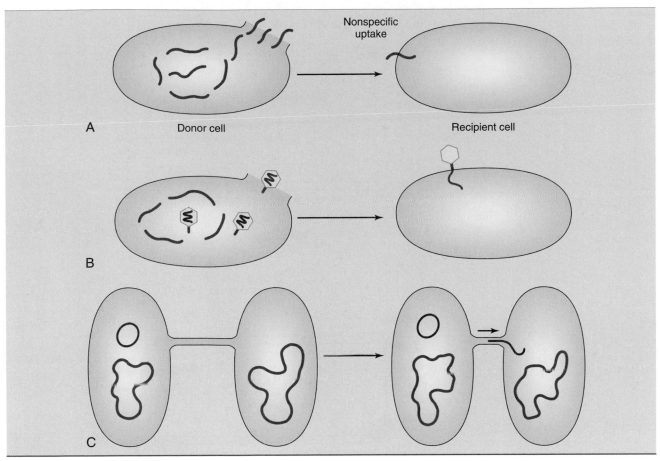

Figure 10.13   Transfer of DNA between bacterial cells. The three mechanisms of DNA transfer shown here are collectively known as "parasexual" processes. **A**, Transformation. **B**, Transduction. **C**, Conjugation.

foreign DNA. For most bacteria, however, including *E. coli*, transformation is a rare event in nature. Special treatments are necessary to achieve transformation of these bacteria in the laboratory.

In **transduction**, a bacteriophage carries a fragment of host cell DNA from cell to cell. The host cell DNA is erroneously packaged into a virus particle, and the virus injects bacterial DNA instead of (or in addition to) viral DNA into the next host cell.

JUMPING GENES CAN CHANGE THEIR POSITION IN THE GENOME

Bacterial genomes contain mobile genetic elements, but, unlike the retrotransposons of eukaryotes, the "jumping genes" of bacteria do not move through an RNA intermediate.

An insertion sequence is a small mobile element, about 1000 base pairs long, that is framed by inverted repeats of between 9 and 41 base pairs. Most insertion sequences are present in 5 to 30 copies that are identical or nearly identical, including the inverted repeats at their ends. The inverted repeats are flanked by short (4–12 base pairs) direct repeats that differ in different

copies of the insertion sequence and that arise as target site duplications during transposition.

Insertion sequences contain a solitary gene for **transposase**, an enzyme that appears to catalyze most or all of the enzymatic reactions required for transposition. *Figure 10.14* shows a hypothetical mechanism.

The transposase recognizes the inverted repeats of its own insertion sequence. It cannot transpose unrelated insertion sequences with different inverted repeats. Insertion sequences are "selfish DNA" that is of no obvious advantage to the cell. They can cause crippling mutations when they jump into an important gene.

Transposons are insertion sequences with a payload. They contain useful genes in addition to a gene for transposase, for example, genes for antibiotic resistance. In **composite transposons,** the useful genes are flanked not by simple inverted repeats but by insertion sequences (*Fig. 10.15*). Indeed, *any gene that becomes framed by two insertion sequences becomes transposable.*

Transposons can jump back and forth among the bacterial chromosome, plasmids, and bacteriophages. Self-transmissible plasmids can spread them from cell to cell by conjugation, and bacteriophages can spread them by transduction.

Figure 10.14 Hypothetical mechanism for duplicative transposition of a bacterial insertion sequence. *poly I*, DNA polymerase I.

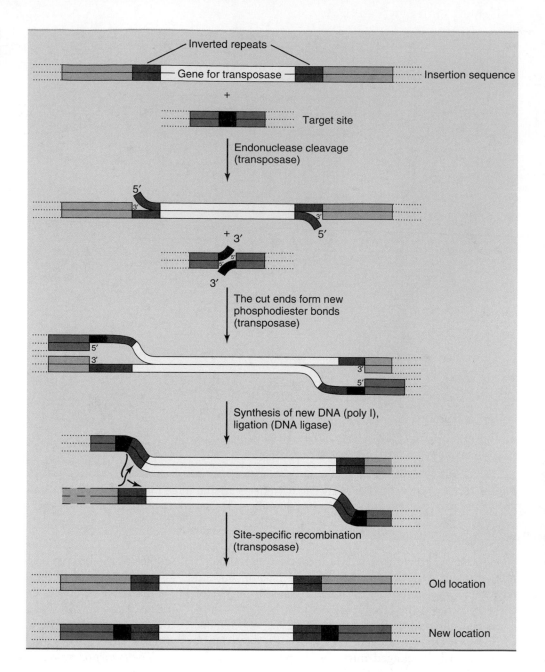

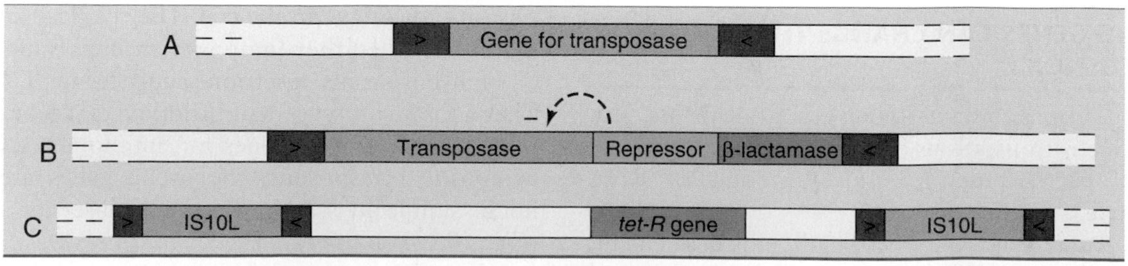

Figure 10.15 Examples of mobile elements in bacteria. **A,** An insertion sequence: a gene for transposase that is flanked by inverted terminal repeat sequences (■). **B,** Transposon Tn3. Besides the transposase gene, this transposon contains both a gene for a repressor that regulates the expression of the transposase gene, and a gene for the penicillin-degrading enzyme β-lactamase. Bacteria carrying this transposon are resistant to penicillin. **C,** Transposon Tn10. This transposon contains a gene for tetracycline resistance (*tet-R* gene). Unlike Tn3, it is not framed by simple inverted repeats but by two identical insertion sequences (IS10L), each of which contains a transposase gene.

SUMMARY

Viruses have no cellular structure and no metabolism, but they can replicate within a host cell by exploiting the host's enzymes, ribosomes, and metabolic energy.

DNA viruses substitute their own genomic DNA for the host cell DNA, directing the synthesis of viral mRNA and viral proteins. RNA viruses substitute their own RNA for the host's mRNA, directing the synthesis of viral proteins without the need for transcription. Retroviruses synthesize a DNA copy of their genomic RNA and integrate it into the host cell genome.

Prokaryotic cells contain many semiautonomous genetic elements. Plasmids are small circular DNA duplexes that function as accessory chromosomes. Some plasmids are infectious, transmitting themselves from cell to cell by conjugation. Insertion sequences and transposons are integrated in the bacterial chromosome, but they are capable of inserting copies of themselves in new locations.

Further Reading

Barré-Sinoussi F: HIV: a discovery opening the road to novel scientific knowledge and global health improvement, *Virology* 397:255–259, 2010.

Hackett PR, Largaespada DA, Cooper LJN: A transposon and transposase system for human application, *Mol Ther* 18:674–683, 2010.

Nikaido H: Multidrug resistance in bacteria, *Annu Rev Biochem* 78:119–146, 2009.

Rasko DA, Sperandio V: Anti-virulence strategies to combat bacterial-mediated infections, *Nat Rev Drug Discov* 9:117–128, 2010.

Sabeti PC, Walsh E, Schaffner SF, et al: The case for selection at CCR5-Δ32, *PLoS Biol* 3(11):e378, 2005.

Weigel LM, Clewell DB, Gill SR, et al: Genetic analysis of a high-level vancomycin-resistant isolate of *Staphylococcus aureus*, *Science* 302:1569–1571, 2003.

QUESTIONS

1. **In order to infect a new host cell, a virus has to bind specifically to a "virus receptor" on the surface of the host cell. In the case of the virus causing AIDS (a retrovirus), this initial interaction involves the viral**

   A. Spike proteins
   B. Reverse transcriptase
   C. Capsid proteins
   D. RNA
   E. Integrase

2. **An inhibitor of reverse transcriptase would be useful to**

   A. Prevent λ phage from integrating into the host cell chromosome
   B. Prevent lytic infection by T4 bacteriophage
   C. Inhibit homologous recombination between two DNAs
   D. Cure rabies, a disease caused by an RNA virus
   E. Cure AIDS, a disease caused by a retrovirus

Chapter 11
DNA TECHNOLOGY

Molecular genetics is the most active field in medical research today, and for good reason. Identification of the genetic risk factors for complex diseases allows us to understand the mechanisms of these diseases and to find targets for treatment. The diagnosis of genetic disease susceptibilities helps in disease prevention, diagnosis of diseases, and choice of treatments. Thus we see the emergence of a "personalized medicine" that is tailored to the patient's genetic constitution. Although diagnosis is the main medical application of molecular genetics, genetic treatment modalities are being explored as well. This chapter introduces the basic toolkit that is used for these applications.

RESTRICTION ENDONUCLEASES CUT LARGE DNA MOLECULES INTO SMALLER FRAGMENTS

The DNA in human chromosomes has lengths of up to 300 million base pairs. For most applications, these unwieldy molecules need to be broken into smaller fragments.

The choice tools for DNA fragmentation are **restriction endonucleases.** *These bacterial enzymes cleave DNA selectively at palindromic sequences of four to eight nucleotides.* The average length of the resulting **restriction fragments** depends on the length of the recognition sequence. For example, an enzyme that recognizes a four-base sequence cleaves on average once every 256 (4^4) nucleotides and creates fragments with an average length of 256 base pairs. An enzyme that recognizes an eight-base sequence creates fragments with an average length of 65,536 (4^8) base pairs. Several hundred restriction endonucleases that recognize different palindromic sequences are available commercially.

Most restriction enzymes make staggered cuts one or two base pairs away from the symmetry axis of their recognition sequence in both strands. Therefore *the double-stranded restriction fragments have short single-stranded ends* (**Fig. 11.1** and *Table 11.1*).

Because the single-stranded overhangs are complementary to one another, *every restriction fragment can anneal (base pair) with any other restriction fragment produced by the same enzyme.* The annealed restriction fragments can be linked covalently by DNA ligase. This

is the most fundamental procedure in **recombinant DNA technology:** the cutting and joining of DNA in the test tube.

Restriction endonucleases are produced by bacteria as a defense against DNA viruses. The bacteria protect susceptible sites in their own genome by methylation, but the unmethylated viral DNA is cut to pieces by the restriction enzyme.

COMPLEMENTARY DNA PROBES ARE USED FOR IN SITU HYBRIDIZATION

The identification of a mutation requires a **molecular probe** that can distinguish the mutation from the normal sequence. *A probe is a single-stranded DNA (or RNA) that is complementary to the target DNA.* To be detectable, the probe must be labeled with either a radioactive isotope or a fluorescent group.

A labeled messenger RNA (mRNA), for example, can be used as a probe. When genomic DNA is digested by a restriction enzyme and then denatured, *the mRNA probe binds to all restriction fragments that contain exon sequences of its gene.* Instead of the mRNA itself, a **complementary DNA (cDNA) probe** made from the mRNA by reverse transcriptase is frequently used.

A cDNA with a strong fluorescent label can be used to detect gene deletions by **fluorescent in situ hybridization (FISH).** A chromosome spread is prepared from a metaphase cell, the chromosomal DNA is denatured, and the probe is applied. *If the gene is present, the probe binds; if it is deleted, the probe does not bind.*

Even interphase cells can be used to detect deletion or aneuploidy with FISH. If the probe for a gene binds to only one spot in the amorphous chromatin, the second copy of the gene is deleted. If it binds to three spots, the gene—or the entire chromosome—is present in three instead of the normal two copies.

DOT BLOTTING IS USED FOR GENETIC SCREENING

The diagnosis of small mutations requires a synthetic **oligonucleotide probe.** *The probe must be at least 17 or 18 nucleotides long* because shorter probes are likely to

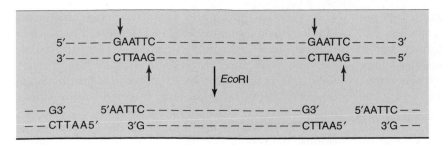

Figure 11.1 Generation of restriction fragments by the restriction endonuclease *Eco*RI. Both strands are cut. Note that the double-stranded DNA fragments have single-stranded ends.

Table 11.1 Examples of Restriction Endonucleases

Enzyme*	Source	Cleavage Specificity	No. of Cleavage Sites on λ Phage DNA†
*Eco*RI	*Escherichia coli* RY 13	5′ G↓A A T T C 3′ 3′ C T T A A↑G 5′	5
*Eco*RII	*E. coli* R 245	5′↓C C T G G 3′ 3′ G G A C C↑ 5′	>35
*Hind*III	*Haemophilus influenzae* R$_d$	5′ A↓A G C T T 3′ 3′ T T C G A↑A 5′	6
*Hae*III	*Haemophilus aegyptius*	5′ G G↓C C 3′ 3′ C C↑G G 5′	>50
*Bam*HI	*Bacillus amyloliquefaciens*	5′ G↓G A T C C 3′ 3′ C C T A G↑G 5′	5

*The first three letters in the name of each enzyme indicates the bacterium from which it is derived.
†The λ phage DNA (see Chapter 10) consists of 48,513 base pairs.

hybridize with multiple sites in the genome. Oligonucleotides of this size can be synthesized by chemical methods.

The identification of a small mutation or polymorphism requires a pair of **allele-specific oligonucleotides** with identical lengths, one complementary to the normal sequence and the other complementary to the mutation. These probes are applied under conditions of high **stringency**. These are conditions of high temperature and/or low ionic strength that destabilize base pairing and permit annealing only if the sequences match precisely. Under conditions of low stringency, the probes would bind irrespective of the mismatch, and discrimination would be impossible.

Dot blotting (*Fig. 11.2*) is a rapid, inexpensive screening test for the detection of small mutations and polymorphisms. The extracted and denatured DNA is applied to two strips of nitrocellulose paper, which binds the single-stranded DNA tightly. One strip is dipped into a solution containing an oligonucleotide probe for the normal sequence, and the other is dipped into a solution with a probe for the mutation. *If only the probe for the normal sequence binds, the patient is homozygous normal. If only the probe for the mutation binds, the patient is homozygous for the mutation. If both probes bind, the patient is heterozygous.*

Cystic fibrosis (CF), for example, is a severe recessively inherited disease that affects 1 in 2500 newborns of European descent. About 4% of the population are heterozygous carriers of a CF mutation, and the risk of two carrier parents having an affected child is 25%.

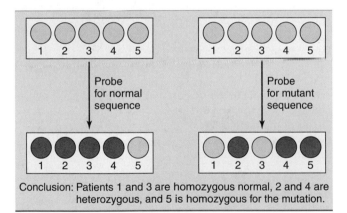

Conclusion: Patients 1 and 3 are homozygous normal, 2 and 4 are heterozygous, and 5 is homozygous for the mutation.

Figure 11.2 Use of dot blotting for diagnosis of a mutation with fluorescent-labeled probes for the normal and the mutated sequence. Denatured DNA from five different individuals is applied to two strips of nitrocellulose paper, each in a single dot. One is dipped into a solution with a probe for the normal sequence, the other into a solution with a probe for the mutant sequence. Excess probe is washed off, and the bound probe is visualized under the ultraviolet lamp.

In theory, CF is easy to prevent. All that is needed is to screen the whole population for CF mutations, identify all couples at risk, and persuade them to refrain from producing affected children. Other than a child-free lifestyle, the options for these couples include donor gametes, intrauterine or postnatal adoption, prenatal diagnosis with selective termination of affected pregnancies, and preimplantation genetic diagnosis with selective implantation of unaffected embryos.

More than 100 CF mutations are known, but a three–base-pair deletion (ΔPhe^{508} mutation) accounts for 50% to 70% of all CF mutations in the white population. For genetic screening, the DNA of large numbers of people is subjected to dot blotting with three to more than a dozen probes for the most common CF mutations in the local population. This design misses the rare mutations, but 80% to 90% of all CF carriers are identified.

SOUTHERN BLOTTING DETERMINES THE SIZE OF RESTRICTION FRAGMENTS

Southern blotting (named after Ed Southern, who developed the method in 1975) provides information not only about the presence of a mutation but also about the length of the restriction fragment carrying the mutation.

As shown in *Figure 11.3*, restriction fragments obtained from genomic DNA are separated by electrophoresis in a cross-linked agarose or polyacrylamide gel. *This method separates the restriction fragments by their size rather than their charge/mass ratio.* Small fragments move fast, and large fragments move slowly because they are retarded by the gel.

The DNA is denatured by dipping the gel into a dilute sodium hydroxide solution, and then is transferred ("blotted") to nitrocellulose paper to which it binds tightly. *A replica of the gel with its separated restriction fragments is made on the nitrocellulose.*

The desired fragment is identified by dipping the nitrocellulose paper in a neutral solution of the probe and washing off the excess unbound probe. Multiple fragments can be identified by using probes for different target sequences that are labeled with different fluorescent groups.

Northern blotting is a similar procedure for the analysis of RNA rather than DNA. **Western blotting** is a

Figure 11.3 Identification of restriction fragments by Southern blotting. Only the restriction fragments with sequence complementarity to the probe are seen in the last step. This method provides two important pieces of information. It shows whether the genomic DNA contains sequences with complementarity to the probe, and it shows the approximate length of the restriction fragment carrying these sequences. *UV,* Ultraviolet.

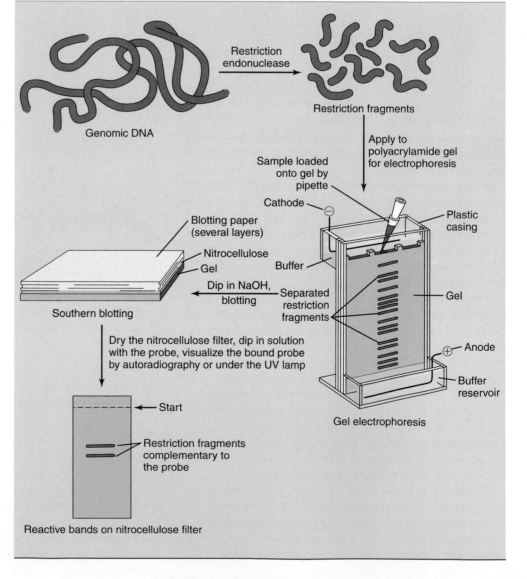

method for the separation of polypeptides that are then analyzed by monoclonal antibodies.

DNA CAN BE AMPLIFIED WITH THE POLYMERASE CHAIN REACTION

Southern blotting requires about 10 μg of DNA. This amount can be obtained from 1 ml of blood or from 10 mg of chorionic villus biopsy material. When less than this amount is available for analysis, the DNA has to be amplified with the **polymerase chain reaction (PCR)**.

The procedure (shown in *Figure 11.4*) uses a heat-stable DNA polymerase such as **Taq polymerase**. This enzyme is derived from *Thermus aquaticus,* a thermophilic bacterium that was originally isolated from a hot spring in Yellowstone National Park. It functions best at temperatures close to 60°C and can survive repeated heating to 90°C.

Like other DNA polymerases, Taq polymerase requires a primer. To amplify a defined section of genomic DNA, *a pair of oligonucleotide primers that are complementary to the ends of the targeted DNA on both strands is used.* The primers are added to the DNA in very large (>10^8-fold) molar excess, along with Taq polymerase and the precursors deoxy-ATP (dATP), deoxy-GTP (dGTP), deoxy-CTP (dCTP), and deoxy-TTP (dTTP). *This mix is repeatedly heated to 90°C in order to denature the target DNA and cooled to 60°C for annealing of the primers and polymerization.*

The target DNA is replicated in each cycle, and a single DNA molecule can be amplified to more than one million copies in about 1 hour. The resulting **PCR product** is a blunt-ended, double-stranded DNA that has the primers incorporated at its ends. It can be analyzed either by electrophoresis alone or by the use of allele-specific probes.

PCR has been used to amplify DNA from buccal smears, from single hairs sent to the laboratory in the mail or found at the scene of a crime, and even for sequencing of the Neanderthal genome from 40,000-year-old bones. However, it is difficult to reliably amplify DNA sequences longer than three kilobases. Individual exons can be amplified easily, but most genes are too large to be amplified in one piece. One limitation is that the Taq polymerase has no proofreading 3′-exonuclease activity. Therefore it misincorporates bases at a rate of about 1 every 5000 to 10,000 base pairs.

PCR IS USED FOR PREIMPLANTATION GENETIC DIAGNOSIS

PCR is especially useful in **prenatal diagnosis.** *The aim of prenatal diagnosis is the detection of severe fetal defects, with the option of terminating affected pregnancies.* Fetal cells can be obtained by chorionic villus sampling at about 10 weeks of gestation or by amniocentesis at about 16 weeks. In this context, PCR is used to obviate the time-consuming culturing of fetal cells.

Preimplantation genetic diagnosis is a high-tech alternative to prenatal diagnosis. The embryo is produced by in vitro fertilization (IVF) and allowed to grow to the 8- or 16-cell stage. At this point, *a single cell is removed from the embryo to supply the DNA for the diagnostic test.* This does not impair further development of the embryo. Up to one dozen embryos are obtained in a single IVF cycle. All of them are subjected to the diagnostic test, and only the healthy ones are implanted.

PCR with nested primers is used to amplify DNA from a single cell. In this procedure, a section of the target DNA is amplified, and the amplification product is subjected to a second round of PCR with a more closely spaced primer pair.

Figure 11.5 shows the use of PCR with nested primers for preimplantation diagnosis of the ΔPhe^{508} mutation. This three–base-pair deletion is readily identified by PCR followed by gel electrophoresis because the mutated sequence yields a PCR product three base pairs shorter than normal. However, base substitutions cannot be identified by electrophoresis alone. They require the application of allele-specific probes to the PCR product.

PCR can detect deletions of entire exons or genes. For example, **Duchenne muscular dystrophy** is a fatal X-linked recessive muscle disease caused by deletions in the gene for the muscle protein dystrophin. With 79 exons scattered over more than two million base pairs of DNA, the dystrophin gene is the largest gene in the human genome. Most patients have large deletions that remove one or several exons from the gene.

Figure 11.6 shows how these deletions are identified by amplification of deletion-prone exons. *If one of the target exons is deleted, its PCR product is absent.*

ALLELIC HETEROGENEITY IS THE GREATEST CHALLENGE FOR MOLECULAR GENETIC DIAGNOSIS

All patients with sickle cell disease have the same mutation. Therefore a single pair of allele-specific oligonucleotide probes is sufficient for molecular diagnosis. However, this is an unusual situation. More commonly, any **loss-of-function mutation** that prevents the synthesis of a functional protein product will cause disease. In some diseases, such as CF, a small number of mutations accounts for a large majority of the cases. Therefore most carriers can be identified with a small assortment of oligonucleotide probes, one for each common mutation.

In the worst cases, most or all mutations for the disease are rare. In the X-linked clotting disorder **hemophilia B,** for example, more than 2000 different mutations in the gene for clotting factor IX have been observed in different patients. This degree of **allelic**

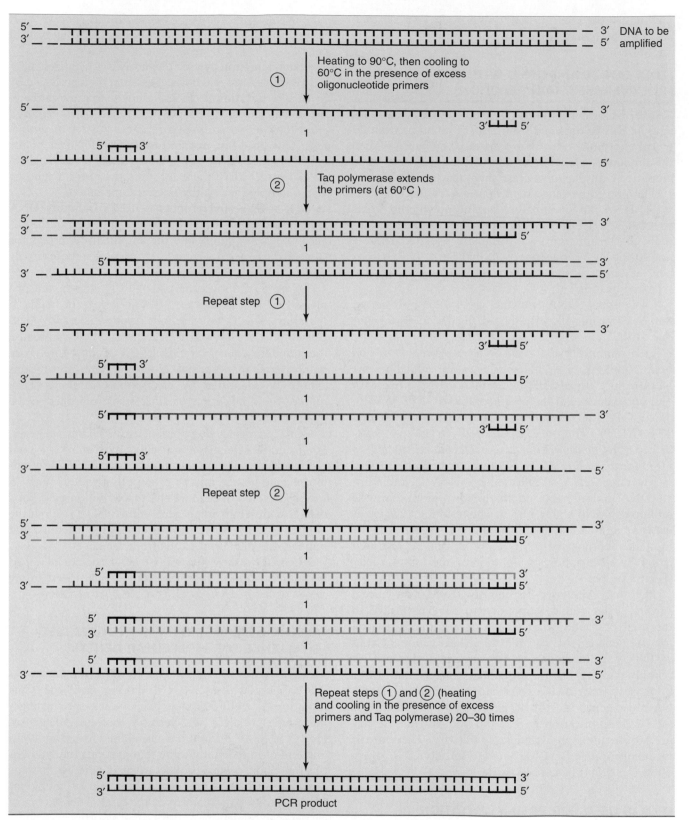

Figure 11.4 Polymerase chain reaction (PCR). The sequence to be amplified is defined by the 5′ ends of the oligonucleotide primers. The primers base pair with the heat-denatured DNA strands. The Taq polymerase catalyzes DNA polymerization at 60°C and survives a temperature of 90°C during heat denaturation of the DNA. Neither primer nor Taq polymerase needs to be added during repeated cycles of heating and cooling. In theory, the amount of DNA between the primers doubles during each cycle of heating and cooling. ⌴⌴⌴, Oligonucleotide primer.

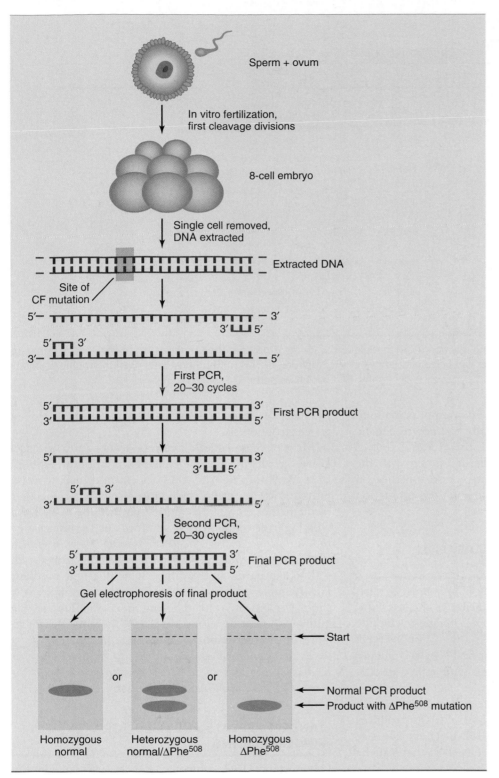

Figure 11.5 Use of polymerase chain reaction (PCR) with nested primers for preimplantation diagnosis of the ΔPhe^{508} cystic fibrosis mutation. This three-base-pair deletion results in a PCR product three nucleotides shorter than normal. The two PCR products can be separated by gel electrophoresis.

Within the figure:

Sperm + ovum

In vitro fertilization, first cleavage divisions

8-cell embryo

Single cell removed, DNA extracted

Extracted DNA

Site of CF mutation

First PCR, 20–30 cycles

First PCR product

Second PCR, 20–30 cycles

Final PCR product

Gel electrophoresis of final product

Start

or   or

Normal PCR product
Product with ΔPhe^{508} mutation

Homozygous normal

Heterozygous normal/ΔPhe^{508}

Homozygous ΔPhe^{508}

heterogeneity makes the use of allele-specific oligonucleotide probes impractical. There are three ways to obviate this problem:

1. *Mismatch scanning*. This is done by amplifying the exons of the gene and hybridizing the PCR products from the patient with the corresponding products from the normal gene. The mismatch can be detected either by chemical reagents that cleave selectively at the site of the mismatch or by electrophoresis under partially denaturing conditions.

2. *Gene sequencing*. Sequencing all exons of the gene is becoming popular because of rapid advances in sequencing technology.

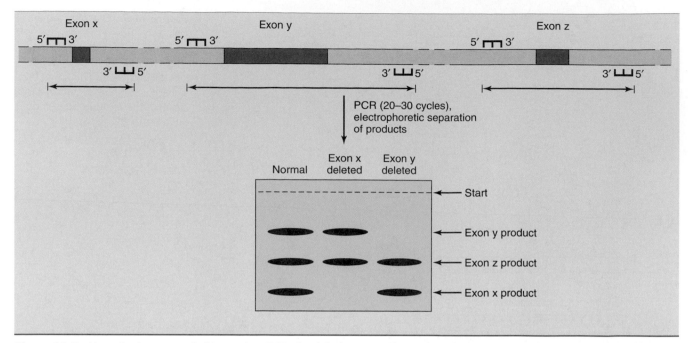

Figure 11.6 Use of polymerase chain reaction (PCR) for deletion scanning. Note that the primer pairs are designed to generate PCR products of different lengths that can be separated by gel electrophoresis. This method has been used to amplify deletion-prone exons in patients with Duchenne muscular dystrophy. ▪, Exons; ⊔⊔, primer.

3. *Linkage analysis.* In this case, no attempt is made to identify the mutation. Instead, a known genetic marker that is located next to the mutated gene is analyzed. The mutation is inherited along with the marker simply because they are close together on the same DNA molecule, and meiotic recombination between the gene and the marker is very rare.

NORMAL POLYMORPHISMS ARE USED AS GENETIC MARKERS

A polymorphism is defined as any DNA sequence variant for which the population frequency of the less common allele is more than 1%. **Single-nucleotide polymorphisms (SNPs)** are the most common type. There are more than 15 million SNPs in the human genome. They can be analyzed with allele-specific probes or with DNA microarrays.

Some SNPs obliterate or create a cleavage site for a restriction endonuclease. This subset of SNPs produces **restriction-site polymorphisms (RSPs)**. They give rise to restriction fragments of different sizes that can be separated easily by gel electrophoresis.

Microsatellite polymorphisms are even more useful. These are tandemly repeated sequences with, in most cases, two to four nucleotides in the repeat unit and a total length well below 1000 base pairs (*Fig. 11.7, B*). The number of repeat units, and therefore the length of the microsatellite, varies among people. *Whereas SNPs and RSPs have only two alleles, the most useful microsatellites have more than two alleles.* Polymorphic microsatellites produce restriction fragments and PCR products of different length that can be separated by gel electrophoresis.

Most of these genetic markers do not cause disease. However, when a disease-causing mutation arises next to a polymorphic site on the chromosome, disease mutation and normal polymorphism travel together through the generations until they get divorced by a crossing-over in meiosis. Therefore *the inheritance of the mutation can be traced by tracing the inheritance of the polymorphic markers with which it is associated.*

Linkage patterns are different in different families. For example, the same mutation can arise next to a short variant of a neighboring microsatellite in one family and next to a long variant of the same microsatellite in another family. Therefore *linkage cannot be used for population screening; it can be used only for studies of families in which the genotypes of one or more affected individuals are known.*

TANDEM REPEATS ARE USED FOR DNA FINGERPRINTING

Polymorphic DNA sequences can be used to identify criminals and, as has happened in many cases, for exonerating prisoners who had been wrongly convicted. This application is called **DNA fingerprinting.** Any polymorphism can be used, but microsatellite polymorphisms are most useful for DNA fingerprinting.

DNA fingerprinting can be performed with Southern blotting or PCR (*Fig. 11.8*). Southern blotting requires a substantial amount of DNA, for example, from a drop of seminal fluid from a sex offender.

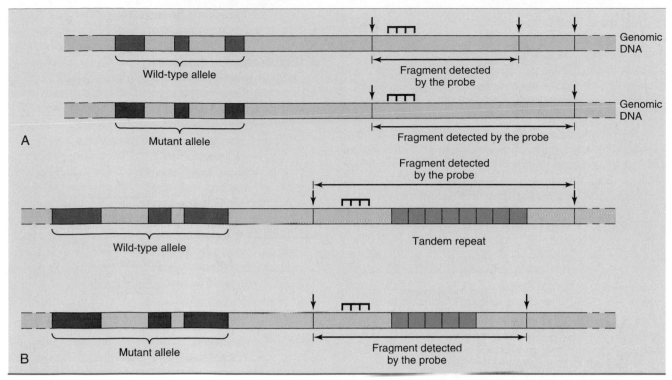

Figure 11.7 Use of restriction-site polymorphisms and polymorphic tandem repeats for linkage analysis. **A,** A restriction-site polymorphism is caused by a base substitution in the recognition site of a restriction endonuclease. In this example, the normal ("wild-type") allele is linked to the shorter fragment, and the mutant allele is linked to the longer fragment. **B,** Polymorphic microsatellites are especially useful because more than two alleles (repeat lengths) occur in the population. In this example, the mutant allele of the heterozygote will be transmitted to the children together with the shorter fragment. ↓, Cleavage by the restriction endonuclease; ⊓⊓, probe used to detect the polymorphism.

PCR is used when only a small amount of DNA is available, for example, from a single hair of the murderer stuck under the victim's fingernail. However, because of its high sensitivity, PCR is more vulnerable to contamination by extraneous DNA. This could put the laboratory technician at risk for being wrongly convicted!

Another use of polymorphic microsatellites is paternity testing. Unlike the time-honored method of blood group typing, DNA tests allow an almost 100% accurate determination of paternity, unless the candidate fathers are monozygotic twins.

DNA MICROARRAYS CAN BE USED FOR GENETIC SCREENING

Dot blotting tests for only one or a few mutations or polymorphisms at a time. **DNA microarrays,** also known as "DNA chips," permit simultaneous testing of up to one million genetic variants.

An **oligonucleotide microarray** is prepared from a glass slide that is subdivided into up to one million little squares. Through photochemical methods, *oligonucleotide probes with a length of 20 to 60 nucleotides are synthesized on each square.* Each square receives a different oligonucleotide that is complementary to a short stretch of genomic DNA. Different probes are made for the alternative alleles of a polymorphic site.

Fluorescent-labeled genomic DNA fragments that are applied to the microarray hybridize primarily with the exact complementary probe but not the probe for the alternative allele. For example, when one square of the microarray has a probe for the sickle cell mutation and another has a probe for the corresponding normal sequence, normal DNA produces substantially more fluorescence on the square for the normal sequence. DNA from a sickle cell patient produces substantially more fluorescence on the square with the probe for the sickle cell mutation, and the DNA of a heterozygote produces about equal fluorescence on both. However, more imaginative methods are being explored as well (*Fig. 11.9*).

Copy number variations are diagnosed with **array-based comparative genomic hybridization** (*Fig. 11.10*). In this method the probes on the microarray do not need to be directed at polymorphic sites. They only need to be targeted at sequences that are spaced more or less evenly across the genome. Patient DNA and reference DNA are labeled with different-colored fluorescent groups, and equal amounts of the two DNAs are mixed. After application to the microarray, both kinds of fluorescence are about equally strong on most of

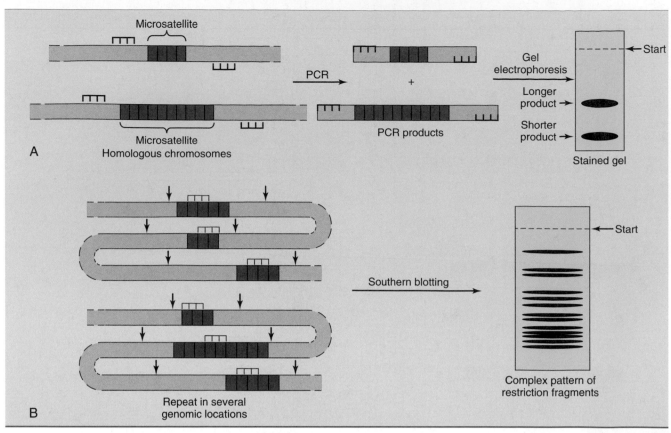

Figure 11.8 Use of polymorphic tandem repeats for DNA fingerprinting. **A,** Microsatellites consist of dinucleotides, trinucleotides, or tetranucleotide repeats. They are used for single-locus DNA fingerprinting with the polymerase chain reaction (PCR). Even if the repeat is present in many places throughout the genome, use of the primers ensures that only one of them is amplified. The two homologous chromosomes in each individual will produce two PCR products, and in most cases they will be of different lengths. This method does not require a probe because the PCR products can be identified directly by staining the gel after electrophoresis. **B,** Longer tandem repeats (also called minisatellites) that are present in a limited number of genomic locations can be used for multilocus DNA fingerprinting. The DNA is fragmented with a frequently cutting restriction endonuclease. After Southern blotting, the fragments are detected with a probe for the repeat sequence itself. If, for example, the repeat is present in 20 genomic locations, gel electrophoresis will show a unique pattern of up to 40 bands. ⊓⊓, Primer; ⊓⊓⊓, probe; ↓, restriction site.

Figure 11.9 Experimental method for microarray-based single-nucleotide polymorphism (SNP) genotyping. Note that the fluorescent-labeled dideoxynucleotides (ddATP, ddCTP, ddGTP, ddTTP) are incorporated by the DNA polymerase but also cause immediate chain termination, similar to their use in DNA sequencing (see **Fig. 11.13**). The immobilized oligonucleotides on the DNA chip are complementary to those that were incubated with the genomic DNA.

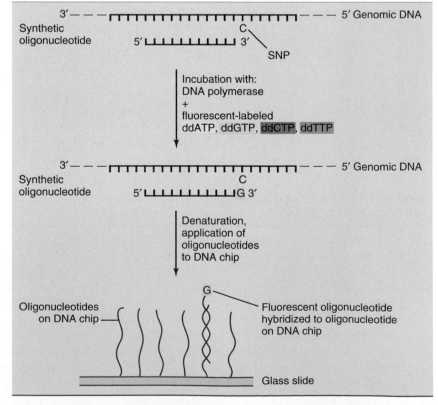

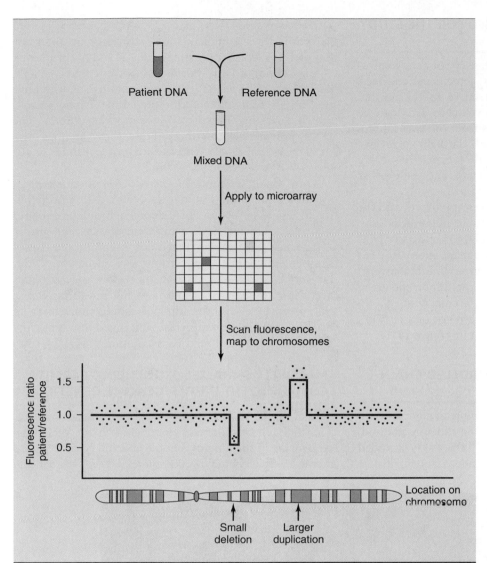

Figure 11.10 Use of comparative genome hybridization for detection of duplications and deletions. Patient DNA and control DNA are labeled with different fluorescent dyes. A deletion in the patient reduces the fluorescence of patient DNA relative to reference DNA by 50%, and a duplication enhances this ratio by 50%.

the squares. However, in places where the patient has a deletion, the fluorescence from the reference DNA is stronger; and where the patient has a duplication, the patient DNA produces the stronger fluorescence.

CLINICAL EXAMPLE 11.1: Molecular Diagnosis of Mental Retardation

Mental deficiency can have many different causes. Environmental causes include trauma, intrauterine infections, hypoxia, prematurity, and severe jaundice at birth. Genetic causes include single-gene disorders, aberrations in chromosome number, and chromosomal rearrangements.

Traditionally, the cause of mental deficiency could be identified in only about half of the patients. Chromosomal deletions, translocations, and duplications involving more than about three million base pairs can be identified in a **banded karyotype** by observing stained chromosomes under the microscope. Such large aberrations are the cause of mental retardation in 3% to 4% of patients.

Another 5% to 6% of patients are found to have smaller genomic aberrations that are not detected with a banded karyotype but are found by **fluorescent in situ hybridization** (**FISH**) with fluorescent probes directed at frequently affected sites in the genome. In this method, the fluorescent probe is applied to the chromosome spread and is identified under the microscope.

Array-based comparative genomic hybridization detects another 4% to 7% of patients. Thus it appears that overall between 12% and 18% of mentally retarded patients owe their condition to genomic aberrations that involve one or several genes. Genomic abnormalities are more likely to be found in mentally retarded patients who also have physical abnormalities.

DNA MICROARRAYS ARE USED FOR THE STUDY OF GENE EXPRESSION

Microarrays are also used for the study of gene expression. For example, in cancer cells, some genes are overactive and others are silenced relative to the normal tissue from which the cancer developed. This can be studied by extracting the mRNAs from the two sources and turning them into cDNA with the help of reverse transcriptase. The cDNAs from the normal tissue are equipped with a green fluorescent tag, and the cDNAs from the tumor with a red fluorescent tag.

The cDNAs from the two sources are mixed, and the mix is applied to a microarray that has oligonucleotides or cDNAs complementary to the cDNAs under study. If the expression of a gene is increased in the tumor, the red fluorescence is stronger than the green fluorescence; if the gene's expression is reduced in the tumor, the green fluorescence is stronger. In theory, a chip with 30,000 squares can test for the expression of each of a person's 30,000 genes. An example is shown in **Figure 11.11**.

DNA IS SEQUENCED BY CONTROLLED CHAIN TERMINATION

Whole-genome sequencing is becoming an alternative to array-based genetic diagnosis. In the **dideoxy method**, the DNA to be sequenced is used in a single-stranded form. A short oligonucleotide primer is annealed to a sequence in this DNA, and a DNA polymerase is used to synthesize a complementary strand of up to a few hundred nucleotides, starting at the 3′ end of the primer.

In addition to the normal substrates dATP, dGTP, dTTP and dCTP, each test tube contains small quantities of all four **dideoxyribonucleoside triphosphates**, which lack the 3′-hydroxyl group (**Fig. 11.12**). The DNA polymerase can incorporate these analogs into the DNA, but *DNA synthesis cannot continue in the absence of a 3′-hydroxyl group*.

Only small amounts of the dideoxyribonucleotides are added, so chain termination occurs with a probability of less than 1% in each step. Each dideoxyribonucleotide is labeled with a different fluorescent group. Automated sequencing machines separate the newly synthesized chains by electrophoresis in narrow capillaries. This produces a string of closely spaced bands according to the chain lengths of the products, whose fluorescence reveals the kind of dideoxynucleotide at their 3′ end. The fluorescence is scanned automatically by a laser beam and read by a computer (**Fig. 11.13**).

MASSIVELY PARALLEL SEQUENCING PERMITS COST-EFFICIENT WHOLE-GENOME GENETIC DIAGNOSIS

The dideoxy method was good enough for the initial sequencing of the human genome and still is the standard method implemented by commercial DNA sequencing

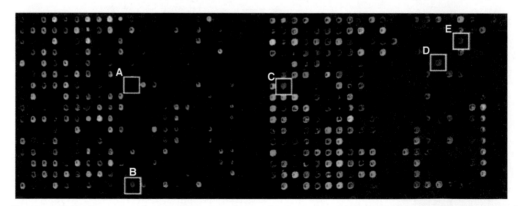

Figure 11.11 Section of a microarray showing a comparison of messenger RNA (mRNA) levels in fibroblasts (*green*) and rhabdomyosarcoma cells (*red*).

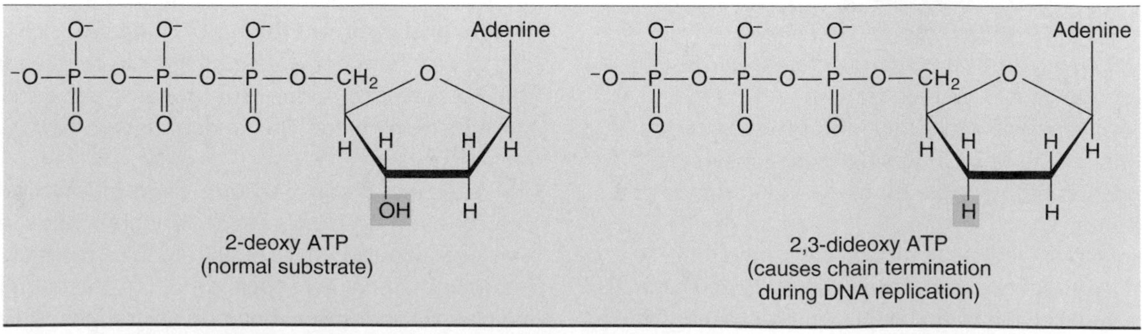

Figure 11.12 Structure of a dideoxynucleoside triphosphate. DNA polymerases can incorporate a dideoxynucleotide into a new DNA strand, but further chain growth is prevented by lack of a free 3′-hydroxyl group. *ATP*, Adenosine triphosphate.

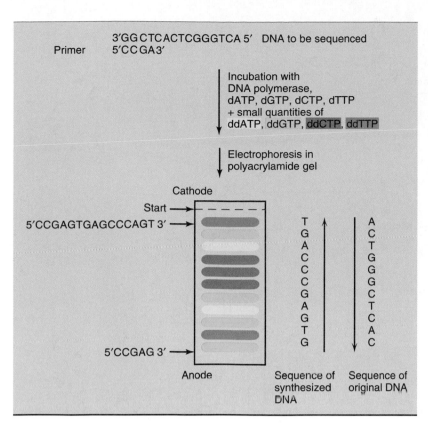

Figure 11.13 DNA sequencing with the dideoxy method. Each of the four dideoxynucleotides (ddATP, ddCTP, ddGTP, ddTTP) is labeled with a different fluorescent tag. They are added with a large excess of the deoxynucleotides dATP, dCTP, dGTP, and dTTP.

machines. However, the ultimate aim is the diagnostic use of whole-genome sequencing at a cost not much higher than $1000 per genome.

This aim is pursued by miniaturization of procedures and by running thousands to millions of sequencings in parallel. The sequence reads are aligned in the computer. In most techniques, DNA is amplified on a solid surface, such as a glass slide (*Fig. 11.14, A*) or the surface of microbeads. Amplification is followed by sequencing, which usually is done by synthesis of a complementary strand (*Fig. 11.14, B*).

Several commercial sequencing systems are entering the marketplace. Whether whole-genome sequencing will make the diagnostic use of DNA microarrays obsolete in the not-too-distant future remains to be seen.

PATHOGENIC DNA VARIANTS ARE LOCATED BY GENOME-WIDE ASSOCIATION STUDIES

The diagnosis of genetic disease risks requires knowledge of disease-related genes. Although the molecular causes of many single-gene disorders are known in some detail, little is known about the genetic risk factors for "multifactorial" diseases, which include the majority of all diseases encountered in medical practice.

The **common disease—common polymorphism hypothesis** proposes that most genetic risk factors are common genetic variations that each makes a small contribution to the disease risk. These genetic variants are identified with a type of case-control study known as a **genome-wide association (GWA) study.**

The prime tool for the GWA study is the DNA microarray. Typically, more than 1000 patients with a multifactorial disease such as myocardial infarction, stroke, asthma, or Alzheimer disease ("cases") are genotyped along with several thousand unaffected individuals ("controls"). Genotyping for up to one million SNPs is routine in these studies. An SNP is associated with the disease if one of its alleles is significantly over-represented or underrepresented in cases relative to controls. The statistical significance level must be strictly defined because with measurement of hundreds of thousands of SNPs, some will be highly associated with the disease simply by chance.

Some of the correctly identified SNPs may themselves be causal contributors to disease risk. More likely, however, they are merely associated with a causal DNA variant located nearby on the chromosome. This nonrandom association is called **genetic linkage.**

Linkage occurs because every new pathogenic mutation arises on a single chromosome that already has its own fingerprint of SNPs and other polymorphisms left and right of the site of the mutation. New mutation and preexisting polymorphisms are inherited together through the generations simply because they are close together on the same DNA molecule. In the course of many generations, however, genetic linkage slowly decays because of crossing-over in meiosis.

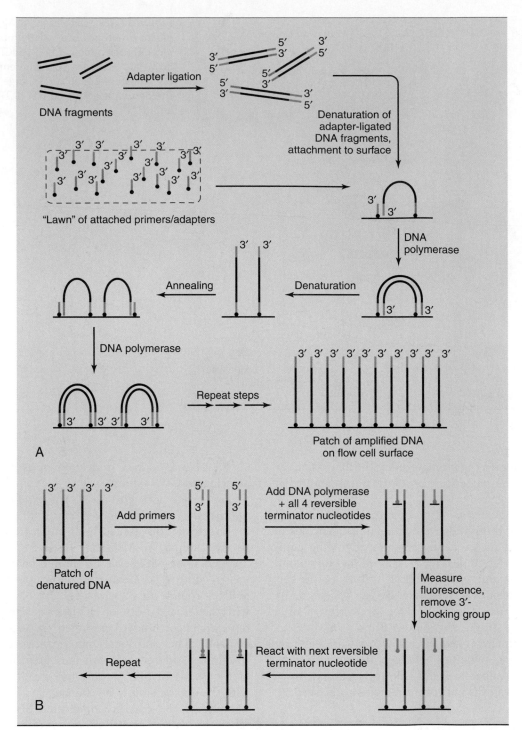

Figure 11.14 A "next generation" procedure for massively parallel DNA sequencing. **A,** Amplification step. DNA fragments are equipped with adapters at both ends. The adapters of a single DNA fragment bind to complementary primers that are attached to a slide. A patch of this DNA is generated by "bridge amplification." **B,** Sequencing-by-synthesis step. A mix of nucleotide analogs that have both a fluorescent label and a blocked 3'-hydroxyl group is added. The fluorescence is scanned before the 3' blocking group is removed for the next step of synthesis.

As a consequence, population-based GWA studies are promising only for disease-associated variants that originated in a single individual dozens to hundreds of generations ago and have already spread to a substantial percentage of the population, either by chance or by natural selection. *Such variants usually will have a small effect on the disease risk because highly pathogenic mutations are quickly removed by natural selection.*

The alternative **mutational load hypothesis** assumes that pathogenic mutations, some of them having a rather large effect, arise by chance in every generation but are removed continuously by purifying selection. Because these pathogenic mutations are short lived, they show consistent linkage patterns only in affected families or small inbred populations, but not in large, heterogeneous populations. *This type of genetic risk factor cannot be investigated by population-based GWA studies but is best studied with whole-genome sequencing.*

To date, GWA studies can explain only a small percentage of the genetic disease risk for any major multifactorial disease. Studies that use whole-genome sequencing will be the next step in this research program.

GENOMIC DNA FRAGMENTS CAN BE PROPAGATED IN BACTERIAL PLASMIDS

Molecular cloning is the propagation and multiplication of selected DNAs in microorganisms. Most methods use a **cloning vector** that is derived from a plasmid or bacteriophage or is constructed de novo ("from scratch") as an artificial chromosome. *Cloning requires the covalent joining of the foreign DNA with the vector DNA.*

Figure 11.15 shows the cloning of human DNA with a plasmid-derived cloning vector. Resistance genes for tetracycline and ampicillin in the cloning vector serve

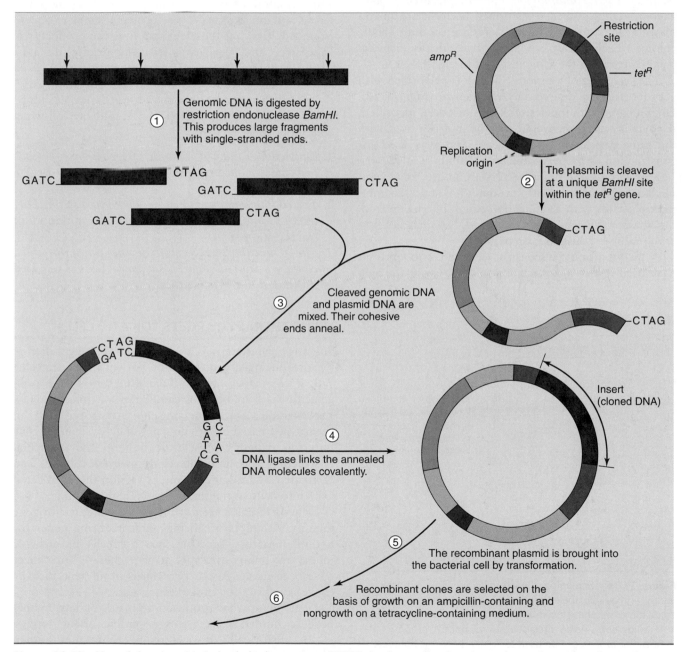

Figure 11.15 Use of the plasmid-derived cloning vector pBR322. In the application shown here, the tetracycline resistance (*tet^R*) gene is destroyed during cloning, but the ampicillin resistance (*amp^R*) gene remains intact. Bacteria transformed by a recombinant plasmid can be selected because they can grow in the presence of ampicillin but not tetracycline.

as **selectable markers** that permit the selective survival of vector-containing bacteria on antibiotic-containing media.

The same restriction endonuclease is used to fragment the human DNA into large pieces of many thousand base pairs and to cleave the vector at a single site in the tetracycline resistance gene. Plasmid DNA and human DNA are mixed in the test tube, and their cohesive ends anneal spontaneously. DNA ligase is added, and *plasmid DNA and human DNA are covalently linked into a circle.* The recombinant plasmids are spirited into the bacteria by transformation.

*A **genomic library** is a large collection of transformed bacteria, each containing a random piece of human genomic DNA.* When transformed bacteria are spread on an agar plate, individual bacteria grow into visible colonies. Each colony is a **clone** of genetically identical bacteria carrying the same insert of foreign DNA.

The **screening** of a genomic library is performed with a probe for the desired DNA sequence (**Fig. 11.16**). Once a clone with the desired DNA has been identified, the vector can be recovered and the insert excised with the same restriction endonuclease that was used for construction of the recombinant plasmid.

Many kinds of cloning vectors are in use. For example, **bacterial artificial chromosomes** are large recombinant plasmids with a replication origin borrowed from the F factor. They are used to clone DNA pieces of several hundred thousand base pairs.

A **cDNA library** is constructed from mRNAs that have been reverse transcribed into cDNA with the help of reverse transcriptase. It contains only the *expressed* DNA of a cell type or tissue. For example, a cDNA library from bone marrow contains many clones with the cDNAs for hemoglobin α- and β-chains, whereas a cDNA library from the pancreas contains many cDNAs for pancreatic zymogens.

EXPRESSION VECTORS ARE USED TO MANUFACTURE USEFUL PROTEINS

Many human proteins can be used as therapeutic agents. They include hormones such as insulin, growth hormone, and erythropoietin, blood clotting factors, and mediators of immune responses such as the interferons and interleukins. These proteins can be extracted from cadavers, but the yields are low, the products are expensive, and they can transmit deadly diseases. Therefore *many therapeutic proteins now are produced with the help of genetically engineered bacteria.*

The effective transcription and translation of cloned DNA requires an **expression vector,** and the following conditions must be met:

1. *Only cDNA and not genomic DNA can be expressed in bacteria.* Bacteria cannot splice introns out of a transcript.
2. *The coding sequence must be joined to a strong bacterial promoter.* This is required for initiation of transcription.
3. *The 5'-untranslated region of the transcript must contain a Shine-Dalgarno sequence.* This is required for initiation of translation.

GENE THERAPY TARGETS SOMATIC CELLS

Somatic gene therapy is an attempt at treating a disease by introducing a gene into the patient's somatic cells. *This strategy does not manipulate the germ line.* Monogenic diseases are obvious candidates for this approach. For example, Duchenne muscular dystrophy can, in theory, be treated by bringing an intact dystrophin gene into the patient's muscle fibers, and the bronchial obstruction and lung infections in cystic fibrosis can be treated by bringing an intact version of the affected gene into cells of the patient's lung epithelium.

Genetic diseases are not the only candidates for gene therapy. Attempts are being made to bring genes for antiinflammatory proteins into the cells of arthritic joints, and many attempts at gene therapy for cancer have been made. About two thirds of all gene therapy trials have been for cancer treatment.

Gene therapy has produced no magic bullets, mainly because human cells are xenophobic about foreign DNA. Historically, most foreign DNAs that human cells encountered have been viruses. Therefore foreign DNA is not allowed to cross the plasma membrane and the nuclear envelope, and watchful DNases are

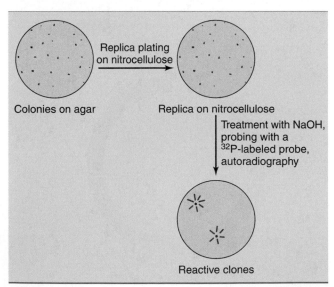

Figure 11.16 Screening of bacterial clones in a genomic library with a radiolabeled probe. Only the clones (colonies) that contain the matching insert bind the probe and are identified by autoradiography. As an alternative to radioactive probes, fluorescent probes can be used to screen genomic libraries. Fluorescent probes can be detected directly under the ultraviolet lamp, without the need for autoradiography. *32P*, Radioactive phosphorus.

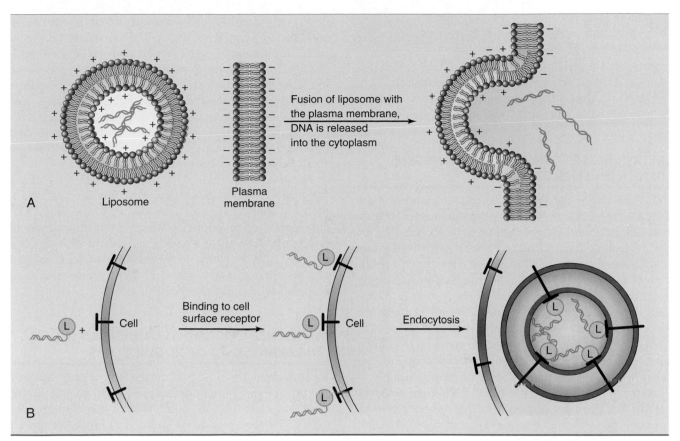

Figure 11.17 Physical methods of gene delivery. **A,** The foreign gene is enclosed in a liposome. To facilitate fusion of the liposome with the plasma membrane, the liposome is constructed in large part from cationic lipids. **B,** The foreign gene is covalently linked to a ligand that is taken up by receptor-mediated endocytosis. Only cells possessing the receptor for the ligand are transformed. Viral proteins that disrupt the endosome membrane can be added as well, to prevent routing of the DNA to the lysosomes. *L,* Ligand; T, receptor.

lurking at every corner. Methods have been developed to facilitate the cellular uptake of foreign DNA (*Fig. 11.17*), but none has been notably efficient.

Even if a therapeutic gene reaches the cytoplasm, uptake into the nucleus is limited, and in the nucleus, stable integration into the genome is a rare event.

VIRUSES ARE USED AS VECTORS FOR GENE THERAPY

Viruses are already well designed to bring their genes into the host cell. In theory, all that is needed for gene therapy is to replace one or more of the viral genes by the therapeutic **transgene** and have it ferried into the cell by the virus. This process of virus-mediated gene transfer is called **transfection.**

DNA viruses can be used for this purpose. Adenoviruses, for example, are minor respiratory pathogens in humans. It is possible to replace some nonessential viral genes by an intact gene for the chloride channel that is defective in cystic fibrosis (CF). The virus will bring this transgene into the cells of the respiratory epithelium of CF patients, where it is expressed as long as the virus is present. However, *DNA viruses do not normally integrate themselves into the host cell DNA.* Therefore the therapeutic benefits are transient.

Also, viral proteins and virus particles are still produced by the vector. This damages the cells and alerts the adaptive immune system to produce antibodies against the virus and destroy the virus-infected cells. However, these vectors can be produced in quantity, and they are able to infect nondividing cells.

CLINICAL EXAMPLE 11.2: Risks of Gene Therapy

In 2000, a trial of gene therapy for an X-linked form of severe combined immunodeficiency was started in France. The white blood cells of the patients were treated with a retroviral vector containing the functional version of the defective gene in vitro and then reinserted into the body. The initial results were promising, and most of the 10 affected children in the trial improved.

In 2002, excitement gave way to alarm when two of the children developed a leukemia-like disease with abnormal proliferation of lymphocytes. In these two children, the retroviral vector had inserted next to the

Continued

CLINICAL EXAMPLE 11.2: Risks of Gene Therapy—cont'd

promoter of a growth-promoting cellular gene, thereby turning it into a cancer-promoting oncogene (see Chapter 18). This greatly enhanced the expression of the cellular gene and caused abnormal cell proliferation.

RETROVIRUSES CAN SPLICE A TRANSGENE INTO THE CELL'S GENOME

Retroviruses are the most popular vectors for somatic gene therapy because they integrate themselves into the host cell genome as part of their normal lifecycle. The retroviral vectors that are used for gene therapy contain the long terminal repeats of a "real" retrovirus, but except for a portion of the *gag* gene that doubles as a packaging signal, *the viral genes are replaced by the transgene*. Therefore the vector can produce neither viral proteins nor virus particles. Retroviral vectors can carry inserts of up to 9000 base pairs, enough to code for a large protein. The transgenes are intronless constructs that are produced from a cDNA or are chemically synthesized.

Retroviral vectors are produced in cultured cells that contain the genomes of two defective retroviruses. One contains the viral genes but no packaging signal; the other is the vector with transgene and packaging signal but no viral genes. These cells produce virus particles, but only the vector RNA is packaged into the virus together with reverse transcriptase and integrase (*Fig. 11.18*).

Retroviral gene transfer is not very efficient. Even in cell cultures, fewer than 10% of the cells are transfected in most experiments. Because most other retroviruses lack a nuclear localization signal and therefore can infect only dividing cells, many retroviral vectors are constructed from lentiviruses, the retroviral family to which human immunodeficiency virus (HIV) belongs.

Gene therapy still is experimental. It is most promising in cases where transfection of a small number of cells is sufficient to cure the disease and tightly regulated gene expression is not required. For example, clotting factor deficiencies such as hemophilia potentially can be treated by bringing an intact copy of the affected gene into a small percentage of liver cells.

However, gene therapy for diabetes with a transgene for insulin would be difficult because expression of the gene would have to be responsive to the blood glucose level. In hemoglobinopathies, the transgene would have to be brought into a substantial fraction of bone marrow cells in which it would have to be expressed at appropriate levels and during the right stages of erythrocyte maturation.

ANTISENSE OLIGONUCLEOTIDES CAN BLOCK THE EXPRESSION OF ROGUE GENES

Some diseases are caused not by the lack of a normal gene but by the expression or overexpression of an undesirable gene. In cancers, for example, growth-stimulating genes either are overexpressed or mutated to produce superactive proteins. These genes are called **oncogenes** (see Chapter 18). In theory, *cancer growth can be blocked by inhibiting the expression of oncogenes in the malignant cells*. Similarly, *viral diseases can be treated by inhibiting the expression of essential viral genes*.

Antisense technology makes use of oligonucleotides that are complementary to an undesirable mRNA. By hybridizing with the mRNA, the antisense oligonucleotide

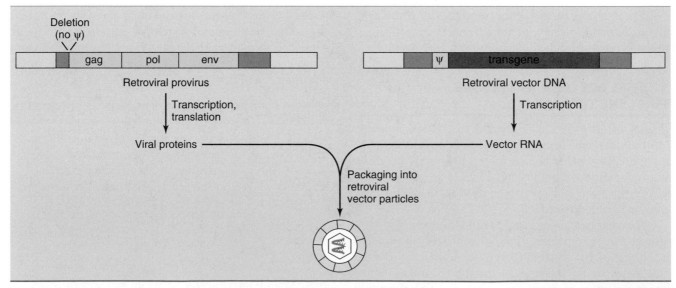

Figure 11.18 Construction of a retroviral vector for gene therapy. Both the retroviral provirus and the retroviral vector DNA are integrated in the producer cell genome. The vector RNA is packaged with the proteins produced by the retroviral provirus. The provirus RNA cannot be packaged because it lacks the packaging signal. ▢, Viral genes; ▪, long terminal repeat; ▪, foreign gene to be transferred; Ψ, packaging signal; gag, pol, and env, normal retroviral genes.

blocks translation and, in many cases, induces the cleavage of the mRNA by **RNase H.** Ordinarily, this cellular enzyme cleaves the RNA strand in a DNA-RNA hybrid. It participates in primer removal during DNA replication, and it is part of the cell's defenses against viral infections.

Antisense agents must have a length of at least 18 to 20 nucleotides to achieve sufficient selectivity for their target sequence, and *nuclease-resistant oligonucleotide analogs are commonly used. Figure 11.19* shows some examples. However, very high doses of these rather expensive oligonucleotides would have to be used because of their poor uptake into cells.

Another approach exploits the natural process of **RNA interference.** It uses short pieces of *double-stranded* RNA with a length of 20 to 25 base pairs that is complementary to a site in the undesirable mRNA and acts as a small interfering RNA (**siRNA**). Alternatively, a short hairpin RNA (**shRNA**) can be used that is processed to a siRNA by the nucleases drosha and dicer. One of the RNA strands becomes bound to the Ago2 protein in the RNA-induced silencing complex (RISC), which then cleaves the targeted mRNA (see Chapter 7).

In theory, a single double-stranded RNA molecule can direct the enzyme to destroy thousands of mRNA molecules carrying the same sequence. Effectively, *the antisense oligonucleotide tricks the cell into treating its own mRNA as an invading RNA virus.*

GENES CAN BE ALTERED IN ANIMALS

The functions of genes can be studied by genetic modifications in laboratory animals, usually mice. Three approaches can be used.

1. **Knockout** is selective disruption of a normal gene in the germ line. It produces **knockout mice,** whose phenotype reveals the biological function of the knocked-out gene.
2. **Knockin** is the insertion of a gene that is not normally present in the genome. It produces **transgenic animals.**
3. **Knockdown** is achieved by preventing the translation of an mRNA, without changing the genome. Unlike the other methods, which are performed in the zygote or early embryo, gene knockdown is done in adult mice. The genome remains unchanged, and the manipulation is reversible.

All three methods are used to create animal models of human diseases. Transgenic animals are used not only in research but also in "pharming." For example, cattle and sheep that secrete human hormones, clotting factors, or other therapeutic proteins in their milk have been produced.

Knockout mice and transgenic mice can be produced with DNA constructs that have sequence homology with the targeted gene (*Fig. 11.20*). These constructs

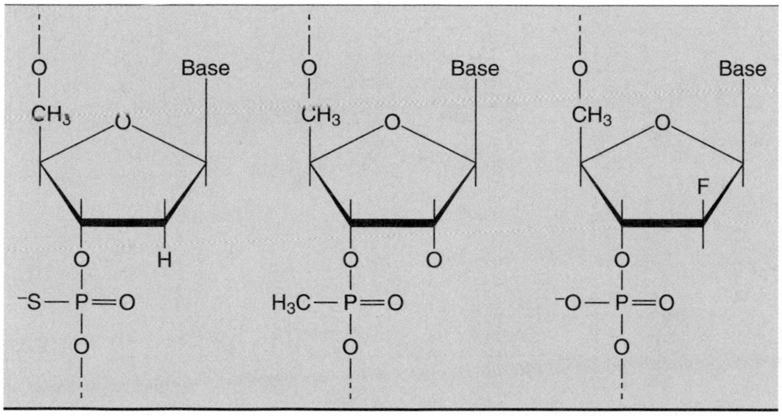

Figure 11.19 Structural modifications in experimentally used antisense oligonucleotides. These modifications are intended to make the oligonucleotides resistant to nucleases, facilitate their uptake into cells, or increase their affinity for their mRNA targets.

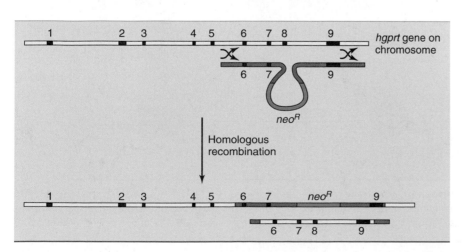

Figure 11.20 Disruption of the gene for hypoxanthine-guanine phosphoribosyltransferase (*hgprt*) in embryonic stem cells. The disrupting DNA is incorporated into the *hgprt* gene through homologous recombination with the chromosomal DNA. A neomycin resistance gene (*neo^R*) is included in the disruption probe as a selectable marker. Only cells that have incorporated this gene are able to grow on a neomycin-containing medium.

have to be brought into the zygote or cultured embryonic stem cell by injection or electroporation, and their integration into the genome depends on the cellular enzymes for homologous recombination.

Three procedures are available for the production of knockout mice and transgenic mice (*Fig. 11.21*).

1. *The foreign gene is injected into the oocyte.* After fertilization in the test tube, the zygote is implanted into a foster animal and grown into a genetically modified animal.
2. *The foreign gene is engineered into cultured embryonic stem cells, followed by injection of the engineered stem cells into an embryo at the blastocyst stage.* Because embryonic stem cells are totipotent, they can contribute to all tissues of the developing embryo. After implantation in a foster animal, the embryo develops into a chimeric animal. *If some of the engineered stem cells contribute to the germ line, the genetic modification can be transmitted to the animal's descendants.* Although the genetic change initially is present in the heterozygous state, it can be made homozygous by classic breeding. This is currently the major method for production of genetically modified animals.
3. *The gene is engineered into embryonic stem cells whose nuclei are then transferred into enucleated oocytes.* The cloned animals that are produced with this method have the genetic modification in all their cells.

Reversible gene knockdown is achieved by bringing either single-stranded or double-stranded RNA into cells of the adult animal. Double-stranded RNAs are especially effective because they exploit the natural mechanism of RNA interference.

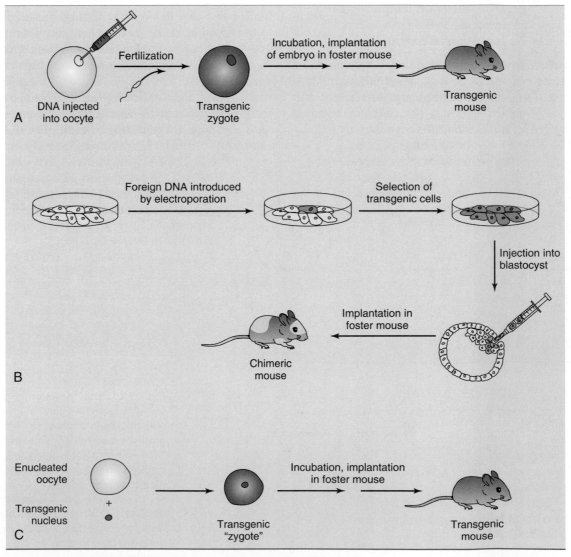

Figure 11.21 Three methods for the production of genetically modified animals. **A,** Foreign DNA is injected into the oocyte. **B,** Cultured embryonic stem cells are genetically modified. These cells are injected in the inner cell mass of a developing embryo at the blastocyst stage to produce a chimeric animal. **C,** Reproductive cloning with the nucleus of a genetically modified embryonic stem cell.

TISSUE-SPECIFIC GENE EXPRESSION CAN BE ENGINEERED INTO ANIMALS

The tissue-specific expression of an artificially introduced gene is determined in large part by its promoter. For example, a genetic engineer who wants to make humans capable of cellulose digestion could combine a cellulase gene from a snail or a fungus with a signal sequence and the promoter of the gene for trypsinogen or some other pancreatic zymogen. After introduction into the germ line, the cellulase would be secreted by the pancreas.

Gene knockouts can be made tissue specific with the help of **loxP** sites. The loxP site is a 34–base-pair palindromic sequence that is recognized by the **Cre recombinase,** an integrase enzyme from a bacteriophage. It acts somewhat like a spliceosome but with DNA rather than RNA as a substrate. *Cre recombinase cuts out the DNA between two loxP sites and splices together the flanking DNA.*

Figure 11.22 shows a procedure that has been used to knock out the gene for the insulin receptor specifically in adipose tissue. The transgenic mice have exon 4 of the insulin receptor gene flanked with loxP sites. They also have the cre gene under the control of a promoter that permits gene expression only in adipose tissue.

The Cre recombinase does no harm to the normal DNA in adipose cells, which does not contain any loxP sites. Only exon 4 of the insulin receptor gene is cut out of the genome.

The resulting mice cannot make insulin receptors in adipose tissue. Therefore their adipose tissue cannot respond to insulin. However, they are not diabetic because the insulin receptor is intact in all other tissues. These mice are very lean, and they live longer than normal laboratory mice.

A similar result can be achieved with an **antisense gene** whose RNA is complementary to the targeted mRNA, or an artificial gene whose RNA product is processed to a siRNA. For example, an antisense gene for the insulin receptor with an adipose tissue specific promoter would prevent the synthesis of the insulin receptor in adipose tissue without destroying the insulin receptor gene.

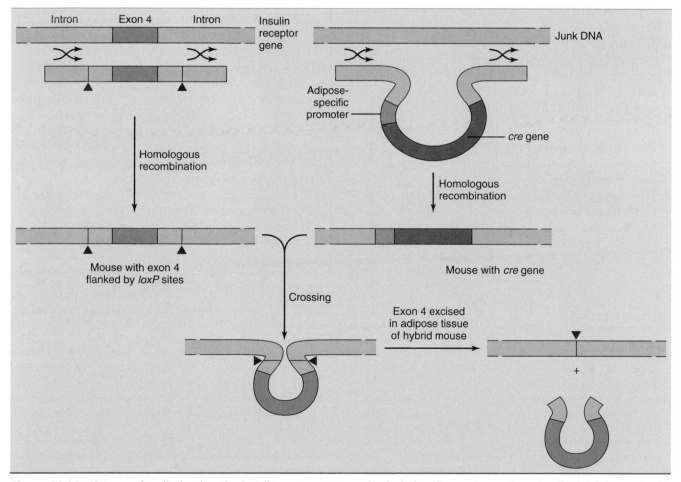

Figure 11.22   Strategy for eliminating the insulin receptor gene selectively in adipose tissue. A strain of mice is created with *loxP* sites (▲) flanking one of the exons (exon 4) of the insulin receptor gene. Another strain is created with the *cre* gene under the control of an adipose tissue selective promoter. When these two strains are crossed to create mice with both kinds of genetic modification, the Cre recombinase excises exon 4 only in adipose tissue.

PRODUCTION OF TRANSGENIC HUMANS IS TECHNICALLY POSSIBLE

In theory, transgenic humans can be produced with the methods shown in *Figure 11.21*. However, the risk of genetic and developmental abnormalities would be unacceptably high.

Methods of **gene repair** are under investigation. Gene repair is attempted by injecting the oocyte or zygote with a rather long DNA molecule that contains the normal counterpart of the defective gene. In order to facilitate homologous recombination between this external DNA and the mutated gene, a highly selective **zinc finger nuclease** is injected along with the corrective DNA. These enzymes are constructed by fusing a nuclease with a series of zinc fingers that are highly selective for a sequence in the defective gene. The aim is to cleave the defective DNA and replace it with functional DNA by exploiting the cellular mechanism for homologous double-strand break repair (see Chapter 9). This method is not (yet) safe for use in humans because the nuclease can wreak havoc by cleaving DNA outside the defective gene.

Human artificial chromosomes might be a safer way of making better people. These chromosomes contain centromeres, telomeres, and replication origins, along with splice sites for the insertion of gene cassettes. The desired genes are inserted, and the chromosome is injected into the nucleus of the oocyte or zygote during in vitro fertilization. Genes that people might wish to give to their children include the following:

1. *Life-prolonging genes.* Some genetic manipulations in animals, including the adipose-selective insulin receptor knockout shown in *Figure 11.22*, are known to prolong life.
2. *Tumor suppressor genes.* These are normal genes for DNA repair or negative controls on mitosis whose homozygous inactivation contributes to cancer. For example, transgenic mice with an extra copy of the tumor suppressor gene *p53* (see Chapter 18) have a substantially reduced cancer risk. Many tumor suppressor genes exist, and having one or two extra copies of each could protect people from cancer.
3. *Genes that antagonize age-related changes.* For example, accumulation of β-amyloid in Alzheimer disease (see Chapter 1) might be preventable by a brain-expressed antisense gene for the amyloid precursor protein.

Human artificial chromosomes can be equipped with loxP sites left and right of the centromere and a *cre* gene controlled by a germline-specific promoter. In that case, *the centromere will be cut out and the chromosome will be destroyed in the germ line, preventing its transmission to the next generation.* When deciding about their children's genes, parents will certainly want to give them not their own outdated chromosome but the most recent model!

SUMMARY

Highly efficient methods are available for fragmentation of DNA, cloning of fragments in bacteria, enzymatic amplification, and DNA sequencing.

The most important applications of molecular genetic techniques in medicine are genotyping and diagnosis of genetic diseases. People can be tested for recessive disease genes and for genes that predispose to multifactorial diseases. Prenatal and preimplantation genetic diagnoses are possible, and whole populations can be screened for problematic genes. DNA microarrays can be used to test for thousands of mutations and genetic polymorphisms in a single procedure, and even whole-genome sequencing is becoming affordable as a diagnostic procedure.

Somatic cell gene therapy and RNA interference are being investigated for therapeutic use. Germline gene modifications have not yet been attempted in humans, although whole armies of knockout mice and transgenic animals have been created.

Further Reading

Barrett JB, Clayton DG, Concannon P, et al: Genome-wide association study and meta-analysis find that over 40 loci affect risk of type 1 diabetes, *Nat Genet* 41:703–707, 2009.

Beaudet AL, Belmont JW: Array-based DNA diagnostics: let the revolution begin, *Annu Rev Med* 59:113–129, 2008.

Bentley DR, Balasubramanian S, Swerdlow HP, et al: Accurate whole human genome sequencing using reversible terminator chemistry, *Nature* 456:53–59, 2008.

Blüher M, Kahn BB, Kahn CR: Extended longevity in mice lacking the insulin receptor in adipose tissue, *Science* 299:572–573, 2003.

Bonetta L: RNA-based therapeutics: ready for delivery? *Cell* 136:581–584, 2009.

Branda CS, Dymecki SM: Talking about a revolution: the impact of site-specific recombinases on genetic analyses in mice, *Dev Cell* 6:7–28, 2004.

Büning H, Perabo L, Coutelle O, et al: Recent developments in adeno-associated virus vector technology, *J Gene Med* 10:717–733, 2008.

Castanotto D, Rossi JJ: The promises and pitfalls of RNA-interference-based therapeutics, *Nature* 457:426–433, 2009.

Chiu RWK, Cantor CR, Lo YMD: Non-invasive prenatal diagnosis by single molecule counting technologies, *Trends Genet* 25:324–331, 2009.

Cho YS, Go MJ, Kim YJ, et al: A large-scale genome-wide association study of Asian populations uncovers genetic factors influencing eight quantitative traits, *Nat Genet* 41:527–534, 2009.

Choi M, Scholl UI, Ji W, et al: Genetic diagnosis by whole exome capture and massively parallel DNA sequencing, *Proc Natl Acad Sci U S A* 106:19096–19101, 2009.

Coombs A: The sequencing shakeup, *Nat Biotechnol* 26:1109–1112, 2008.

Daetwyler HD, Villanueva B, Woolliams JA: Accuracy of predicting the genetic risk of disease using a genome-wide approach, *PLoS ONE* 3(10):e3395, 2008.

Edelstein ML, Abedi MR, Wixon J: Gene therapy trials worldwide to 2007—an update, *J Gene Med* 9:833–842, 2007.

Friedman JM: High-resolution array genomic hybridization in prenatal diagnosis, *Prenat Diagn* 29:20–28, 2009.

Friedman JM, Adam S, Arbour L, et al: Detection of pathogenic copy number variants in children with idiopathic intellectual disability using 500 K SNP array genomic hybridization, *BMC Genomics* 10:526, 2009.

Garcia-Cao I, Garcia-Cao M, Martin-Caballero J, et al: "Super p53" mice exhibit enhanced DNA damage response, are tumor resistant and age normally, *EMBO J* 21:6225–6235, 2002.

Gupta PK: Single-molecule DNA sequencing technologies for future genomics research, *Trends Biotechnol* 26:602–611, 2008.

Harbers M: The current status of cDNA cloning, *Genomics* 91:232–242, 2008.

Hindorff LA, Sethupathy P, Junkins HA, et al: Potential etiologic and functional implications of genome-wide association loci for human diseases and traits, *Proc Natl Acad Sci U S A* 106:9362–9367, 2009.

Kahvejian A, Quackenbush J, Thompson JF: What would you do if you could sequence everything? *Nat Biotechnol* 26:1125–1133, 2008.

Korn JM, Kuruvilla FG, McCarroll SA, et al: Integrated genotype calling and association analysis of SNPs, common copy number polymorphisms and rare CNVs, *Nat Genet* 40:1253–1260, 2008.

Ku CS, Loy EY, Pawitan Y, et al: The pursuit of genome-wide association studies: where are we now? *J Hum Genet* 55:195–206, 2010.

Li B, Leal SM: Discovery of rare variants via sequencing: implications for the design of complex trait association studies, *PLoS Genet* 5(5):e100048, 2009.

Manolio TA, Collins FS, Cox NJ, et al: Finding the missing heritability of complex diseases, *Nature* 461:747–753, 2009.

Mardis ER: Next-generation DNA sequencing methods, *Annu Rev Genomics Hum Genet* 9:387–402, 2008.

Metzker ML: Sequencing technologies—the next generation, *Nat Rev Genet* 11:31–45, 2010.

Morozova O, Marra MA: From cytogenetics to next-generation sequencing technologies: advances in the detection of genome rearrangements in tumors, *Biochem Cell Biol* 86:81–90, 2008.

Mott R: Finding the molecular basis of complex genetic variation in humans and mice, *Philos Trans R Soc Lond B Biol Sci* 361:393–401, 2006.

Sabatti C, Service SK, Hartikainen A-L, et al: Genome-wide association analysis of metabolic traits in a birth cohort from a founder population, *Nat Genet* 41:35–46, 2009.

Shen F, Huang J, Fitch KR, et al: Improved detection of global copy number variation using high density, non-polymorphic oligonucleotide probes, *BMC Genet* 9:27, 2008.

Shendure J, Ji H: Next-generation DNA sequencing, *Nat Biotechnol* 26:1135–1143, 2008.

Spits C, Sermon K: PGD for monogenic disorders: aspects of molecular biology, *Prenat Diagn* 29:50–56, 2009.

Stankiewicz P, Beaudet AL: Use of array CGH in the evaluation of dysmorphology, malformations, developmental delay, and idiopathic mental retardation, *Curr Opin Genet Devel* 17:182–192, 2007.

Stock G: *Redesigning humans: choosing our children's genes*, London, 2002, Profile Books.

Tucker T, Marra M, Friedman JM: Massively parallel sequencing: the next big thing in genetic medicine, *Am J Hum Genet* 85:142–154, 2009.

Vissers LELM, de Vries BBA, Veltman JA: Genomic microarrays in mental retardation: from copy number variation to gene, from research to diagnosis, *J Med Genet* 47:289–297, 2010.

QUESTIONS

1. **To sequence a piece of DNA with the dideoxy method, you will probably want to use**

   A. A pair of primers
   B. Reverse transcriptase
   C. Southern blotting
   D. Fluorescent-labeled deoxyribonucleotides
   E. Fluorescent-labeled dideoxyribonucleotides

2. **You have been instructed by the U.S. Department of Health and Human Services to screen the whole population of New York City for the presence of the sickle cell mutation. What method would be best for this project?**

   A. Southern blotting with allele-specific probes
   B. PCR, with electrophoretic separation of the products
   C. Linkage analysis with closely linked RSPs or SNPs
   D. cDNA microarrays
   E. Dot blotting

3. **Retroviral vectors are more popular for somatic gene therapy than other viral vectors because**

   A. They replicate faster than most other viruses
   B. They contain several copies of their DNA genome in the virus particle
   C. They can integrate themselves into the host cell DNA
   D. Their replication is more accurate than that of most other viruses
   E. Their DNA has extensive sequence homology with normal cellular DNA

4. The steps of classic Southern blotting include (1) denaturation of DNA with alkali, (2) electrophoresis in a cross-linked agarose or polyacrylamide gel, (3) application of a probe, (4) treatment of DNA with a restriction endonuclease, and (5) blotting of DNA to nitrocellulose paper. The correct sequence of these steps is

A. $1 \rightarrow 4 \rightarrow 2 \rightarrow 5 \rightarrow 3$
B. $4 \rightarrow 3 \rightarrow 1 \rightarrow 2 \rightarrow 5$
C. $1 \rightarrow 5 \rightarrow 2 \rightarrow 3 \rightarrow 4$
D. $4 \rightarrow 2 \rightarrow 1 \rightarrow 5 \rightarrow 3$
E. $2 \rightarrow 1 \rightarrow 5 \rightarrow 4 \rightarrow 3$

5. If you want to use genetically engineered bacteria for the production of human growth hormone, you need all of the following ingredients except

A. A cDNA obtained by the reverse transcription of growth hormone mRNA
B. A bacterial promoter sequence
C. A DNA sequence that codes for a bacterial ribosome-binding sequence
D. Genomic DNA of the growth hormone gene
E. Restriction endonucleases

6. PCR-based procedures are often preferred over Southern blotting for the prenatal diagnosis of genetic diseases after amniocentesis or chorionic villus sampling. Why?

A. PCR requires less DNA; therefore, lengthy cell culturing may not be necessary.
B. PCR requires less technical skill than Southern blotting and therefore is less costly.
C. PCR is less sensitive to contamination by extraneous DNA and therefore is less prone to false positive results.
D. Unlike Southern blotting, PCR does not require DNA from many family members.
E. Unlike Southern blotting, PCR does not require any knowledge of the DNA sequence in and around the affected gene.

7. The classic PCR procedure (without probes) can be used to

A. Amplify the whole dystrophin gene with its 79 exons and 78 introns in one piece
B. Diagnose the sickle cell mutation after amniocentesis
C. Diagnose HIV infection in people with risky lifestyles

D. Detect point mutations in a gene whose sequence is unknown
E. Perform all of the above

8. In order to genotype a skin color gene in DNA from a 30,000-year-old Neanderthal skeleton, you will definitely have to use

A. Southern blotting with allele-specific probes
B. In situ hybridization
C. PCR
D. Oligonucleotide microarrays
E. Linkage with closely linked microsatellite polymorphisms

9. Linkage studies with closely linked microsatellite polymorphisms are the preferred diagnostic method for the detection of heterozygous carriers of recessive disease genes when

A. There is allelic heterogeneity, and it is not known which mutation in a known disease gene causes the disease in a family
B. There is locus heterogeneity, and it is not known which gene is mutated in an affected family
C. No case of the disease has so far occurred in the family
D. Population-wide screening is intended
E. The exact molecular nature of the mutation is known

10. In order to compare the expression of a large number of genes in rhabdomyosarcoma cells with gene expression in normal skeletal muscle, you have isolated mRNA from the two sources by affinity chromatography on an oligo-dT column. The most direct method for comparing the two mRNA patterns would be

A. PCR with nested primers
B. Dot blotting
C. Cloning in bacteria
D. Southern blotting
E. Northern blotting

11. Alternatively, the mRNAs from the tumor and normal cells can be compared using

A. Allele-specific amplification
B. Expression cloning
C. In situ hybridization
D. cDNA microarrays
E. RNA interference

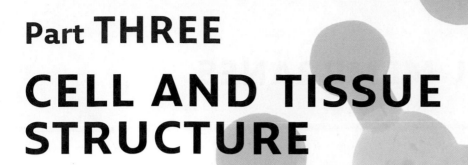

Part THREE
CELL AND TISSUE STRUCTURE

Chapter 12
BIOLOGICAL MEMBRANES

All cells are surrounded by a **plasma membrane**, and eukaryotes (but not prokaryotes) have membrane-bounded **organelles** as well.

The terms *plasma membrane* and *cell wall*, so often confused by students, refer to very different structures. The plasma membrane is as thin and fragile as a soap bubble, yet it forms an effective diffusion barrier. It consists of lipids and proteins.

The cell wall, on the other hand, is strong and stiff and maintains the shape of the cell. Plants and bacteria have a cell wall that is made of tough polysaccharides such as cellulose or peptidoglycan, but humans do not. Human cells are kept in shape by the **cytoskeleton** instead, and human tissues derive mechanical strength from the **extracellular matrix.** This chapter introduces the structure and properties of cellular membranes.

MEMBRANES CONSIST OF LIPID AND PROTEIN

Under the electron microscope, a biological membrane in cross-section looks like a railroad track, with a lightly stained layer sandwiched between two deeply stained layers. This structure, with a total diameter of 8 nm, is formed from two layers of lipids.

The membrane lipids are **amphiphilic** or **amphipathic.** This means that *hydrophilic and hydrophobic parts are combined in the same molecule.* **Phospholipids** contain a phosphate group in their hydrophilic part, and **glycolipids** contain covalently attached carbohydrate. Based on their chemical building blocks, three classes of membrane lipids can be distinguished: **phosphoglycerides, sphingolipids,** and **cholesterol.**

Membranes contain proteins as well as lipids. *Lipids form the structural backbone of the membrane, and proteins are in charge of specific functions.* These functions include enzymatic activities, regulated transport, ion permeability and excitability, contact with structural proteins, and transmission of physiological signals. Therefore the protein/lipid ratio is highest in membranes with high metabolic activity, such as the inner mitochondrial membrane (*Fig. 12.1*).

PHOSPHOGLYCERIDES ARE THE MOST ABUNDANT MEMBRANE LIPIDS

Phosphoglycerides account for more than half of all lipids in most membranes (see *Fig. 12.1*). Their parent compound is **phosphatidic acid,** or **phosphatidate.** It looks similar to a triglyceride but with the third fatty acid of the triglyceride replaced by phosphate:

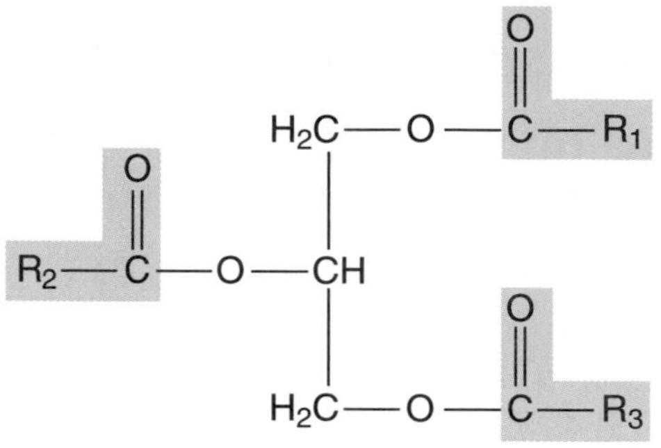

Triglyceride

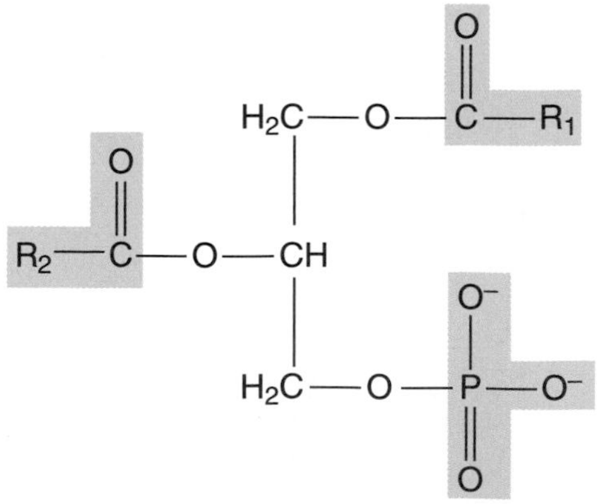

Phosphatidate

The major membrane phosphoglycerides have a second alcohol bound to the phosphate group in phosphatidic acid, and they are named as derivatives of phosphatidic acid (phosphatidyl-) (*Fig. 12.2*).

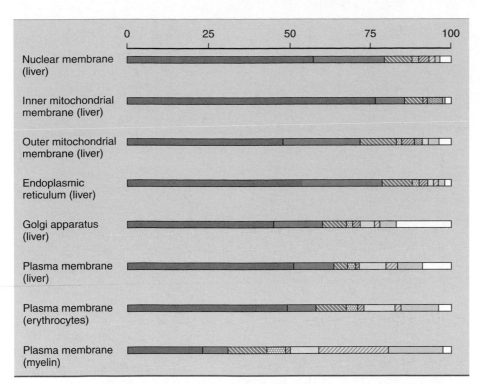

Figure 12.1 Composition of biological membranes. ■, Protein; ▨, phosphatidyl choline; ▨, phosphatidyl ethanolamine; ▨, phosphatidyl serine; ▨, phosphatidyl inositol; ▨, cardiolipin; ▨, sphingomyelin; ▨, glycolipids; □, cholesterol; □, others.

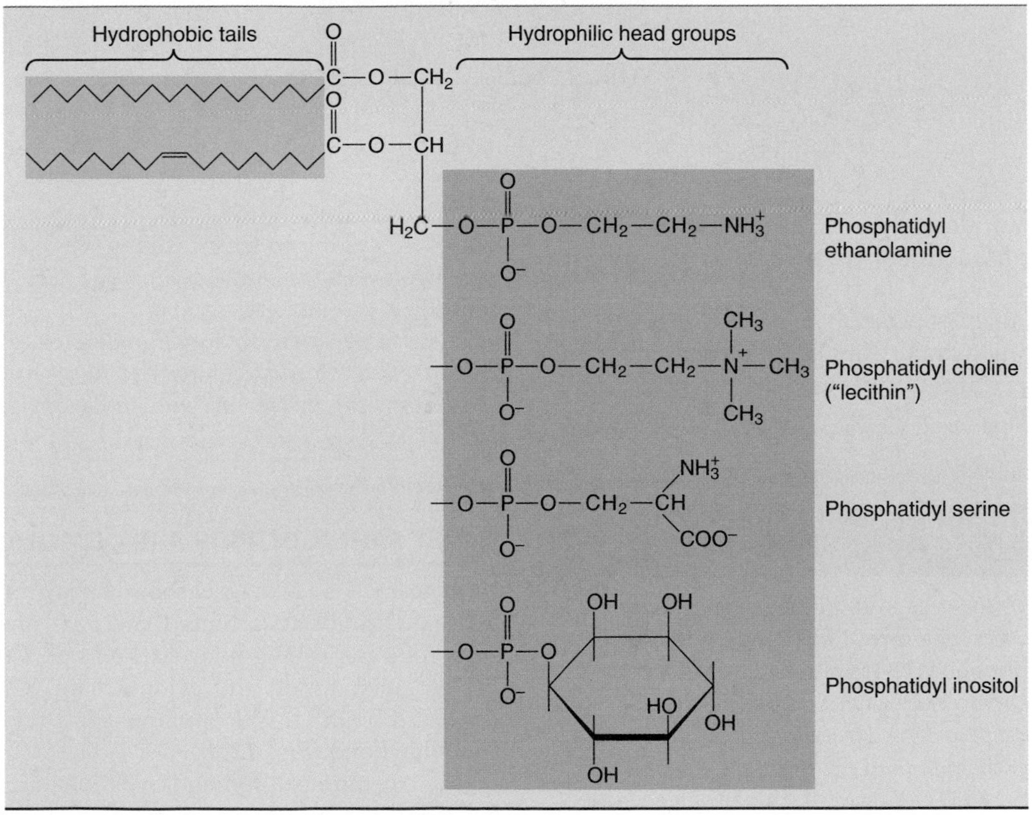

Figure 12.2 Structures of the most common phosphoglycerides.

The variable alcohol that is bound to the phosphate either is charged or has a high hydrogen bonding potential. *Together with the negatively charged phosphate, it forms the hydrophilic head group of the molecule, whereas the fatty acids form two hydrophobic tails.*

The fatty acid in position 1 usually is saturated, and that in position 2 is unsaturated.

Two less common phosphoglycerides are shown in **Figure 12.3**. **Cardiolipin** (diphosphatidylglycerol) is common only in the inner mitochondrial membrane.

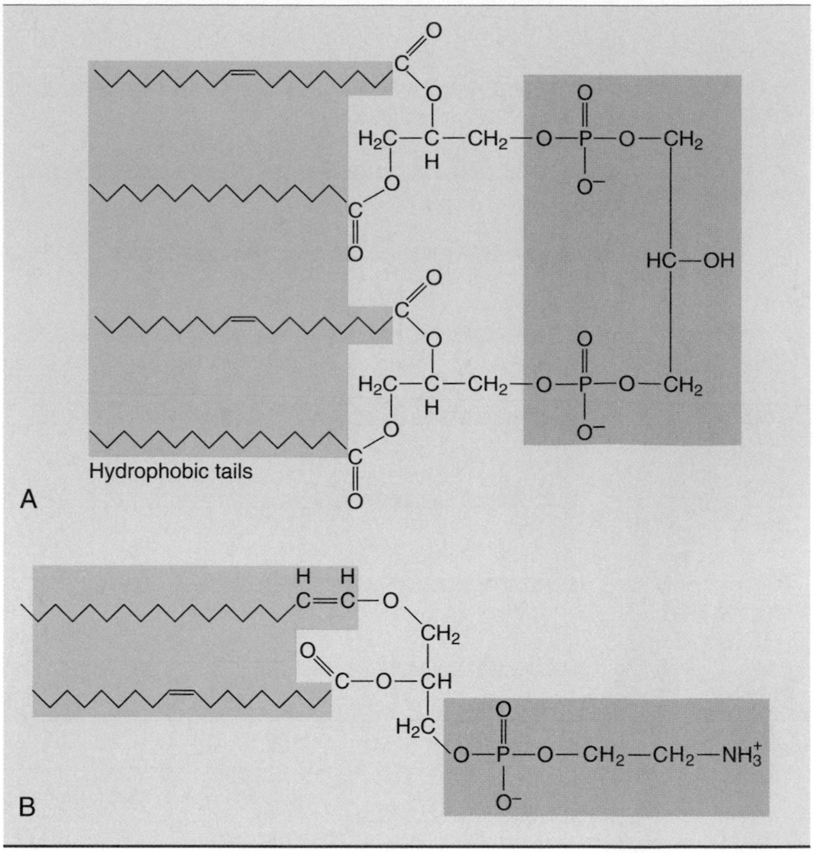

Figure 12.3 Structures of cardiolipin and plasmalogen. **A,** Cardiolipin, a major lipid of the inner mitochondrial membrane. **B,** Ethanolamine plasmalogen. Plasmalogens account for up to 10% of the phospholipid in muscle and nervous tissue and are present in most other tissues as well.

The widespread **plasmalogens,** usually with ethanolamine in their head group, are defined by the presence of an α-β unsaturated fatty alcohol, rather than a fatty acid residue, in position 1. In addition to their function as membrane lipids, phospholipids can play other specialized roles in the body (*Clinical Example 12.1*).

CLINICAL EXAMPLE 12.1: Respiratory Distress Syndrome

The type II alveolar cells in the lungs secrete **lung surfactant,** which is a mix of lipid and protein with **dipalmitoyl phosphatidylcholine** (dipalmitoyl lecithin) as its main component. *Dipalmitoyl phosphatidylcholine reduces the surface tension by forming a monolayer on the thin fluid film that lines the alveolar walls* (see **Fig. 12.6D**). Without it, the alveoli collapse and breathing becomes difficult.

Preterm infants who are born with insufficient lung surfactant develop **respiratory distress syndrome,** a condition that is responsible for 15% to 20% of neonatal deaths in the Western Hemisphere. For the timing of elective deliveries, the maturity of the fetal lungs is determined by measuring the lecithin/sphingomyelin (L/S) ratio in amniotic fluid. The L/S ratio initially is low but rises to about 2 or a little higher sometime between 30 and 34 weeks of gestation. Infants who are born before their lungs have sufficient surfactant can be treated with surfactant administered by inhaler.

MOST SPHINGOLIPIDS ARE GLYCOLIPIDS

Sphingosine is an 18-carbon amino alcohol with hydroxyl groups at carbons 1 and 3, an amino group at carbon 2, and a long hydrocarbon tail. **Ceramide** consists of sphingosine and a long-chain (C-18 to C-24) fatty acid bound to the amino group of sphingosine by an amide bond (*Fig. 12.4*).

The membrane sphingolipids contain a variable hydrophilic head group covalently bound to the C-1 hydroxyl group of ceramide. *Like the phosphoglycerides, the sphingolipids have two hydrophobic tails.* One is a fatty acid residue, and the other is the hydrocarbon tail of sphingosine.

Sphingomyelin (*Fig. 12.5*), which has the same head group as phosphatidylcholine in *Figure 12.2*, is the only important phosphosphingolipid. All other sphingolipids are glycolipids. The most complex glycosphingolipids are the **gangliosides.** They contain between one and four residues of the acidic sugar derivative **N-acetylneuraminic** acid (NANA) in terminal positions of their oligosaccharide chain:

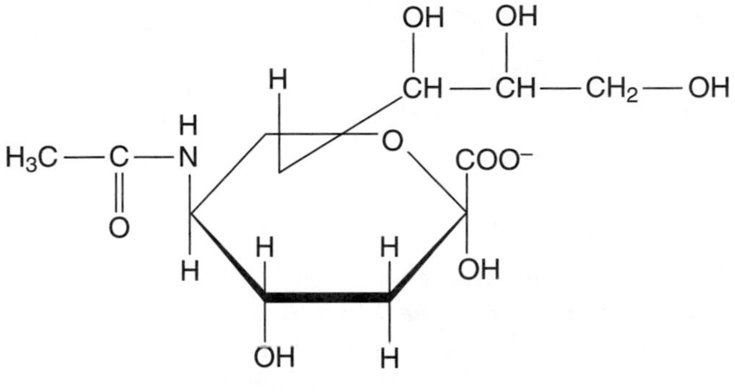

N-Acetylneuraminic acid
(NANA)

Glycosphingolipids are most abundant in the outer leaflet of the plasma membrane, where their carbohydrate heads face the extracellular environment. Sphingomyelin and galactocerebroside (the latter partly in a sulfated form) are important constituents of myelin, and gangliosides and galactocerebroside are most abundant in the gray matter of the brain.

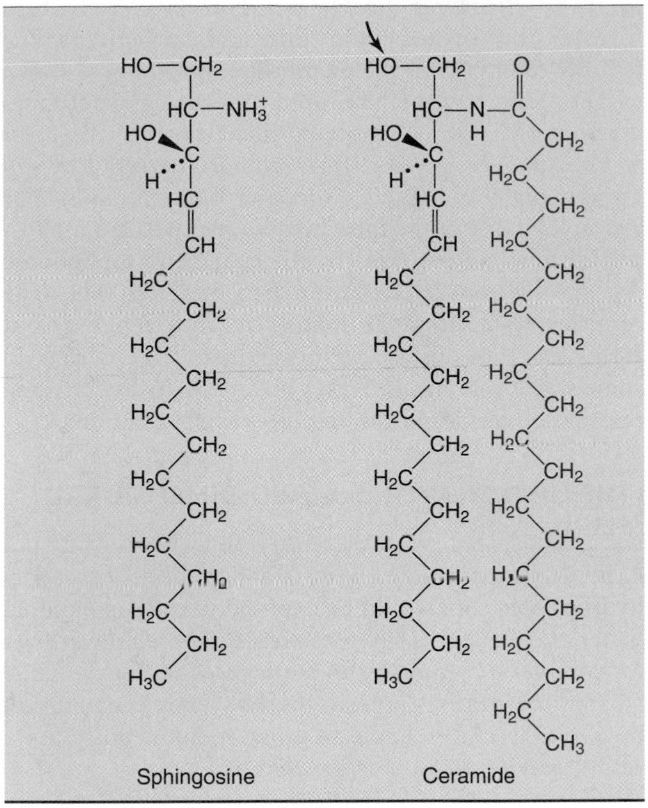

CHOLESTEROL IS THE MOST HYDROPHOBIC MEMBRANE LIPID

Cholesterol is structurally more rigid than the other membrane lipids, with a stiff **steroid ring system** instead of wriggly hydrocarbon tails; and instead of a stately hydrophilic head group, only a puny hydroxyl group is present at one end of the molecule:

Figure 12.4 Structures of sphingosine and ceramide. The fatty acid residues in ceramide often are very long (C-20 to C-24). The hydroxyl group of ceramide that is substituted in the sphingolipids is marked by an *arrow.*

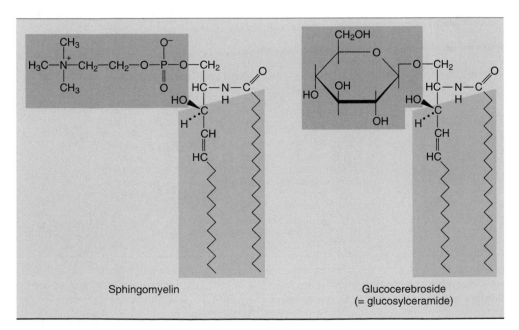

Figure 12.5 Two types of sphingolipid. Sphingomyelin is a phosphosphingolipid, and glucocerebroside is a glycosphingolipid.

Sphingomyelin

Glucocerebroside
(= glucosylceramide)

With this structure, *cholesterol is by far the least water-soluble membrane lipid.* Also, unlike the other membrane lipids, *cholesterol alone cannot form membrane-like structures; it occurs only as a minor component in membranes whose basic structure is formed by other lipids.*

Cholesterol accounts for 10% or more of the total lipid only in the plasma membrane and the Golgi membrane. It is prominent only in animals. Plants have **phytosterols** instead, and most bacteria have no sterols at all. Therefore *a vegan diet is cholesterol free.*

MEMBRANE LIPIDS FORM A BILAYER

The hydrophilic head groups of the membrane lipids interact with water, whereas the hydrophobic tails avoid water. Rather than dissolving in water as individual molecules, the membrane lipids form noncovalent aggregates (*Fig. 12.6*).

Most polar lipids, including ordinary detergents, form globular **micelles**. **Monolayers** form only at aqueous/nonaqueous interfaces (e.g., between water and air), whereas **bilayers** are surrounded by water on both sides. *All biological membranes contain a lipid bilayer as their structural backbone.* The bilayer is held together by hydrophobic interactions between the hydrocarbon tails of the membrane lipids.

The geometry of the lipid molecules determines whether a bilayer or a globular micelle forms. *A bilayer is formed only if the cross-sectional area of the head groups matches that of the hydrophobic tails.* For example, if one of the fatty acids is removed from phosphatidylcholine (lecithin) by the enzyme **phospholipase A₂**, the hydrophobic portion becomes too thin. The resulting **lysolecithin** no longer fits into a bilayer but forms micelles instead. Phospholipase A₂ occurs in some snake venoms. It causes hemolysis by hydrolyzing phosphoglycerides in the red blood cell membrane.

THE LIPID BILAYER IS A TWO-DIMENSIONAL FLUID

A lipid bilayer cannot exist as a flat sheet because its hydrophobic core would be exposed to the surrounding water at the edges. Therefore *pieces of lipid bilayer tend to close in on themselves to form vesicles.* For the same reason, any tear or hole in the bilayer is energetically unfavorable and is liable to close spontaneously. As a result, *membranes are self-sealing.*

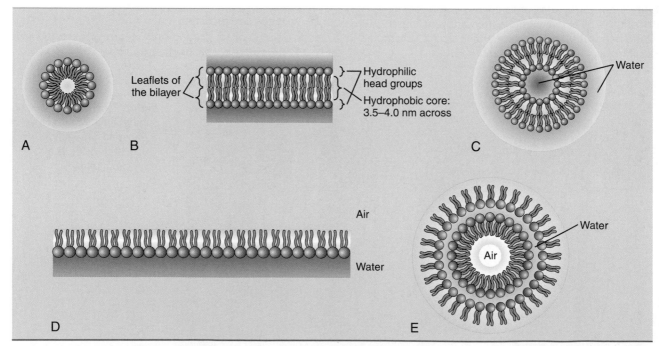

Figure 12.6 Behavior of polar lipids in water. **A,** A *micelle* is a small, spherical structure with a hydrophilic surface and a hydrophobic core. **B,** A *bilayer* is the prototype of a biological membrane. As in the micelle, the hydrophilic head groups are on the surface and the hydrophobic tails are buried in the center. **C,** A *liposome* is the prototype of a membrane-bounded vesicle. It forms spontaneously from a lipid bilayer. **D,** A *monolayer* forms at the interface between water and air. **E,** A *soap bubble* consists of two monolayers enclosing a thin water film.

Lipid bilayers are easily deformed even by slight forces. The hydrophobic tails of the lipids can merrily wriggle around, and *each molecule is free to diffuse laterally in the plane of the bilayer*. Lateral diffusion proceeds at a speed of about 2 µm/s in artificial bilayers.

When a synthetic lipid bilayer that contains only one lipid is cooled, it "freezes" at a well-defined temperature. Above the phase transition, the lipids move around like people on a busy town square, but below the transition they are immobile like a platoon of soldiers standing at attention.

Real membranes contain a mixture of many different lipids along with proteins, and the phase transition is gradual. *At ordinary body temperature, membranes behave like a viscous liquid.*

Long, saturated fatty acid chains in the membrane lipids make the membrane more rigid because they align themselves in parallel, forming multiple van der Waals interactions. Unsaturated fatty acids destabilize this orderly alignment because their *cis* double bonds introduce kinks in the hydrocarbon chain (*Fig. 12.7*).

Therefore *a high content of unsaturated fatty acid residues makes the membrane more fluid.*

Animals adjust their membrane fluidity by varying the fatty acid composition of their membrane lipids. For example, cold-water fish have more unsaturated fatty acids in their membranes than do tropical fish. This maintains optimal membrane fluidity at frigid temperatures, and it makes cold-water fish a valuable dietary source of polyunsaturated fatty acids.

Because of its stiff ring system, *cholesterol tends to make membranes more rigid.* However, it also inserts itself between the fatty acid chains and prevents their crystallization. In this respect, it acts like an impurity that decreases the melting point of a chemical.

THE LIPID BILAYER IS A DIFFUSION BARRIER

To penetrate a lipid bilayer, a substance has to pass from the aqueous solution through the region of the hydrophilic head groups, then across the hydrophobic core and out between the head groups on the opposite side.

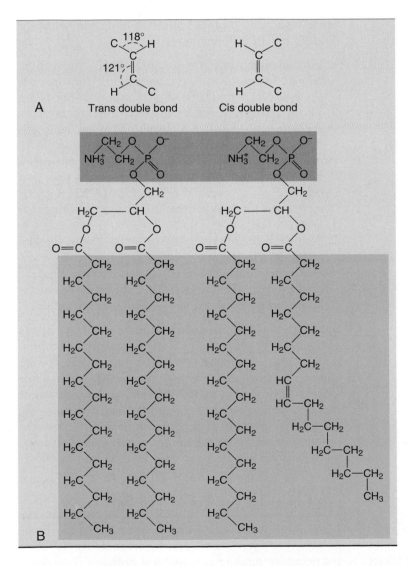

Figure 12.7 Effect of a *cis* double bond on the array of fatty acid chains in the hydrophobic core of the lipid bilayer. **A,** The geometry of *trans* and *cis* double bonds. There is no free rotation around the bond, and all four substituents of the double-bonded carbons are in the same plane. The double bonds in natural fatty acids are always in *cis* configuration. **B,** A phospholipid with an unsaturated fatty acid in the lipid bilayer (right side).

Water-soluble substances such as inorganic ions, sugars, amino acids, and proteins cannot penetrate the bilayer because they do not dissolve in lipid. Breakage of their interactions with water would require too much energy. Triglycerides and other water-insoluble lipids also cannot pass because they form fat droplets that are repelled by the hydrophilic head groups. Only small molecules that are at least somewhat soluble in both lipid and water can pass freely.

Oxygen, carbon dioxide, and other gases diffuse freely across membranes, but *most nutrients, metabolic intermediates, and coenzymes are water soluble and cannot cross the lipid bilayer* (**Fig. 12.8**). Because inorganic ions cannot cross, *the electrical conductivity of lipid bilayers is very low*. Real membranes contain ion channels, formed by membrane proteins, which regulate ion permeabilities and thereby membrane potential and excitability.

Many nutrients and metabolic products are transported by specialized membrane carriers. Some drugs are sufficiently hydrophobic for passive diffusion across the lipid bilayer, but highly water-soluble drugs cannot enter cells or penetrate the blood-brain barrier. When a drug contains ionizable groups, only the uncharged form passively crosses membranes. However, many hydrophilic drugs can commandeer a nutrient or metabolite transporter protein to move across membranes. This process is important not only for the absorption of drugs from the intestine but also for the metabolism and excretion of drugs by the liver and kidney.

Some very small lipophilic molecules dissolve in the lipid bilayer and increase its fluidity. Inhalation anesthetics such as ether, chloroform, halothane, and even ethanol have this property.

MEMBRANES CONTAIN INTEGRAL AND PERIPHERAL MEMBRANE PROTEINS

Proteins account for about half of the total mass in most membranes. *Membrane proteins are globular proteins*. According to the **fluid-mosaic model** of membrane structure (**Fig. 12.9**), they associate with the lipid bilayer in different ways:

1. **Integral membrane proteins** are embedded in the lipid bilayer. In most cases, *the polypeptide traverses the lipid bilayer by means of a **transmembrane helix***. This is a stretch of α-helix, about 25 amino acids long, that consists mainly of hydrophobic amino acid residues. *The nonpolar side chains of these amino acids interact with the membrane lipids*. Some integral membrane proteins traverse the lipid bilayer only once, but others crisscross several times (**Fig. 12.10**). Integral membrane proteins can be dissolved only with detergents that destroy the lipid bilayer.

2. **Peripheral membrane proteins** interact with integral membrane proteins or the hydrophilic head groups of the membrane lipids, but they do not traverse the lipid bilayer. They can be detached from the membrane by manipulating pH or salt concentration.

Some proteins are tethered to the outer surface of the plasma membrane by a covalently bound glycophospholipid anchor. Trehalase on intestinal microvilli (see Chapter 19), alkaline phosphatase on osteoblasts (see Chapter 14), and carcinoembryonic antigen (a tumor marker) are prominent examples. Some proteins on the cytoplasmic surface of the plasma membrane and the organelle membranes achieve the same result with covalently bound fatty acids or isoprenoids (**Fig. 12.11**).

MEMBRANES ARE ASYMMETRICAL

Membrane proteins can diffuse laterally in the plane of the membrane, although their mobility is often restricted by binding to structural proteins. Transverse

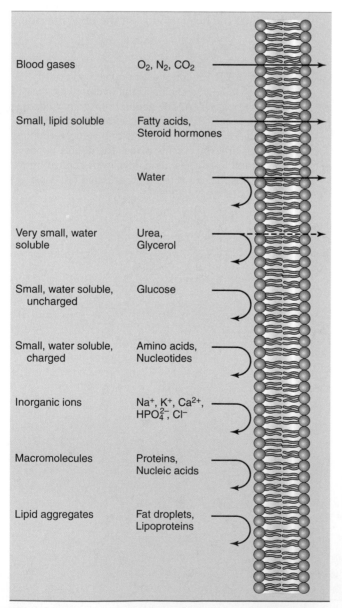

Blood gases	O_2, N_2, CO_2
Small, lipid soluble	Fatty acids, Steroid hormones
	Water
Very small, water soluble	Urea, Glycerol
Small, water soluble, uncharged	Glucose
Small, water soluble, charged	Amino acids, Nucleotides
Inorganic ions	Na^+, K^+, Ca^{2+}, HPO_4^{2-}, Cl^-
Macromolecules	Proteins, Nucleic acids
Lipid aggregates	Fat droplets, Lipoproteins

Figure 12.8 Permeability properties of a typical lipid bilayer.

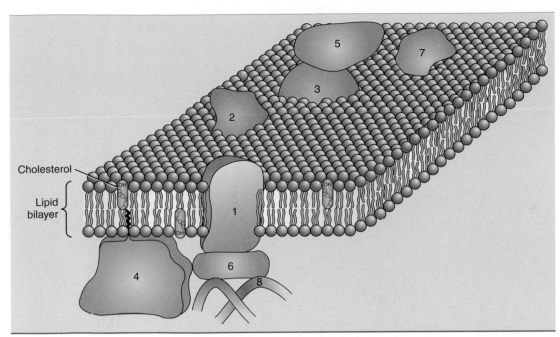

Figure 12.9   The fluid-mosaic model of membrane structure. *1, 2, 3,* Integral membrane proteins traversing the lipid bilayer; *4,* protein anchored by a covalently bound lipid (myristyl, farnesyl, or geranylgeranyl); *5, 6,* peripheral membrane proteins bound to integral membrane proteins; *7,* peripheral membrane protein adsorbed to the head groups of membrane lipids; *8,* cytoskeletal protein attached to a peripheral membrane protein.

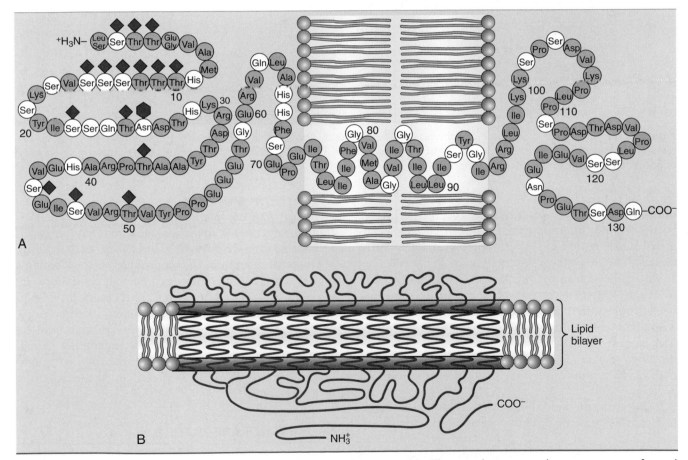

Figure 12.10   Examples of membrane-spanning integral membrane proteins. The membrane-spanning segments are formed by nonpolar α-helices. **A,** Glycophorin A, a major protein of the erythrocyte membrane. ⊙, Nonpolar residues; ⊙, charged residues. ◆, *O*-linked carbohydrate; ⬣, *N*-linked carbohydrate. **B,** Band 3 protein, another major protein of the red blood cell membrane. The polypeptide consists of 929 amino acid residues and traverses the membrane approximately a dozen times. It is present in a dimeric form, functioning as an anion channel and as an attachment point for cytoskeletal proteins.

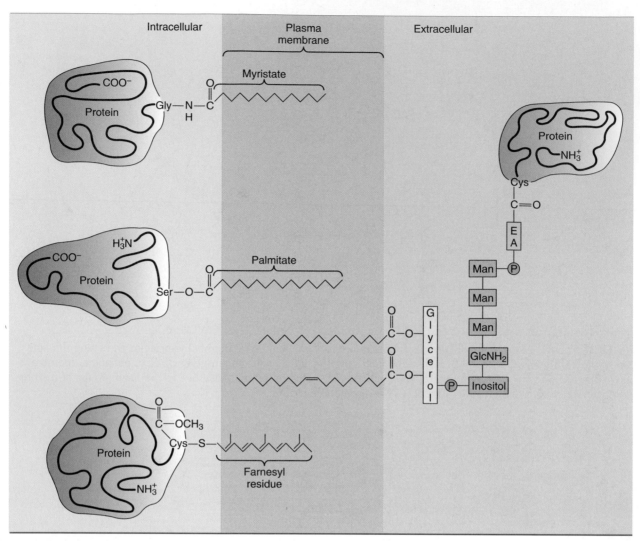

Figure 12.11 Attachment of proteins to the plasma membrane by covalently bound lipids. The structure of the glycosyl phosphatidylinositol anchor shown on the **right** varies somewhat in different membrane proteins. *EA*, Ethanolamine; *GlcNH2*, nonacetylated glucosamine; *Man*, D-mannose.

diffusion ("flip-flop") of membrane proteins has never been observed. In erythrocytes, for example, the asymmetrical orientation of the membrane proteins is maintained throughout the 120-day lifespan of the cell.

The same is true for membrane lipids. To flip-flop from one leaflet of the bilayer to the other, the polar head group of the lipid has to abandon its interactions with water molecules and neighboring head groups to dive across the hydrophobic core. Only cholesterol flip-flops spontaneously, but lipids with large hydrophilic head groups require the assistance of specialized proteins.

As a result, the lipid distribution in biological membranes is asymmetrical. Plasma membranes, for example, contain most of their phosphatidylethanolamine, phosphatidylserine, and phosphatidylinositol in the cytoplasmic leaflet and most of their glycolipids, phosphatidylcholine, and sphingomyelin in the exoplasmic leaflet (*Fig. 12.12*).

In the plasma membrane, the carbohydrate portions of glycolipids and glycoproteins face the extracellular space (see *Fig. 12.10, A*). The carbohydrate portions of membrane glycoproteins and glycolipids are constructed on their protein or lipid core by enzymes in the endoplasmic reticulum and Golgi apparatus. Being located in the lumen of these organelles, *the enzymes form the carbohydrates only on the noncytoplasmic surface of the membrane.* When Golgi-derived vesicles fuse with the plasma membrane, the carbohydrate is placed on the exoplasmic face (*Fig. 12.13*).

MEMBRANES ARE FRAGILE

All noncovalent structures are fragile. Biological membranes are especially vulnerable to agents that disrupt hydrophobic interactions. *Exposed membranes are destroyed by detergents and nonpolar organic solvents.*

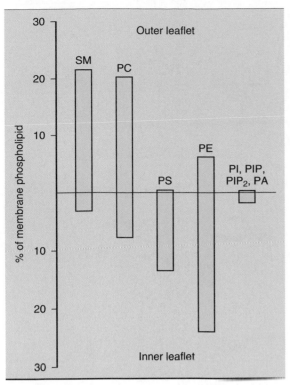

Figure 12.12 Distribution of phospholipids in the outer and inner leaflets of the erythrocyte membrane. *PA*, Phosphatidic acid; *PC*, phosphatidylcholine; *PE*, phosphatidylethanolamine; *PI*, phosphatidylinositol; *PIP*, phosphatidylinositol 4-phosphate; *PIP₂*, phosphatidylinositol 4,5-bisphosphate; *PS*, phosphatidylserine; *SM*, sphingomyelin.

Phenol, ethanol, and cationic detergents act as disinfectants by disrupting the membranes of microorganisms.

Crystalline materials damage membranes mechanically. Crystals of hemoglobin S damage the erythrocyte membrane in sickle cell disease (see Chapter 9), crystals of sodium urate damage the membranes of phagocytic cells in patients with gouty arthritis (see Chapter 28), and ice crystals damage the cells of frostbitten limbs (*Clinical Example 12.2*).

CLINICAL EXAMPLE 12.2: Cryopreservation

The preservation of cells and tissues in the frozen state (cryopreservation) is difficult. Freezing and thawing do not destroy proteins and nucleic acids, but they can destroy cellular membranes. This is in part because of osmotic stress and in part because the relentlessly growing ice crystals pierce the membranes.

Quick freezing of dispersed cells or small tissue samples in the presence of antifreeze avoids the formation of large ice crystals. Sperm and embryos are routinely preserved by quick freezing in 10% glycerol. The cryopreservation of oocytes is more difficult, although it is becoming routine in fertility clinics.

However, complete organs cannot be cryopreserved because their large heat capacity makes quick freezing impossible. The same applies to entire human bodies.

A patient with an incurable disease would be ill advised to jump into liquid nitrogen in the hope that someone will thaw him someday when a cure for his disease has been found.

MEMBRANE PROTEINS CARRY SOLUTES ACROSS THE LIPID BILAYER

In a few biological membranes, most notably the outer mitochondrial membrane, membrane proteins form **pores** that allow the passage of all small, water-soluble molecules. Usually, however, passive diffusion is limited to lipid-soluble molecules that are able to cross the lipid bilayer.

Channels are more selective than pores. They have a gate with a binding site for a specific solute and are permeable only for that solute. Inorganic ions are moved across membranes through channels. These channels can be regulated, for example, by a neurotransmitter that binds to the channel (see Chapter 17) or by the membrane potential.

Transporters, also known as **membrane carriers**, work somewhat like channels but undergo conformational changes during the transport cycle (*Fig. 12.14*). Carrier-mediated transport is called **facilitated diffusion** if it is passive and **active transport** if it requires metabolic energy (*Table 12.1*). Carrier-mediated transport is distinguished from simple diffusion by three important features:

1. **Substrate specificity.** Because the substrate must bind noncovalently to the carrier, *transport depends on the proper fit between substrate and carrier*. The glucose transporter in red blood cells, for example, transports D-glucose but not L-glucose, and it has markedly reduced affinities for other hexoses such as D-mannose and D-galactose.
2. **Saturability.** The rate of passive diffusion is directly proportional to the concentration gradient, but *carrier-mediated transport is limited by the number of carriers in the membrane* (*Fig. 12.15*).
3. **Specific inhibition and physiological regulation.** Carriers, like enzymes, can be inhibited. Glucose transport into erythrocytes, for example, is competitively inhibited by various glucose analogs. Membrane transport can also be a rate-limiting and regulated step in metabolic pathways. For example, the carrier that brings glucose into muscle and adipose tissue (but not erythrocytes) is activated by insulin.

TRANSPORT AGAINST AN ELECTROCHEMICAL GRADIENT REQUIRES METABOLIC ENERGY

Like chemical reactions, *membrane transport is driven by the free energy change* ΔG [see Equation (5) in Chapter 4]. However, the situation is less complex because *there is no*

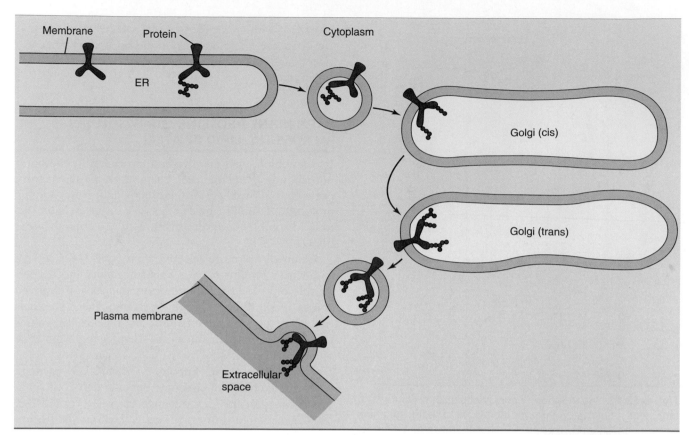

Figure 12.13 Placement of a glycoprotein in the plasma membrane. Note that the luminal surface of the organelles corresponds to the exoplasmic face of the plasma membrane. Glycolipids are synthesized the same way, with their carbohydrate initially facing the lumen of the endoplasmic reticulum (*ER*) and Golgi apparatus.

Figure 12.14 Facilitated diffusion of glucose across the erythrocyte membrane. There is no external energy source, so the net transport is down the concentration gradient. All steps in this cycle are reversible. A net transport of glucose into the cell takes place only because glucose is consumed in the cell, thereby maintaining a concentration gradient.

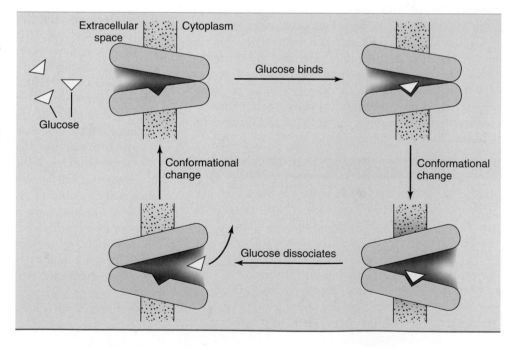

enthalpy change ($\Delta H = 0$), and the process is purely entropy driven. For an uncharged molecule, the driving force ΔG for the transfer of a molecule from a compartment with the concentration c_1 to a compartment with the concentration c_2 is given by the equation

$$(1) \quad \Delta G = R \times T \times \ln\frac{c_2}{c_1} = 2.303 \times R \times T \times \log\frac{c_2}{c_1}$$

where R = gas constant (1.987×10^{-3} kcal $\times$ mol^{-1} $\times$ K^{-1}) and T = absolute temperature. It now is possible

Table 12.1 Transport of Small Molecules and Inorganic Ions across Biological Membranes

Type of Transport	Carrier Required	Transport against Gradient	Metabolic Energy Required	ATP Hydrolysis	Example
Passive diffusion	−	−	−	−	Steroid hormones, many drugs
Facilitated diffusion	+	−	−	−	Glucose in RBCs and blood-brain barrier
Active transport	+	+	+	+	Na^+,K^+-ATPase, Ca^{2+}-ATPase
Secondary active transport	+	+	+	−	Sodium cotransport of glucose in kidney and intestine

ATP, Adenosine triphosphate; ATPase, adenosine triphosphatase; RBC, red blood cell.

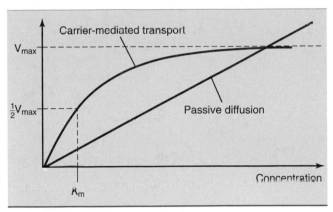

Figure 12.15 Saturability of carrier-mediated transport. We assume that the substrate moves from a compartment with variable concentration (concentration on the x-axis) to a compartment where its concentration is zero. This corresponds to the assumption of negligible product concentration in Michaelis-Menten kinetics. Compare this graph with Figure 4.6. V_{max} depends on the number of carriers in the membrane and the number of molecules transported per second. K_m, Michaelis constant; V_{max}, maximal reaction rate.

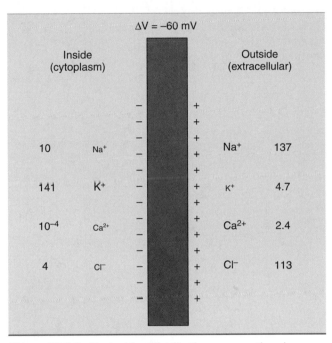

Figure 12.16 Typical ion distributions across the plasma membrane. All concentrations are in (mmol/L). ΔV, Membrane potential.

to calculate the energy required to pump 1 mol of an uncharged molecule against a 10-fold concentration gradient ($c_2/c_1 = 10$) at 25°C (298K):

$$\Delta G = 2.303 \times 1.987 \times 10^{-3} \frac{kcal}{mol \times K} \times 298\ K \times \log 10$$

$$= +1.36\ kcal/mol$$

For an ion, the energy requirement depends not only on the concentration gradient but also on the membrane potential:

(2) $\quad \Delta G = \left[2.303 \times R \times T \times \log\frac{C_2}{C_1} \right] + [Z \times F \times \Delta V]$

where Z = charge of the ion, F = Faraday constant (23.062 kcal $\times V^{-1} \times mol^{-1}$), and ΔV = membrane potential in volts.

By substituting the values of ***Figure 12.16*** into ***Equation (2)***, it is possible, for example, to calculate the energy required to pump a sodium ion out of the cell:

$$\Delta G = 2.303 \times 1.987 \times 10^{-3} \frac{kcal}{mol \times K} \times 298\ K$$

$$\times \log\frac{137}{10} + 1 \times 23.062 \frac{kcal}{V \times mol} \times 0.06\ V$$

$$= 1.545 \frac{kcal}{mol} + 1.384 \frac{kcal}{mol} = +2.929\ kcal/mol$$

Equation (2) defines the **electrochemical gradient** for ions. The electrochemical gradient is large for ions such as Na^+ and Ca^{2+}, for which the two components of ***Equation (2)*** have the same sign, and small for ions such as K^+ and Cl^-, for which they have opposite signs.

ACTIVE TRANSPORT CONSUMES ATP

The **sodium/potassium (Na^+,K^+) pump** maintains the normal gradients of sodium and potassium across the plasma membrane. It is a glycoprotein with two α-subunits and two β-subunits. Each α-subunit has about 10 transmembrane α-helices, and three of them participate in the formation of the gated channel. These three helices are amphipathic, with hydrophobic amino acid residues facing the lipid bilayer and hydrophilic ones lining the channel.

Figure 12.17 shows the transport cycle. In its "inside-open" conformation, the gated channel exposes three Na⁺-binding sites to the cytoplasm. Na⁺ binding triggers phosphorylation of an aspartate side chain, which flips

the channel into the "outside-open" conformation. This conformation has low affinity for Na⁺ and high affinity for K⁺. Therefore the three Na⁺ ions diffuse into the extracellular space, and two K⁺ ions bind. This triggers dephosphorylation of the aspartate side chain. The channel flips back into the inside-open conformation, which has low affinity for K⁺ and high affinity for Na⁺. K⁺ is released into the cytoplasm, Na⁺ again binds, and the process is repeated.

Figure 12.17 Transport cycle of Na⁺,K⁺-ATPase. *Asp*, Aspartate; P_i, inorganic phosphate.

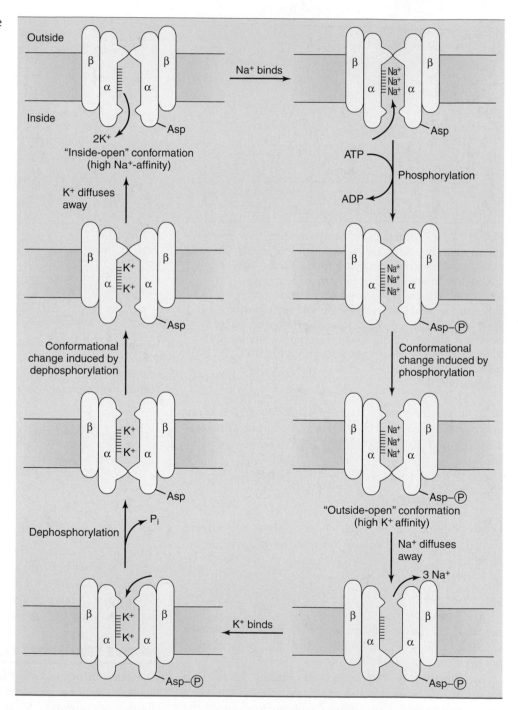

During each transport cycle, three Na^+ ions are transported out of the cell, two K^+ ions are transported into the cell, and one ATP molecule is consumed. Because of the net transport of an electrical charge, this transport is called **electrogenic.**

Most cells spend at least 10% of their metabolic energy for sodium/potassium pumping. In the brain this proportion is as high as 70% because sodium movements into neurons during membrane depolarization need to be balanced by sodium pumping.

The **calcium pump** that accumulates calcium in the sarcoplasmic reticulum of muscle fibers uses the same transport mechanism as the sodium/potassium pump. It constitutes almost 90% of the total membrane protein in the sarcoplasmic reticulum of skeletal muscle and consumes close to 10% of the total metabolic energy in resting muscle.

SODIUM COTRANSPORT BRINGS MOLECULES INTO THE CELL

The coupled transport of two substrates by the same carrier is called **cotransport.** If, as in the case of the sodium/potassium pump, the two substrates are transported in opposite directions, the mechanism is called **antiport.** If they are transported in the same direction, it is called **symport.**

In **sodium cotransport,** the carrier transports a molecule or inorganic ion into the cell together with a sodium ion. Sodium moves down its steep electrochemical gradient, and this drives the uphill transport of the cotransported substrate. *This type of transport does not hydrolyze ATP but depends on the maintenance of the sodium gradient by the sodium/potassium pump.* Therefore it is characterized as **secondary active transport.**

Sodium cotransport is used for the absorption of glucose and amino acids in the intestinal mucosa and their reabsorption in the kidney tubules (*Fig. 12.18*). Kidneys and intestines often use the same sodium cotransporter, and many inherited transport defects are therefore expressed in both organs.

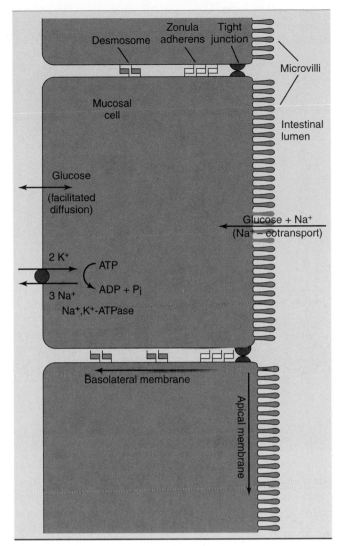

Figure 12.18 Absorption of glucose in the brush border of the small intestine. The apical (luminal) membrane and the basolateral (serosal) membrane of the epithelial cells are physiologically different. The tight junctions between adjacent cells prevent not only the diffusion of solutes around the cells but also the lateral diffusion of membrane proteins. Therefore different sets of carriers are present in the two parts of the plasma membrane. P_i, Inorganic phosphate.

CLINICAL EXAMPLE 12.3: Cardiotonic Steroids

The contraction of the myocardium, like that of skeletal muscle, is triggered by calcium. *The higher the intracellular calcium concentration, the greater is the force of contraction.* Myocardial cells regulate their intracellular calcium stores by pumping calcium out of the cell in exchange for sodium. Thus *the extrusion of excess calcium from the cell requires a sodium gradient* (*Fig. 12.19*).

The sodium gradient depends on the sodium/potassium pump. Steroidal glycosides from the plant

Digitalis purpurea L. inhibit the sodium/potassium pump, weaken the sodium gradient, and thereby impair the removal of calcium from the cell. The excess calcium is pumped into the sarcoplasmic reticulum, which stores it for release into the cytoplasm during contraction. This increases the force of contraction (positive inotropic effect). Digitalis glycosides are still used for treatment of congestive heart failure, but they are very toxic because they cause fatal cardiac arrhythmias at high doses.

Continued

CLINICAL EXAMPLE 12.3: Cardiotonic Steroids—cont'd

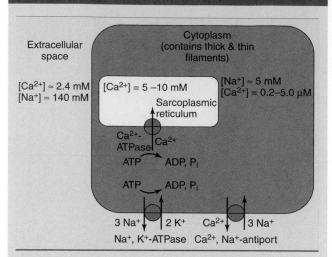

Figure 12.19 Regulation of the intracellular calcium concentration in myocardial cells. Cardiotonic steroids (digitalis) reduce the sodium gradient and therefore the effectiveness of the Ca^{2+}/Na^+ antiporter in the plasma membrane. P_i, Inorganic phosphate.

SUMMARY

The structural core of biological membranes is a bilayer that consists of amphipathic lipids: phosphoglycerides, sphingolipids, and cholesterol. Integral membrane proteins are embedded in the lipid bilayer, and peripheral membrane proteins are attached to its surface. Most integral membrane proteins traverse the lipid bilayer in the form of a transmembrane α-helix.

Whereas the lipid bilayer forms a diffusion barrier for water-soluble solutes, membrane proteins are in charge of specialized functions. Some membrane proteins are enzymes, and others form structural links with the cytoskeleton and the extracellular matrix or are components of signaling pathways.

The carriers that transport hydrophilic substrates across the membrane form gated channels across the lipid bilayer. Some types of carrier-mediated transport are passive, and others are driven by the hydrolysis of ATP, either directly or indirectly.

Further Reading

Engel A, Gaub HE: Structure and mechanics of membrane proteins, *Annu Rev Biochem* 77:127–148, 2008.

Fadeel B, Xue D: The ins and outs of phospholipid asymmetry in the plasma membrane: roles in health and disease, *Crit Rev Biochem Mol Biol* 44:264–277, 2009.

Giacomini KM, Huang SM, Tweedie DJ, et al: Membrane transporters in drug development, *Nat Rev Drug Discov* 9: 215–236, 2010.

Kaplan JH: Biochemistry of Na, K-ATPase, *Annu Rev Biochem* 71:511–535, 2002.

Kinoshita T, Fujita M, Maeda Y: Biosynthesis, remodeling and functions of mammalian GPI-anchored proteins: recent progress, *J Biochem* 144:287–294, 2008.

Lingwood D, Simons K: Lipid rafts as a membrane-organizing principle, *Science* 327:46–50, 2010.

Neumann S, van Meer G: Sphingolipid management by an orchestra of lipid transfer proteins, *Biol Chem* 389: 1349–1360, 2008.

QUESTIONS

1. **The selective transport of molecules and inorganic ions across the membrane requires a "gated channel" across the lipid bilayer. The most typical structural feature of these gated channels is**

   A. Several segments of antiparallel β-pleated sheet structure
   B. Glycolipids forming the inner lining of the channel
   C. Lipids that form a covalent bond with the transported solute
   D. Several amphipathic α-helices forming the channel
   E. Nonpolar α-helices forming the channel

2. **Which of the following characteristics applies to the lipids in biological membranes?**

   A. Triglycerides and phosphoglycerides are the most abundant lipids in most membranes.
   B. Most glycerol-containing lipids are glycolipids.
   C. Cholesterol is common in the nuclear and inner mitochondrial membranes but not in the plasma membrane of most cells.
   D. The glycolipids of the plasma membrane are found in the outer leaflet of the bilayer.
   E. Membranes in the brain have a high phosphoglyceride content but only very small amounts of sphingolipids.

3. **The transport of glucose across the capillary endothelium of cerebral blood vessels ("blood-brain barrier") is achieved by facilitated diffusion. This means that**

A. Specific inhibition of cerebral glucose uptake is not possible

B. The cerebral glucose uptake is always directly proportional to the concentration gradient for glucose across the endothelium

C. The inhibition of ATP synthesis in the endothelial cells will prevent glucose uptake into the brain

D. As long as glucose is only consumed but not produced in the brain, the cerebrospinal fluid glucose concentration is always less than the blood glucose concentration

E. There is no upper limit to the amount of glucose that can be taken up by the brain

4. **Many properties of biological membranes depend on the structure of the lipid bilayer. Typical features of lipid bilayers include**

A. Impermeability for small inorganic ions such as sodium and protons

B. Rapid exchange of phospholipids between the two leaflets of the bilayer

C. High electrical conductivity

D. Lack of lateral mobility of membrane lipids at normal body temperature

E. Permeability for proteins

Chapter 13
THE CYTOSKELETON

As diffusion barriers, biological membranes form the boundary between the cell and its surroundings, and they form compartments within eukaryotic cells. However, they do not give the cell its shape. They do not provide structural strength, resistance to mechanical stress, or resilience to deformation. These properties require a network of cellular fibers known collectively as the **cytoskeleton.**

In addition to giving the cell its shape and mechanical strength, the cytoskeleton has two additional functions: intracellular transport and cell motility. Transport of proteins and organelles down the axons of neurons, amoeboid movement of phagocytic cells, beating of cilia and flagella, and muscle contraction all are specialized functions of the cytoskeleton.

THE ERYTHROCYTE MEMBRANE IS REINFORCED BY A SPECTRIN NETWORK

Erythrocytes travel about 300 miles during their 120-day life, part of this through tortuous capillaries in which they suffer mechanical deformation. They can survive this only because their membrane is reinforced by a meshwork of fibers formed by the proteins **α-spectrin** and **β-spectrin.** Each spectrin monomer consists of spectrin repeats, a domain of 106 amino acids

that forms a coiled coil of three intertwined α-helices. It is repeated (with variations) 20 times in the α-chain and 17 times in the β-chain (*Fig. 13.1*).

Spectrin forms an antiparallel dimer, with an α-chain and a β-chain lying side by side. These α-β dimers condense head to head to form a tetramer, which is a long, wriggly, wormlike molecule with a contour length of 200 nm and a diameter of 5 nm. The ends of the spectrin tetramer are bound noncovalently to short (35-nm) actin filaments. This interaction is facilitated by two other proteins: **band 4.1 protein** (so named after its migration in gel electrophoresis) and **adducin.** By binding several spectrin tetramers, *the actin filaments form the nodes of a two-dimensional network* that can be likened to a fishing net or a piece of very thin, flexible chicken wire (*Fig. 13.2, B*).

The spectrin network is anchored to the membrane by the peripheral membrane protein **ankyrin,** which itself is bound to the integral membrane protein **band 3 protein.** This binding is stabilized by **band 4.2 protein** (pallidin). The actin microfilaments are attached to the membrane mainly through **band 4.1 protein** and the integral membrane protein **glycophorin.** The erythrocyte membrane skeleton is important because inherited defects in its components give rise to hemolytic anemias (*Clinical Example 13.1*).

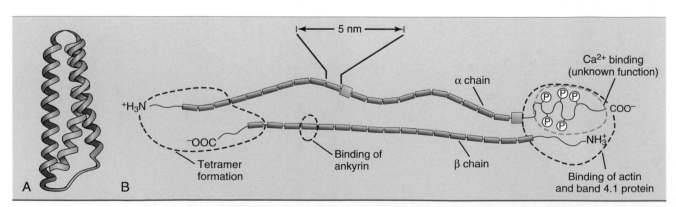

Figure 13.1   **A,** The spectrin repeat consists of three α-helical coiled coils with a total of 106 amino acid residues. **B,** Structure of a spectrin dimer consisting of an α-chain and β-chain, which have 20 and 17 spectrin repeats, respectively.

Hereditary spherocytosis is defined by the presence of erythrocytes that are spherical instead of biconcave. *Mild anemia can result because the spherocytes are fragile and are easily trapped and destroyed in the spleen.*

Most patients with hereditary spherocytosis have primary defects in ankyrin, β-spectrin, or band 3 protein. The amount of spectrin is always reduced because any spectrin that is not tied into the membrane skeleton falls prey to proteolytic enzymes during erythrocyte maturation.

In **hereditary elliptocytosis,** the erythrocytes are ellipsoidal rather than spherical. Mutations in the genes for band 4.1 protein or α-spectrin are the most common causes.

With a prevalence of 1 in 5000 each, spherocytosis and elliptocytosis are the most common inherited hemolytic anemias in many countries. Seventy-five percent of cases are inherited as autosomal dominant traits. Splenectomy cures the anemia in most patients.

KERATINS ARE THE MOST IMPORTANT STRUCTURAL PROTEINS OF EPITHELIAL TISSUES

Epithelial cells receive most of their structural support from **keratin,** which is one of several classes of **intermediate filaments.** In addition to its role in living epithelia, the keratin cytoskeleton of dead cells forms hair, fingernails, and the horny layer of the skin.

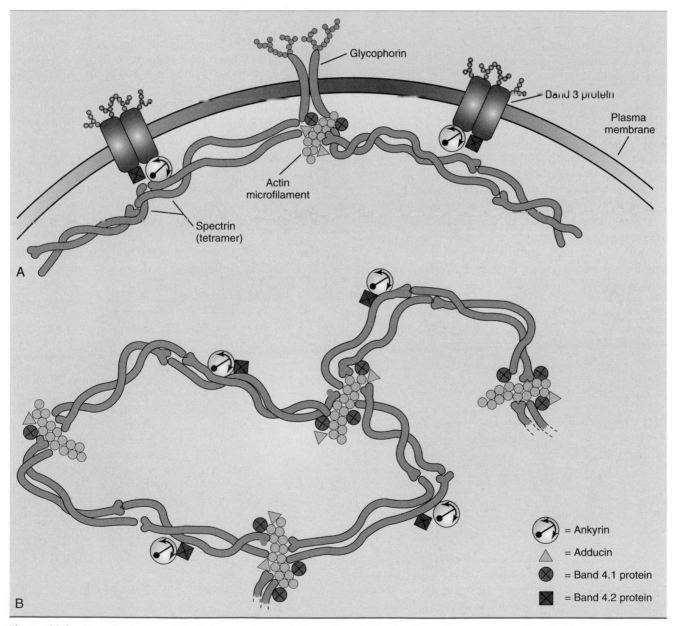

Figure 13.2 Hypothetical model of the membrane skeleton in red blood cells. **A,** Transverse section. **B,** Tangential section.

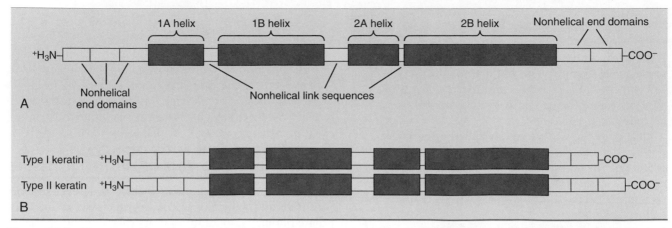

Figure 13.3 Structure of keratin, the major intermediate filament protein of epithelial tissues. **A,** Domain structure of a single polypeptide (type I keratin). The central, mostly α-helical part consists of approximately 310 amino acids. **B,** Parallel heterodimer formed from a type I and a type II keratin polypeptide.

All keratins contain long stretches of α-helix interrupted by short nonhelical segments (**Fig. 13.3, A**). The two different types are the acidic (type I) and the basic (type II) keratins. Each comes in about 15 different variants. *They form heterodimers, with a type I polypeptide forming a **coiled coil** with a type II polypeptide* (**Fig. 13.3, B**). The α-helices of the two keratins make contact through hydrophobic amino acid side chains on one edge of each helix. Typical keratin fibrils contain between 12 and 24 of these heterodimers in a staggered array.

Different keratins are expressed in different cell types. The basal layer of the epidermis forms K14 as the major type I keratin and K5 as the major type II keratin. In the more mature cells of the spinous and granular layers, keratins K10 and K1 are the major type I and type II keratins, respectively (**Fig. 13.4**).

Single-layered epithelia express keratins 18, 19, and/or 20 (type I) and keratins 7 and 8 (type II). Various other keratin pairs are expressed in the cells that form hair and nails.

Several intermediate filament proteins other than the keratins are expressed in various cell types (**Table 13.1**). *All of them are dynamic structures that are assembled and disassembled continuously.*

The **lamins** are the only intermediate filament proteins that are found in the nucleus rather than the cytoplasm. They form a supporting fiber network under the nuclear envelope. During mitosis, the lamins become phosphorylated by the cell cycle–induced protein kinase Cdk1. This leads to the disassembly of the fibers and the collapse of the nuclear envelope (see Chapter 18).

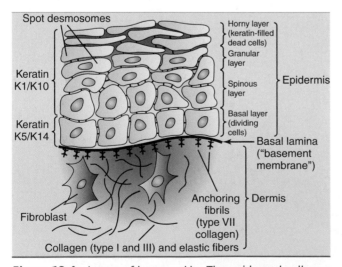

Figure 13.4 Layers of human skin. The epidermal cells are held together by numerous spot desmosomes. These spot desmosomes are attachment points for the intracellular keratin filaments.

Table 13.1 Major Types of Intermediate Filament Proteins*

Protein	Tissue or Cell Type
Keratin	Epithelial cells, hair, nails
Vimentin	Embryonic tissues, mesenchymal cells, most cultured cells
Desmin	Myocardium, at Z disk in skeletal muscle
Glial fibrillary acidic protein	Astrocytes, Schwann cells
Peripherin	Neurons of PNS
α-Internexin	Neurons of CNS
Neurofilament proteins (NF-L, NF-M, NF-H)	Neurons of CNS and PNS
Lamin	Nucleus of all nucleated cells.

CNS, Central nervous system; *PNS,* peripheral nervous system.
*All of these proteins have the general structure depicted in **Figure 13.3**, for keratin.

CLINICAL EXAMPLE 13.2: Skin Blistering Diseases

A blister forms when the epidermis detaches from the dermis. Therefore any condition that weakens the boundary between dermis and epidermis leads to abnormal blistering.

Epidermolysis bullosa (EB) is a group of dominantly inherited skin blistering diseases in which even mild mechanical stress damages the dermal-epidermal junction. It comes in all degrees of severity, from mild forms with occasional blistering to severe forms that are fatal shortly after birth.

The classic forms of EB are caused by point mutations in the genes of keratin K14 or keratin K5, which are expressed in the basal cells of the epidermis. Therefore *shear forces easily destroy the basal cell layer but leave the overlying cells intact.*

Point mutations in the genes for K1 and K10, the major keratins of the spinous and granular cell layers, cause **epidermolytic hyperkeratosis**, a dominantly inherited type of skin disease with scaling, hyperkeratosis, and blistering.

CLINICAL EXAMPLE 13.3: Laminopathies

Mutations that affect the lamins of the nuclear lamina, especially the predominant lamin A, cause an astonishing spectrum of disease. **Hutchinson-Gilford progeria** is an extremely rare syndrome of premature aging, with an incidence of about 1 in 5 million live births. Although normal at birth, patients present with failure to thrive at 1 or 2 years, followed by signs of premature aging: hair loss, osteoporosis, loss of subcutaneous fat, atherosclerosis. Most patients die of myocardial infarction or stroke at age 12 to 14 years. The usual mutation in this disease is a point mutation that activates a cryptic splice site, creating a messenger RNA (mRNA) that is missing 150 nucleotides and a lamin A protein that is missing 50 amino acids.

Different mutations in the lamin A gene cause different diseases, including subtypes of limb girdle and Emery-Dreifuss muscular dystrophies, cardiomyopathies, lipodystrophies, skin disorders, and peripheral neuropathy.

The mechanisms by which lamin mutations cause so many seemingly unrelated syndromes is not known. The lamins interact not only with each other and with proteins of the inner nuclear membrane but also with core histones and many other components of chromatin. In addition to mechanical fragility of the nucleus, deranged gene expression is a possible mechanism.

ACTIN FILAMENTS ARE FORMED FROM GLOBULAR SUBUNITS

All cells contain **microfilaments** that are formed by the polymerization of globular **actin** subunits. Collectively, the six isoforms of actin that occur in different tissues are among the most abundant types of protein in the human body. In most cells, the microfilaments are concentrated under the plasma membrane where they form the gel-like cortex of the cytoplasm. *When actin monomers polymerize into microfilaments, the cytoplasm turns into a gel; when they disassemble, the cytoplasm turns into a viscous liquid.*

The loose subunits are called **G-actin** (G for globular). They have a molecular weight (MW) of 42,000 and a nucleotide binding site that is occupied by ATP or ADP. These subunits can polymerize into a filament in which two strands are coiled gently around one another (**Fig. 13.5**). *Microfilaments are dynamic structures that can be assembled and disassembled continuously.*

The two ends of the actin filament are not equivalent. At the **positive (+) end,** addition and dissociation of actin monomers are fast. At the opposite end, the **negative (−) end,** both processes are slow. The bound nucleotide is also important. *ATP-actin binds strongly to other actin monomers and tends to add to the microfilament, whereas ADP-actin binds weakly and tends to break away from the microfilament.*

The large majority of free actin monomers in the cytoplasm contain a bound ATP. This form adds to the + end of the microfilament. In the microfilament, however, the ATP is hydrolyzed. When the concentration of G-actin is

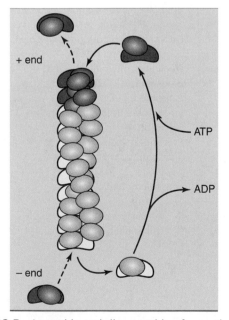

Figure 13.5 Assembly and disassembly of an actin microfilament. The filament grows at the + end and is disassembled at the − end. ○, Actin monomer with bound ADP; ◗, actin monomer with bound ATP.

high, the addition of new actin monomers to the + end is faster than the hydrolysis of the bound ATP. As a result, the last subunits at the + end are in the ATP form, whereas the rest of the microfilament is in the ADP form. *This filament tends to grow at the + end and frizzle away at the − end.*

Cells have a bloated bureaucracy of proteins to regulate the formation, growth, and dissolution of microfilaments. Some initiate the formation of a new microfilament, some anchor the filaments to membranes or cytoskeletal structures, and others bundle them into networks or parallel arrays (*Table 13.2*).

Many specialized cellular functions depend on microfilaments, including

1. Muscle contraction
2. Amoeboid motility
3. Phagocytosis
4. Contraction of intestinal microvilli
5. Formation of the cleavage furrow during mitosis
6. Shape change of activated platelets
7. Outgrowth of dendrites and axons in developing neuroblasts

Actin-dependent processes are inhibited by **cytochalasin B,** a fungal metabolite that prevents actin polymerization by capping the + end of the growing microfilament. **Phalloidin,** another fungal toxin, prevents the depolymerization of actin filaments. These agents change

Table 13.2 Proteins That Regulate Actin Microfilaments

Protein	Function
Thymosin	Binds free actin monomers, making them unavailable for polymerization
Profilin	Delivers actin monomers to growing microfilaments
ARP complex	Nucleates microfilaments at the − end
Formin	Binds to the + end of microfilaments, promotes elongation
Tropomyosin	Strengthens microfilaments, regulates their length
Caldesmon, Troponin	Prevents myosin from binding to actin/tropomyosin
Spectrin, Fodrin, Filamin	Link microfilaments into a gel
α-Actinin, Fimbrin, Villin	Link microfilaments into parallel bundles
Talin, Myosin-1, Catenin, Vinculin, α-Actinin	Link microfilaments to the plasma membrane
Cap Z	Caps and stabilizes the + end of microfilaments
Tropomodulin	Caps and stabilizes the − end of microfilaments
Gelsolin	Cuts microfilaments

the shapes of many cells, inhibit cell motility, and prevent the outgrowth of axons from ganglia.

STRIATED MUSCLE CONTAINS THICK AND THIN FILAMENTS

Amoeboid motion, phagocytosis, and muscle contraction all require the interaction of actin microfilaments with the ATPase **myosin.** Various forms of myosin are present in most cells, but only the myosin of muscle (myosin II) forms stable fibers. These are the **thick filaments,** in contrast to the **thin filaments** that are formed from actin.

A skeletal muscle fiber has a diameter of 20 to 50 μm and a length of 1 to 40 mm. It is functionally divided into **myofibrils** that run lengthwise through the muscle fiber (*Fig. 13.6, A*). Each myofibril is cylindrical in shape, about 0.6 μm in diameter, and surrounded by cisternae of the sarcoplasmic reticulum.

The myofibrils are organized into **sarcomeres** by transverse partitions known as **Z disks.** Invaginations of the plasma membrane form the **transverse (T) tubules,** which reach each sarcomere at the level of the Z disk. The T tubules are in close apposition to the cisternae of the sarcoplasmic reticulum that envelop the sides of the sarcomere.

The + ends of the thin filaments (7-nm diameter) are attached to the Z disk, and their capped − ends protrude toward the center of the sarcomere. The thick filaments (16-nm diameter) are suspended in the center of the sarcomere, overlapping with the thin filaments. *The length of the filaments does not change during contraction, but the thick and thin filaments slide along each other* (see *Fig. 13.6, B* and *C*). This shortens the sarcomere by about 30%.

The thin filaments of skeletal muscle contain tropomyosin and troponin in addition to actin. **Tropomyosin** is a long coiled coil of two α-helical polypeptides that winds along the microfilament near the groove between the two actin strands. **Troponin** consists of the three globular subunits **Tn-T** (tropomyosin binding), **Tn-I** (inhibitory, actin binding), and **Tn-C** (calcium binding). This complex is spaced at regular intervals of 38.5 nm along the thin filament, corresponding to the length of the tropomyosin dimer (*Fig. 13.7*). *Troponin makes the thin filament sensitive to calcium.*

MYOSIN IS A TWO-HEADED MOLECULE WITH ATPASE ACTIVITY

The myosin of skeletal muscle contains one pair of heavy chains (MW 230,000 each) and two pairs of light chains (MW 16,000 and 20,000) (*Fig. 13.8, A*). The carboxyl terminal 60% of the two heavy chains forms an α-helical coiled coil with a length of 130 nm and a diameter of 2 nm. *This coiled coil bundles the myosin into the thick filaments.*

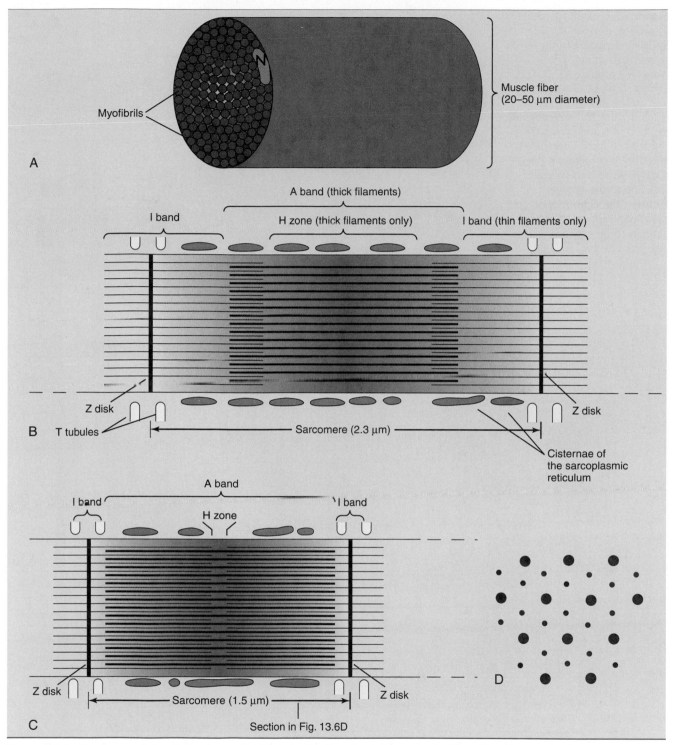

Figure 13.6 Structure of the skeletal muscle fiber. **A,** Section through a muscle fiber. The fiber has a diameter of 20 to 50 μm and is surrounded by the plasma membrane (sarcolemma). Its nuclei (*N*, up to 100 per fiber) are located peripherally, and the mitochondria are interspersed between the myofibrils. More than 100 myofibrils (diameter 0.6–1.0 μm) run the length of the muscle fiber. **B,** Sarcomere structure of the myofibril in the relaxed state. **C,** The sarcomere in the contracted state. **D,** Cross-section through the overlap zone of thick and thin filaments. The filaments are neatly packed, with each thick filament surrounded by six thin filaments and each thin filament surrounded by three thick filaments.

Figure 13.7 Thin filaments of skeletal muscle. **A,** Simplified model of thin filament structure. The troponin complex (*Tn-C, Tn-I,* and *Tn-T*) binds to a specific site on the dimeric tropomyosin (*TM*) molecule. **B,** Position of tropomyosin (*T*) in the relaxed state (low [Ca^{2+}]) and during contraction (high [Ca^{2+}]). When tropomyosin moves into the groove between the actin monomers, the myosin-binding sites on actin become exposed.

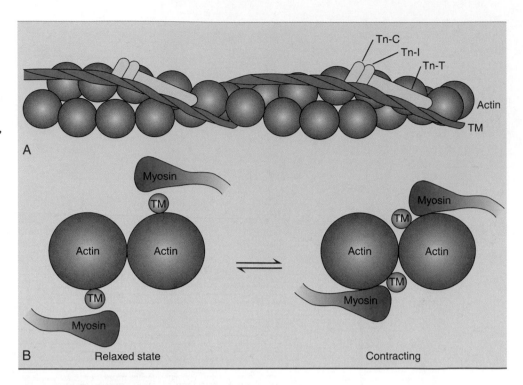

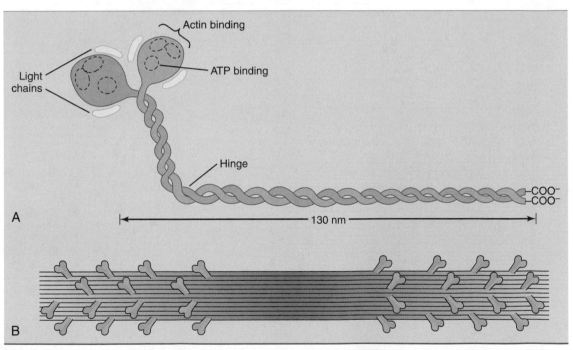

Figure 13.8 Structure of myosin and the thick filaments. **A,** Structure of a single myosin molecule. **B,** Structure of the thick filaments in skeletal muscle. The globular heads of myosin are on the surface of the filament. Its center consists only of the fibrous tails and therefore is without globular heads. The packed tails have a diameter of 10.7 nm.

Together with the light chains, the amino terminal ends of the two heavy chains form two globular heads (see **Fig. 13.8, A**). *The myosin heads hydrolyze ATP very fast when they are in physical contact with actin,* but ADP and inorganic phosphate remain tightly bound to the catalytic site and prevent the access of further ATP molecules.

The thick filament consists of 300 to 400 myosin molecules whose heads protrude in all directions (see **Fig. 13.8, B**). In the middle of the filament the molecules are bundled tail to tail; therefore, this central portion has no heads. A hinge region in the myosin tail functions as a joint, allowing the myosin heads to wag back and forth on the surface of the thick filament.

MUSCLE CONTRACTION REQUIRES CALCIUM AND ATP

In resting muscle, the myosin-binding sites on actin are blocked by tropomyosin (see *Fig. 13.7, B*). Removal of tropomyosin from these sites requires the binding of calcium to the troponin complex. Therefore *the muscle fiber can contract only when the cytoplasmic calcium level rises substantially above its resting level of 10^{-7} mol/L.*

During nerve stimulation, the neurotransmitter acetylcholine depolarizes the membrane of the skeletal muscle fiber. This depolarization is transmitted into the interior of the fiber by the T tubules. The T tubules are in contact with the sarcoplasmic reticulum, and *membrane depolarization triggers the release of calcium from the sarcoplasmic reticulum.*

Within a few milliseconds the cytoplasmic calcium level rises up to 100-fold, and four Ca^{2+} ions bind to troponin C on the thin filaments. *Calcium binding triggers a conformational change in the troponin complex that pulls tropomyosin from the myosin-binding sites of actin* (see *Fig. 13.7, B*).

The myosin heads, each with a tightly bound ADP, now bind to the exposed actin of the thin filaments (*Fig. 13.9*). Actin binding causes release of the bound ADP and phosphate. This triggers a conformational change in the myosin that pulls the thick filament about 7 nm along the thin filament. ATP is required to detach the myosin head from actin but then is rapidly hydrolyzed to ADP and phosphate.

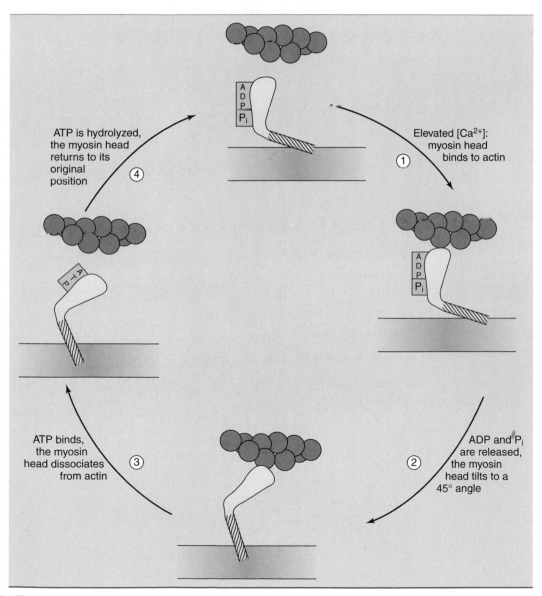

Figure 13.9   The mechanism of muscle contraction. In this model, the conformational change of the myosin molecule ("power stroke") is induced by binding of the myosin head to the thin filament and the subsequent release of ADP and inorganic phosphate (P_i). ATP is needed to detach the myosin head from the thin filament and prepare it for another stroke.

CLINICAL EXAMPLE 13.4: Rigor Mortis

Binding of the myosin heads to the thin filaments requires calcium, and their dissociation from the thin filaments requires ATP. In death, the cytoplasmic Ca^{2+} concentration rises while ATP is depleted. Therefore the myosin heads bind to the thin filaments but cannot dissociate in the absence of ATP. The resulting stiffness of the muscles is called **rigor mortis**.

THE CYTOSKELETON OF SKELETAL MUSCLE IS LINKED TO THE EXTRACELLULAR MATRIX

Dystrophin is a distant relative of spectrin that is found under the plasma membrane of skeletal, cardiac, and smooth muscle. It is a large protein with 3685 amino acids, containing an actin-binding domain, 24 spectrin repeats, a calcium-binding domain, and a carboxyl-terminal domain for membrane attachment (*Fig. 13.10*).

Dystrophin constitutes only 0.002% of the total muscle protein, but it is essential for the structural integrity of the muscle fiber. It binds to a set of membrane proteins known as the **dystroglycan complex.** These membrane proteins bind to proteins of the basal lamina. *They form the link between the cytoskeleton and the extracellular matrix.* The connection between cytoskeleton and extracellular matrix is essential for the structural integrity of the muscle fiber, and inherited defects in any of its components can cause degenerative muscle diseases (see *Fig. 13.10, B,* and *Clinical Example 13.5*).

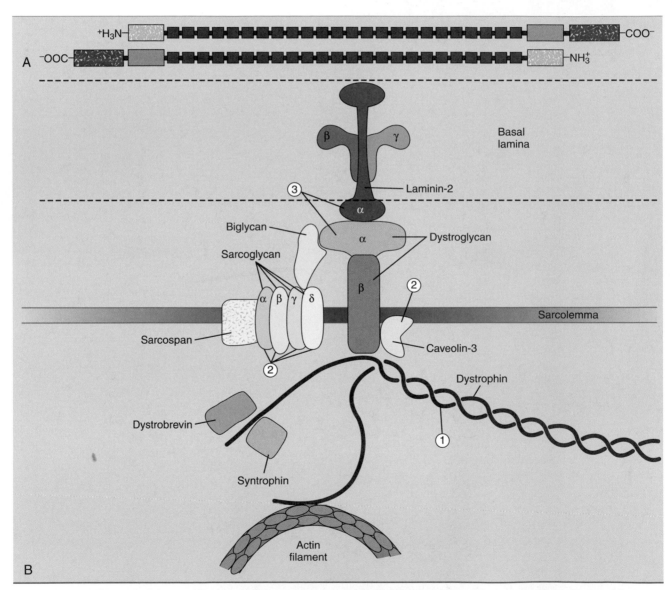

Figure 13.10 Structure of dystrophin, the major component of the membrane skeleton in muscle fibers. Dystrophin is thought to form an antiparallel dimer. **A,** Domain structure of dystrophin. ▨, Actin-binding domain; ▧, calcium-binding domain; ▨, membrane attachment; ▪, spectrin repeat. **B,** Dystrophin-associated proteins in the sarcolemma. These proteins link the cytoskeleton to the extracellular matrix. Disease associations: ① Duchenne and Becker muscular dystrophies; ② limb girdle muscular dystrophy; ③ congenital muscular dystrophy.

CLINICAL EXAMPLE 13.5: Duchenne Muscular Dystrophy

Muscular dystrophies are inherited diseases that lead to destruction of skeletal muscle. **Duchenne muscular dystrophy (DMD)** is the deadliest and most common form. It is caused by X-linked recessive mutations in the gene for dystrophin and affects about 1 in 4000 male births. The patients develop muscle weakness and muscle wasting in early childhood, are wheelchair bound by age 10 to 12 years, and die of respiratory or cardiac failure usually before age 20 years.

Most patients with DMD have deletions that eliminate one or more exons of the dystrophin gene. The gene has 79 exons, so the mutation rate is quite high. Because affected males do not reproduce and the gene can be transmitted only through unaffected female carriers, many patients have a new mutation. Milder mutations in the dystrophin gene that permit survival into adulthood are diagnosed as **Becker muscular dystrophy.**

Patients with DMD are prime candidates for gene therapy. Skeletal muscle fibers have multiple nuclei, and getting the gene into only one or a few of them might well be sufficient. However, the large size of the gene makes the construction of vectors difficult. Many other muscular dystrophies have been described and are summarized in **Table 13.3.**

Table 13.3 Muscular Dystrophies*

Disease	Affected Protein	Inheritance	Clinical Course
Duchenne muscular dystrophy	Dystrophin	XR	Normal at birth, muscle weakness beginning age 2–3 years, death at age 15–22 years
Becker muscular dystrophy	Dystrophin	XR	Like Duchenne muscular dystrophy, but later onset and survival into adulthood
Limb girdle muscular dystrophy	Sarcoglycan or lamin-A/C	AR	Muscle weakness beginning at age 3–10 years, variable severity, mainly shoulders and hips
Congenital muscular dystrophy	Laminin α-2 chain or integrin α7	AR	Lethal in infants
Emery-Dreifuss muscular dystrophy	Emerin or lamin-A/C	XR, AD or AR	Slowly progressive muscle wasting, contractures, cardiac arrhythmias

AD, Autosomal dominant; *AR*, autosomal recessive; *XR*, X-linked recessive.
*These diseases are caused by inherited defects in structural muscle proteins.

MICROTUBULES CONSIST OF TUBULIN

Microtubules are thick hollow tubes with an outer diameter of 24 nm, an inner diameter of 14 nm, and a length up to several micrometers. They are important for the *maintenance of cell shape* and for many kinds of *intracellular transport*. During mitosis, for example, microtubules serve as ropes to pull the chromosomes to opposite poles of the cell, and in neurons they are used as railroad tracks to ship vesicular organelles from the perikaryon to the nerve terminals.

Microtubules form when globular dimers of **α-tubulin** and β-tubulin (MW 53,000 each) polymerize into a helical array with 13 protein subunits per turn (*Fig. 13.11*). Like the actin microfilaments, microtubules have a + end where new subunits are added and a − end where subunits break off. Like actin, tubulin binds a nucleotide that facilitates polymerization. This nucleotide is not ATP but guanosine triphosphate (GTP), and it hydrolyzes to guanosine diphosphate (GDP) after polymerization. As a result, *microtubules can rapidly be assembled and disassembled as needed.*

Microtubule-dependent transport requires proteins that translate the hydrolysis of ATP into sliding movement along the side of the microtubule. **Dyneins** move

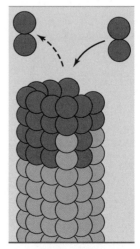

Figure 13.11 End of a microtubule. GTP-ligated tubulin (●) adds to the end of the microtubule. GTP-ligated tubulin has a greater propensity for polymerization than does the GDP-ligated tubulin (○) that is formed by the hydrolysis of the bound GTP in the microtubule.

organelles and proteins from the + end to the − end of the microtubule, and **kinesins** move things in the opposite direction. In the axons of neurons, for example, where all microtubules have the same orientation, kinesins move vesicles from the cell body toward the nerve terminals, and dyneins move things in the opposite direction at a speed of up to 25 cm/day (3 μm/s).

Colchicine, the poison of autumn crocus, blocks the polymerization of tubulin. It inhibits microtubule-dependent processes, including mitosis.

EUKARYOTIC CILIA AND FLAGELLA CONTAIN A 9 + 2 ARRAY OF MICROTUBULES

Cilia and flagella are hairlike cell appendages that are capable of beating or swirling motion (***Fig. 13.12***). Ciliated cells are found in the epithelia of the bronchial tree, upper respiratory tract, and fallopian tubes. The only flagellated cell in humans is the sperm cell. Cilia are about 6 μm long, and the sperm flagellum is about 40 μm long.

The skin of cilia and flagella is an extension of the plasma membrane, and their skeleton consists of microtubules: two single microtubules in the center, and nine double microtubules in the periphery. The double microtubules consist of a circular A fiber and a crescent-shaped B fiber (***Fig. 13.13***). Unlike the cytoplasmic microtubules that are assembled and dismantled as needed, *the microtubules of cilia and flagella are permanent structures.*

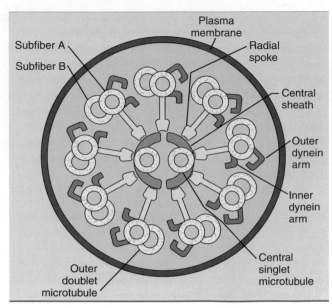

Figure 13.13 Cross-section through a cilium or flagellum. All eukaryotic (but not prokaryotic) cilia and flagella have this general structure.

The A subfiber of the doublet microtubules extends two arms that are formed by the protein **dynein**. The outer dynein arm has three globular heads, and the inner arm has either two or three. *The dynein heads use the energy of ATP hydrolysis to walk along the B subfiber of a neighboring doublet microtubule.* Thus dynein plays the same role in flagellar movement that myosin plays in muscle contraction. Even the role of ATP is similar in the two systems. ATP is needed to dissociate the dynein heads from the neighboring B subfiber, as it is needed to dissociate the myosin heads from the thin filament.

CLINICAL EXAMPLE 13.6: Immotile Cilia Syndrome

Defects in dynein or other microtubule-associated proteins of cilia and flagella result in **immotile cilia syndrome**, also known as **Kartagener syndrome**. Patients with this rare recessively inherited disease (incidence at birth: 1:20,000 to 1:60,000) suffer from frequent infections of the bronchi and nasal sinuses. The epithelium in these locations is covered by a mucus blanket with a thickness of about 5 μm. Most inhaled particles and microorganisms get caught on this glue trap and are moved up the bronchi and the trachea by coordinated ciliary beating. This "mucus elevator" removes 30 to 40 g of mucus from the bronchial system every day.

Male patients with this syndrome are infertile because their sperm cells are paralyzed. The fertility of affected females is reduced as well, presumably for lack of ciliary movement in the fallopian tubes. The most surprising (and still unexplained) observation, however, is that 50% of all patients with immotile cilia syndrome have complete situs inversus (left-right inversion of the internal organs).

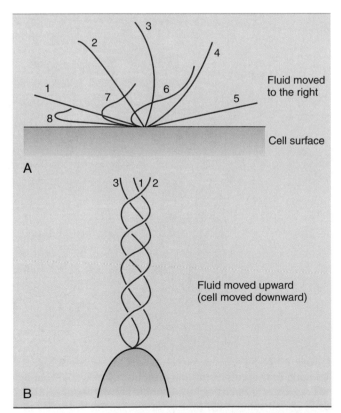

Figure 13.12 Motile patterns of cilia and flagella. **A,** Cilium. **B,** Flagellum. Sperm flagella beat 30 to 40 times per second.

CELLS FORM SPECIALIZED JUNCTIONS WITH OTHER CELLS AND WITH THE EXTRACELLULAR MATRIX

The cells of solid tissues form specialized sites of contact with neighboring cells and with structural proteins of the extracellular matrix.

Anchoring junctions link the cytoskeleton either with the cytoskeleton of a neighboring cell or with the extracellular matrix. All anchoring junctions contain a transmembrane protein, which is a protein of the **cadherin** family in cell-cell junctions and an **integrin** in cell-matrix junctions. The transmembrane protein connects to either microfilaments or intermediate filaments through an adapter protein.

Table 13.4 lists the composition of the four kinds of anchoring junction. The **zonula adherens** ("belt desmosome," *Fig. 13.14*) is the most characteristic anchoring junction in single-layered epithelia. In intestinal mucosal cells, for example, it forms a belt that encircles the cells. Ordinary desmosomes do not form a belt, but they form spot welds between the cells. Unlike the zonula adherens, they are linked to intermediate filaments rather than actin filaments. In the epidermis, they connect the keratin filaments of neighboring cells.

The integrins of **hemidesmosomes** and **focal adhesions** link the cell to collagen, laminin, fibronectin, and other proteins of the extracellular matrix. For example, epidermal cells of the skin are glued to the basal lamina by hemidesmosomes.

CLINICAL EXAMPLE 13.7: Pemphigus

Whereas some serious skin diseases are inherited (see *Clinical Example 13.2*), others are caused by autoimmunity. In the serious disease **pemphigus**, antibodies are formed against a cadherin in the epidermis. This leads to disruption of the desmosomes that hold the epidermal cells together, resulting in blistering and epidermal fragility.

Table 13.4 Four Types of Anchoring Junction

	Adherens Junction	Desmosome
Contact with	Neighboring cell	Neighboring cell
Transmembrane protein	Cadherin	Cadherin
Cytoskeletal attachment	Microfilaments	Intermediate filaments
Intracellular adapter protein	Catenin, vinculin, plakoglobin	Desmoplakin, plakoglobin
	Focal Adhesion	**Hemidesmosome**
Contact with	Extracellular matrix	Extracellular matrix
Transmembrane protein	Integrin	Integrin
Cytoskeletal attachment	Microfilaments	Intermediate filaments
Intracellular adapter proteins	Talin, vinculin, filamin	Plectin

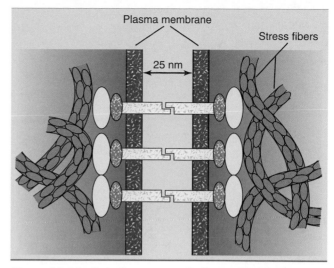

Figure 13.14 Belt desmosome ("adherens junction"). The major adhesive membrane protein is E-cadherin (□). E-cadherin is bound to β-catenin or plakoglobin (◉) on the cytoplasmic side of the membrane, and these are bound to α-catenin (◐), which interacts with actin microfilaments ("stress fibers"). Spot desmosomes have a similar molecular architecture but are linked to intermediate filaments rather than microfilaments.

Tight junctions form a continuous belt around the cells of single-layered epithelia. The intestinal epithelium, for example, has an **apical surface** to absorb nutrients from the lumen and a **basolateral surface** to transfer the nutrients from the cell to the extracellular fluid and the blood. These two surfaces have different sets of membrane carriers, and those of the apical membrane must be prevented from mixing with those of the basolateral membrane.

The barrier between the two surfaces is formed by the tight junctions: a network of long strands formed by the integral membrane proteins **claudin** and **occludin** (*Fig. 13.15*). *The tight junction forms a seal that prevents the diffusion of many water-soluble molecules through the narrow clefts between the epithelial cells.* Because the protein strands cut through the lipid bilayer, *it also forms the boundary between the apical and basolateral membrane by preventing the lateral diffusion of membrane proteins and membrane lipids.*

The tightness of tight junctions differs in different tissues. For example, those in the intestine are 10,000 times more permeable for small cations such as sodium than are those in the urinary bladder.

Gap junctions are clusters of small channels that interconnect the cytoplasm of neighboring cells. Each half-channel is formed by six subunits of the transmembrane protein **connexin** (*Fig. 13.16*). With a diameter of 2 nm, *gap junctions allow the passage of molecules up to a molecular weight of approximately 1200 D.* Because they are permeable to inorganic ions, *gap junctions can transmit membrane depolarization from cell to cell.* Myocardial contraction, for example, depends on the electrical coupling of the cells by gap junctions.

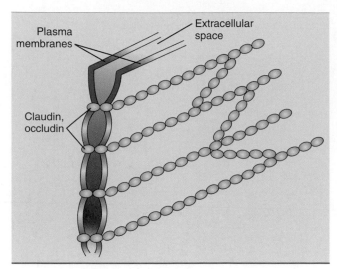

Figure 13.15 Tight junction. The junctional proteins (claudin, occludin) form a tight seal that restricts the diffusion of water-soluble molecules and ions through the narrow clefts of extracellular space between the cells. The proteins prevent the lateral diffusion of membrane proteins and membrane lipids as well. Therefore the cell can maintain different protein and lipid compositions on the two sides of the tight junction.

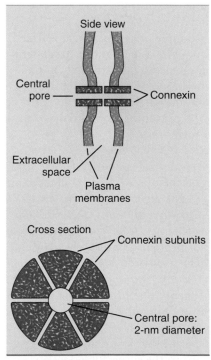

Figure 13.16 Gap junction. In the "open" state, the central pore allows the passage of solutes with molecular weights up to about 1200 D.

Gap junctions close when the cytoplasmic calcium level rises. This happens when a cell dies. In this situation, the surrounding cells have to sever their trade relations with the dying neighbor to maintain their own ion gradients and to prevent a unidirectional drain of their metabolites.

Many different connexins occur in human tissues that are encoded by separate genes. For example, mutations in the gene for connexin-26, which is expressed mainly in the inner ear, are the most common cause of recessively inherited deafness.

SUMMARY

Cytoskeletal fibers are formed either by the bundling of fibrous proteins (keratin, myosin) or by the polymerization of globular protein subunits (tubulin, actin). They participate in the maintenance of cell shape, cell motility, and intracellular transport.

Microfilaments consist of polymerized actin. They determine the physical consistency of the cytoplasm, interact with proteins of the membrane skeleton such as spectrin and dystrophin, and form links with specialized cell-cell and cell-matrix adhesions. They are essential for most kinds of cell motility and are most prominent in muscle fibers, where they form the thin filaments.

Intermediate filaments give structural support to the cell. The most important class are the keratins, which guarantee the integrity of skin and other epithelia.

Microtubules are large hollow tubes of polymerized tubulin. They participate in intracellular transport processes, and they form the skeleton of cilia and flagella.

Further Reading

Arin MJ: The molecular basis of human keratin disorders, *Hum Genet* 125:355–373, 2009.

Burridge K, Wennerberg K: Rho and rac take center stage, *Cell* 116:167–179, 2004.

Calderwood DA, Shattil SJ, Ginsberg MH: Integrins and actin filaments: reciprocal regulation of cell adhesion and signaling, *J Biol Chem* 275:22607–22610, 2000.

Capell BC, Collins FS: Human laminopathies: nuclei gone genetically awry, *Nat Rev Genet* 7:940–951, 2006.

Dalkilic I, Kunkel LM: Muscular dystrophies: genes to pathogenesis, *Curr Opin Genet Dev* 13:231–238, 2003.

Goldman YE: Wag the tail: structural dynamics of actomyosin, *Cell* 93:1–4, 1998.

Michele DE, Campbell KP: Dystrophin-glycoprotein complex: post-translational processing and dystroglycan function, *J Biol Chem* 278:15457–15460, 2003.

Perez-Moreno M, Jamora C, Fuchs E: Sticky business: orchestrating cellular signals at adherens junctions, *Cell* 112:535–548, 2003.

Pollard TD, Borisy GG: Cellular motility driven by assembly and disassembly of actin filaments, *Cell* 112:453–465, 2003.

Rankin J, Ellard S: The laminopathies: a clinical review, *Clin Genet* 70:261–274, 2006.

Reisler E, Egelman EH: Actin structure and function: what we still do not understand, *J Biol Chem* 282:36133–36137, 2007.

Weis WI, Nelson WJ: Re-solving the cadherin-catenin-actin conundrum, *J Biol Chem* 281:35593–35597, 2006.

QUESTIONS

1. **Some cytoskeletal fibers are formed from globular protein subunits. This type of fiber includes the**

   A. Intermediate filaments and actin microfilaments
   B. Thick and thin filaments of skeletal muscle
   C. Microtubules and the thick filaments of skeletal muscle
   D. Keratin filaments in the skin and the thick filaments of skeletal muscle
   E. Actin microfilaments and microtubules

2. **Colchicine is a plant alkaloid that prevents the formation of microtubules. This drug is most likely to inhibit**

   A. The mechanical integrity of the horny layer of the skin
   B. Mitosis
   C. Muscle contraction
   D. The electrical coupling between myocardial cells
   E. The contraction of intestinal microvilli

3. **The structural integrity of the epidermis depends critically on the presence of**

   A. Keratin filaments and zonula adherens
   B. Actin microfilaments and tight junctions
   C. Keratin filaments and desmosomes
   D. Myosin filaments and gap junctions
   E. Keratin filaments and tight junctions

4. **Recurrent respiratory infections in children can have many causes. One possibility that you should consider in a child who presented with repeated bouts of bronchitis and sinusitis is an inherited defect in the protein**

   A. Dynein
   B. Tropomyosin
   C. Connexin
   D. Keratin
   E. Dystrophin

Chapter 14
THE EXTRACELLULAR MATRIX

The cells of soft tissues such as liver, brain, and epithelia are separated only by narrow clefts about 20 nm wide. The mechanical properties of these tissues are determined by the cytoskeleton and by specialized cell-cell adhesions.

Connective tissues, in contrast, consist mainly of extracellular matrix. *The mechanical properties of these tissues are determined by the composition of the extracellular matrix.* Several building materials contribute to the extracellular matrix (*Fig. 14.1*):

1. **Collagen fibers** are ropelike structures that give the tissue tensile strength.
2. **Elastic fibers** have the properties of rubber bands and give elasticity to the tissue.
3. **Proteoglycans** and **hyaluronic acid** have a gel-like or slimy consistency. They are major constituents of the amorphous ground substance.
4. **Multiadhesive glycoproteins** are the glue that holds fibers and cells together.

4-hydroxyproline   3-hydroxyproline

5-hydroxylysine

COLLAGEN IS THE MOST ABUNDANT PROTEIN IN THE HUMAN BODY

Collagen accounts for 25% to 30% of the total body protein in adults, making it the most abundant protein in the human body. As is evident from *Table 14.1*, *collagen is most abundant in strong, tough connective tissues.*

Humans have 28 different collagens and 42 genes encoding collagen chains. Some collagens form fibrils, but others, including the important type IV collagen in basement membranes, form extended networks. Others either are membrane proteins or are found on the surface of collagen fibrils (*Table 14.2*).

Type I collagen is by far the most abundant collagen in the body. It has a most unusual amino acid composition, with 33% glycine and 10% proline. It also contains 0.5% 3-hydroxyproline, 10% 4-hydroxyproline, and 1% 5-hydroxylysine:

Table 14.1 Approximate Collagen Contents of Different Tissues, Expressed as Percentage of the Dry Weight

Tissue	Collagen Content (%)
Demineralized bone*	90
Tendons	80-90
Skin†	50-70
Cartilage	50-70
Arteries	10-25
Lung	10
Liver	4

*Bone from which the inorganic components (mostly calcium phosphates) have been removed by acid treatment.
†Mostly in the dermis. The major structural proteins of the epidermis are the keratins (see Chapter 13).

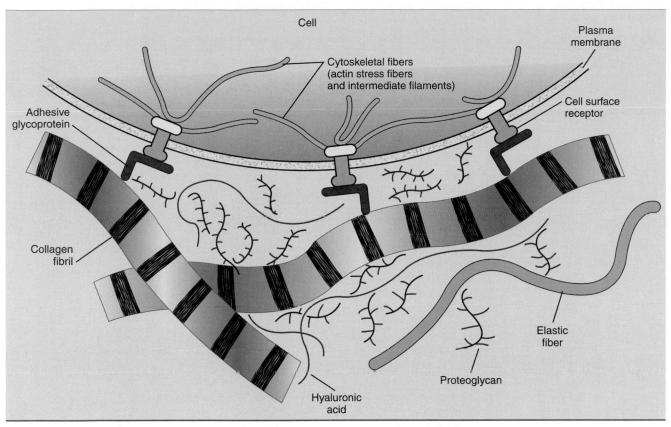

Figure 14.1 Major constituents of the extracellular matrix. Collagen fibers and elastic fibers are required for tensile strength and elasticity, respectively. The amorphous ground substance is formed from proteoglycans, adhesive glycoproteins, and the polysaccharide hyaluronic acid. The extracellular matrix is linked to the cytoskeleton through proteins in the plasma membrane.

These hydroxylated amino acids are not represented in the genetic code. Therefore they must be synthesized posttranslationally from prolyl and lysyl residues in the polypeptide.

Collagen is deficient in some of the nutritionally essential amino acids, such as isoleucine, phenylalanine/tyrosine, and the sulfur amino acids. Thus, Jell-O (**gelatin** is denatured collagen) is not a good source of dietary protein.

Collagen contains a small amount of carbohydrate, most of it linked to the hydroxyl group of hydroxylysine in the form of a Glu-Gal disaccharide. The carbohydrate content of the fibrillar collagens is low (0.5%–1% in types I and III), but it is higher in some of the nonfibrillar types (14% in type IV).

TROPOCOLLAGEN MOLECULE FORMS A LONG TRIPLE HELIX

The basic structural unit of collagen fibrils, the **tropocollagen** molecule, consists of three intertwined polypeptides (*Fig. 14.2*). In type I collagen, this three-stranded rope contains two different polypeptides, each with about 1050 amino acids: two copies of the $\alpha_1(I)$ chain and one copy of the $\alpha_2(I)$ chain. The structural formula is $[\alpha_1(I)]_2\alpha_2(I)$. *These polypeptides have very unusual amino acid sequences, with glycine in every third position.*

Each of the three polypeptides in tropocollagen forms a **polyproline type II helix,** which is very different from the familiar α-helix (see Chapter 2). The α-helix is a compact right-handed helix with 3.6 amino acids per turn and a rise per amino acid of 0.15 nm. The polyproline helix, however, is an extended left-handed helix with three amino acids per turn. With a rise of 0.30 nm per amino acid, it is twice as extended as the α-helix.

The glycine residues are in every third position of the amino acid sequence; therefore, *all glycine residues are on the same side of the helix.* Unlike the α-helix, the polyproline helix is not stabilized by hydrogen bonds between peptide bonds but by steric repulsion of the bulky proline and hydroxyproline side chains.

The three helical polypeptides of the tropocollagen molecule are wound around each other in a right-handed triple helix. Like the β-pleated sheet (see Chapter 2), this superhelical structure is held together by hydrogen bonds between the peptide bonds of the interacting polypeptides. The contacts are formed by that edge of the polyproline helix that has the glycine residues. Only glycine is small enough to permit close contact between the polypeptides. The whole molecule has a length of 300 nm and a diameter of 1.5 nm.

Table 14.2 Collagens

Type	Composition	Most Common Structural Features	Tissue Distribution
I	$[\alpha_1(I)]_2, \alpha_2(I)$	67-nm-banded fibrils	Most abundant type, in most connective tissues
II	$[\alpha_1(II)]_3$	67-nm-banded fibrils	Cartilage, vitreous humor
III	$[\alpha_1(III)]_3$	67-nm-banded fibrils	Fetal tissues, skin, blood vessels, lungs, uterus, intestine, tendons, fresh scars
IV	$[\alpha_1(IV)]_2, \alpha_2(IV)*$	Globular C-terminal end domain; forms a branched network	All basement membranes
V	$[\alpha_1(V)]_2, \alpha_2(V)†$	67-nm-banded fibrils	Most tissues, minor component associated with type I collagen
VI	$\alpha_1(VI), \alpha_2(VI), \alpha_3(VI)$	C- and N-terminal globular domains; forms a network	Most tissues, including cartilage
VII	$[\alpha_1(VII)]_3$	Forms anchoring fibrils	Under basement membranes in dermis and bladder
VIII	$[\alpha_1(VIII)]_2, \alpha_2(VIII)$	Short helix, globular end domains, forms a network	Formed by endothelial cells, in Descemet membrane
IX	$\alpha_1(IX), \alpha_2(IX), \alpha_3(IX)$	With bound dermatan sulfate	On surface of type II collagen fibrils in cartilage
X	$[\alpha_1(X)]_3$	Similar to type VIII	Calcifying cartilage
XI	$\alpha_1(XI), \alpha_2(XI), \alpha_3(XI)$	67-nm-banded fibrils	Cartilage
XII	$[\alpha_1(XII)]_3$	Many globular domains	On surface of type I collagen fibrils
XIII	$[\alpha_1(XIII)]_3 (?)$	With transmembrane domain	Minor collagen in skin, intestine
XIV	$[\alpha_1(XIV)]_3$	Associated with fibrils	Like type XII
XV	$[\alpha_1(XV)]_3 (?)$	Multiple triple-helix domains with interruptions	Capillaries, testis, kidney, heart
XVI	$[\alpha_1(XVI)]_3 (?)$	Associated with collagen fibrils	Dermis, kidney
XVII	$[\alpha_1(XVII)]_3$	With transmembrane domain	Hemidesmosomes of skin
XVIII	$[\alpha_1(XVIII)]_3 (?)$	Multiple triple-helix domains with interruptions	Liver, kidney, skeletal muscle
XIX	$[\alpha_1(XIX)]_3 (?)$	On surface of collagen fibrils	In basement membrane

*Tissue-specific $\alpha_3(IV)$, $\alpha_4(IV)$, $\alpha_5(IV)$, and $\alpha_6(IV)$ chains also occur.
†A less abundant $\alpha_3(V)$ chain is also often present.

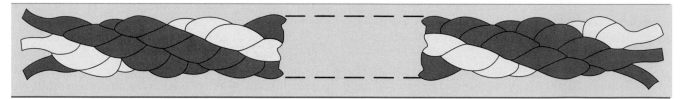

Figure 14.2 Triple-helical structure of collagen. The tropocollagen molecule has a length of approximately 300 nm and a diameter close to 1.5 nm. In the typical fibrillar collagens, only short terminal portions of the polypeptides (the telopeptides) are not triple helical.

COLLAGEN FIBRILS ARE STAGGERED ARRAYS OF TROPOCOLLAGEN MOLECULES

Collagen types I, II, III, V, and XI form cross-striated fibrils with diameters between 10 and 300 nm and a length of many hundreds of micrometers, containing hundreds or even thousands of tropocollagen molecules in cross-section. The tropocollagen molecules in the fibrils form a characteristic staggered array in which the end of one molecule extends 67 nm beyond that of its neighbor and with gaps of approximately 35 nm between the ends of successive molecules (*Fig. 14.3*). This staggered array gives collagen a characteristic cross-striated appearance under the electron microscope. More often than not, a single fibril contains more than one type of collagen.

Collagen fibrils have great tensile strength, and a fibril 1 mm in diameter would be able to carry a weight of about 10 kg. This tensile strength is fully exploited in tendons in which the fibrils are aligned in parallel. Collagen is also durable, with lifespans ranging from several weeks (blood vessels, fresh scars) to many years (bone).

Collagen degradation is initiated by an extracellular collagenase that cleaves a single peptide bond about three fourths down the length of the triple helix. The resulting fragments unravel spontaneously and are further degraded by other proteases. Intact, triple-helical collagen is very resistant to common proteases such as pepsin and trypsin.

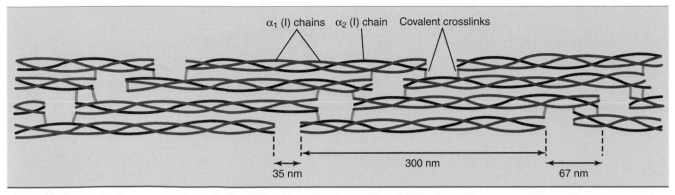

Figure 14.3 Typical staggered array of tropocollagen molecules in the collagen fibril. The telopeptides participate in covalent cross-linking.

COLLAGEN IS SUBJECT TO EXTENSIVE POSTTRANSLATIONAL PROCESSING

Like all extracellular proteins, *collagen is processed through the secretory pathway* (see Chapter 8). The ribosomes on the rough endoplasmic reticulum (ER) synthesize **pre-procollagen**, which contains amino- (N-) and carboxyl- (C-) terminal propeptides in addition to the 1050 amino acids of tropocollagen. The propeptides have neither the unusual amino acid composition nor the triple-helical structure of tropocollagen. In the α_1(I) chain of type I collagen, the propeptides measure approximately 170 amino acids at the amino end and 220 at the carboxyl end. The propeptides are needed to initiate the formation of the triple helix in the ER and to prevent premature fibril formation.

The steps in the processing of type I collagen (*Fig. 14.4*) are as follows:

1. Removal of a signal sequence of approximately 25 amino acids converts pre-procollagen to **procollagen.**
2. Disulfide bonds are formed in the propeptides.
3. 4-Hydroxyproline, 3-hydroxyproline, and 5-hydroxylysine are formed by three different enzymes.
4. Some of the 5-hydroxylysyl residues become glycosylated. Uridine diphosphate (UDP)-galactose and UDP-glucose are the precursors.
5. The triple helix forms in the C→N terminal direction. Interchain disulfide bonds in the C-terminal propeptides initiate this process. Because the hydroxylating and glycosylating enzymes act only on the non–triple-helical polypeptides, any delay in triple helix formation or any imperfection of the triple-helical structure is likely to cause overhydroxylation and overglycosylation.
6. Procollagen is secreted. Only triple-helical procollagen is secreted. Improperly coiled molecules are degraded.
7. The propeptides are removed by extracellular proteases. This leaves triple-helical tropocollagen molecules with short nonhelical **telopeptides** at both ends. The α_1(I) chains, for example, have a helical sequence of 1014 amino acids, an N-terminal

telopeptide of 16 amino acids, and a C-terminal telopeptide of 26 amino acids.
8. After removal of the propeptides, tropocollagen molecules assemble into fibrils.
9. The molecules in the fibril become cross-linked. Covalent cross-linking is initiated by the oxygen-dependent, copper-containing enzyme **lysyl oxidase,** which forms allysine and hydroxyallysine residues in the gaps between the ends of tropocollagen molecules. These aldehyde-containing products form a variety of covalent cross-links by reacting nonenzymatically with other allysyl residues, unmodified lysyl and hydroxylysyl residues, and sometimes histidyl residues (*Fig. 14.5*).

COLLAGEN METABOLISM IS ALTERED IN AGING AND DISEASE

The meat of young animals is soft and tender, whereas that of old animals is tough and unpalatable. The reason is that *the collagen of old animals and humans has more covalent cross-links than that of the young.* In addition, the amount of collagen, relative to the proteins of parenchymal cells, increases with age. The gourmet knows, of course, that actin and myosin taste much better than collagen!

CLINICAL EXAMPLE 14.1: Scurvy

The hydroxylation of prolyl and lysyl side chains in procollagen requires ascorbic acid (vitamin C). As a result, patients with vitamin C deficiency **(scurvy)** form a collagen with insufficient hydroxyproline that denatures spontaneously at body temperature. Most of the abnormal collagen is degraded in the cell because it fails to form the secretable triple-helical structure. This leads to a generalized hemorrhagic tendency, loose teeth, poor wound healing, rupture of scar tissue, and other signs of connective tissue weakness.

Collagen synthesis is stimulated by injury, with fibroblasts creeping to the edge of the wound and into the blood clot to form abundant collagen. *Scars consist mainly of types I and III collagen.* The same can

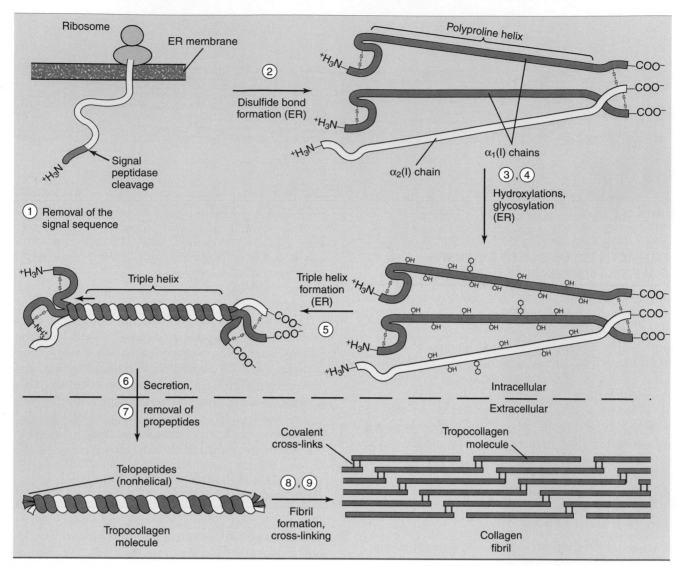

Figure 14.4 Posttranslational processing of type I collagen, the most abundant fibrillar collagen. *ER*, Endoplasmic reticulum.

happen after the death of parenchymal cells in tissues such as liver, spleen, kidneys and ovaries. In **liver cirrhosis,** for example, dead hepatocytes are replaced by fibrous connective tissue.

Collagen synthesis is also stimulated at sites of bacterial infection. This prevents the spread of the infection, and the bacteria become walled off in a localized **abscess.** This defense mechanism is not always successful. *Some pathogenic bacteria secrete collagenases that degrade tropocollagen.* Anaerobic bacteria of the genus *Clostridium* use this trick to spread far and wide through the tissues. They cause **gas gangrene,** an especially severe form of wound infection.

MANY GENETIC DEFECTS OF COLLAGEN STRUCTURE AND BIOSYNTHESIS ARE KNOWN

Many inherited abnormalities in the structure or posttranslational processing of collagen chains are known.

Mutations in the type I collagen genes cause bone diseases because virtually all of the collagen in bone is type I collagen (see *Clinical Example 14.2*). Most other tissues contain type I collagen along with type II (cartilage) or type III collagen (skin, blood vessels, hollow viscera).

Ehlers-Danlos syndrome typically presents with *stretchy skin and loose joints.* The "India rubber man" who could bend and twist himself in incredible shapes and package himself into tiny boxes had Ehlers-Danlos syndrome. The price for this virtuosity is a fragile skin that bruises easily. Even small wounds heal poorly, with the formation of characteristic "cigarette paper" scars. The classic forms are caused by defects in type V collagen, but numerous other clinical types are caused by different molecular lesions (*Table 14.3*).

Structural defects of type III collagen result in the arterial form of Ehlers-Danlos syndrome. This disease can lead to the rupture of large blood vessels, the colon, or the gravid uterus. These tissues are rich in type III collagen.

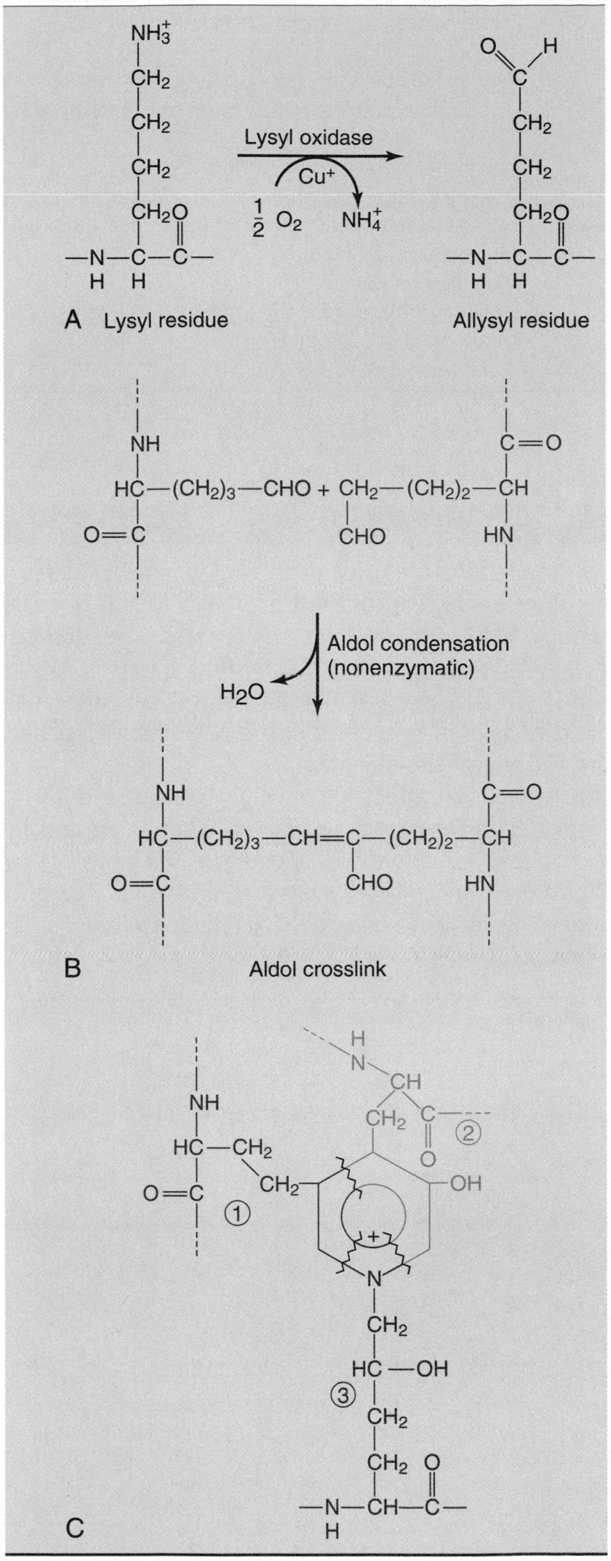

Figure 14.5 Covalent cross-linking of collagen. **A,** Lysyl oxidase reaction. **B,** Aldol cross-link in collagen. **C,** An "advanced" type of covalent cross-link in collagen formed from allysine ①, hydroxyallysine ②, and hydroxylysine ③.

Abnormalities of type II, IX, X, and XI collagen result in **chondrodysplasias.** These diseases affect endochondral bone formation and lead to skeletal deformities and dwarfism. The most important type,

diagnosed as **spondyloepiphyseal dysplasia,** leads to dwarfism, joint degeneration, and ocular abnormalities of variable severity.

Type VII collagen forms anchoring fibrils at the dermal-epidermal junction that anchor the basement membrane to the underlying dermis. The absence of this collagen causes the dystrophic variety of **epidermolysis bullosa.** Its clinical manifestations are similar to those of the keratin defects described in Chapter 13.

ELASTIC FIBERS CONTAIN ELASTIN AND FIBRILLIN

Human tissues must be able to revert to their original shape after mechanical deformation. This requires elastic fibers with properties similar to those of little rubber bands. The elastic fibers of the extracellular matrix have two components: an inner core of amorphous **elastin** and a layer of 10-nm **microfibrils** surrounding the elastin. Elastin is the most abundant protein in arteries. It accounts for 50% of the dry weight of the aorta.

In addition to a high content of hydrophobic amino acids, elastin is rich in glycine (31%), alanine (22%), and proline (11%). Some 4-hydroxyproline (1%) is present, but there is no hydroxylysine. *Like collagen, elastin contains covalent cross-links that are derived from allysine.* Therefore lysyl oxidase is required for the synthesis of elastin as well as collagen. The covalent cross-links of elastin are similar to those of collagen except for **desmosine,** which is present in elastin but not collagen:

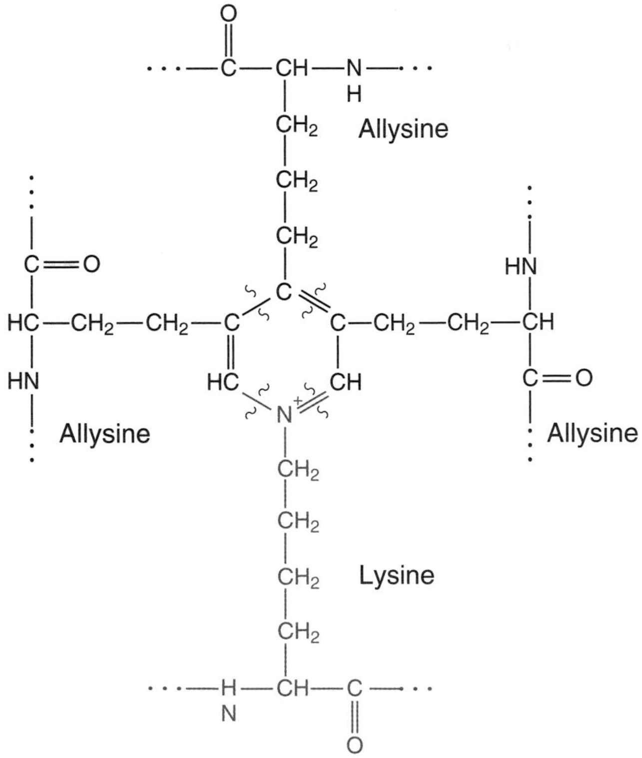

Table 14.3 Collagen Diseases

Disease	Inheritance	Affected Collagen	Signs and Symptoms
Osteogenesis imperfecta	AD (most)	I	Brittle bones, blue sclera, deafness
Ehlers-Danlos syndrome			
Types 1 (gravis) and 2 (mitis)	AD	V	Hyperextensible skin, easy bruising, "cigarette paper" scars, hypermobile joints, more severe in the gravis type
Type III (hypermobile type)	AD	Not known	Joint hypermobility, no scarring
Type IV (arterial type)	AD	III	Rupture of arteries and bowel, gravid uterus
Type VI (ocular, scoliotic type)	AR	(Lysyl hydroxylase)	Extensible skin, joint hypermotility, ocular fragility
Type VII (arthrochalasis type)	AD	I*	Joint hypermobility, hip dislocation
Spondyloepiphyseal dysplasia	AD	II	Short-limbed dwarfism
Bethlem myopathy	AD (most)	VI	Proximal muscle weakness, distal contractures
Epidermolysis bullosa dystrophica	AD or AR	VII	Abnormal skin blistering
Fuchs endothelial corneal dystrophy		VIII	Visual Impairment

AD, Autosomal dominant; *AR*, autosomal recessive.
*Failure to remove the *N*-terminal propeptides.

CLINICAL EXAMPLE 14.2: Osteogenesis Imperfecta

Osteogenesis imperfecta (OI) is characterized by *brittle bones ("glass bones") and frequent fractures.* In the mildest forms the patient has only occasional fractures, but in the most severe forms the patient dies shortly after birth with severe fractures and skeletal deformities. Extraskeletal manifestations can include blue discoloration of the sclera, hearing loss, and poor tooth development. The incidence of OI is about 1 in 10,000, and the inheritance is autosomal dominant in most cases.

OI is caused by mutations in the genes for the α_1 and α_2 chains of type I collagen. More than 200 different OI mutations are known, many of them point mutations that replace a glycine residue by another amino acid.

These mutations are most damaging when they occur near the carboxyl end of the triple helix. This is because the triple helix forms in the C→N terminal direction (see Fig. 14.4). The amino acid substitution arrests coiling, resulting in overhydroxylation and overglycosylation of amino acid residues located in the N-terminal direction from the site of the mutation.

Mutations that affect the α_1 chain are worse than those affecting the α_2 chain. The α_1 chain is present in two copies in the triple helix. Therefore, 75% rather than 50% of the tropocollagen molecules in the heterozygous patient have at least one defective chain and are degraded (**Fig. 14.6**).

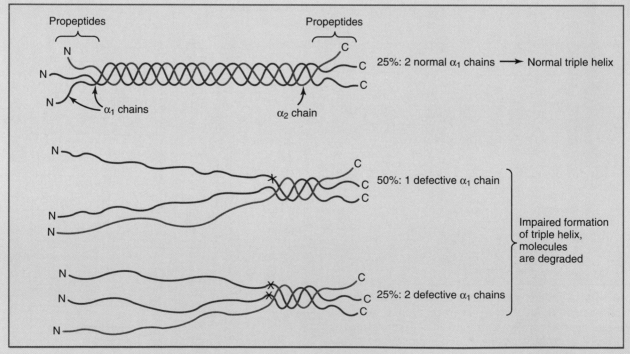

Figure 14.6 Amino acid substitutions in the α_1 chain of type I collagen are "included" mutations. The abnormal polypeptide initially is included in the molecule, but molecules with at least one abnormal chain are nonfunctional and/or are degraded. Heterozygotes form 50% normal and 50% abnormal α_1 chains, but 75% of the triple-stranded molecules contain at least one abnormal chain and therefore are useless. A similar heterozygous mutation in the gene for the α_2 chain would disrupt only 50% of the molecules and cause a milder disease.

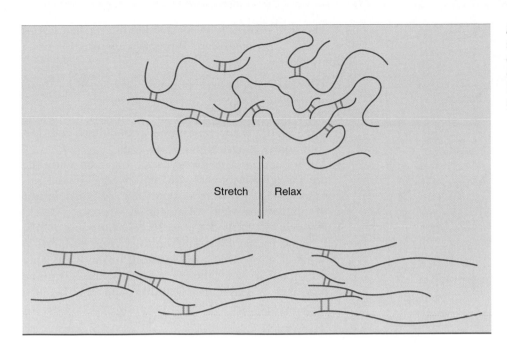

Stretch | Relax

Figure 14.7 Model for the structure of elastin. Elastic recoil during relaxation is thought to depend on hydrophobic interactions between amino acid side chains in the polypeptide.

Little is known about the molecular basis for elastin's elasticity. According to one model, the protein is held in a somewhat disordered but compact shape by weak hydrophobic interactions between amino acid side chains. Stretch loosens these interactions while the elastin network is still held together by the covalent cross-links (***Fig. 14.7***).

CLINICAL EXAMPLE 14.3: Alport Syndrome

Like other collagens, type IV collagen of basement membranes consists of three polypeptide chains, but the helical structure is disrupted at many positions to create bends. Six genetically different polypeptides can contribute to various forms of type IV collagen.

One chain, the α_5(IV) chain (encoded by the *COL4A5* gene), is defective in most patients with **Alport syndrome.** This X-linked condition presents with hematuria and proteinuria, and it leads to renal failure in most male and some female patients. Hearing loss is another frequent complication. The incidence of Alport syndrome is about 1 in 10,000 in many populations, and nearly 300 different mutations in the *COL4A5* gene have been identified in different families.

Some patients have mutations not in the *COL4A5* gene but in the *COL4A3* or *COL4A4* gene encoding the α_3(IV) and α_4(IV) chains of type IV collagen. In these cases, the inheritance is autosomal recessive or, less commonly, autosomal dominant. Thus, as in osteogenesis imperfecta (see Clinical Example 14.2), mutations in different genes can cause the disease. These are examples of **locus heterogeneity.**

CLINICAL EXAMPLE 14.4: Marfan Syndrome

Microfibrils play multiple roles in connective tissues, even apart from their role as constituents of elastic fibers. The most important microfibril protein, **fibrillin-1,** is defective in **Marfan syndrome.** Patients with this rare dominantly inherited condition (incidence of 1 in 10,000 births) are unusually tall, with long, spidery fingers (arachnodactyly); the lens is displaced (ectopia lentis); and the media of the large arteries is abnormally weak. Many patients die suddenly in midlife after rupture of their dilated aorta.

HYALURONIC ACID IS A COMPONENT OF THE AMORPHOUS GROUND SUBSTANCE

Glycosaminoglycans (GAGs) are unbranched acidic polysaccharides that consist of repeating disaccharide units. One of their building blocks is always an amino sugar. The other is, in most cases, a uronic acid. Uronic acids are hexoses in which C-6 is oxidized to a carboxyl group (***Fig. 14.8***).

Hyaluronic acid consists of glucuronic acid and N-acetylglucosamine, held together by β-glycosidic bonds that favor an extended conformation (***Fig. 14.9***). With more than 10,000 disaccharide units, it is the largest of all GAGs. Its negative charges bind plenty of water and cations, and, as a result, *hyaluronic acid forms viscous solutions at low concentrations and a hydrated gel at high concentrations.*

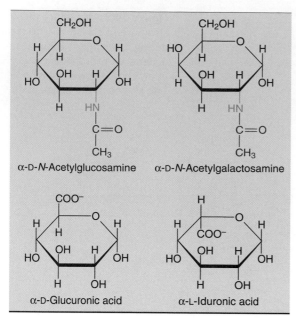

Figure 14.8 Amino sugars and uronic acids are the most common building blocks of the glycosaminoglycans. In the amino sugars, the hydroxyl group at C-2 of the hexose is replaced by an amino group. This amino group is most often acetylated and sometimes sulfated. In the uronic acids, C-6 of the hexose is oxidized to a carboxyl group. *N*-Acetylglucosamine and *N*-acetylgalactosamine are the most common amino sugars, and glucuronic acid and iduronic acid (C-5 epimer of glucuronic acid) are the most common uronic acids. The amino sugars, but not the uronic acids, are also common in glycoproteins and glycolipids. The D and L series of monosaccharides are designated according to the absolute configuration at the asymmetrical carbon farthest away from the carbonyl carbon; hence, the C-5 epimer of D-glucuronic acid belongs to the L series.

Hyaluronic acid is present in the extracellular matrix of all tissues. **Wharton jelly** in the umbilical cord is a hyaluronate-based gel. The **vitreous body** of the eye is a gel of sodium hyaluronate with an interspersed network of type II collagen fibrils. **Synovial fluid** is a lubricant that contains 0.3% hyaluronic acid along with a glycoprotein.

SULFATED GLYCOSAMINOGLYCANS ARE COVALENTLY BOUND TO CORE PROTEINS

GAGs other than hyaluronic acid carry sulfate groups in the form of sulfate esters and, sometimes, in amide bond with the nitrogen of the amino sugar. These sulfate groups contribute additional negative charges. *The sulfated GAGs are much shorter than hyaluronic acid, and they are covalently bound to amino acid side chains in a core protein.*

The core protein with its covalently attached GAGs is called a **proteoglycan.** Proteoglycans are found in many places:

1. They are major components of the amorphous ground substance of connective tissues.
2. Some proteoglycans reside in the plasma membrane (**Fig. 14.10**). They contain heparan sulfate and, less commonly, chondroitin sulfate.
3. *Mucus contains proteoglycans.* Together with the **mucins** (glycoproteins with abundant O-linked oligosaccharides), proteoglycans are responsible for the slimy consistency of mucus secretions.
4. *Heparin is formed by mast cells and basophils.* It has anticoagulant and lipid-clearing properties. When it is released together with histamine during inflammatory and allergic reactions, the histamine increases vascular permeability and the heparin prevents excessive fibrin formation in the interstitial space.

CARTILAGE CONTAINS LARGE PROTEOGLYCAN AGGREGATES

Approximately two thirds of the dry weight of cartilage is collagen (mainly types I and II). Most of the rest is a large proteoglycan called **aggrecan.** Aggrecan has a core protein of 2316 amino acids. Two globular domains at the amino end are followed by a keratan sulfate domain, a large chondroitin sulfate domain, and finally another globular domain at the carboxyl end (**Fig. 14.11**).

The aggrecan molecule looks like a test tube brush, with approximately 100 chondroitin sulfate chains and 50 to 80 keratan sulfate chains extending from the core protein in all directions. These sprawling, hydrated GAGs fill a large volume. In all, aggrecan has a molecular weight of approximately 2×10^6 D and a length of 400 nm (0.4 μm).

Aggrecan molecules, as their name implies, are gregarious. Large **proteoglycan aggregates** are formed when the N-terminal domains of the core protein bind noncovalently to hyaluronic acid. This binding is reinforced by a small, noncovalently bound link protein (**Fig. 14.12**). Spaced about 40 nm apart, a single hyaluronic acid molecule binds up to a few hundred aggrecan molecules. These aggregates have a molecular weight of 1 to 5×10^8 D and a length of a few micrometers. The volume occupied by a single proteoglycan aggregate is larger than a bacterial cell!

Proteoglycan aggregates are responsible for the elasticity, resilience, and gel-like properties of cartilage. Collagen fibers make it resistant to stretch and shear forces.

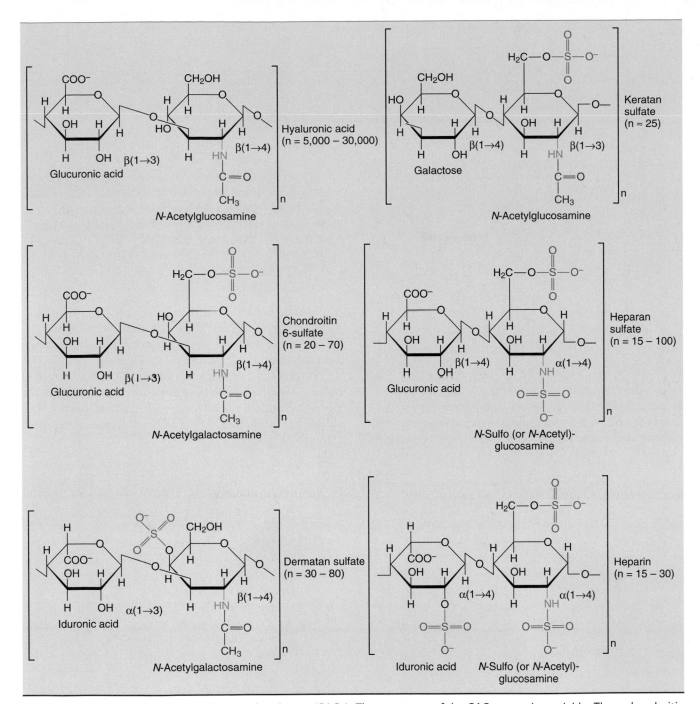

Figure 14.9 The most important glycosaminoglycans (GAGs). The structures of the GAGs are quite variable. Thus, chondroitin 4-sulfate has a sulfate on C-4 rather than C-6 of the amino sugar; dermatan sulfate contains some glucuronic acid besides iduronic acid, and the sulfate of the amino sugar may be either on C-4 or on C-6; heparan sulfate contains some iduronic acid besides glucuronic acid; and heparin contains both glucuronic acid and iduronic acid.

PROTEOGLYCANS ARE SYNTHESIZED IN THE ER AND DEGRADED IN LYSOSOMES

Like "ordinary" glycoproteins, proteoglycans are processed through the secretory pathway. *The core protein is made by ribosomes on the rough ER, and the polysaccharides are constructed in the ER and Golgi apparatus.* The precursors of the GAG chains are nucleotide-activated sugars (*Fig. 14.13*).

The polysaccharide chains are modified enzymatically after formation of the glycosidic bonds. Iduronic acid is formed by the epimerization of glucuronic acid, and sulfate groups are introduced by the transfer of sulfate from **phosphoadenosine phosphosulfate (PAPS)**:

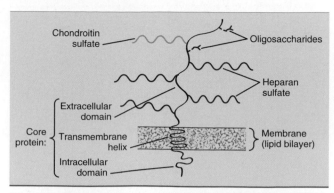

Figure 14.10 Structure of a surface proteoglycan that is present in the plasma membrane of many epithelial cells. Note that more than one glycosaminoglycan (GAG) may be present and that *N-* or *O-*linked oligosaccharides may be present as well.

PAPS is derived from ATP. *It provides an activated sulfate for sulfation reactions much as ATP provides an activated phosphate for phosphorylation reactions.*

At the end of their lifecycle, *the extracellular proteoglycans are endocytosed and sent to the lysosomes.*

Many different enzymes have to cooperate in their degradation. The complete degradation of heparan sulfate, for example, requires three different exoglycosidases, four sulfatases, and an acetyl transferase.

The polysaccharide chains of the GAGs are degraded by the stepwise removal of monosaccharides from the nonreducing end. Only hyaluronic acid and chondroitin sulfate can be degraded by a lysosomal endoglycosidase ("hyaluronidase").

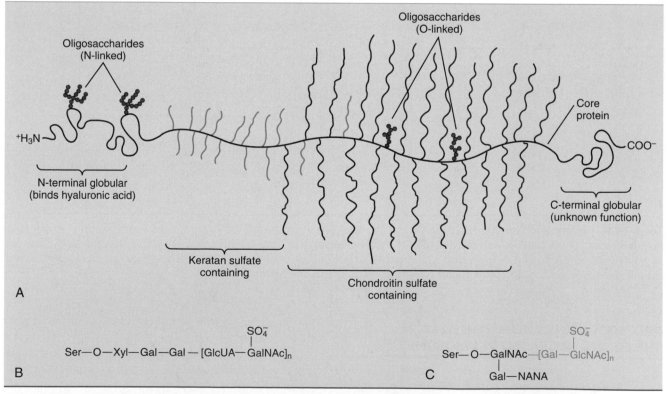

Figure 14.11 Structure of aggrecan, the major proteoglycan of cartilage. **A**, Overall structure (schematic). **B**, Covalent attachment of chondroitin sulfate to serine side chains in aggrecan. The xylose-galactose-galactose linker sequence has been found in other proteoglycans as well. **C**, Covalent attachment of keratan sulfate to serine (sometimes threonine) side chains in aggrecan. In some other proteoglycans, keratan sulfate is bound *N-*glycosidically to asparagine rather than *O-*glycosidically to serine. *NANA, N-*acetylneuraminic acid.

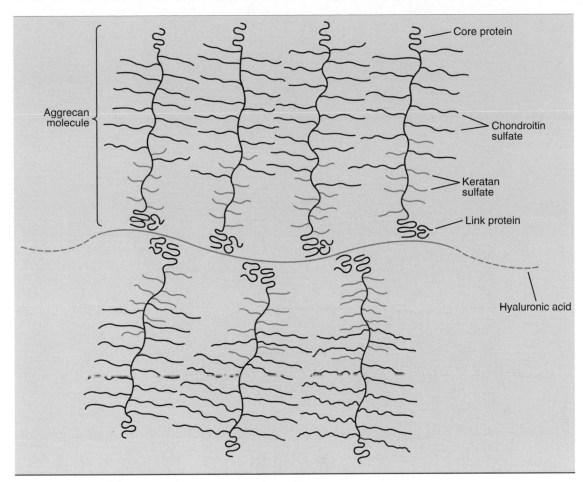

Figure 14.12   Structure of the proteoglycan aggregate in cartilage.

MUCOPOLYSACCHARIDOSES ARE CAUSED BY DEFICIENCY OF GLYCOSAMINOGLYCAN-DEGRADING ENZYMES

The deficiency of only one of the required lysosomal enzymes can interrupt the ordered sequence of GAG degradation. As a result, *the undegraded GAGs accumulate in the lysosomes.* Partially degraded polysaccharide appears in blood and urine, where it can be demonstrated in diagnostic tests.

The result is a type of **lysosomal storage disease** called **mucopolysaccharidosis.** "Mucopolysaccharide" is an obsolete name for GAG, but "glycosaminoglyca-nosis" does not seem to sound right. Some features of the mucopolysaccharidoses (*Table 14.4*) should be emphasized:

1. *The enzyme deficiency is generalized, affecting all organ systems.* Unlike many other metabolic enzymes, lysosomal enzymes do not have tissue-specific isoenzymes.

2. *Inheritance is autosomal recessive or X-linked recessive.* This means that heterozygotes, which typically have half of the normal enzyme activity, are healthy. Heterozygotes can be identified by measuring the enzyme activity in cultured leukocytes, fibroblasts, or amniotic cells.

3. *Many mucopolysaccharidoses exist in both severe and mild forms.* Total absence of the enzyme activity leads to severe disease, whereas enzymes with greatly reduced activity lead to milder disease. The difference between types IH and IS (see *Table 14.4*) is an example.

4. *Most mucopolysaccharidoses are not apparent at birth.* Signs and symptoms develop gradually as more and more mucopolysaccharide accumulates.

5. *Defects in the degradation of keratan sulfate and dermatan sulfate cause skeletal deformities and other connective tissue abnormalities.* Accumulation of these GAGs leads to coarse facial features ("gargoylism"), short stature, corneal clouding, hearing loss, joint stiffness, valvular heart disease, obstructive lung disease, and hepatosplenomegaly. All of these problems are caused by the buildup of GAGs in the tissues.

6. *Only defects leading to the accumulation of heparan sulfate cause mental retardation and neurological degeneration.* Heparan sulfate is the only important GAG in the central nervous system.

7. *Chondroitin sulfate and hyaluronic acid do not accumulate* because they can also be degraded by lysosomal hyaluronidase, an endoglycosidase.

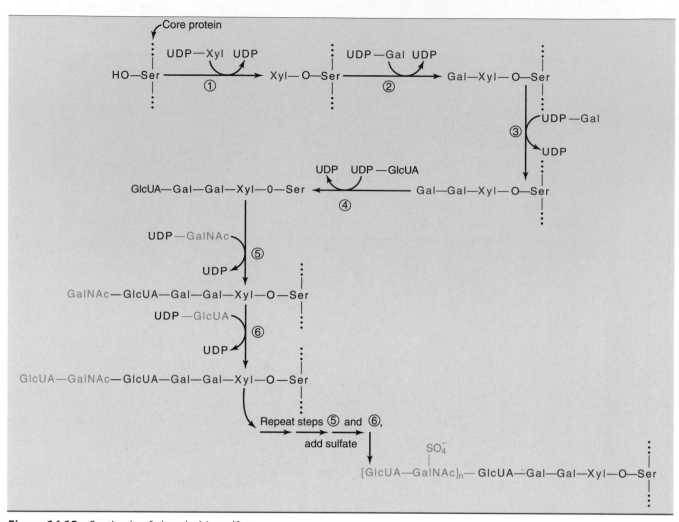

Figure 14.13 Synthesis of chondroitin sulfate.

Table 14.4 Mucopolysaccharidoses

Systematic Name	Common Name	Inheritance	Enzyme Deficiency	GAG(s) Affected	Clinical Features
IH	Hurler	AR	α-L-Iduronidase (complete deficiency)	Dermatan sulfate, heparan sulfate	Skeletal deformities, dwarfism, corneal clouding, hepatosplenomegaly, valvular heart disease, mental retardation, death at ≤10 years
IS	Scheie	AR	α-L-Iduronidase (partial deficiency)	Dermatan sulfate, heparan sulfate	Corneal clouding, stiff joints, normal intelligence and lifespan
II	Hunter	XR	Iduronate sulfatase	Dermatan sulfate, heparan sulfate	Similar to Hurler but no corneal clouding; death at 10–15 years
IIIA	Sanfilippo A	AR	Heparan-N-sulfatase	Heparan sulfate	Severe to profound mental retardation, mild physical abnormalities
IIIB	Sanfilippo B	AR	α-N-Acetyl-glucosaminidase		
IIIC	Sanfilippo C	AR	Acetyl-CoA: α-glucosaminide acetyltransferase		
IIID	Sanfilippo D	AR	N-Acetylglucosamine 6-sulfatase		
IVA	Morquio A	AR	Galactose 6-sulfatase	Keratan sulfate	Corneal clouding, normal intelligence
IVB	Morquio B	AR	β-Galactosidase		
VI	Maroteaux-Lamy	AR	N-Acetylgalactosamine 4-sulfatase	Dermatan sulfate	Severe skeletal deformities, corneal clouding, normal intelligence
VII	Sly	AR	β-Glucuronidase	Dermatan sulfate, heparan sulfate	Skeletal deformities, hepatosplenomegaly

AR, Autosomal recessive; *CoA*, coenzyme A; *GAG*, glycosaminoglycan; *XR*, X-linked recessive.

The mucopolysaccharidoses are rare diseases, with a combined incidence of approximately 1 in 10,000 to 1 in 20,000.

BONE CONSISTS OF CALCIUM PHOSPHATES IN A COLLAGENOUS MATRIX

Bone consists of approximately 10% water, 20% organic materials, and 70% inorganic salts. *The organic matrix is mainly type I collagen, and the inorganic salts are derived from calcium phosphate* $[Ca_3(PO_4)_2]$. Hydroxyapatite, $3[Ca_3(PO_4)_2] \cdot Ca(OH)_2$, is the major inorganic component. There are also considerable amounts of Mg^{2+}, Na^+, CO_3^{2-}, F^-, and citrate.

Other metal ions can be incorporated into this "bone salt." Sr^{2+}, for example, can take the place of Ca^{2+} in the crystal lattice. Radioactive ^{90}Sr, formed during nuclear blasts, can stay in bone for many years, causing damage to the rapidly dividing cells of the bone marrow.

During bone formation, the organic matrix is deposited first. Mineralization begins with the formation of insoluble $CaHPO_4 \cdot 2H_2O$ in the gaps between the ends of tropocollagen molecules in the collagen fibrils. This salt is slowly converted into the even less soluble hydroxyapatite.

Plasma and extracellular fluid are supersaturated with the components of bone salt, but crystallization is prevented by the presence of inorganic pyrophosphate. In bone, pyrophosphate is destroyed by the enzyme **alkaline phosphatase** on the surface of osteoblasts. Patients with a recessively inherited deficiency of alkaline phosphatase suffer from **hypophosphatasia.** They have poor bone mineralization similar to rickets.

In pathological situations, bones become demineralized whenever either the calcium or the phosphate concentration in the plasma and the extracellular medium is reduced. For example, **rickets** (vitamin D deficiency, see Chapter 29) reduces the availability of calcium. **Hypophosphatemia**, also known as **vitamin D–resistant rickets,** is an inherited defect of renal phosphate reabsorption that impairs bone mineralization because it reduces the serum phosphate level.

The solubility of the bone salt increases profoundly at slightly reduced pH. Therefore *chronic acidosis leads to bone demineralization*. Patients with renal failure develop bone demineralization due to a combination of impaired vitamin D metabolism and an incompletely compensated metabolic acidosis.

Impaired formation of the organic matrix leads to brittle bones that break easily. **Osteoporosis** is a common age-related disorder that is associated with reduced synthesis of type I collagen. Low collagen leads to poor mineralization and abnormal fractures. Osteoporosis can be treated with estrogens or androgens and with supplements of calcium and vitamin D.

Metastatic calcification is the inappropriate deposition of insoluble calcium salts in soft tissues. It is caused by prolonged periods of hypercalcemia or hyperphosphatemia.

BASEMENT MEMBRANES CONTAIN TYPE IV COLLAGEN, LAMININ, AND HEPARAN SULFATE PROTEOGLYCANS

The "basement membrane" is not a biological membrane but a thin, translucent sheet of extracellular matrix with a thickness of 60 to 100 nm. Epithelial cells rest on a basement membrane, and large cells such as muscle fibers and adipocytes are surrounded by it (*Fig. 14.14*).

The **type IV collagen** of basement membranes contains the familiar triple helix, but it cannot form fibrils because the triple helix is interrupted at about 20 sites. There is also a globular, nonhelical domain at the

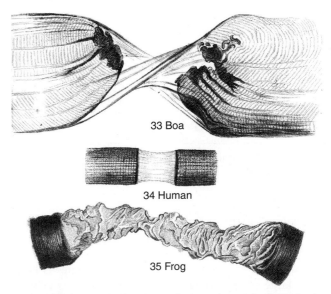

33 Boa

34 Human

35 Frog

Figure 14.14 Early drawings of severed muscle fibers in the boa constrictor, human, and frog, showing the translucent basement membrane.

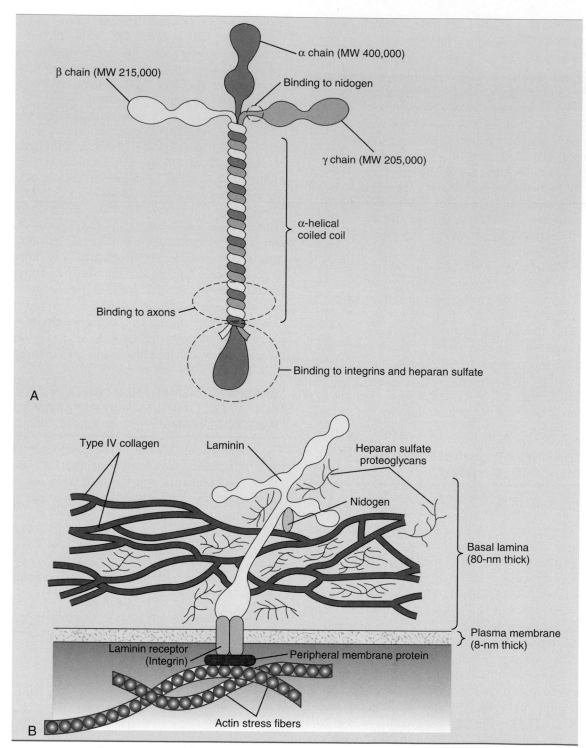

Figure 14.15 Laminin and structure of basal lamina. **A**, Structure of laminin. **B**, Hypothetical position of laminin on the cell surface. *MW*, Molecular weight.

C-terminus of the polypeptide. *Instead of fibrils, type IV collagen forms an irregular two-dimensional network in the basement membrane.*

Another component of basement membranes is **laminin,** a large cross-shaped glycoprotein consisting of three intertwined polypeptides (***Fig. 14.15***). Laminin has binding sites for integrin receptors on the cell surface, for

type IV collagen, heparan sulfate proteoglycans, and the basement membrane glycoprotein entactin (nidogen). *Laminin holds together the components of the basement membrane and mediates interactions with the overlying cells.*

Laminin is more than glue. *By binding to integrin receptors, laminin triggers physiological responses in the* cells. Some cell types proliferate or change their shape in response to laminin binding, and epithelial cells spread on laminin-coated surfaces. In this respect, *laminin acts like a hormone or growth factor that triggers physiological responses by binding to cell surface receptors.*

In addition to laminin and type IV collagen, basement membranes contain heparan sulfate proteoglycans, which influence the permeability of the basement membrane for soluble proteins. This is most important in the double-thickness basement membrane of the renal glomerulus. *This "membrane" retains the negatively charged plasma proteins, whereas cationic proteins of equal size can pass.* It behaves as if it had pores that are lined by negative charges. Almost all plasma proteins have isoelectric points well below the normal blood pH of 7.4 and therefore are negatively charged. A reduced heparan sulfate content of the glomerular basement membrane (e.g., in diabetic patients) can lead to proteinuria.

FIBRONECTIN GLUES CELLS AND COLLAGEN FIBERS TOGETHER

Fibronectin is the most abundant multiadhesive protein in connective tissues, and it even circulates in the plasma in a concentration of about 30 mg/100 mL. It is a very large protein, formed from two similar polypeptides of about 2500 amino acids each that are linked by disulfide bonds near their carboxyl end (*Fig. 14.16*).

Humans have only one fibronectin gene, but tissue-specific isoforms are formed by differential splicing of

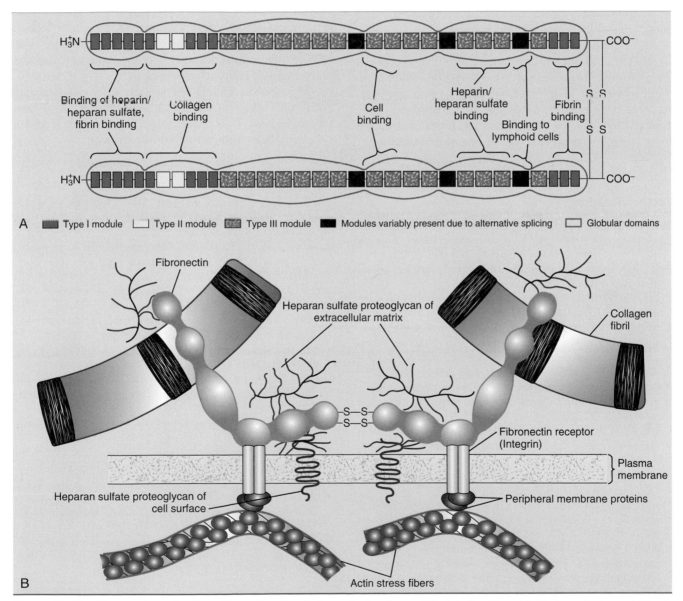

Figure 14.16 Fibronectin and cell-to-fiber adhesion. **A,** Domain structure of fibronectin. The cell-binding site is surprisingly small, with the sequence Arg-Gly-Asp-Ser as the minimal required structure. As a result of alternative splicing, the binding site for lymphoid cells is present in some but not all fibronectins. **B,** Hypothetical position of fibronectin on the cell surface.

the transcript. Plasma fibronectin is a soluble dimer, but tissue fibronectin forms disulfide-bonded fibrils. Different parts of fibronectin bind to cell surface receptors, heparan sulfate proteoglycans, fibrillar collagens, and fibrin. Through these interactions, *fibronectin glues the cells to the fibrous meshwork of the extracellular matrix.*

Fibronectin is formed from three different types of sequences called modules that are, with much variation, repeated many times. *These modules are encoded by separate exons.* Sequences homologous to the type I and type II modules are also present in some other, unrelated proteins. Apparently, *the fibronectin gene was assembled by exon shuffling and exon duplication.*

During embryonic development, fibronectin is necessary for the migration of cells along fibrous tracks. During wound healing, it is incorporated into the fibrin clot and even becomes covalently cross-linked to fibrin. This enmeshed fibronectin attracts fibroblasts and endothelial cells during wound healing.

Many malignant cells are devoid of surface-bound fibronectin, although they possess fibronectin receptors. *The binding of these receptors to tissue fibronectin facilitates metastasis.* In animal experiments, tumor metastasis could be reduced by treatment with synthetic peptide analogs that bind to the integrin receptors of itinerant tumor cells and prevent their binding of fibronectin.

SUMMARY

The extracellular matrix of connective tissue contains fibers embedded in an amorphous ground substance. The most abundant fiber type is formed from collagen, a long ropelike molecule consisting of three intertwined polypeptides. The many types of collagen differ in their structure, properties, and tissue distribution.

Collagen is synthesized from a larger precursor called procollagen, which is processed in the secretory pathway and extracellularly. Several inherited connective tissue diseases are caused by abnormalities of collagen.

The amorphous ground substance consists of proteoglycans, hyaluronic acid, and multiadhesive glycoproteins. Hyaluronic acid and proteoglycans are highly hydrated, with a mucilaginous or gel-like consistency. Cells interact with the extracellular matrix through cell surface receptors of the integrin type. These interactions not only play mechanical roles; they also regulate cellular responses.

Mucopolysaccharidoses are caused by deficiencies of lysosomal enzymes for the degradation of glycosaminoglycans. These diseases cause connective tissue abnormalities and/or mental impairment.

Further Reading

Bateman JF, Boot-Handford RP, Lamande SR: Genetic diseases of connective tissues: cellular and extracellular effects of ECM mutations, *Nat Rev Genet* 10:173–183, 2009.

Brady RO: Enzyme replacement for lysosomal diseases, *Annu Rev Med* 57:283–296, 2006.

Dean JCS: Marfan syndrome: clinical diagnosis and management, *Eur J Hum Genet* 15:724–733, 2007.

Gleghorn L, Ramesar R, Beighton P, et al: A mutation in the variable repeat region of the aggrecan gene (*AGC1*) causes a form of spondyloepiphyseal dysplasia associated with severe, premature osteoarthritis, *Am J Hum Genet* 77:484–490, 2005.

Itano N: Simple primary structure, complex turnover regulation and multiple roles of hyaluronan, *J Biochem* 144:131–137, 2008.

Kawasaki K, Buchanan AV, Weiss KM: Biomineralization in humans: making the hard choices in life, *Annu Rev Genet* 43:119–142, 2009.

Malinda KM, Kleinman HK: The laminins, *Int J Biochem Cell Biol* 28:957–959, 1996.

Morava E, Guillard M, Lefeber DJ, et al: Autosomal recessive cutis laxa syndrome revisited, *Eur J Hum Genet* 17:1099–1110, 2009.

Nguyen TV, Center JR, Eisman JA: Pharmacogenetics of osteoporosis and the prospect of individualized prognosis and individualized therapy, *Curr Opin Endocrinol Diabetes Obesity* 15:481–488, 2008.

Parish CR, Freeman C, Hulett MD: Heparanase: a key enzyme involved in cell invasion, *Biochim Biophys Acta* 1471:M99–M108, 2001.

Ramirez F, Dietz HC: Extracellular microfibrils in vertebrate development and disease processes, *J Biol Chem* 284:14677–14681, 2009.

Sanes JR: The basement membrane/basal lamina of skeletal muscle, *J Biol Chem* 278:12601–12604, 2003.

Shoulders MD, Raines RT: Collagen structure and stability, *Annu Rev Biochem* 78:929–958, 2009.

Silbert JE, Sugumaran G: Biosynthesis of chondroitin/dermatan sulfate, *IUBMB Life* 54:177–186, 2002.

Streuli CH, Akhtar N: Signal co-operation between integrins and other receptor systems, *Biochem J* 418:491–506, 2009.

Tammi MI, Day AJ, Turley EA: Hyaluronan and homeostasis: a balancing act, *J Biol Chem* 277:4581–4584, 2002.

Tatham AS, Shewry PR: Elastomeric proteins: biological roles, structures and mechanisms, *Trends Biochem Sci* 25:567–571, 2000.

Watanabe H, Yamada Y, Kimata K: Roles of aggrecan, a large chondroitin sulfate proteoglycan, in cartilage structure and function, *J Biochem* 124:687–693, 1998.

Weigel PH, DeAngelis PL: Hyaluronan synthases: a decade-plus of novel glycosyltransferases, *J Biol Chem* 282:36777–36781, 2007.

QUESTIONS

1. In a home for handicapped children, you see an 11-year-old girl who is only 90 cm tall, is wheelchair bound, and has multiple limb deformities. The nurse tells you that the girl has "glass bones" and had suffered severe fractures on many occasions. Most likely, this girl has a mutation in a gene for

   A. Type I collagen
   B. Type III collagen
   C. Elastin
   D. Fibronectin
   E. Fibrillin

2. Besides the ubiquitous type I collagen, cartilage contains large quantities of

   A. Type III collagen and fibronectin
   B. Type VII collagen and elastin
   C. Elastin and hyaluronic acid
   D. Type III collagen and laminin
   E. Type II collagen and proteoglycans

3. A first-semester medical student presents with follicular hyperkeratosis (gooseflesh), numerous small subcutaneous hemorrhages, and loose teeth. He reports that for the past 4 months, he has been living only on canned foods, spaghetti, and soft drinks. The process that is most likely impaired in this student is

   A. Removal of propeptides from procollagen
   B. Hydroxylation of prolyl and lysyl residues in procollagen
   C. Formation of allysine residues in collagen
   D. Formation of covalent cross-links between allysine and lysine residues in collagen
   E. Formation of desmosine in elastin

4. Some mucopolysaccharidoses cause only connective tissue problems. In others, however, the patients have mental deficiency. Mental deficiency is most likely to occur in diseases with impaired breakdown of

   A. Hyaluronic acid
   B. Chondroitin sulfate
   C. Dermatan sulfate
   D. Heparan sulfate
   E. Keratan sulfate

5. Poor bone mineralization can be expected in all of the following situations *except*

   A. Increased intestinal absorption of dietary calcium
   B. Increased renal excretion of inorganic phosphate
   C. Deficiency of alkaline phosphatase in bone
   D. Chronic acidosis

Part FOUR
MOLECULAR PHYSIOLOGY

Chapter 15

PLASMA PROTEINS

When blood is centrifuged in the presence of an anticoagulant, the pellet of blood cells occupies between 40% and 50% of the total volume. The remainder is a clear, yellowish fluid called **plasma**. When clotting is induced before centrifugation (e.g., by stirring the blood with a toothpick in the absence of an anticoagulant), the resulting fluid is called not plasma but **serum**. It has the same composition as plasma except for the absence of fibrinogen and some other clotting factors that are consumed during clotting.

Plasma contains approximately 0.9% inorganic ions, 0.8% small organic molecules (more than half of this is lipid), and 7% protein (*Table 15.1*). A pink coloration of the plasma suggests hemolysis, either in the patient or, more often, in the test tube as a result of careless handling. A milky appearance, or the formation of a fatty layer during centrifugation, shows the presence of chylomicrons, which are small fat droplets that appear in the plasma after a fatty meal. A turbid appearance in the fasting state suggests a hypertriglyceridemia with elevated very-low-density lipoprotein.

Plasma contains about a dozen major and innumerable minor proteins. They participate in regulation of the blood volume, transport of nutrients and hormones, blood clotting, and defense against infections. This chapter describes the most important plasma proteins, their functions, and their abnormalities in diseases.

THE BLOOD pH IS TIGHTLY REGULATED

Most biomolecules contain ionizable groups that are subject to protonation and deprotonation. Consequently, all biological processes are pH dependent. *The pH of plasma is approximately 7.40 in arterial blood and 7.35 in venous blood.* The difference is caused by the higher concentration of carbonic acid in venous blood. Carbonic acid forms spontaneously from carbon dioxide and water, but the reaction is accelerated dramatically by the enzyme **carbonic anhydrase** in erythrocytes:

$$\underset{\text{anhydrase}}{\overset{\text{Carbonic}}{}} \qquad \overset{\text{Spontaneous}}{}$$
$$CO_2 + H_2O \rightleftharpoons H_2CO_3 \rightleftharpoons HCO_3^- + H^+$$

At 37°C and pH 7.4, there are approximately 800 molecules of dissolved CO_2 and 16,000 molecules of HCO_3^- for every molecule of H_2CO_3. The apparent pK for the overall reaction $CO_2 + H_2O \rightarrow HCO_3^- + H^+$ is 6.1. Thus the bicarbonate system acts as an effective buffer in the neutral to slightly acidic pH range.

Carbonic acid/bicarbonate is the most important physiological buffer system in the body. It is important because CO_2 and HCO_3^- are present in high concentrations in the interstitial and intracellular compartments as well as the plasma (*Fig. 15.1*). In addition, *the CO_2 level can be regulated by the lungs and the HCO_3^- level by the kidneys.*

Phosphate groups provide an additional buffer system:

$$H_3PO_4 \overset{H^+}{\underset{}{\rightleftharpoons}} H_2PO_4^- \overset{H^+}{\underset{}{\rightleftharpoons}} HPO_4^{2-} \overset{H^+}{\underset{}{\rightleftharpoons}} PO_4^{3-}$$
$$pK = 6.8$$

The phosphate buffer is important only in the intracellular compartments, in which both inorganic phosphate and organically bound phosphate are plentiful.

Proteins provide additional buffering capacity through the ionizable groups in their side chains and their free amino and carboxyl termini.

ACIDOSIS AND ALKALOSIS ARE COMMON IN CLINICAL PRACTICE

Even small deviations from the normal blood pH lead to severe disturbances. An arterial pH lower than 7.35 is called **acidemia**, and an arterial pH exceeding 7.45 is called **alkalemia**. The pathological states leading to these outcomes are called **acidosis** and **alkalosis**, respectively.

Respiratory acidosis is caused by the abnormal retention of CO_2, and **respiratory alkalosis** is caused by hyperventilation. For example, a doubling in the rate of alveolar ventilation raises the blood pH from 7.40 to 7.62, and a 50% reduction in alveolar ventilation lowers the blood pH from 7.40 to 7.12 (*Fig. 15.2*).

Table 15.1 Reference Values for Some Plasma Constituents

Plasma Constituent	Reference Value
Gases and Electrolytes	
pO_2 arterial	95-100 mmHg
CO_2 arterial	21-28 mmol/L
CO_2 venous	24-30 mmol/L
HCO_3^-	21-28 mmol/L
Cl^-	95-103 mmol/L
Na^+	136-142 mmol/L
K^+	3.8-5.0 mmol/L
Ca^{2+} (total)	2.3-2.74 mmol/L
Mg^{2+}	0.65-1.23 mmol/L
pH	7.35-7.44
Metabolites	
Glucose (fasting)	3.9-6.1 mmol/L (70-110 mg/dl)
Ammonia	7-70 μmol/L (12-120 μg/dl)
Urea nitrogen	2.9-8.2 mmol/L (8-23 mg/dl)
Uric acid	0.16-0.51 mmol/L (2.7-8.5 mg/dl)
Creatinine	53-106 μmol/L (0.6-1.2 mg/dl)
Bilirubin (total)	2-20 μmol/L (0.1-1.2 mg/dl)
Bile acids	0.3-3 mg/dl
Lipids (total)	400-800 mg/dl
Acetoacetic acid	20-100 μmol/L (0.2-1 mg/dl)
Acetone	50-340 μmol/L (0.3-2 mg/dl)
Proteins	
Total protein	6-8 g/dl
Albumin	3.2-5.6 g/dl (52%-65% of total)
α_1-Globulins	0.1-0.4 g/dl (2.5%-5% of total)
α_2-Globulins	0.4-1.2 g/dl (7%-13% of total)
β-Globulins	0.5-1.1 g/dl (8%-14% of total)
γ-Globulins	0.5-1.6 g/dl (12%-22% of total)

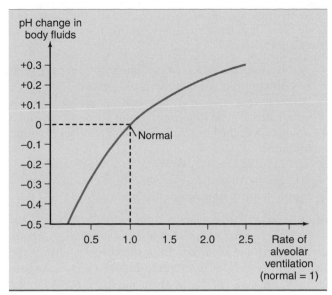

Figure 15.2 pH change in plasma and extracellular fluids in response to changes in alveolar ventilation.

Metabolic acidosis is caused either by the overproduction of an organic acid or by failure of the kidneys to excrete excess acid. The normal urinary pH varies between 4.0 and 7.0, depending on the need to excrete excess protons. Conversely, **metabolic alkalosis** is caused by the abnormal loss of acids from the body (e.g., as a result of excessive vomiting).

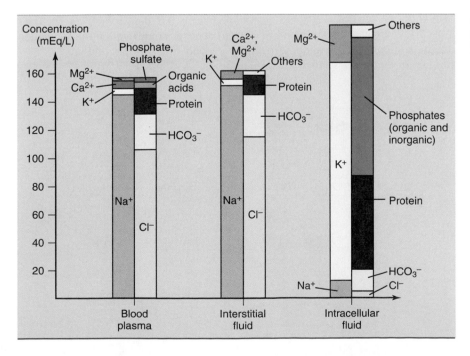

Figure 15.1 Ionic compositions of blood plasma, interstitial fluid, and intracellular fluid.

Whenever the blood pH is abnormal, the body uses three lines of defense in an attempt to restore a normal blood pH:

1. The buffer systems act immediately to prevent excessive fluctuations of the blood pH.
2. Alveolar ventilation increases in acidosis and decreases in alkalosis. The respiratory center in the medulla oblongata of the brain responds to pH and CO_2 within minutes.
3. The kidneys excrete excess H^+ in acidosis and excess HCO_3^- in alkalosis. This is a long-term mechanism that acts on a time scale of hours to days.

Measurement of the plasma total carbon dioxide (CO_2 + H_2CO_3 + HCO_3^-) distinguishes between metabolic and respiratory acidosis. In respiratory acidosis, the total carbon dioxide is elevated because CO_2 retention is, by definition, the cause of the acidosis. In metabolic acidosis, it is reduced because the patient hyperventilates in an attempt to eliminate excess carbonic acid. The converse applies to alkalosis.

PLASMA PROTEINS ARE BOTH SYNTHESIZED AND DESTROYED IN THE LIVER

Immunoglobulins are synthesized by plasma cells, but *most other plasma proteins are made by the liver.* The liver synthesizes about 25 g of plasma proteins every day, which accounts for nearly 50% of the total protein synthesis in the liver.

With the important exception of albumin, *most plasma proteins are glycoproteins.* Their N-linked oligosaccharides end with sialic acid (*N*-acetylneuraminic acid) bound to galactose. A typical plasma protein remains in the circulation for several days, and during this time the terminal sialic acid residues are gradually chewed off by endothelial neuraminidases (*Fig. 15.3*). After the loss of the sialic acid, the exposed galactose at the end of the oligosaccharide binds to an **asialoglycoprotein receptor** on the surface of hepatocytes,

followed by receptor-mediated endocytosis and lysosomal degradation.

ALBUMIN PREVENTS EDEMA

Electrophoresis is the most important method for the separation of plasma proteins in the clinical laboratory (*Fig. 15.4*). It usually is performed at alkaline pH on a solid or semisolid support such as cellulose acetate foil or an agarose gel. *This method separates the proteins by their charge/mass ratio.* Five fractions can be identified by staining and densitometric scanning: albumin, and the α_1-, α_2-, β-, and γ-globulins.

Of these five fractions, *only the albumin peak consists of a single major protein.* Albumin is a single tightly packed polypeptide with 585 amino acids, without covalently bound carbohydrate. Its compact shape minimizes its effect on plasma viscosity. In general, compact proteins do not increase the plasma viscosity to the same extent as more elongated proteins of the same molecular weight (MW).

Albumin has a half-life of 17 days in the circulation. With its MW of 66,000 D and acidic isoelectric point (p*I*), it is able to avoid renal excretion, but it does cross the vascular endothelium of most tissues to some extent. Therefore it is present in interstitial fluid and lymph, but at lower concentrations than in the plasma.

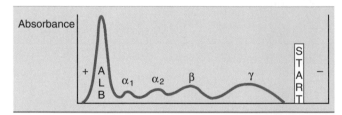

Figure 15.4 Electrophoretic separation of plasma proteins on cellulose acetate foil at pH 8.6, densitometric scan. The electrophoretic pattern depends somewhat on the separation conditions, including support medium, pH, and ionic strength. *ALB,* Albumin.

Figure 15.3 Terminal sialic acid residues (*Sia*) of plasma glycoproteins are removed slowly by endothelial neuraminidases. The exposed terminal galactose residues (*Gal*) mediate binding to the hepatic asialoglycoprotein receptor.

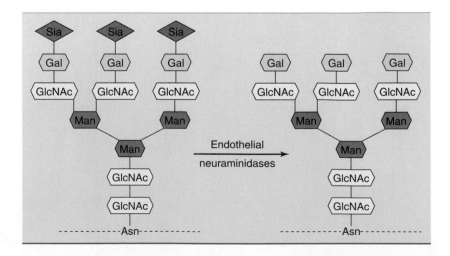

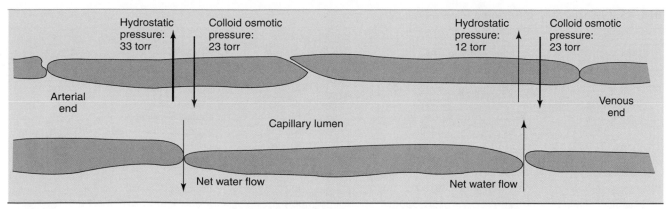

Figure 15.5 Importance of the colloid osmotic pressure for fluid exchange across the capillary wall. A net flow of water into the interstitium is observed at the arterial end of the capillary. This is balanced by a net flow into the capillary at its venous end.

Because the interstitial fluid volume is far larger than the plasma volume (12% and 4.5% of body volume, respectively), the total amount of albumin in the interstitial spaces slightly exceeds that in the vascular compartment. This albumin is returned to the blood by the lymph.

Although albumin accounts for only 60% of the total plasma protein, it provides 80% of the colloid osmotic pressure. This is because the colloid osmotic pressure depends on the amount of water and electrolytes that a protein attracts to its surface, and albumin is one of the most hydrophilic plasma proteins.

The colloid osmotic pressure is necessary to prevent edema. The hydrostatic pressure of the blood forces fluid from the capillaries into the interstitial spaces, and the colloid osmotic pressure of the plasma proteins is required to pull the fluid back into the capillaries (*Fig. 15.5*).

Usually, edema develops when the albumin concentration drops below 2.0 g/dl. Other possible causes of edema include an increase in capillary permeability, venous obstruction, impaired lymph flow, and congestive heart failure with increased venous pressure.

ALBUMIN BINDS MANY SMALL MOLECULES

Fatty acids, thyroxine, cortisol, heme, bilirubin, and many other metabolites bind noncovalently to albumin. Even approximately half the serum calcium and magnesium are albumin bound. Many drugs bind to serum albumin as well. In these cases, *only the free, unbound fraction of a drug is pharmacologically active.* Being noncovalent, albumin binding is reversible:

$$\text{Albumin} \cdot \text{Drug} \rightleftharpoons \text{Albumin} + \text{Drug}$$

The dissociation constant K_D for the release of the drug from albumin is defined as

$$(1) \quad K_d = \frac{[\text{Alb}] \times [\text{Drug}]}{[\text{Alb} \cdot \text{Drug}]}$$

This can be rearranged as

$$(2) \quad \frac{[\text{Drug}]}{[\text{Alb} \cdot \text{Drug}]} = \frac{K_d}{[\text{Alb}]}$$

As long as the molar concentration of albumin is far higher than that of the drug, the concentration of free, unbound albumin [Alb] approximates the total serum albumin concentration. *Equation (2)* indicates that in a patient whose albumin concentration is only half of normal, the ratio of free drug/bound drug is doubled. This is important because only the fraction of the drug that is not protein bound in the plasma equilibrates freely with the tissues. Therefore *it is not the total drug concentration, but the concentration of the unbound drug, that determines the biological response.*

If the patient has severe hypoalbuminemia, an otherwise desirable plasma level of a drug may actually be in the toxic range because an increased fraction of the drug is in the biologically active, unbound form. The commonly used laboratory tests for plasma drug levels do not distinguish between the free and bound fractions.

SOME PLASMA PROTEINS ARE SPECIALIZED CARRIERS OF SMALL MOLECULES

Many of the proteins listed in *Table 15.2* are specialized binding proteins that ferry endogenous substances through the blood.

Transthyretin, also called **prealbumin** because it moves slightly ahead of albumin during electrophoresis, participates in retinol transport. The liver releases stored retinol into the blood as a noncovalent complex with **retinol-binding protein (RBP)**. RBP is a small protein of only 182 amino acids (MW 21,000), which has to bind to the larger transthyretin (MW 62,000) to avoid renal excretion.

Transthyretin also binds thyroid hormones. However, the major transport protein for these hormones is **thyroxine-binding globulin (TBG)**, which binds thyroxine

Table 15.2 Characteristics of Some Plasma Proteins

Protein	Fraction	Concentration (mg/dl)	Molecular Weight (D)	Properties
Transthyretin	Prealbumin	15–35	62,000	Retinol transport, binds T_4
Albumin	Albumin	4000–5000	66,000	Colloid osmotic pressure, binding protein
Retinol-binding protein	α_1	3–6	21,000	Retinol transport
α_1-Antiprotease	α_1	200–400	54,000	Protease inhibitor
Thyroxine-binding globulin	α_1	<1.0	58,000	Major binding protein for T_3 and T_4
Transcortin	α_1	3–3.5	52,000	Binds glucocorticoids
α-Fetoprotein	α_1	0.002 (adults) 200–400 (fetus)		Elevated in adults with hepatoma
Ceruloplasmin	α_2	20–40	132,000	Contains copper
α_2-Macroglobulin	α_2	150–350	725,000	Protease inhibitor
Haptoglobin	α_2	50–300	100,000*	Binds hemoglobin
Transferrin	β	200–400	80,000	Binds iron
Hemopexin	β	50–120	60,000	Binds heme
Fibrinogen	β	150–400	340,000	Clot formation
C-reactive protein	γ	<0.2	125,000	Acute-phase reactant
Immunoglobulins	γ	700–1500	150,000–850,000	Very heterogeneous

T_3, Triiodothyronine; T_4, thyroxine.
*One genetic variant forms higher-molecular-weight polymers (>200,000 D).

with 100 times higher affinity than does transthyretin. An increased level of TBG leads to an increased level of total circulating thyroid hormone, whereas its congenital absence leads to abnormally low levels. In both cases, however, the patient is healthy because the level of the free, unbound hormone is kept in the physiological range by homeostatic mechanisms.

Steroid hormones have two binding proteins: **transcortin** for glucocorticoids, and **sex hormone–binding globulin** for androgens and estrogens. *Only the unbound fraction of the hormone determines the biological response.* Therefore variable levels of the binding proteins can complicate the interpretation of hormone levels measured in the clinical laboratory. What the laboratory measures routinely is the concentration of the total (free + protein-bound) hormone, but the strength of the biological response depends only on the unbound fraction.

The hormone-binding proteins buffer the plasma concentration of the free, unbound hormone, in the same way that a pH buffer buffers the concentration of free protons.

Haptoglobin and **hemopexin** are binding proteins with a very different function. After intravascular hemolysis, the hemoglobin that is released from the ruptured erythrocytes dissociates into α-β dimers that are too small (MW 33,000 D) to escape renal excretion. *To prevent the loss of hemoglobin with its valuable iron, the hemoglobin binds to haptoglobin, and any free heme binds to hemopexin.* These complexes are cleared by phagocytic cells and hepatocytes, respectively (***Fig. 15.6***).

Because haptoglobin is degraded along with its bound hemoglobin, *the serum haptoglobin level is depressed in all hemolytic conditions,* sometimes to near zero.

Haptoglobin does not bind the myoglobin that is released from damaged muscles. Therefore *the haptoglobin level is normal in muscle diseases.* Because the common laboratory tests for "blood" in the urine do not distinguish between hemoglobin and myoglobin, measurement of serum haptoglobin can distinguish between hemoglobinuria and myoglobinuria.

DEFICIENCY OF α_1-ANTIPROTEASE CAUSES LUNG EMPHYSEMA

The proteolytic cascades that normally occur during blood clotting and immune responses are modulated by circulating protease inhibitors. Some of these inhibitors are very selective, but others inhibit a large number of proteases.

α_2-**Macroglobulin** binds a great variety of proteases and even forms covalent bonds with them. These protease-inhibitor complexes are ingested by phagocytes, followed by lysosomal degradation. α_2-Macroglobulin is considered a backup protease inhibitor that comes into play when more selective inhibitors fail.

α_1-**Antiprotease** is also known as α_1-**protease inhibitor** or α_1-**antitrypsin**. It inhibits many serine proteases, with highest affinity for elastase from white blood cells. In the laboratory, its activity is measured as the **trypsin inhibitory capacity** (TIC).

More than 75 genetic variants of α_1-antiprotease are known. One of them, the Z allele, codes for a protein that cannot be secreted from the hepatocytes in which it is synthesized. Some ZZ homozygotes succumb to neonatal hepatitis or infantile cirrhosis, presumably because the accumulating protein damages the hepatocytes. Those who escape serious liver damage are prone to lung emphysema.

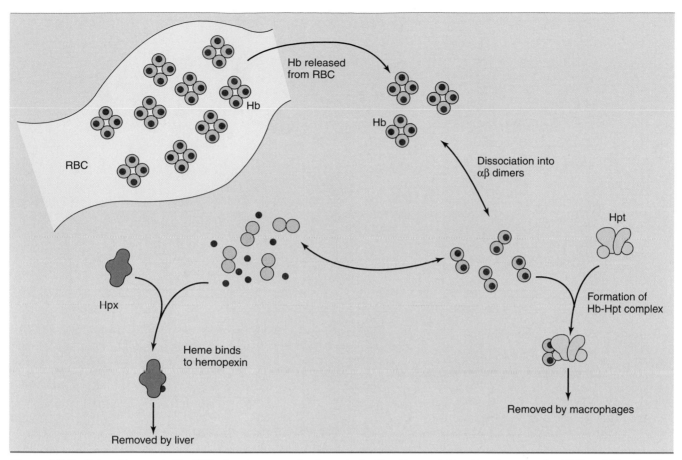

Figure 15.6 Fate of hemoglobin (*Hb*) after intravascular hemolysis. *Hpt*, Haptoglobin; *Hpx*, hemopexin; *RBC*, red blood cell.

Ordinarily, emphysema is caused by the smoldering inflammation of chronic bronchitis and is seen mainly in long-term smokers. Chronic inflammation destroys the septa of the lung alveoli, reducing the surface area available for gas exchange.

The observation of early-onset lung emphysema in individuals with α_1-antiprotease deficiency suggests that *excessive proteolytic activity contributes to tissue damage in chronic bronchitis*. Macrophages and neutrophils spill lysosomal proteases during phagocytosis. These proteases must be kept in check by α_1-antiprotease, which is present not only in the blood but also in bronchial secretions and interstitial fluid. The lungs are especially vulnerable to out-of-control proteases because they are exposed to inhaled bacteria and other foreign particles that must be scavenged continuously by neutrophils and alveolar macrophages.

α_1-*Antiprotease can be inactivated by smoking.* An essential methionine residue in the protein becomes oxidized to methionine sulfoxide by components of cigarette smoke. This contributes to the development of chronic bronchitis and emphysema in smokers, even those without a genetic defect in the protease inhibitor system.

The prevalence of α_1-antiprotease deficiency in the white population of the United States is about 1 in 7000. Eighty percent of these patients eventually will develop emphysema, many at an early age. Treatment is strict avoidance of smoking. α_1-Antiprotease can be administered by intravenous injection or by inhaler to the lungs.

LEVELS OF PLASMA PROTEINS ARE AFFECTED BY MANY DISEASES

Plasma protein electrophoresis is a valuable aid in the diagnosis of many diseases. *Figure 15.7* summarizes some typical patterns.

Acute-phase reactants are plasma proteins whose levels change within 1 or 2 days after acute trauma or surgery, and especially during infections and inflammation (*Table 15.3*). Their synthesis is controlled by stress hormones and cytokines that are released in these conditions. The albumin peak is reduced, whereas the α_2 peak is often increased because one of its major components, haptoglobin, is a positive acute-phase reactant.

The most sensitive acute-phase reactant is **C-reactive protein.** Its plasma level rises up to 100-fold in bacterial infections and to a lesser degree in some other stressful conditions. C-reactive protein binds avidly to some bacterial polysaccharides and seems to participate in the innate immune response.

γ-Globulins are increased in many chronic diseases, including infections, malignancies, and liver cirrhosis.

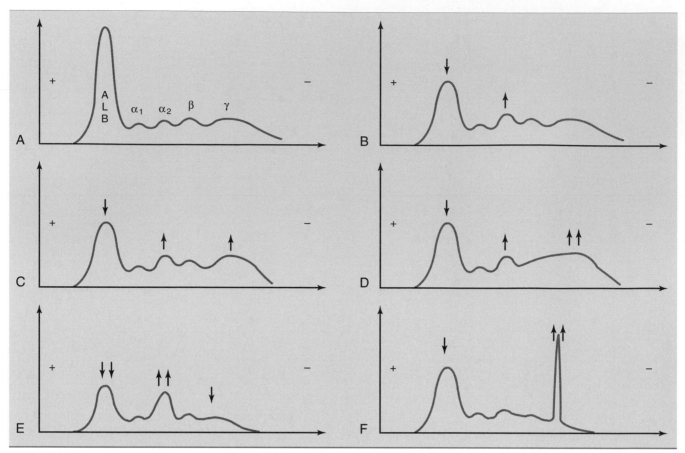

Figure 15.7 Plasma protein electrophoresis in various disease states. **A,** Normal. *ALB,* Albumin. **B,** Immediate response pattern. **C,** Delayed response pattern. **D,** Liver cirrhosis. **E,** Protein-losing conditions (nephrotic syndrome, protein-losing enteropathy). **F,** Monoclonal gammopathy ("paraprotein").

Table 15.3 Acute-Phase Reactants*

Protein	Fraction	Response
Albumin	Albumin	↓
α_1-Acid glycoprotein	α_1	↑↑
α_1-Antiprotease	α_1	↑
Ceruloplasmin	α_2	(↑)
Haptoglobin	α_2	↑↑
α_2-Macroglobulin	α_2	↓
Fibrinogen	β/γ	↑
C-reactive protein	β/γ	↑↑↑

*The levels of these plasma proteins are either elevated or reduced in many acute illnesses.

The nonselective stimulation of immunoglobulin synthesis in these conditions is called **polyclonal gammopathy.**

Nephrotic syndrome is caused by damage to the glomerular basement membrane in the kidneys. As a result, plasma proteins, especially those of low MW, are lost in the urine. The albumin peak and most of the globulin peaks are depressed, but the α_2 peak is increased. The α_2-macroglobulin in this fraction is so large (MW 725,000 D) that it is retained while the smaller plasma proteins are lost.

Similar patterns of decreased albumin and increased α_2-globulin are seen in protein-losing enteropathy, when plasma proteins are lost through a large inflamed area in the intestine, and in extensive burns, when plasma proteins seep through the denuded body surface.

Abnormalities in the concentrations of minor plasma proteins cannot be divined from the electrophoretic pattern and have to be determined by sensitive immunological methods. For example, **α-fetoprotein** is synthesized in the fetal liver but occurs in only trace amounts in normal adult blood. Its levels are increased in most patients with hepatocellular carcinoma. Effectively, the cancer cells revert to a fetal phenotype that entails α-fetoprotein production in addition to rapid proliferation. More importantly, *α-fetoprotein is used for the prenatal diagnosis of open neural tube defects.* In these severe malformations, α-fetoprotein leaks from the fetal blood into amniotic fluid and even into the maternal blood (*Fig. 15.8*).

BLOOD COMPONENTS ARE USED FOR TRANSFUSIONS

Blood transfusions necessitate blood group matching, and there is a risk of transmitting acquired immunodeficiency syndrome (AIDS), hepatitis, and other diseases.

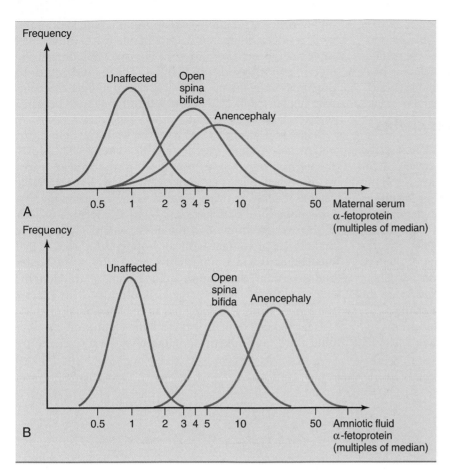

Figure 15.8 Use of α-fetoprotein in amniotic fluid for the diagnosis of neural tube defects in the fetus. Maternal serum can be screened for α-fetoprotein (**A**), and suspect results are followed up by amniocentesis (**B**).

Also, not every patient requires the same blood component. An anemic patient needs red blood cells, a patient with nephrotic syndrome needs albumin, a patient with a clotting disorder needs clotting factors or platelets, and a patient with an immunodeficiency can be treated with immunoglobulins. *Table 15.4* lists some of the most important blood products and their uses.

IMMUNOGLOBULINS BIND ANTIGENS VERY SELECTIVELY

The immunoglobulins make up approximately 20% of the total plasma protein. Most move in the γ-globulin region during electrophoresis, but there are immunoglobulins under the β and α₂ peaks as well.

The immunoglobulins function as **antibodies** that bind tightly to **antigens**. An antigen is, by definition, any molecule that induces the formation of a matching antibody. An antigen must fulfill two requirements:

- *It has to be large*, ideally with a MW of greater than 10,000 D.
- *It has to be a foreign molecule.* Except in autoimmune diseases, humans do not form antibodies to components of their own bodies.

Antigen-antibody binding is noncovalent and therefore reversible. *Formation of the antigen-antibody complex initiates the elimination of the antigen.* Phagocytic cells can both endocytose soluble antigen-antibody complexes and phagocytize antibody-coated bacteria and viruses.

Table 15.4 Plasma Components Available for Therapeutic Use

Product	Uses	Comments
Fresh-frozen plasma	Multiple clotting factor deficiencies, liver cirrhosis, disseminated intravascular coagulation	Danger of disease transmission
Cryoprecipitate	Clotting disorders: hypofibrinogenemia, hemophilia, von Willebrand disease	Produced by freezing and thawing of plasma; enriched in fibrinogen, factor VIII, fibronectin
Factor VIII concentrate	Hemophilia A	Some danger of hepatitis transmission
Albumin 5%	Hypovolemic shock	No danger of hepatitis or HIV transmission; no
Albumin 25%	Cerebral edema	blood group antibodies present
Immune serum globulin	Immunodeficiency states affecting B cells; passive immunization against hepatitis, tetanus	For intravenous or intramuscular injection

The most astounding property of antibodies is their diversity. *Every person has more than one million structurally different antibodies, each with its own unique antigen-binding specificity.* This diversity enables the body to recognize and eliminate almost any imaginable antigen.

ANTIBODIES CONSIST OF TWO LIGHT CHAINS AND TWO HEAVY CHAINS

All antibodies have the same general structure, as shown for immunoglobulins of the G1 class (IgG1) in *Figure 15.9*. The molecule consists of four disulfide-bonded polypeptides: two identical heavy chains with MW of 53,000 D each and two identical light chains with MW of 23,000 D each. The molecule has the shape of the letter Y. Each of the two arms of the Y is formed by the amino-terminal half of a heavy chain and a complete light chain. The stem consists of the carboxyl-terminal halves of the two heavy chains.

The light chain has two globular domains, and the heavy chain has four. All domains have a similar higher-order structure, with approximately 110 amino acid residues folded into two blanketlike antiparallel β-pleated sheets (*Fig. 15.10*). The two "blankets" are held together by a disulfide bond. The second and third domains of the heavy chain are separated by a less compact **hinge region,** which forms disulfide bonds between the two heavy chains.

The amino-terminal domains of both the light chain and the heavy chain are the **variable domains.** They form the part of the antibody that binds to the antigen. Most of the variability is concentrated in **hypervariable regions.** There are three hypervariable regions in the variable domain of the light chain, and either three or four in the variable domain of the heavy chain. They are the major sites of contact with the antigen. If a very skilled biochemist could isolate thousands of IgG1 molecules and determine their amino acid sequences individually, she would rarely ever find two molecules with exactly the same amino acid sequence in the variable domains.

The second domain of the light chain and the second, third, and fourth domains of the heavy chain are

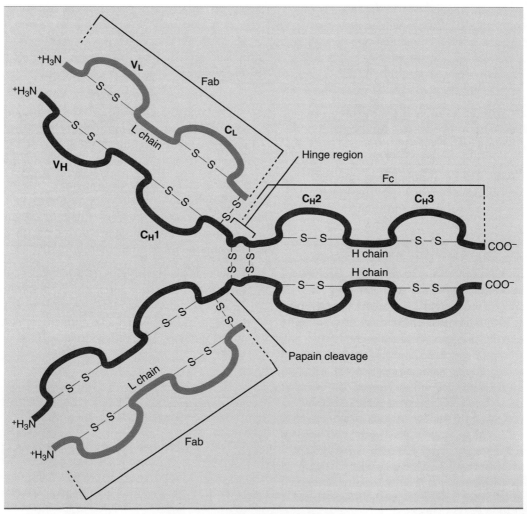

Figure 15.9 Structure of human immunoglobulin G1 (IgG1). Each domain (V_L and C_L in the light [L] chains; V_H, C_H1, C_H2, and C_H3 in the heavy [H] chains) is a globular portion of the molecule, stabilized by an intrachain disulfide bond. *Fab,* Antigen-binding fragment; *Fc,* crystallizable fragment.

the **constant domains.** Several classes of immunoglobulins are defined by the constant domains of their heavy chain. For example, all molecules of the IgG1 class have the same γ1 heavy chain, which is defined by its constant domains. Two kinds of light chain, **κ (kappa)** and **λ (lambda),** are defined by their different constant domains. *Each immunoglobulin molecule has either two κ chains or two λ chains but never one of each.*

The important properties of the immunoglobulins are *antigen binding* and *effector functions.* Effector functions are the events that are triggered by antigen binding, such as complement activation, stimulation of phagocytosis (opsonization), and induction of histamine release from mast cells.

Protease cleavage reveals the allocation of these functions to different regions of the molecule. Papain, a protease from the latex of the papaya plant, cleaves a single peptide bond in the hinge region of IgG1. This generates two types of fragment: two identical **antigen-binding (Fab) fragments,** containing a complete light chain and the amino-terminal half of a heavy chain, and one **crystallizable (Fc) fragment,** consisting of the carboxyl-terminal halves of the two heavy chains. *The Fab fragment binds the antigen, and the Fc fragment determines the effector functions.*

There are two antigen-binding regions in the immunoglobulin molecule, each consisting of the variable domain of a light chain and the variable domain of a heavy chain.

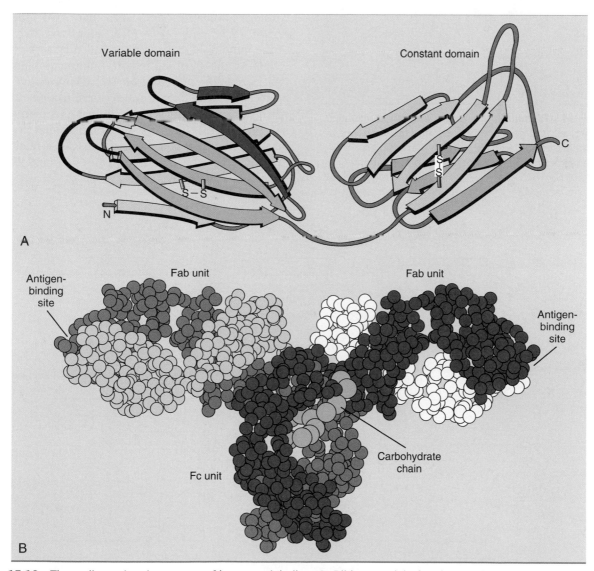

Figure 15.10   Three-dimensional structure of immunoglobulins. **A,** Ribbon model of an immunoglobulin light chain. Each domain contains two "blankets" formed from antiparallel β-pleated sheets (⇨ and ⇨). The interfaces of the two blankets are formed by hydrophobic amino acid side chains, and the structure is reinforced by a single disulfide bond. The variable domain contains two additional β-pleated sheet sequences not present in the constant domain (➡). The antigen binds to three loops (▬) that are formed by the hypervariable regions. **B,** Three-dimensional structure of an immunoglobulin G molecule. In this immunoglobulin class, *N*-linked oligosaccharides participate in the interactions between the heavy chains. *Fab,* Antigen-binding fragment; *Fc,* crystallizable fragment.

Therefore large insoluble aggregates can be formed from soluble antigen and antibody molecules. This is called **precipitation.** It works best with equimolar concentrations of antigen and antibody (*Fig. 15.11*).

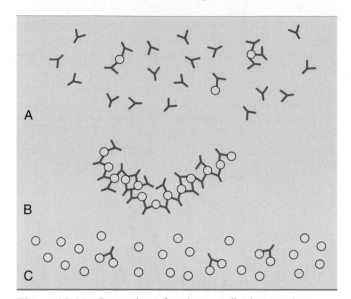

Figure 15.11 Formation of antigen-antibody complexes.
A, Antibody excess: small complexes, no precipitation.
B, Equivalence zone: large complexes, precipitation.
C, Antigen excess: small complexes, no precipitation.

When the antigen is on a cell surface, the two antigen-binding sites can combine with antigen on different cells, thereby gluing the cells together. This is called **agglutination.** It is observed when blood cells are mixed with an antiserum to a blood group antigen.

DIFFERENT IMMUNOGLOBULIN CLASSES HAVE DIFFERENT PROPERTIES

The five major classes of immunoglobulin are defined by their heavy chains: immunoglobulin G (IgG) has γ-chains; immunoglobulin M (IgM), μ-chains; immunoglobulin A (IgA), α-chains; immunoglobulin D (IgD), δ-chains; and immunoglobulin E (IgE), ε-chains. IgG has four subclasses containing four slightly different γ-chains with about 95% sequence homology in their constant domains, and IgA has two subclasses. *Figure 15.12* and *Table 15.5* summarize the features of the immunoglobulin classes and subclasses.

IgG is the most abundant immunoglobulin. *Only IgG crosses the placental barrier.* Maternal IgG has to protect the fetus from intrauterine infections at a time when the fetus is not yet able to make its own antibodies (*Fig. 15.13*). The flip side of placental transfer is that any maternal IgG antibody against a fetal antigen can enter the fetal blood and cause damage. In **rhesus**

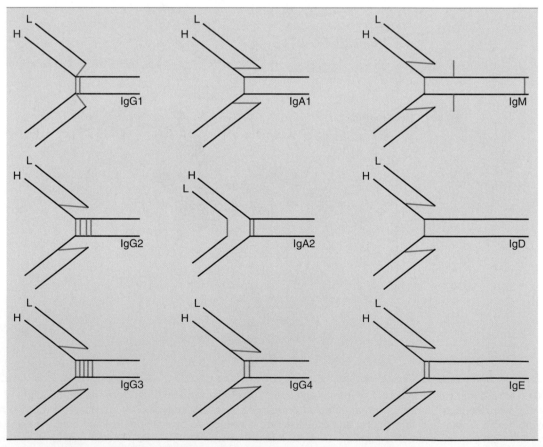

Figure 15.12 Structural features of the different immunoglobulin classes and subclasses. Immunoglobulins M (*IgM*) and E (*IgE*) have four rather than three constant domains. Note the variability in the locations of the interchain disulfide bonds. *H,* Heavy chain; *IgA, IgD,* and *IgG,* immunoglobulin A, D, and G, respectively; *L,* light chain; —, disulfide bonds.

incompatibility, a maternal IgG antibody against the fetal rhesus blood group antigen causes severe hemolysis in the fetus.

IgM is a disulfide-bonded pentamer that contains a small polypeptide known as the **J chain** (*Fig. 15.14*). In many infections, IgM antibodies are formed within 1 week but return to baseline after convalescence. IgG is formed more slowly but remains elevated for a long time. Vaccinations are meant to induce the formation of IgG, not IgM, antibodies.

IgA is the most abundant immunoglobulin in external secretions, including tears, saliva, bronchial mucus, intestinal and genitourinary secretions, and milk. Secretory IgA is synthesized in submucosal lymphatic tissues, including the tonsils in the throat and the Peyer patches in the intestine. It is secreted as a dimer, with a J chain and a noncovalently bound **secretory component.** The secretory component is derived from the membrane receptor that triggers transcytosis of the IgA across the mucosa (*Fig. 15.15*).

Table 15.5   Properties of the Different Immunoglobulin Classes

Immunoglobulin (Ig) Class	IgG	IgM	IgA	IgD	IgE
H-chain class	γ	μ	α	δ	ε
H-chain subclasses	γ1, γ2, γ3, γ4	—	α1, α2	—	—
Polymeric forms	—	Pentamer	Monomer, dimer, or trimer (serum), dimer (secreted)	—	—
Molecular weight (D)	150,000	950,000	180,000 (monomer) 400,000 (secreted)	180,000	190,000
Carbohydrate content (%)	2–3	12	7–11	9–14	12
Serum concentration (mg/dl)	1200	120	200	3	0.005
Serum half-life (days)	21	5	6	3	2
Complement fixation (classic)	++*	+++	–	–	–
Binding to monocytes/ macrophages	++†	+	–	–	+
Binding to neutrophils	+‡	—	++	–	–
Binding to mast cells	–	–	–	–	+++
Secretion across epithelia	–	–	+++	–	–
Placental transfer	+++	–	–	–	–

Binding to monocytes/macrophages and neutrophils is important for the stimulation of phagocytosis, and binding to mast cells is important for the stimulation of histamine release during allergic responses.
*Except IgG4.
†Except IgG2.
‡IgG1 and IgG3 only.

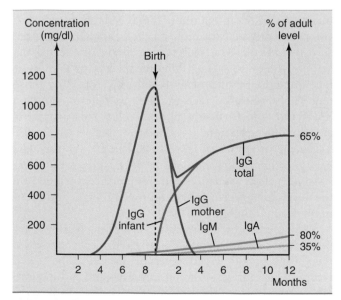

Figure 15.13 Levels of immunoglobulins before and after birth. The fetus depends almost entirely on maternal immunoglobulin G. *H,* Heavy chain; *L,* light chain.

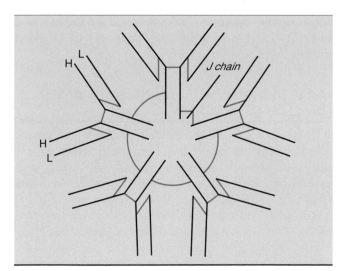

Figure 15.14 Structure of immunoglobulin M (IgM), which is present as a pentamer of molecular weight 900,000 D in the serum. IgM on the surface of B cells, however, is present in a monomeric form. —, Disulfide bonds.

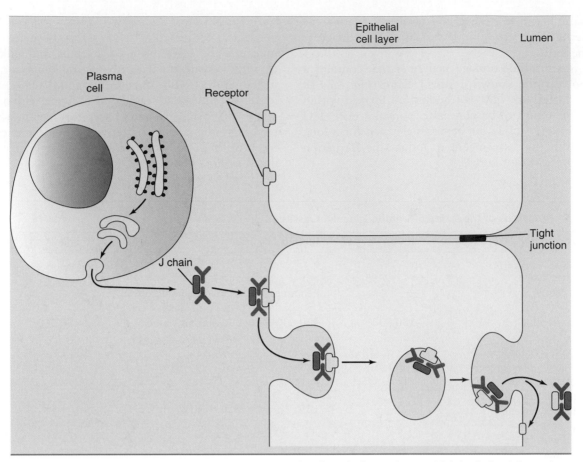

Figure 15.15 Synthesis of secretory immunoglobulin A (IgA). The dimeric form of IgA, which is derived from plasma cells in submucosal lymphatic tissue, is transported across the epithelial cell by transcytosis after binding to a cell surface receptor. On the luminal surface, the extracellular domain of the receptor is cleaved from the membrane-spanning domain and remains bound to the secreted IgA as the "secretory component."

IgE is the most troublesome immunoglobulin. *IgE mediates allergic reactions.* It binds avidly to the surface of basophils and mast cells, where it functions as an antigen receptor. *Binding of the antigen to surface IgE induces the release of stored histamine from the cell.* Most allergic symptoms are mediated by the released histamine, and most antiallergic drugs act by blocking the effects of histamine on its target cells.

ADAPTIVE IMMUNE RESPONSES ARE BASED ON CLONAL SELECTION

B lymphocytes do not secrete their antibody but deposit it in their plasma membrane. Each B cell produces only one antibody, but there are millions of B cells, each making an antibody with distinctive antigen-binding specificity. *This surface immunoglobulin makes the B cell responsive to antigen, much as a hormone receptor makes a cell responsive to a hormone (**Fig. 15.16**).*

The surface antibody is anchored in the membrane through a transmembrane helix near the C-terminus of the heavy chain that is missing in the secreted antibody. This structural feature results from the optional use of a small exon at the 3′ end of the immunoglobulin gene (**Fig. 15.17**).

B cells become activated by the binding of antigen to their surface antibody and by exposure to helper T cells. The activated B cell proliferates and produces a clone of antibody-secreting **plasma cells.** It can also produce **memory cells** that maintain the B-cell phenotype but can proliferate and form plasma cells after future exposure to antigen. The secreted antibody of the plasma cell has the same antigen-binding specificity as the surface immunoglobulin of its B cell ancestor. Only those few B cells whose surface antibody matches the antigen proliferate and turn into plasma cells. This process is called **clonal selection.**

During proliferation, *the B cell can change the class of its antibody without changing its antigen-binding specificity.* IgM is always the first surface antibody on the developing B cell. IgM is followed by IgD and eventually by IgG, IgA, or IgE.

The T cells, which constitute 70% of the lymphocytes in humans, do not produce antibodies. They possess a membrane-bound **T-cell receptor** instead. The T-cell receptor has antigen-binding domains and is functionally equivalent to the surface antibodies of B cells. *Only B lymphocytes and T lymphocytes possess antigen receptors on their surface that enable them to respond*

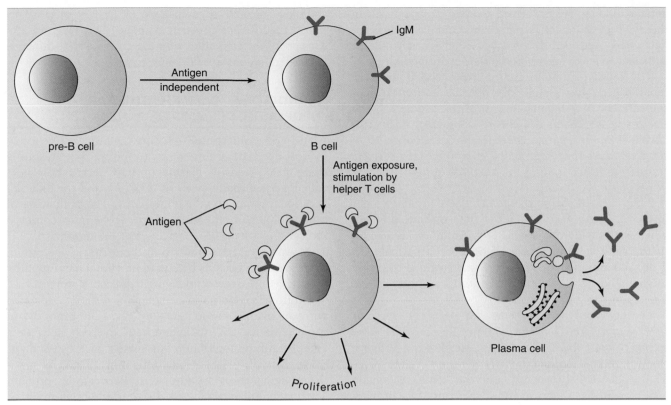

Figure 15.16 Differentiation of a B lymphocyte. Class switching can occur either before or after antigen exposure. *IgM*, Immunoglobulin M.

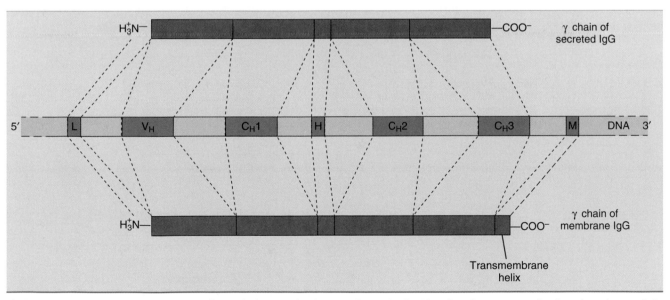

Figure 15.17 Intron-exon structure of a γ-chain gene is shown schematically. The signal sequence, the four domains, and the hinge region are encoded by separate exons. The exon for the membrane attachment region (*M*) is included in membrane-bound immunoglobulin G (*IgG*) but not in secreted IgG. Exon *L* (for leader) encodes the signal sequence.

specifically to a matching antigen. They constitute the **adaptive immune system,** in contrast to the **innate immune system** of phagocytic cells. Phagocytes respond to conserved microbial surface constituents by means of **Toll-like receptors** on their surface, without the need for prior antigen exposure.

IMMUNOGLOBULIN GENES ARE REARRANGED DURING B-CELL DEVELOPMENT

How can humans make millions of different antibodies even though they have only 30,000 genes in their genome? This task is not as formidable as it seems because the antigen-binding site is formed by two polypeptides. In theory, 1000 different heavy chains and 1000 different light chains, encoded by a total of 2000 genes, would be sufficient to make one million different antibodies.

The immunoglobulin chains are encoded by three separate gene clusters: one for κ light chains (on chromosome 2), one for λ light chains (on chromosome 22), and one for heavy chains (on chromosome 14). *Each gene cluster contains separate genes for the variable and constant domains that have to be combined into a single transcription unit coding for a complete light chain or heavy chain.*

Figure 15.18 shows the gene cluster for the κ light chain. A single gene codes for the constant domain, which starts with amino acid 109. Amino acids 1 to 95 of the variable domain are encoded by a **variable (V) gene,** and amino acids 96 to 108 are encoded by a tiny **joining (J) gene.** The germline contains a library of five J genes and about 35 V genes.

During B-cell development, *one of the V genes is selected at random from the library of V genes and spliced to one of the J genes.* This forms a single-exon V/J gene that is transcribed along with the constant domain gene. The sequence between V/J and the constant domain gene is treated as an intron and spliced out of the primary transcript.

The heavy chain genes are assembled the same way, but the heavy chain gene cluster contains a set of approximately 30 **diversity (D) genes** in addition to the V, J, and C_H genes (*Fig. 15.19*). During class switching, the complete variable domain gene (V/D/J) is successively joined to different constant domain genes (*Fig. 15.20*). This produces antibodies with the same variable domains but different constant domains.

MONOCLONAL GAMMOPATHIES ARE NEOPLASTIC DISEASES OF PLASMA CELLS

Abnormal proliferation of a single plasma cell leads to overproduction of a single antibody. The resulting sharp peak seen on plasma protein electrophoresis is called a **paraprotein** (see *Fig. 15.7, F*), and the disorder is called a **monoclonal gammopathy.** The evaluation of monoclonal gammopathies is one of the most common indications for plasma protein electrophoresis.

Paraproteins are common in the geriatric age group. They are diagnosed as **benign monoclonal gammopathy** as long as no signs of malignant disease are present.

Multiple myeloma is a malignant disease associated with an overproduced IgG, IgA, or IgD antibody. In some patients, the malignant cells overproduce not a complete immunoglobulin but loose κ or λ light chains that eventually are excreted in the urine. These overproduced light chains are known as **Bence Jones protein.** The malignant plasma cells thrive in the bone marrow, where they cause bone pain and abnormal fractures.

Waldenstrom macroglobulinemia is a malignant disease with overproduction of an IgM antibody. Because of its high MW of 900,000 D, this IgM antibody causes a dangerous increase of blood viscosity.

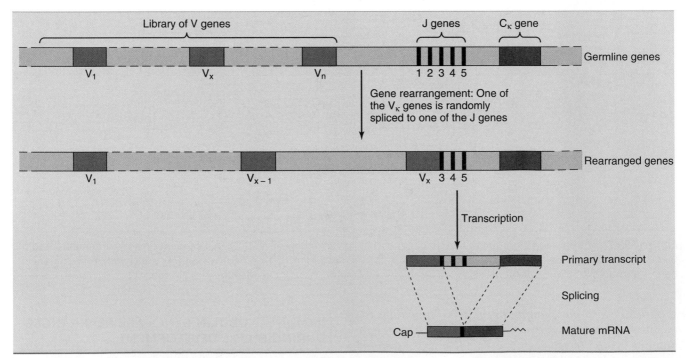

Figure 15.18 Rearrangement and expression of the κ light chain genes. The gene rearrangement takes place early in the development of B lymphocytes, before any antigen exposure. During the gene rearrangement, the intervening DNA (in this case, the DNA between genes V_x and J3) is deleted.

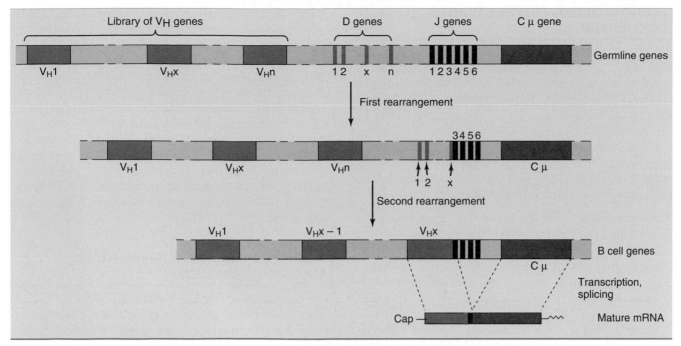

Figure 15.19 Rearrangements of heavy chain genes in developing B lymphocytes. The process is similar to the rearrangement of κ light chains shown in **Figure 15.18**, but an additional small gene, the D (diversity) gene, contributes in addition to the V (variable), J (joining), and C (constant domain) genes. The introns in the Cμ gene are not shown.

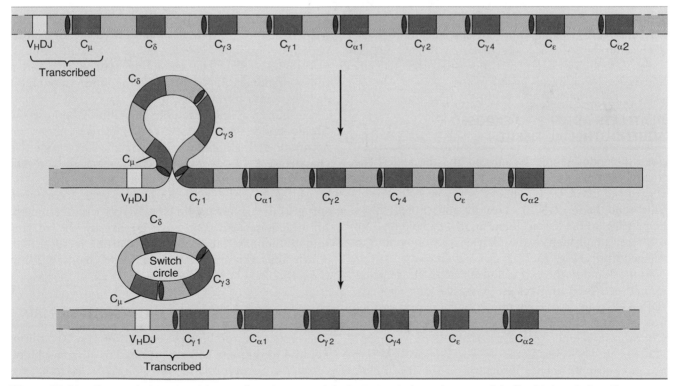

Figure 15.20 Class switching, in this case from immunoglobulin M (μ-chain) to immunoglobulin G1 (γ₁-chain). Class switching takes place after the rearrangements shown in **Figures 15.18** and **15.19**. It can be triggered by cytokines that are released from activated T lymphocytes. The intervening genes (in this case, μ, δ, and γ₃) are released as a cyclic product known as a "switch circle." Each gene is preceded by a switch region (◖). Recombination takes place between the switch regions of two CH genes.

BLOOD CLOTTING MUST BE TIGHTLY CONTROLLED

Blood clotting is essential to prevent excessive blood loss after injury, but it has to remain limited to sites of damage. Sometimes an abnormal clot, or **thrombus**, forms in an intact blood vessel. Indeed, *thrombus formation is the critical event in each of the three major causes of cardiovascular death: myocardial infarction, stroke, and venous thromboembolism.* Therefore blood clotting must be regulated precisely to prevent excessive bleeding while avoiding thrombosis. These are the major characters in the drama of blood coagulation, or **hemostasis**:

1. **Endothelial cells** inhibit blood clotting. Some of the proteins and heparan sulfate proteoglycans in their membrane inhibit the clotting cascade, and they form prostacyclin and nitric oxide, which prevent platelet activation.
2. **Subendothelial tissues** contain membrane proteins and extracellular matrix proteins that are not normally in contact with the blood. When the endothelium is damaged, platelets and clotting factors bind to these proteins and become activated in the process.
3. **Platelets** become activated when they bind to subendothelial tissue. The activated platelets are docking sites for clotting factors, which become activated on the platelet surface.
4. **Clotting factors** are plasma proteins that form a proteolytic cascade, activating each other by selective proteolytic cleavages. This cascade ends with the formation of insoluble fibrin from soluble fibrinogen. The clotting factors are designated by Roman numerals. The subscript letter "a" denotes the proteolytically activated form of the clotting factor.

PLATELETS ADHERE TO EXPOSED SUBENDOTHELIAL TISSUE

When the endothelium is damaged and the underlying extracellular matrix is exposed to the blood, platelets bind to the extracellular matrix with the help of **von Willebrand factor (vWF)**. This plasma protein glues the platelets to the extracellular matrix by binding both to a receptor protein in the platelet membrane and to collagen fibrils (*Fig. 15.21*).

As they bind to the extracellular matrix, the platelets become activated and release a wealth of chemicals: ADP; ATP; 5-hydroxytryptamine; calcium; and various proteins, including fibrinogen, vWF, factor V, factor XIII, thromboxane, platelet-derived growth factor (PDGF), and platelet factor 4. The released clotting factors contribute to the formation of the fibrin clot, thromboxane constricts the blood vessels, PDGF helps in wound healing, and platelet factor 4 prevents the formation of an active thrombin inhibitor from heparin and antithrombin III as discussed later and shown in Fig. 15.27.

During activation, a receptor for fibrinogen becomes exposed on the platelet membrane. *Fibrinogen binds to this receptor and glues the platelets together.* This process is called **platelet aggregation**. Even the membrane lipids become rearranged during platelet activation. Phosphatidyl serine, in particular, which is normally concentrated in the inner leaflet of the plasma membrane, flip-flops to the outer leaflet, where it helps in the binding of prothrombin and other clotting factors.

The importance of the platelet plug is shown by the observation that *patients with unusually low platelet counts (<40,000/µl) develop spontaneous hemorrhages.* Normal platelet counts range between 100,000 and 400,000/µl.

INSOLUBLE FIBRIN IS FORMED FROM SOLUBLE FIBRINOGEN

The platelet plug alone is sufficient to seal very small lesions, but larger injuries require the formation of a fibrin clot. **Fibrin** is not a constituent of normal blood, but its precursor **fibrinogen** circulates at concentrations averaging 300 mg/dl. With MW of 340,000 D, it is larger than most plasma proteins, and it is more elongated, with dimensions of 9×45 nm. Its three polypeptides, designated Aα, Bβ, and γ, are present in two copies each. The overall structure of fibrinogen is shown in *Figure 15.22*.

*The protease **thrombin** converts fibrinogen to fibrin.* Thrombin cleaves two peptide bonds near the amino termini of the Aα and Bβ chains, releasing two small peptides: fibrinopeptides A (20 amino acids) and B (18 amino acids). The remaining protein is called a **fibrin monomer**. Once formed, the fibrin monomers aggregate into fibrous structures.

Fibrinogen is more soluble than fibrin because the fibrinopeptides are studded with negative charges on aspartate and glutamate side chains. These negative charges keep fibrinogen molecules apart and prevent the formation of fibrous aggregates.

Although insoluble, the fibrin monomers form only a soft gel rather than a solid clot. For structural strength, fibrin requires covalent cross-linking by the enzyme **transglutaminase** (also known as **clotting factor XIII$_a$**), which links glutamine and lysine side chains in fibrin (*Fig. 15.23*).

THROMBIN IS DERIVED FROM PROTHROMBIN

The protease **thrombin** converts fibrinogen into fibrin. Because fibrin must never be formed in an intact blood vessel, *thrombin formation must be restricted to the site of the injury.* Therefore thrombin circulates in the blood as the inactive precursor **prothrombin**. The cleavage of prothrombin by **factor X$_a$** is required to generate active thrombin and a catalytically inactive N-terminal fragment (*Fig. 15.24*).

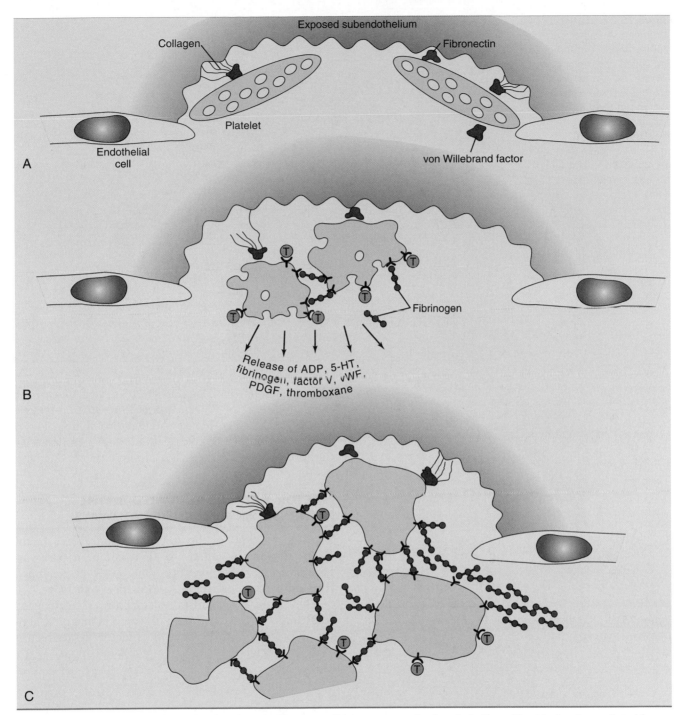

Figure 15.21 Formation of the platelet plug. **A,** Platelets adhere to exposed subendothelium. The binding is mediated by von Willebrand factor (*vWF*), but direct binding to tissue fibronectin or other tissue components may be important as well. **B,** Platelets become activated after binding to the subendothelial tissue and exposure to thrombin (*T*), resulting in shape change and degranulation. Functional fibrinogen receptors are assembled on the cell surface. **C,** Continued thrombin exposure, together with some of the released mediators (ADP, thromboxane), activates more and more platelets. The platelets are glued together by fibrinogen, and the platelet plug forms. The action of thrombin on fibrinogen forms insoluble fibrin, and the platelets become enmeshed in the fibrin clot. *5-HT,* 5-hydroxytryptamine; *PDGF,* platelet-derived growth factor.

This amino-terminal fragment contains 10 residues of **γ-carboxyglutamate,** which is formed by the post-translational modification of glutamate residues in the endoplasmic reticulum of hepatocytes. The enzyme catalyzing this reaction requires **vitamin K.**

Unlike glutamate, γ-carboxyglutamate is a strong calcium chelator. *Through γ-carboxyglutamate and its bound calcium, prothrombin becomes anchored to phosphatidyl serine on the surface of activated platelets.* Also factor X_a contains γ-carboxyglutamate and binds to activated

Figure 15.22 Structure of fibrinogen. **A,** Schematic representation of fibrinogen. The coiled coil regions, each 150 to 160 nm in length, are formed by three α-helical portions of the Aα, Bβ, and γ chains. **B,** Aggregation of fibrin monomers. **C,** Transglutaminase (factor XIII$_a$) strengthens the clot by forming covalent cross-links.

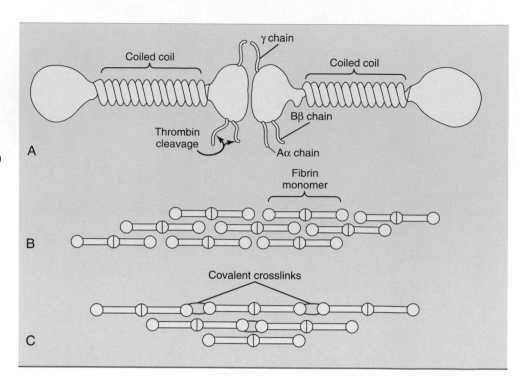

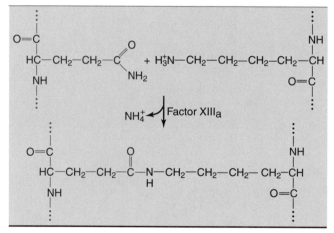

Figure 15.23 Covalent cross-linking of fibrin by factor XIII$_a$ (transglutaminase).

platelets, along with its activator protein **factor V$_a$** (**Fig. 15.25**). *Factor X$_a$ activates prothrombin on the surface of the activated platelet.* Active thrombin no longer adheres to the platelet lipids, but it becomes enmeshed in the fibrin network, in which it retains its enzymatic activity.

FACTOR X CAN BE ACTIVATED BY THE EXTRINSIC AND INTRINSIC PATHWAYS

The last reactions of the clotting cascade, from factor X$_a$ to fibrin, are called the **final common pathway.** However, factor X$_a$, like thrombin, has to be generated from an inactive precursor by proteolytic cleavage.

The main mechanism of factor X activation (**Fig. 15.26**) is the **extrinsic pathway.** The factor X activating protease in this pathway is **factor VII$_a$,** which is

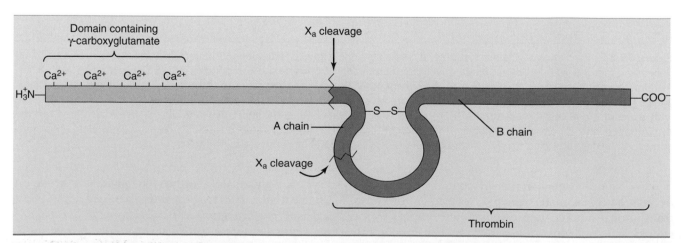

Figure 15.24 Structure of prothrombin. Cleavage by factor X$_a$ produces thrombin (308 amino acids) and a catalytically inactive amino-terminal fragment (274 amino acids).

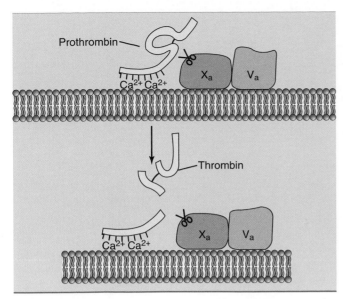

Figure 15.25 Activation of prothrombin by factor X_a on the surface of the platelet membrane. The membrane phospholipids facilitate the reaction by bringing prothrombin and factor X_a together on the surface of the lipid bilayer, and factor V_a enhances the catalytic activity of factor X_a.

formed from inactive factor VII by thrombin or factor X_a. However, proteolytic activation is not sufficient. Factor VII_a is active only in the presence of **tissue factor** (also known as **factor III**), a membrane glycoprotein on cells of subendothelial tissue. *Tissue factor and factor VII come into contact only after vascular injury.* In the presence of calcium, factor VII quickly binds to tissue factor, either before or after its activation to factor VII_a.

The **intrinsic pathway** derives its name from the fact that it can be induced in the test tube in the absence of an "extrinsic" tissue component, requiring only factors already present in the blood. However, *the intrinsic pathway becomes activated only on contact with a negatively charged surface.* The glass of a test tube offers a negatively charged surface, as does the exposed extracellular matrix in the body.

The initiating reactions of the intrinsic pathway are known as **contact-phase activation.** They require two proteases, **kallikrein** and **factor XII_a,** which activate each other on the exposed extracellular matrix. This requires the activator protein **high-molecular-weight kininogen (HMW-K).**

Factor XII_a activates factor XI, factor XI_a activates factor IX, and factor IX_a activates factor X. This last reaction requires the activator protein **factor VIII_a.** The complex of factors VIII_a and IX_a is called the **tenase complex** (the enzyme that activates factor ten).

γ-Carboxyglutamate is present not only in prothrombin and factor X but also in factors VII and IX. Therefore all these clotting factors are targeted to activated platelets. This design keeps clotting highly localized. *The initiating reactions are triggered by components of the exposed subendothelial tissue, and the final steps require activated platelets.*

NEGATIVE CONTROLS ARE NECESSARY TO PREVENT THROMBOSIS

Figure 15.26 shows that the clotting cascade has several elements of *positive feedback*: kallikrein and factor XII_a activate each other, factor XI_a acts on its own precursor to produce more XI_a, and thrombin activates factors V, VII, VIII, and XI in the earlier steps of the cascade. These positive feedback loops permit a quick response to injury, but without inhibitory controls, the process would progress until all blood vessels were filled with solid fibrin.

Protease inhibitors provide negative controls by inactivating clotting factors that have escaped from the site of injury. Most clotting factors can be inactivated by the nonselective inhibitors α_1-antiprotease and α_2-macroglobulin. More important is **antithrombin III** (*Fig. 15.27*), which inhibits most proteases of the intrinsic and final common pathways (*Table 15.6*).

Table 15.6 Properties of the Blood Clotting Factors

Factor	Functions in	Protease Precursor	Molecular Weight (D)	Plasma Concentration (mg/dl)	Vitamin K Dependent	Heparin Inhibited	Activated by
Fibrinogen (I)	Common pathway	No	330,000	150–400	No	No	Thrombin
Prothrombin (II)	Common pathway	Yes	72,000	8–9	Yes	Yes	X_a
V	Common pathway	No	330,000		No	No	Thrombin
X	Common pathway	Yes	59,000	0.6	Yes	Yes	I X_a, VII_a
XIII	Common pathway	No*	320,000		No	No	Thrombin
VII	Extrinsic pathway	Yes	50,000	0.05	Yes	No	Thrombin, X_a
VIII	Intrinsic pathway	No	330,000	0.02	No	No	Thrombin,
IX	Intrinsic pathway	Yes	57,000	0.4	Yes	Yes	XI_a, VII_a
XI	Intrinsic pathway	Yes	160,000	0.5	No	Yes	Thrombin, XI_a, XII_a
XII	Intrinsic pathway	Yes	76,000	3	No	Yes	Kallikrein
Prekallikrein	Intrinsic pathway	Yes	82,000	4	No	No	XII_a
High-molecular-weight kininogen	Intrinsic pathway	No	108,000	7–10	No	No	—

*Yields a fibrin cross-linking enzyme.

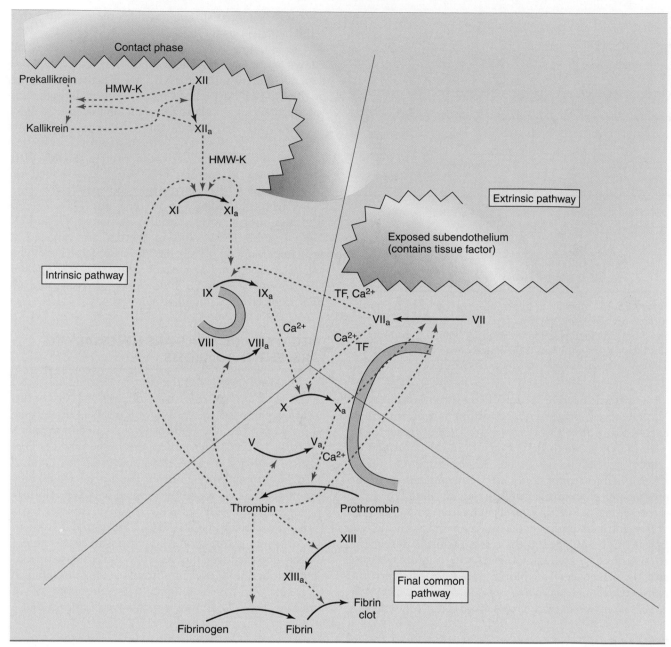

Figure 15.26 Blood clotting system. *Dashed arrows* indicate proteolytic activation. (▨) Surface of activated platelets. *HMW-K,* High-molecular-weight kininogen; *TF,* tissue factor.

Antithrombin III is stimulated by the glycosaminoglycan **heparin.** A specific positioning of sulfate groups on the polysaccharide chains of heparin is necessary for antithrombin III activation. This required structure is present in about 30% of all heparin molecules and in a small proportion of the heparan sulfate chains on the surface of endothelial cells. *Therefore the action of antithrombin III is facilitated by contact with intact endothelial cells in vivo.*

A different anticoagulant mechanism is used by **thrombomodulin (*Fig. 15.28*),** a protein on the surface of endothelial cells that binds circulating thrombin. Once bound to thrombomodulin, thrombin no longer cleaves fibrinogen and the other clotting factors. It activates **protein C** instead. Activated protein C is a protease that acts as a powerful anticoagulant by degrading factors V_a and VIII_a. This action of protein C is stimulated by **protein S.** Because thrombomodulin is present on intact endothelium, *this mechanism prevents the encroachment of clot formation on areas with an intact endothelial lining.*

Some patients with thrombotic disorders have inherited deficiencies of anticoagulant proteins. Abnormalities of factor V (*Clinical Example 15.1*), antithrombin III, protein C, and protein S have been observed repeatedly. They cause venous thrombosis even in heterozygotes.

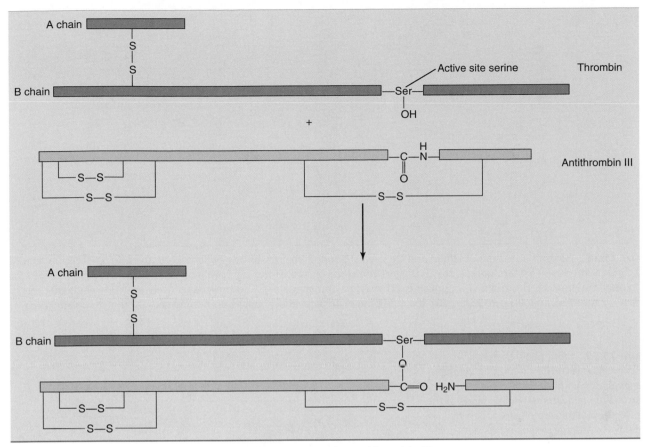

Figure 15.27   Proposed mechanism for inhibition of thrombin by antithrombin III.

CLINICAL EXAMPLE 15.1: Factor V$_{Leiden}$

Genetic variants of clotting factors can affect the risk of thrombosis. The most common variant of this kind, present in 4% of Europeans, is factor V$_{Leiden}$. It is a single amino acid substitution (Arg→Gln in position 506) in factor V that makes this factor resistant to inactivation by activated protein C. The risk of thrombosis is increased twofold to threefold in heterozygotes and eightfold to 12-fold in homozygotes. Tests for this mutation are commonly done in the clinical laboratory and in direct-to-consumer genetic test kits.

Plasminogen can also be activated by **urokinase**, a protease that is present in normal urine and in blood and extracellular matrix. **Streptokinase** is a bacterial protein (from streptococci) that activates plasminogen allosterically, without proteolytic cleavage.

Streptokinase, urokinase, and tPA are used as thrombolytic agents. For example, acute myocardial infarction is caused by thrombus formation on an atherosclerotic plaque in a coronary artery. Thrombolytic therapy can limit the size of the infarction if it is administered within 1 hour after vascular occlusion, before the damage has become irreversible.

PLASMIN DEGRADES THE FIBRIN CLOT

A blood clot is an ephemeral structure that must be removed during wound healing. The major enzyme of fibrin degradation is the protease **plasmin**. Its inactive precursor **plasminogen**, which circulates in the plasma in a concentration of 10 to 20 mg/dl, binds with high affinity to the fibrin clot. This fibrin-bound plasminogen can be activated by **tissue-type plasminogen activator (tPA)**, a serine protease that also binds avidly to fibrin. tPA does not require proteolytic activation, but its activity is minimal in the absence of fibrin. Therefore *active plasmin is formed only in the fibrin clot where it is needed* (**Fig. 15.29**).

HEPARIN AND THE VITAMIN K ANTAGONISTS ARE IMPORTANT ANTICOAGULANTS

All γ-carboxyglutamate containing clotting factors (prothrombin, VII, IX, X) depend on calcium. Therefore *removal of calcium prevents clotting*. The calcium chelators citrate, oxalate, and ethylenediaminetetraacetic acid (EDTA) are used to inhibit clotting in the test tube, but this strategy cannot work in the living body. The blood calcium level must be kept constant, and a dose of a calcium chelator that is sufficient to prevent clotting would kill the patient.

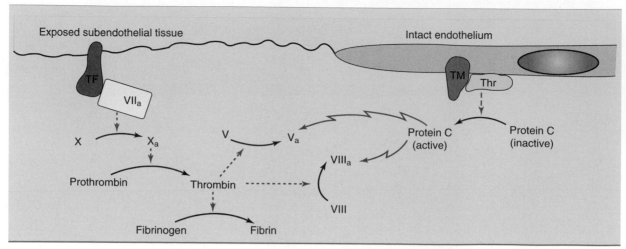

Figure 15.28 Roles of intact endothelium and exposed subendothelial tissue are evident when the effects of tissue factor (*TF*) and thrombomodulin (*TM*) are compared. TF triggers the clotting system through the extrinsic pathway (compare **Fig. 15.26**). TM blocks the process. Thrombin (*Thr*), which is otherwise a "procoagulant," becomes effectively an "anticoagulant" after binding to thrombomodulin. *Dashed arrows* indicate proteolytic activation; *jagged arrows* indicate proteolytic inactivation.

Figure 15.29 Fibrinolytic system. Plasminogen (*PLG*) is a circulating zymogen that binds to the fibrin clot. Tissue-type plasminogen activator (*tPA*) also binds to the clot, where it activates plasminogen by proteolytic cleavage, exposing its active site (✂). Urokinase activates circulating plasminogen by proteolysis, whereas the bacterial protein streptokinase (*Str*) activates plasminogen without proteolytic cleavage, by inducing a conformational change in the zymogen.

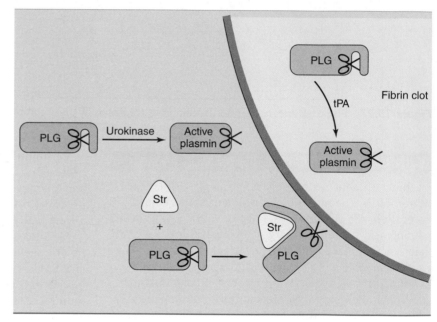

Heparin, acting through antithrombin III, inhibits clotting both in vivo and in vitro. *Heparin is used as a short-acting injectable anticoagulant.* It is not absorbed in the intestine and therefore is not orally active. A low-molecular-weight form of heparin is more commonly used now.

Coumarin, warfarin, and **dicumarol** are competitive antagonists of vitamin K. *They prevent the formation of γ-carboxyglutamate* in factors VII, IX, and X. These drugs act in the endoplasmic reticulum of hepatocytes, where the clotting factors are made. Therefore they cannot prevent clotting in the test tube. In addition, because the vitamin K–dependent clotting factors have plasma half-lives of 1 to 5 days, several days of treatment are required before the old, normal clotting factors are replaced by the abnormal, uncarboxylated factors that are produced in the presence of the drug.

New anticoagulants include **direct thrombin inhibitors** and **factor X_a inhibitors,** which bind competitively to the respective active site of each clotting enzyme. **Aspirin** has anticoagulant activity by blocking platelet activation through inhibition of thromboxane A_2 synthesis (see Chapter 16). Other drug strategies for inhibiting platelet activation and aggregation include blocking the platelet ADP receptor and preventing the interaction of the platelet surface glycoprotein IIb/IIIa complex with fibrinogen and vWF.

The function of the blood clotting system can be assessed with various clotting tests:

1. **Bleeding time.** Bleeding time is measured after a standardized small skin prick lesion in the fingertip or earlobe. *Bleeding time is prolonged in platelet disorders.*
2. **Activated partial thromboplastin time.** Citrated plasma is treated with a combination of kaolin, a phospholipid preparation, and excess calcium. The kaolin activates the contact factors of the intrinsic pathway, and the phospholipid substitutes for platelet membranes. *This procedure tests the functioning of the intrinsic and final common pathways.* It can be used to monitor the heparin effect.
3. **Prothrombin time.** A tissue factor–containing extract from the brain or lungs is added to citrated plasma along with excess calcium. *The prothrombin time is prolonged in deficiencies of the extrinsic and final common pathways.* It is used routinely to monitor patients receiving treatment with coumarin-type anticoagulants.

CLINICAL EXAMPLE 15.2: Rat Poison

Most rat poisons are coumarin-type anticoagulants. These drugs have no immediate toxicity. Therefore rats will eat the poison repeatedly until they die from internal hemorrhage several days later. Poisons with immediate toxicity invariably cause a conditioned taste aversion in rats (as well as humans) after a first exposure to a nonlethal dose.

An accidental ingestion of coumarin-based rat poisons should be treated with oral or injected vitamin K. The prothrombin time should be monitored daily, and a transfusion of fresh-frozen plasma or clotting factor concentrates may be required if a prolonged prothrombin time is found.

CLOTTING FACTOR DEFICIENCIES CAUSE ABNORMAL BLEEDING

Hemophilia A is a serious X-linked bleeding disorder that affects approximately one in 10,000 males. It is caused by a *complete or near-complete deficiency of factor VIII,* one of the components of the intrinsic pathway (see *Fig. 15.26*).

Unlike patients with platelet disorders, hemophiliac patients rarely have spontaneous hemorrhages. They have prolonged bleeding from small wounds. More serious is repeated bleeding into joints, which leads to arthritis. Bleeding into muscle tissue, usually after minor trauma, can lead to muscle necrosis followed by fibrosis and contractures. Bleeding episodes can be treated with cryoprecipitate, factor VIII concentrate, or recombinant factor VIII. These treatments can be used prophylactically but are quite expensive.

Factor IX deficiency (**hemophilia B**) causes the same clinical manifestations as hemophilia A. This is expected because factors VIII and IX are required for the same reaction. Factor XI deficiency causes a milder bleeding disorder, and deficiencies of factor XII, prekallikrein, or HMWK do not cause abnormal bleeding, although the activated partial thromboplastin time is prolonged.

Deficiencies in the final common pathway tend to be more serious than those in the intrinsic pathway. The absence of fibrinogen (**afibrinogenemia**) causes a severe clotting disorder that is often fatal in childhood. The same is true for deficiencies of prothrombin, factor V, and factor X. These clotting factor deficiencies are inherited as recessive disorders.

CLINICAL EXAMPLE 15.3: Von Willebrand Disease

von Willebrand factor has two biological functions: It mediates platelet adhesion to the extracellular matrix, and it binds factor VIII in the plasma, preventing its degradation. Inherited abnormalities of vWF are common but are asymptomatic in most cases. In about 1 of 8000 people the defect is serious enough to cause abnormal bleeding, with signs that mimic either platelet dysfunction or hemophilia. This condition, diagnosed as von Willebrand disease, is the most common bleeding disorder in most populations. The inheritance is autosomal dominant in most cases. Treatment is based on injections of cryoprecipitate or vWF-containing factor VIII concentrates.

TISSUE DAMAGE CAUSES RELEASE OF CELLULAR ENZYMES INTO BLOOD

Intracellular enzymes leak out into the blood whenever a cell dies, so trace amounts of them are always present in the plasma. Once released into the blood, the tissue enzymes have half-lives between 1 day and 1 week (*Table 15.7*).

Cell death is the most common cause of elevated plasma enzyme levels. In other cases, metabolic stress raises the permeability of the plasma membrane. Enzymes

Table 15.7 Plasma Half-Lives of Some Enzymes

Enzyme	T$_{1/2}$ (Days)
Plasma cholinesterase*	12–14
Lactate dehydrogenase	6.8
Alanine transaminase	6.3
Aspartate transaminase	2.0
Creatine kinase	1.4

*This enzyme normally is secreted into the blood by the liver.

leak out, although the cells survive. Cancerous tumors can raise enzyme levels because the tumor cells provide an expanded tissue source of the enzyme and because tumor-invaded tissues are destroyed.

Those enzymes that are present only in one organ or tissue are the most useful for diagnosis, but few enzymes meet this requirement. The enzymes of the major metabolic pathways, in particular, are present in most cells of the body.

Fortunately, *many enzymes occur as tissue-specific isoenzymes.* These are structurally different enzymes that catalyze the same reaction. They can be separated from each other by electrophoresis, and they have different kinetic properties and sensitivity to inhibitors.

In the clinical laboratory, the maximal reaction rate (V_{max}) of the enzyme is determined with saturating concentrations of its substrates at fixed temperature and pH. V_{max} is proportional to the amount of the enzyme (see Chapter 4). Enzyme activities can be expressed in **international units** (IU). *One international unit corresponds to the amount of enzyme that catalyzes the conversion of one micromole (μmol) of substrate to product per minute.*

SERUM ENZYMES ARE USED FOR THE DIAGNOSIS OF MANY DISEASES

The levels of only a limited number of enzymes are determined on a routine basis in most clinical laboratories (*Table 15.8*). The most important of these are as follows.

Plasma Cholinesterase

Plasma cholinesterase is one of the few diagnostically important enzymes whose major place of residence is in the plasma. It differs from the acetylcholinesterase at cholinergic synapses (see Chapter 16) by its broader substrate specificity. Its physiological role is uncertain, but it can inactivate some drugs, including succinylcholine and cocaine.

Plasma cholinesterase is also used for the diagnosis of **organophosphate poisoning.** Organophosphates, which are used as pesticides and nerve gases, inhibit not only the acetylcholinesterase at cholinergic synapses but also the plasma cholinesterase.

CLINICAL EXAMPLE 15.4: Inactivation of Succinylcholine

Succinylcholine is a short-acting muscle relaxant that is used as an adjunct in general anesthesia. It is inactivated by plasma cholinesterase but not by the acetylcholinesterase at cholinergic synapses. *Approximately 1 in 300 otherwise normal people is at least partially deficient in plasma cholinesterase. The patient can develop fatal apnea after a standard dose of succinylcholine.* Therefore a determination of plasma cholinesterase may be prudent before the patient is exposed to succinylcholine.

Table 15.8   Changes in Serum Enzyme Levels in Different Diseases

Enzyme	Viral Hepatitis	Biliary Obstruction	Muscular Dystrophy	Acute Myocardial Infarction	Acute Pancreatitis	Neoplastic Disease Metastasis to Liver	Neoplastic Disease Metastasis to Bone	Other
Plasma cholinesterase	↓↓	— or ↓	—	—	—	↓↓	—	Organophosphate poisoning
Alanine transaminase	↑↑↑	↑	— or ↑	— or ↑	—	↑	—	
Aspartate transaminase	↑↑↑	↑	↑	↑↑	—	↑↑	—	
Alkaline phosphatase	↑	↑↑↑	—	—	—	↑↑	↑↑↑	Bone diseases, fractures
Acid phosphatase	—	—	—	—	—	—	— or ↑	Prostatic carcinoma
Lactate dehydrogenase	↑	↑	↑↑	↑↑	—	↑↑↑	— or ↑	Megaloblastic anemia, shock
Creatine kinase	—	—	↑↑↑	↑↑	—	—	—	
Lipase	—	—	—	—	↑↑↑	—	— ⎫	Perforation of small intestine
Amylase	—	—	—	—	↑↑↑	—	— ⎭	
γ-Glutamyltransferase	↑	↑↑↑	—	—	—	↑↑	—	

—, No change; ↑, increased; ↓, decreased.

Alanine Transaminase and Aspartate Transaminase

Alanine transaminase (ALT) and aspartate transaminase (AST) are enzymes of amino acid metabolism. They are most abundant in the liver, and leak into the plasma from damaged cells. Therefore *transaminases are used for the diagnosis of liver diseases*. In viral hepatitis, the plasma levels of both enzymes can easily be 20 to 100 times above the upper limit of the normal range. The enzyme elevations are proportional to the extent of the ongoing tissue damage, and they can be demonstrated before fever and jaundice develop. Elevation of ALT is quite specific for liver damage, but AST is also elevated in muscle diseases and acute myocardial infarction.

Alkaline Phosphatase

The enzyme alkaline phosphatase (ALP) is abundant in bone, placenta, intestine, and the hepatobiliary system. Each of these organs contains a different isoenzyme. The bone and liver enzymes are the most abundant in normal serum. The bone enzyme is derived from osteoblasts (see Chapter 14). *ALP rises in bone diseases with increased osteoblastic activity,* such as rickets, osteomalacia, hyperparathyroidism, osteitis deformans, neoplastic diseases with bone metastases, and healing fractures. *The liver enzyme is increased in biliary obstruction.*

γ-Glutamyl Transferase

γ-Glutamyl transferase (GGT) is an enzyme of uncertain function that is most abundant in liver and kidney. *GGT is a sensitive indicator of biliary obstruction,* in which it is elevated along with ALP. GGT synthesis in the liver is induced by many drugs and by alcohol. Therefore elevations of GGT are seen in many alcoholics and in patients taking certain drugs, such as phenobarbital.

Acid Phosphatase and Prostate-Specific Antigen

Acid phosphatase (ACP) and prostate-specific antigen (PSA) are tumor markers used for the diagnosis and follow-up of prostatic cancer. ACP was first described in 1925 as a constituent of normal urine. It soon became evident that its concentration was far higher in male than in female urine and that its major source was the prostate gland. *Serum ACP is elevated in metastatic prostatic cancer.* Because it is normal in most patients with early stages of prostate cancer, it is suitable for follow-up of patients with established disease but not for early diagnosis.

PSA is the best marker for the early diagnosis of prostate cancer. It is a serine protease that is normally secreted into seminal fluid but can also be measured by sensitive immunological methods in the serum. It has high **sensitivity** (about 80% of cancer cases are detected) but low **specificity** (only 50% of those with elevated PSA have cancer). Many patients with benign prostatic hypertrophy have elevated PSA, and prostate cancer is easily overdiagnosed with this marker.

Lactate Dehydrogenase

Lactate dehydrogenase (LDH) is an enzyme of anaerobic glycolysis that is present in all tissues. Therefore its plasma level is elevated in a wide variety of diseases. Fortunately, LDH has tissue-specific isoenzymes. The active enzyme is a tetramer of four equivalent subunits, and there are two different subunits: H (heart) and M (muscle). *These subunits can combine to form five different isoenzymes (Table 15.9).* Isoenzyme 1 (H_4) is fastest and isoenzyme 5 (M_4) is slowest during electrophoresis at pH 8.6.

The isoenzyme patterns of the tissues depend on the relative amounts of H and M subunits produced by the cells. Myocardium and bone marrow produce mainly H subunits, and liver and skeletal muscle produce mainly M subunits. Most other tissues produce both.

Table 15.9 Occurrence of Lactate Dehydrogenase Isoenzymes in Different Tissues

Isoenzyme No.*	Composition	Presence in				
		Myocardium	Erythrocytes	Skeletal Muscle	Liver	Kidney
1	H_4	++++	+++	−	−	+
2	H_3M	++++	+++	−	−	+
3	H_2M_2	+	+	+	+	++
4	HM_3	−	−	++	++	++
5	M_4	−	−	++++	++++	++

H, Heart; *M*, muscle.
*Enzyme 1 has the highest, and enzyme 5 the lowest, anodic mobility on electrophoresis at slightly alkaline pH.

CLINICAL EXAMPLE 15.5: Markers of Acute Myocardial Infarction

The time at which myocardial proteins appear in the blood after acute myocardial infarction (MI) depends on the size of the protein and its binding to intracellular structures. **Myoglobin** is elevated first (within 6 hours) because it is small (MW 17,000) and water soluble. Myoglobin is followed by **creatine kinase (CK)** and **aspartate transaminase (AST)**, two soluble enzymes with MW of 80,000 and 93,000, respectively. **Lactate dehydrogenase (LDH)** rises later because of its higher MW (135,000) and consequently slower diffusion, and it remains elevated for at least 1 week because of its slow clearance from the circulation (see **Table 15.7**).

The cardiac isoforms of the **troponin** subunits (MW 18,000–37,000) are located mainly on the thin filaments, although about 5% is dissolved in the cytoplasm. After acute MI the dissolved troponin leaks out of the dying tissue rapidly, with a sharp plasma peak about 24 hours after the infarction (**Fig. 15.30**). The filament-bound troponin leaks out more slowly during the course of 1 to 2 weeks, maintaining elevated plasma troponin despite its rapid clearance. Myoglobin and troponin are measured with immunological methods.

Figure 15.30 Markers of acute myocardial infarction. *CK*, Creatine kinase; *LDH*, lactate dehydrogenase.

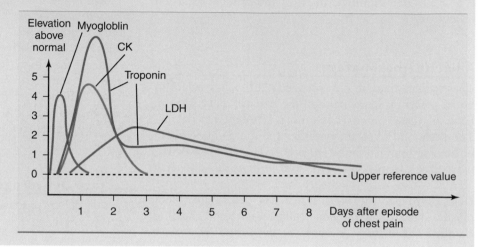

Differential diagnosis requires either the separate determination of the isoenzymes or the simultaneous determination of other enzymes. For example, elevations of isoenzymes 1 and 2, measured 1 or 2 days after an episode of chest pain, suggest myocardial infarction, whereas elevations of isoenzymes 3, 4, and 5 suggest pulmonary infarction. Combined increases of LDH, AST, and creatine kinase (CK) suggest myocardial infarction, whereas elevated LDH with normal AST and CK indicate pulmonary infarction.

Creatine Kinase

Creatine kinase (CK) occurs mainly in muscle tissue, where it catalyzes the reversible reaction

$$Creatine + ATP \rightleftharpoons Creatine\ phosphate + ADP$$

Creatine phosphate serves as a store of high-energy phosphate bonds for contracting muscles (see Chapter 30). Other than muscle tissue, only the brain contains appreciable amounts of CK.

CK is a dimer of two equivalent subunits. Two slightly different monomers occur in the tissues: M subunits in skeletal muscle, and B subunits in brain and smooth muscle. The myocardium contains mainly M but also some B subunits. The two subunits can form three isoenzymes: BB (CK-1), MB (CK-2), and MM (CK-3) (*Table 15.10*).

CK is used for the diagnosis of muscle diseases. Along with LDH, AST, and myoglobin, CK is elevated in dermatomyositis, polymyositis, muscular dystrophies, and after injuries, intramuscular injections, and vigorous physical exercise. CK levels are normal or near normal in patients with neurological motor disorders, such as myasthenia gravis, peripheral neuropathy, and Parkinson disease.

Table 15.10 Isoenzymes of Creatine Kinase

Isoenzymes	Subunit Structure	Electrophoretic Mobility	Present in
CK-1	BB	Fast	Brain
CK-2	BM	Medium	Myocardium
CK-3	MM	Slow	Skeletal muscle, myocardium

CK, Creatine kinase; *B*, brain; *M*, muscle.

Lipase and Amylase

Levels of the digestive enzymes lipase and amylase are elevated in acute pancreatitis. *Their main use is the differential diagnosis in patients who present with severe abdominal pain of sudden onset.* In these "abdominal emergencies," acute pancreatitis must be differentiated from a variety of other disorders, including peptic ulcer disease and cholelithiasis.

Amylase and lipase levels are elevated in some extra-pancreatic diseases as well, including intestinal infarction or perforation, and in peritonitis. Amylase levels can even be elevated in patients with mumps or other forms of parotitis.

SUMMARY

Blood pH and electrolytes must be kept at constant levels by homeostatic mechanisms. The pH is kept constant at 7.4 with the help of the bicarbonate buffer system, which is controlled by the lungs and kidneys. Fluid balance between blood and interstitial spaces depends on the colloid osmotic pressure of the plasma proteins, especially albumin.

The transport of some nutrients and hormones depends on plasma proteins. There are specialized proteins for the transport of steroid and thyroid hormones and even for vitamins and trace minerals, including retinol and iron. The hormone-binding proteins buffer the concentration of the free, unbound hormone in the same way that pH buffers buffer the concentration of free protons.

Immunoglobulins (antibodies) bind foreign macromolecules (antigens). Millions of different antibodies with diverse antigen-binding specificities are produced by B lymphocytes. However, only the few that encounter a matching antigen are mass produced after their B lymphocytes have metamorphosed into antibody-secreting plasma cells.

Blood clotting depends on a cascade of proteolytic activations that culminate in the formation of a fibrin clot from soluble fibrinogen. Blood clotting is subject to complex regulation to ensure that clotting remains limited to areas of injury.

The plasma also contains trace amounts of enzymes and other proteins that usually are intracellular. During tissue damage, these proteins are released into the blood, from which they can be assayed for diagnostic purposes.

Further Reading

Burtis CA, Ashwood ER, editors: *Tietz textbook of clinical chemistry*, ed 3, Philadelphia, 1999, WB Saunders.
Carpenter S, O'Neill LAJ: Recent insights into the structure of Toll-like receptors and post-translational modifications of their associated signalling proteins, *Biochem J* 422:1–10, 2009.
Hedner U, Ezban M: Tissue factor and factor VIIa as therapeutic targets in disorders of hemostasis, *Annu Rev Med* 59:29–41, 2008.
Herr AB, Farndale RW: Structural insights into the interactions between platelet receptors and fibrillar collagen, *J Biol Chem* 284:19781–19785, 2009.
Kampoli A-M, Tousoulis D, Antoniades C, et al: Biomarkers of premature atherosclerosis, *Trends Mol Med* 15:323–332, 2009.
Mackman N: Triggers, targets and treatments for thrombosis, *Nature* 451:914–918, 2008.
Melnikova I: The anticoagulants market, *Nat Rev Drug Discov* 8:353–354, 2009.
Paikin JS, Eikelboom JW, Cairns JA, Hirsh J: New antithrombotic agents—insights from clinical trials, *Nature Rev Cardiology* 7:498–509, 2010.
Teng G, Papavasiliou FN: Immunoglobulin somatic hypermutation, *Annu Rev Genet* 41:107–120, 2007.
Unniraman S, Schatz DG: Strand-biased spreading of mutations during somatic hypermutation, *Science* 317:1227–1230, 2007.
Wood P: Primary antibody deficiency syndromes, *Ann Clin Biochem* 46:99–108, 2009.
Zögg T, Brandstetter H: Activation mechanisms of coagulation factor IX, *Biol Chem* 390:391–400, 2009.

QUESTIONS

1. A complete IgG molecule contains

   A. Two antigen-binding regions
   B. A hinge region between the variable domain and the first constant domain of the heavy chain
   C. One κ light chain and one λ light chain
   D. A J chain
   E. Disulfide bonds between the two light chains

2. During a routine checkup of an asymptomatic middle-aged woman, her level of haptoglobin is found to be extremely low. Other blood values are normal. This finding could indicate

   A. Chronic damage to skeletal muscle
   B. Either liver damage or biliary obstruction
   C. An acute-phase response
   D. Mild chronic hemolysis
   E. Multiple myeloma

3. **A 35-year-old man complains about a chronic cough and poor exercise tolerance. Abnormal breath sounds suggest the presence of emphysema. The man used to smoke moderately for several years but gave up smoking 5 years ago. Which blood test should be performed in this situation?**

   A. Transferrin saturation
   B. Serum creatine kinase
   C. Serum α-fetoprotein
   D. Trypsin inhibitory capacity
   E. Bence Jones protein

4. **Classic hemophilia is caused by an inherited deficiency of clotting factor VIII. This deficiency blocks**

   A. The intrinsic pathway of blood clotting
   B. The extrinsic pathway of blood clotting
   C. The final common pathway of blood clotting
   D. The fibrinolytic system
   E. Contact-phase activation

5. **Patients with nephrotic syndrome have deficiencies of most plasma proteins, but one plasma protein fraction actually is increased. This fraction is**

   A. Albumin
   B. α_1-Globulin
   C. α_2-Globulin
   D. β-Globulin
   E. γ-Globulin

Chapter 16
EXTRACELLULAR MESSENGERS

Cells must respond to their environment. Attachments to neighboring cells and the surrounding extracellular matrix provide signals from the immediate environment, but signals from distant sources have to be transmitted by soluble extracellular messenger molecules.

Hormones are synthesized either by specialized endocrine glands or by "ordinary" tissues such as heart, kidney, intestine, and adipose tissue. They are transported by the blood and induce physiological responses in distant targets.

Paracrine messengers are not transported by the blood but act on neighboring cells in their tissue of origin. Many paracrine messengers also act on the synthesizing cell itself. This is called **autocrine** signaling.

Neurotransmitters are released by neurons at specialized cell-cell contacts called "synapses." Rather than broadcasting a message, they transmit a message between two individual cells.

This chapter describes the metabolism of extracellular messengers. The actions of these agents on their target cells are discussed in Chapter 17.

STEROID HORMONES ARE MADE FROM CHOLESTEROL

The steroids are classic hormones, synthesized in endocrine glands, and transported by the blood. The adrenal steroids regulate energy metabolism (glucocorticoids) and mineral balance (mineralocorticoids), and the gonadal steroids are concerned with sex. *Table 16.1* lists representatives of the major classes of steroid hormones.

All steroid hormones are synthesized from cholesterol. Structural changes that are introduced during hormone synthesis include the following:

1. The side chain at carbon 17 of cholesterol is either shortened to two carbons (progestins, corticosteroids) or lost entirely (androgens, estrogens). This requires **side chain cleavage reactions.**
2. The steroid hormones contain hydroxyl groups and/or keto groups. Only the oxygen atom at C-3 is inherited from cholesterol. Those at C-11 (corticosteroids),

C-17 (glucocorticoids, androgens, estrogens), and C-21 (corticosteroids) have to be introduced by **hydroxylation reactions.**
3. **Mineralocorticoids** have an aldehyde group at C-18.
4. **Estrogens** are distinguished by the aromatic nature of ring A.

PROGESTINS ARE THE BIOSYNTHETIC PRECURSORS OF ALL OTHER STEROID HORMONES

The *precursor relationships* of the steroid hormones can be summarized as follows:

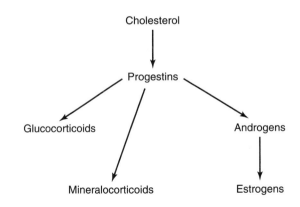

The very first reaction (*Fig. 16.1*) is catalyzed by the mitochondrial **side chain cleavage enzyme,** also known as **desmolase.** It hydroxylates carbons 20 and 22, followed by cleavage of the carbon-carbon bond. This reaction produces **pregnenolone,** which is converted to **progesterone** by a nicotinamide adenine dinucleotide (NAD)-dependent enzyme. Progesterone is the major product of the corpus luteum and the placenta. The other endocrine glands convert pregnenolone and progesterone to other steroid hormones.

The adrenal cortex processes the progestins into **corticosteroids,** including the major glucocorticoid **cortisol** (10–20 mg/day) and the major mineralocorticoid **aldosterone** (0.10–0.15 mg/day). The most important reactions of corticosteroid synthesis (*Fig. 16.2*) are hydroxylations with the overall balance

Table 16.1 Structures of Some Representative Steroids

Steroid Class	Source	Synthesis Stimulated by	Example
Cholesterol	Ubiquitous	—	Cholesterol
Progestins	Corpus luteum,* placenta	LH	Progesterone
Glucocorticoids	Adrenal cortex	ACTH	Cortisol
Mineralocorticoids	Adrenal cortex (zona glomerulosa)	Angiotensin II, ACTH	Aldosterone
Androgens	Leydig cells (major) Adrenal cortex (minor)	LH ACTH	Testosterone
Estrogens	Ovarian follicle (granulosa cells)†	FSH	Estradiol

*Progestins also are released in small quantities by the adrenal cortex and other steroid-producing glands, where they are intermediates in the synthesis of the other hormones.

†Also formed in small quantities in the corpus luteum and by the aromatization of androgens in nonendocrine tissues.

ACTH, Adrenocorticotropic hormone; *FSH,* follicle-stimulating hormone; *LH,* luteinizing hormone.

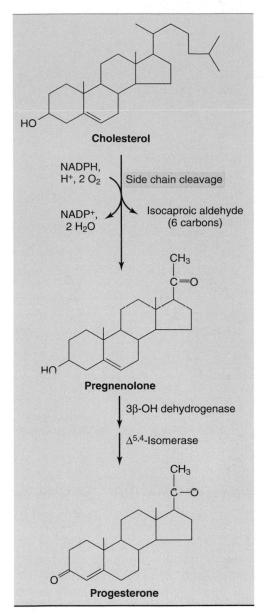

Figure 16.1 Synthesis of progesterone. *NADP⁺, NADPH,* Nicotinamide adenine dinucleotide phosphate.

$$\text{Steroid-H} + O_2 + \text{NADPH} + H^+$$
$$\downarrow \text{P-450}$$
$$\text{Steroid-OH} + \text{NADP}^+ + H_2O$$

These reactions take place in the inner mitochondrial membrane or the endoplasmic reticulum (ER) membrane. They always require the heme-containing subunit **cytochrome P-450.** Molecular oxygen binds to the ferrous heme iron of P-450. An electron is then transferred from NADPH to the heme-bound oxygen, converting the oxygen into a highly reactive form that reacts with the substrate. In the microsomal enzyme complexes (those located in the ER), the electron is transferred through a flavoprotein that contains both flavin adenine dinucleotide (FAD) and flavin mononucleotide (FMN):

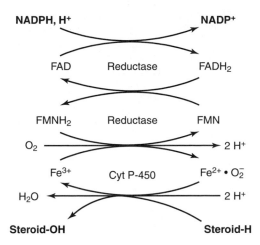

The mitochondrial forms of cytochrome P-450 receive their electrons through an FAD-containing flavoprotein and the iron-sulfur protein **adrenodoxin:**

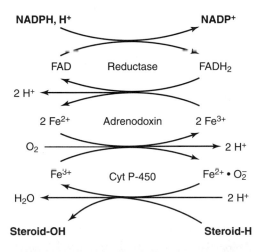

CLINICAL EXAMPLE 16.1: Licorice-Induced Hypertension

The plasma concentration is more than 100 times higher for cortisol than for aldosterone. At this high concentration, cortisol can activate mineralocorticoid receptors in the kidneys and cause the typical mineralocorticoid effects of sodium retention and potassium excretion. This is normally prevented by the NAD⁺-dependent enzyme **11β-hydroxysteroid dehydrogenase** in the kidneys, which converts cortisol to cortisone, which no longer has mineralocorticoid activity (*Fig. 16.3*).

Black licorice candy contains the sweet-tasting glycoside **glycyrrhizic acid,** which is extracted from the root of the licorice tree. Glycyrrhizic acid is hydrolyzed to the aglycone **glycyrrhetinic acid** in the intestine. This product is an inhibitor of 11β-hydroxysteroid dehydrogenase. People who eat excessive amounts of black licorice can develop edema, hypertension, and/or hypokalemia because their kidneys are exposed to the mineralocorticoid effect of

Continued

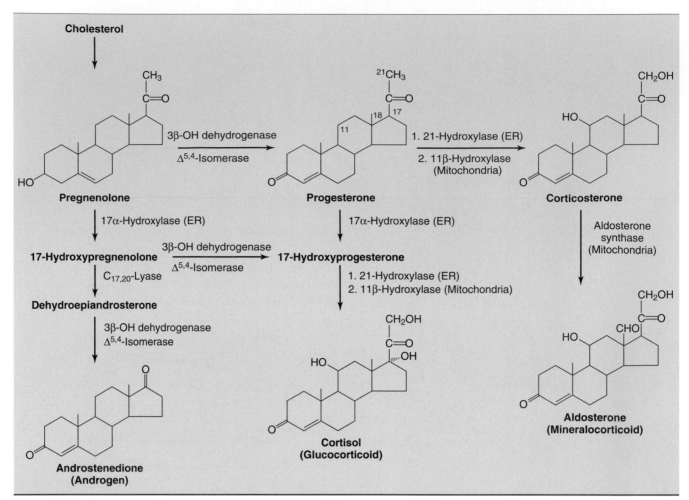

Figure 16.2 Synthesis of adrenal steroids. *ER,* Endoplasmic reticulum.

cortisol. Cortisol levels are elevated during stress. Therefore people who abuse licorice while under stress are most likely to develop these signs.

Licorice extract has medical uses as treatment of peptic ulcer and as a mild laxative. These effects are caused by an unrelated effect of glycyrrhetinic acid in inhibiting the degradation of prostaglandin E.

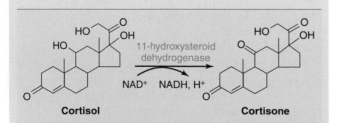

Figure 16.3 Conversion of cortisol to cortisone. Cortisone is a product with little glucocorticoid and no mineralocorticoid activity.

Testosterone is the major testicular androgen. About 5 mg is produced by the Leydig cells in the testis every day. In the target tissues and, to a lesser extent, in the testis itself, testosterone is converted to **dihydrotestosterone (DHT)** by the enzyme **5α-reductase**. The plasma level of DHT is only 10% of the testosterone level, but *DHT is a considerably more potent androgen than is testosterone.* Therefore testosterone acts in part as a precursor, or *prohormone,* of the active hormone DHT.

The adrenal cortex contributes approximately 20 mg of androgen per day. Adrenal androgens include **dihydroepiandrosterone** and **androstenedione,** but only trace amounts of testosterone. The adrenal androgens have a keto group instead of a hydroxy group at C-17 and therefore are far less potent than testosterone, but they are a major source of androgenic activity in females (***Figs. 16.2*** and ***16.4***).

The granulosa cells of the ovarian follicles process testosterone into the potent estrogen **estradiol.** Postmenopausal women no longer make estradiol but still have the weak estrogen **estrone,** which is made from

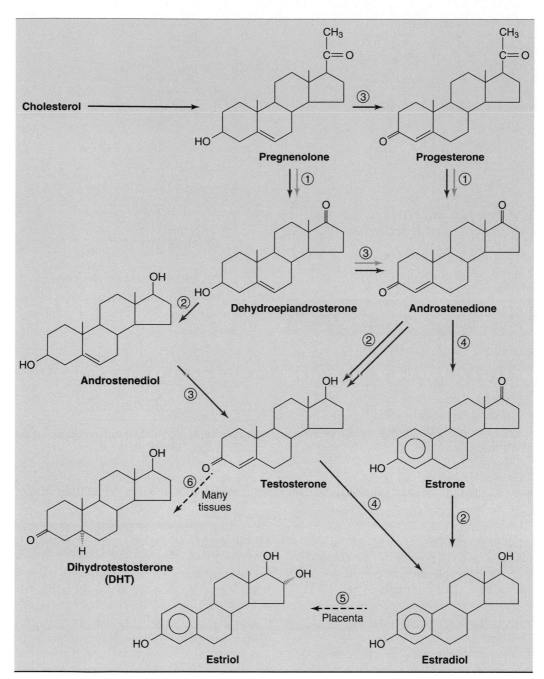

Figure 16.4 Major pathways for synthesis of gonadal steroids. ⟶, All steroid-producing cells; ⟶, ovary, theca cells; ⟶, ovary, granulosa cells; ⟶, testis; ①, 17α-hydroxylase/C$_{17,20}$-lyase; ②, 17β-hydroxysteroid dehydrogenase; ③, 3β-dehydrogenase and Δ^{5,4}-isomerase; ④, aromatase; ⑤, 16α-hydroxylase; ⑥, 5α-reductase.

the adrenal androgen androstenedione. These reactions are catalyzed by the microsomal enzyme system **aromatase.**

Men produce only 65 μg/day of estrone from androstenedione and 45 μg of estradiol from testosterone.

A small quantity of estradiol is synthesized in the testes, but most estrogen in the male is produced in adipose tissue, liver, skin, brain, and other nonendocrine tissues. Therefore *testosterone is a precursor of two other hormones, DHT and estradiol:*

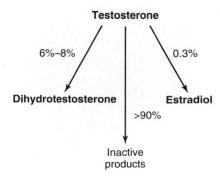

Abnormalities in androgen synthesis lead to disorders of sexual development (*Clinical Examples 16.2* and *16.3*).

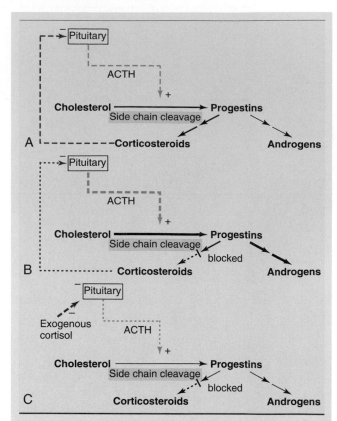

Figure 16.5 Adrenal steroid synthesis in adrenogenital syndrome. **A,** Normal. **B,** Untreated adrenogenital syndrome. **C,** Adrenogenital syndrome treated with cortisol (+ mineralocorticoid). *ACTH,* Adrenocorticotropic hormone.

CLINICAL EXAMPLE 16.2: Congenital Adrenal Hyperplasia

In the adrenal cortex, 21-hydroxylase and 11β-hydroxylase are required for the synthesis of corticosteroids but not androgens (see *Fig. 16.2*). Recessively inherited deficiencies of either of these enzymes leads to **congenital adrenal hyperplasia,** also known as **adrenogenital syndrome** (incidence 1:10,000, 90% of this is 21-hydroxylase deficiency).

Ordinarily, the desmolase reaction in the adrenal cortex is stimulated by adrenocorticotropic hormone (ACTH) from the pituitary gland, and the glucocorticoids inhibit ACTH release. In adrenogenital syndrome, the deficiency of glucocorticoids enhances ACTH release. The excess ACTH causes adrenal hyperplasia and stimulates the desmolase reaction. With the pathway of corticosteroid synthesis blocked, *the overproduced progestins are diverted into androgen synthesis* (*Fig. 16.5*). This disorder produces ambiguous external genitalia in girls and precocious puberty in boys.

Complete or near-complete deficiency of 21-hydroxylase leads to life-threatening hyponatremia and hyperkalemia due to aldosterone deficiency. The opposite is seen in deficiency of 11β-hydroxylase because 11-deoxycorticosterone accumulates. This 21-hydroxylated metabolite acts as a mineralocorticoid, and, because of its high levels, it causes signs of mineralocorticoid excess despite the absence of aldosterone.

Both the virilization and electrolyte imbalances can be cured by orally administered corticosteroids.

CLINICAL EXAMPLE 16.3: 5α-Reductase Deficiency

The recessively inherited deficiency of 5α-reductase prevents the synthesis of dihydrotestosterone (DHT) from testosterone. Affected boys are born with ambiguous external genitalia, although testes and internal wolffian duct structures (epididymis, vas deferens, seminal vesicles) are present. Full virilization takes place only at puberty; therefore, 5α-reductase deficiency is also known as the "penis-at-12 syndrome." This rare disorder shows that *DHT is required for the prenatal development of external male genitalia.*

THYROID HORMONES ARE SYNTHESIZED FROM PROTEIN-BOUND TYROSINE

The thyroid hormones are the only constituents of the human body that contain organically bound iodine:

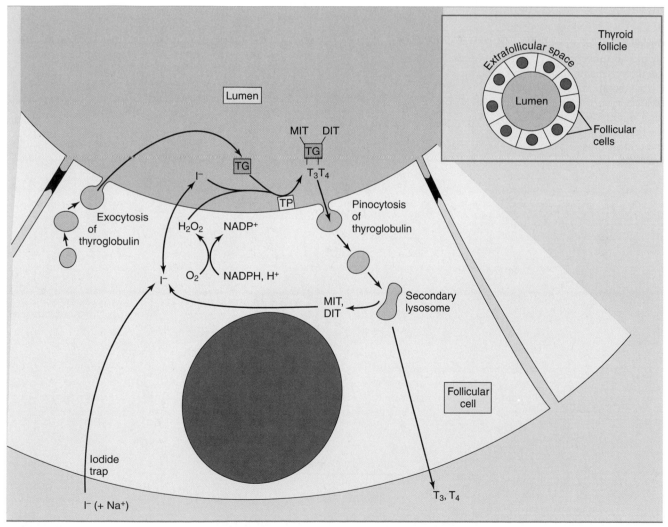

Triiodothyronine
(T₃)

Thyroxine
(T₄)

The typical dietary intake of iodine, in the form of the iodide anion, is approximately 100 μg. Its plasma concentration is only 0.2 μg/dl, but the thyroid gland actively accumulates iodide from the blood by means of sodium cotransport. This carrier is inhibited by several inorganic ions including nitrate, perchlorate, pertechnetate, and isocyanate. Isocyanate is present in some foods, including cabbage and cassava, and can cause goiter when large quantities of these foods are consumed in the context of low dietary iodine.

Iodide enters the lumen of the thyroid follicle by facilitated diffusion from the follicular cells (*Fig. 16.6*). Here it meets the second ingredient for hormone synthesis, **thyroglobulin**. This large glycoprotein (two subunits, $2 \times 330,000$ D) is secreted into the lumen of the thyroid follicle by the follicular cells. Up to 40 tyrosine side chains in thyroglobulin become iodinated, but only 8 to 10 of them are processed to the active hormones.

Figure 16.6 Cellular compartmentation of thyroid hormone synthesis. *DIT*, Diiodotyrosine; *MIT*, monoiodotyrosine; *TG*, thyroglobulin; *TP*, thyroperoxidase.

Iodination of the tyrosine side chains requires the oxidation of iodide by the heme-containing enzyme **thyroperoxidase** on the apical (luminal) surface of the plasma membrane (see *Fig. 16.6*). The iodine reacts with tyrosine side chains, and the coupling of two iodinated tyrosines produces the protein-bound hormones (*Fig. 16.7*).

The hormones are released when thyroglobulin is taken up into the cell by pinocytosis, followed by the complete breakdown of thyroglobulin in lysosomes. The hormones leave the cell, and iodine from iodinated but uncoupled tyrosine is recycled.

More than 99% of triiodothyronine (T_3) and more than 99.9% of thyroxine (T_4) in the blood are bound to plasma proteins. Protein binding protects the hormones from enzymatic attack and renal excretion. Therefore their biological half-lives are remarkably long: 6.5 days for T_4 and 1.5 days for T_3. The T_4 level in the plasma is 50 times higher than the T_3 level (80 ng/ml vs 1.5 ng/ml), but the concentrations of free, unbound hormone are more balanced because T_3 is less extensively bound to plasma proteins than is T_4. *The concentration of the unbound hormone, not the total hormone, determines the biological effects on the tissues.*

Ninety percent of the released hormone is T_4, and 10% is T_3. In the target tissues, some T_4 is converted to active T_3, and some is converted to the inactive reverse T_3 (*Fig. 16.8*). Eighty percent of the circulating T_3 does not come directly from the thyroid gland but is produced from T_4 in peripheral tissues. Of the two hormones, T_3 is about four times more potent than T_4. Therefore T_4 *is a prohormone for the more potent T_3, much as testosterone is a prohormone for the more potent dihydrotestosterone.*

BOTH HYPOTHYROIDISM AND HYPERTHYROIDISM ARE COMMON DISORDERS

The deficiency of thyroid hormone is called **hypothyroidism.** In adults, it is characterized by widespread subcutaneous edema due to excessive amounts of

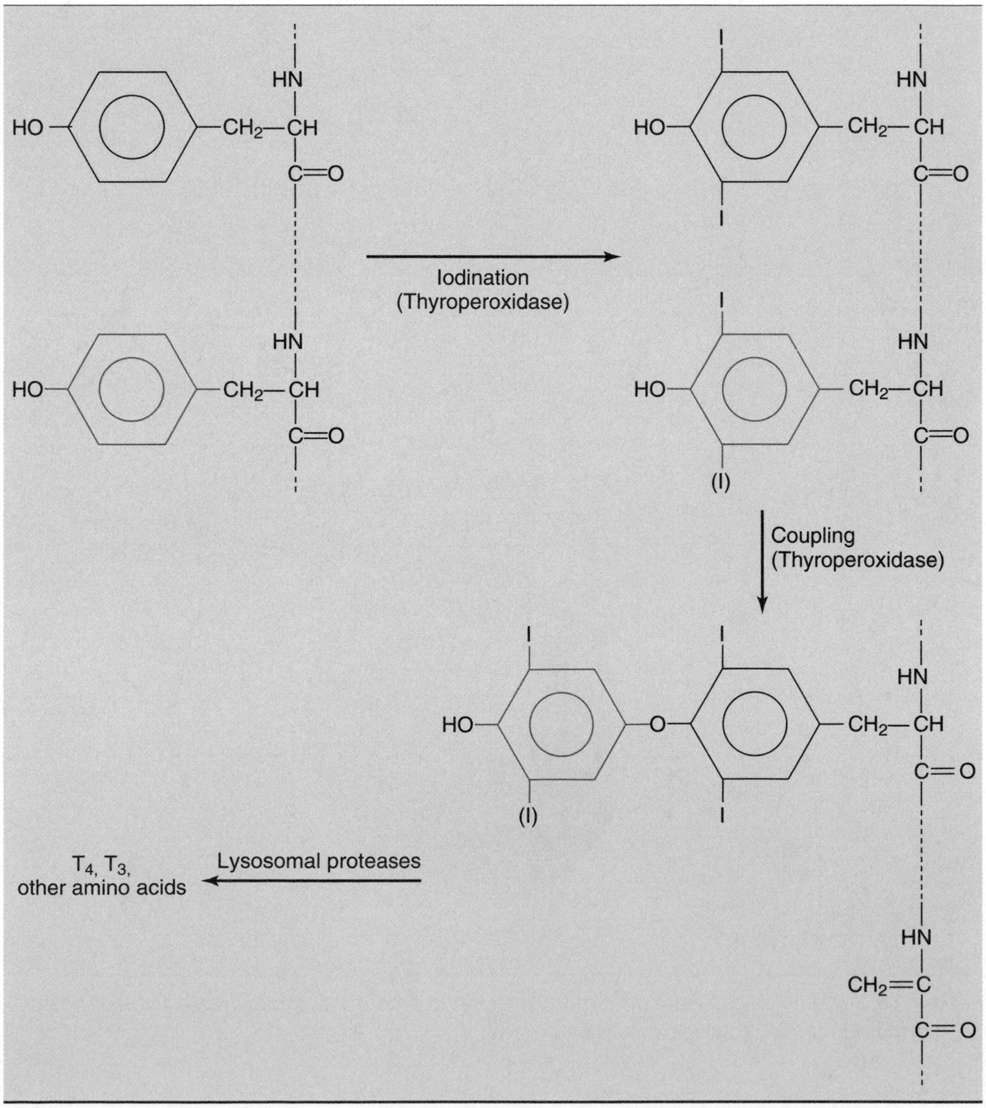

Figure 16.7 Synthesis of thyroid hormones from iodinated tyrosine residues in thyroglobulin. These reactions take place on the luminal surface of the follicular cells in the thyroid gland. T_3, Triiodothyronine; T_4, thyroxine.

Figure 16.8 In its target tissues, thyroxine (T_4) is converted to either the more active triiodothyronine (T_3) or to inactive reverse T_3.

Thyroxine
(T_4)

T_3
(active)

Reverse T_3
(inactive)

hyaluronic acid ("myxedema"), decreased basal metabolic rate, bradycardia, and sluggish thinking. Hypothyroidism in infants leads to severe and irreversible mental deficiency, stunted growth, and multiple physical deformities. This condition is called **cretinism.**

CLINICAL EXAMPLE 16.4: Newborn Screening for Hypothyroidism

Newborn screening for endocrine and metabolic diseases is performed for treatable conditions that would lead to death or disability if left undiagnosed and untreated. Serious congenital hypothyroidism afflicts about 1:4000 newborns. If diagnosed at birth, cretinism can readily be prevented by oral administration of T_4. Therefore neonatal screening for congenital hypothyroidism is routinely performed in all developed parts of the world.

Iodine deficiency causes endemic hypothyroidism in areas of the world where the soil and the plants grown on it are deficient in this mineral. In the Alps, the condition was common until the early years of the twentieth century. Iodine deficiency now is rare in most countries because of the routine use of iodized salt, although there is still an extensive "goiter belt" in the Himalaya Mountains.

Autoimmune thyroiditis, also known as **Hashimoto disease,** is the most common form of adult hypothyroidism in areas with sufficient iodine, with a prevalence of at least 2% in women and 0.4% in men. It is characterized by episodes of inflammation with lymphocytic infiltration that can present with either hypothyroidism or hyperthyroidism. As the thyroid gland is progressively destroyed, lasting hypothyroidism finally develops.

The thyroid gland is stimulated by thyroid-stimulating hormone (TSH) from the pituitary gland. TSH release, in turn, is suppressed by thyroid hormones:

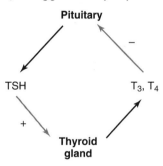

This feedback loop maintains a constant level of thyroid hormone under ordinary conditions. In autoimmune thyroiditis and iodine deficiency, the thyroid gland cannot make its hormones. The thyrotrophs of the pituitary gland are disinhibited, and the TSH level soars. TSH not only stimulates the biochemical steps in thyroid hormone synthesis but also causes hyperplasia of the follicular cells. This condition is called **goiter.**

Graves disease, which afflicts about 1% of women and 0.1% of men, is the most common cause of **hyperthyroidism.** It is an autoimmune disease in which an abnormal immunoglobulin G antibody binds to the TSH receptor. The antibody stimulates the receptor, causing excessive hormone secretion (**thyrotoxicosis**) and enlargement of the gland.

INSULIN IS RELEASED TOGETHER WITH THE C-PEPTIDE

Proteins, glycoproteins, and smaller peptides are the most diverse class of messenger molecules. They include many hormones and neurotransmitters, as well as growth factors and the cytokines that are released by white blood cells during inflammation.

All extracellular signaling proteins are made on the assembly line of the secretory pathway: from ER-bound ribosomes through the ER, Golgi apparatus, and secretory vesicles. *Small peptide hormones are derived from larger polypeptides.* These **prohormones** are processed by endopeptidases in the ER, Golgi apparatus, or secretory vesicles.

The synthesis of insulin in the pancreatic β-cells is an example (*Fig. 16.9*). Mature insulin, which consists of two disulfide-bonded polypeptides with 21 and 30 amino acids, is derived from **preproinsulin,** a single polypeptide with 103 amino acids. The N-terminal 24 amino acids are the signal sequence. They are removed by signal peptidase in the ER. The remaining structure, known as **proinsulin,** is cleaved after paired basic amino acid residues by enzymes in the secretory

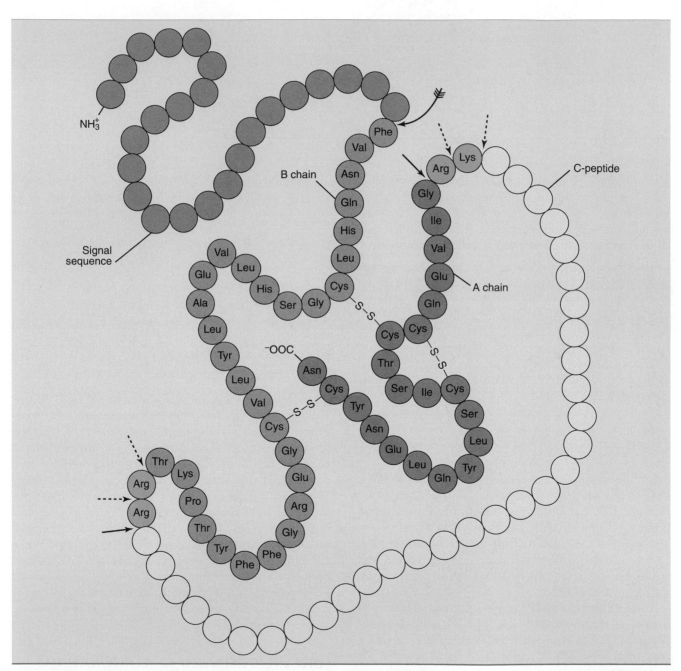

Figure 16.9 Synthesis of insulin from preproinsulin. Mature insulin consists of two disulfide-bonded polypeptides, the A chain and the B chain. During prohormone processing, the signal sequence (●●) and the C-peptide (○○) are removed proteolytically. The proteolytic cleavages are performed by the signal peptidase in the rough endoplasmic reticulum (ER) (⫸→) and by prohormone convertases (⟶) in secretory granules that cleave proinsulin at two sites on the C-terminal side of dibasic residues (Arg-Arg and Lys-Arg). The basic residues are then removed sequentially by carboxypeptidase E/H (--➤).

granules. These cleavages form insulin and a hormonally inactive **C-peptide** (C for connecting).

Being formed in the same secretory vesicle, insulin and C-peptide are released together into the blood. The serum C-peptide level can be determined in the clinical laboratory. With a plasma half-life ($T_{1/2}$) of 30 minutes, C-peptide is longer lived than insulin ($T_{1/2} = $ 4 minutes); therefore, its plasma level is higher. In addition, it can be used to assess β-cell function in diabetic patients who receive insulin injections. Measured insulin can be derived from either injections or the patient's pancreas, but C-peptide reveals the functional state of the patient's pancreas.

PROOPIOMELANOCORTIN FORMS SEVERAL ACTIVE PRODUCTS

Proopiomelanocortin is a prohormone in the corticotroph cells of the anterior pituitary gland. It is a precursor of ACTH, β-endorphin, three forms of melanocyte-stimulating hormone (MSH), and lipotropic hormones that stimulate fat breakdown in adipose tissue.

ACTH and β-lipotropin are the main products in the anterior pituitary gland. They are stored in the same vesicles and are released together in response to the same stimuli. In the pars intermedia of the pituitary gland, ACTH is further processed to α-MSH, whereas β-lipotropin is processed to β-endorphin (*Fig. 16.10*). β-Endorphin is also formed in neurons of the arcuate nucleus of the brain.

Humans form little α-MSH, and most melanocyte-stimulating activity is contained within the larger fragments β-lipotropin, γ-lipotropin, and ACTH.

Hyperpigmentation is a common finding in patients with **Cushing disease** (ACTH-secreting pituitary adenoma). Hyperpigmentation is seen in **Addison disease** (destruction of the adrenal glands) as well, because glucocorticoid deficiency leads to excessive secretion of ACTH and the other proopiomelanocortin-derived hormones.

ANGIOTENSIN IS FORMED FROM CIRCULATING ANGIOTENSINOGEN

Some hormones are produced by proteases in the blood. For example, the vasoconstrictor peptide **angiotensin** is derived from the plasma protein **angiotensinogen**. When the blood pressure in the kidneys is too low, the juxtaglomerular cells release the protease **renin**. Renin cleaves angiotensinogen to form the 10–amino-acid-peptide **angiotensin I**.

Angiotensin I is biologically inactive. It has to be processed to active **angiotensin II** by **angiotensin-converting enzyme,** a protease on the surface of endothelial cells in the lungs. Cleavage by renin is the rate-limiting step in this sequence (*Fig. 16.11*).

Angiotensin II raises the blood pressure by a direct action on vascular smooth muscle and indirectly by enhancing the release of norepinephrine from sympathetic nerve endings and epinephrine from the adrenal medulla. It also stimulates aldosterone secretion from the adrenal cortex. Aldosterone causes a delayed rise in blood pressure by reducing the renal excretion of sodium. Angiotensin II is degraded by endothelial peptidases in less than 1 minute. Some of the fragments have additional biological effects, whereas others are

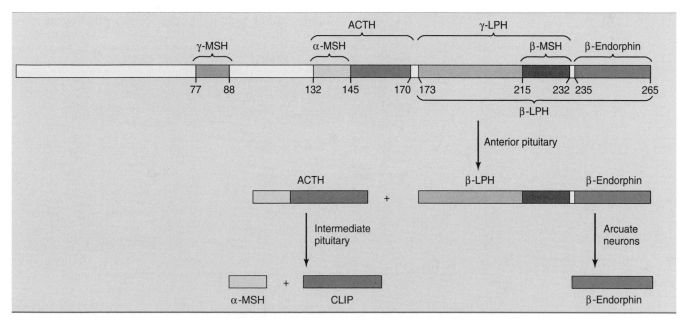

Figure 16.10 Structure and processing of proopiomelanocortin in the pituitary gland. The active fragments are in most cases framed by pairs of basic amino acid residues (not shown here). *ACTH,* Adrenocorticotropic hormone; *CLIP,* hormonally inactive fragment; *LPH,* lipotropic hormone (lipotropin); *MSH,* melanocyte-stimulating hormone.

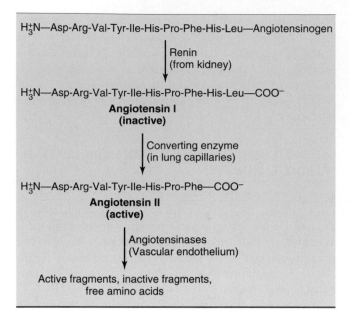

Figure 16.11 Synthesis of angiotensin II from circulating angiotensinogen.

completely inactive. *Most small peptides in the blood are rapidly degraded by peptidases on the surface of capillary endothelial cells.* For example, the lifespans of oxytocin and vasopressin (nine amino acids) are in the 1- to 10-minute range.

CLINICAL EXAMPLE 16.5: Converting Enzyme Inhibitors

Captopril and other inhibitors of angiotensin-converting enzyme (ACE) prevent the conversion of inactive angiotensin I into biologically active angiotensin II. An unrelated function of ACE is the inactivation of the vasodilator peptide bradykinin. Therefore ACE inhibitors simultaneously reduce the level of the vasoconstrictor angiotensin II and raise the level of the vasodilator bradykinin. Cleavage of angiotensinogen by renin is the rate-limiting step in angiotensin synthesis, but renin inhibitors have been introduced into medical practice only recently.

IMMUNOASSAYS ARE THE MOST VERSATILE METHODS FOR DETERMINATION OF HORMONE LEVELS

The plasma concentrations of most hormones are extremely low (*Fig. 16.12*). Therefore very sensitive and specific methods are required for measurement of hormone levels in the clinical laboratory.

The classic procedure is **radioimmunoassay (RIA)**. It requires a specific antibody to the hormone and a radiolabeled version of the hormone containing tritium, radioactive iodine, or some other suitable isotope. When the patient's serum is added to a complex of the antibody with the radiolabeled hormone, *the (unlabeled) hormone in the patient's serum competes with the radioactive hormone for binding to the antibody.*

After incubation for some minutes, the unbound hormone is separated from the hormone-antibody complex. The higher the hormone concentration in the patient's serum, the more radioactive hormone is displaced from the antibody. The principle of this method is illustrated in *Figure 16.13*. RIA is used not only for hormones but also for many low-abundance plasma proteins, for example, C-reactive protein and prostate-specific antigen (see Chapter 15).

RIA procedures are now being replaced by other immunoassay techniques that utilize fluorescence or

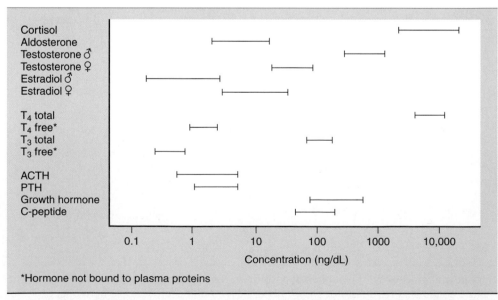

Figure 16.12 Reference ranges for the plasma concentrations of some hormones, logarithmic scale.

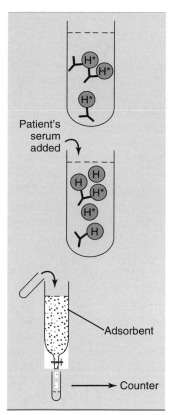

Figure 16.13   General procedure for the radioimmunoassay of a hormone. **Top,** After a specific antibody (Υ) is mixed with the labeled hormone (H*), a radioactive antigen-antibody complex is formed. **Middle,** The patient's serum is added. The unlabeled hormone in the patient's serum (*H*) competes with the labeled hormone for binding to the antibody: Antibody · H* + H ⇌ Antibody · H + H*. **Bottom,** Free hormone and antibody-hormone complex are separated from each other. The radioactivity of the free, unbound hormone is measured. A large amount of hormone in the patient's serum leads to a high specific radioactivity of the free hormone.

chemiluminescence measurements rather than radioactivity. For example, an antibody to a hormone can be immobilized on a solid matrix or plate. The immobilized antibody binds ("catches") the hormone in the patient's sample. After washing, a second antibody, which binds to a second site on the hormone, is added to make an antibody "sandwich." This second antibody has a fluorescent or chemiluminescent tag, or an enzyme, that is covalently attached to it. The amount of the tag or enzyme is a measure of the amount of hormone present. When an attached enzyme is used, the method is referred to as an **enzyme-linked immunosorbent assay** (ELISA). To detect the amount of enzyme present, a substrate is added that can be converted by the enzyme into a fluorescent or chemiluminescent product.

ARACHIDONIC ACID IS CONVERTED TO BIOLOGICALLY ACTIVE PRODUCTS

The **eicosanoids** (from Greek είκοσα meaning "20") are biologically active lipids that are derived from polyunsaturated 20-carbon fatty acids. Any of the three fatty acids shown in *Figure 16.14* can be used as a precursor, but *arachidonic acid is most important because it is far more abundant than the others.* In the cell, these fatty acids are encountered in position 2 of membrane phosphoglycerides, from which they are released by the action of **phospholipase A₂** (*Fig. 16.15*).

Free arachidonic acid can be salvaged by an acyl coenzyme A (CoA) synthetase for reesterification. Alternatively, it can be processed to biologically active products. The **cyclooxygenase pathway** produces prostaglandins, prostacyclin, and thromboxane, whereas the **lipoxygenase pathway** produces leukotrienes (*Fig. 16.16*).

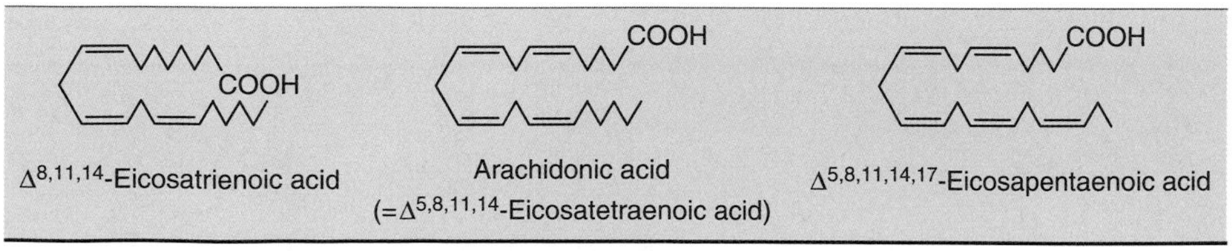

$\Delta^{8,11,14}$-Eicosatrienoic acid

Arachidonic acid
(=$\Delta^{5,8,11,14}$-Eicosatetraenoic acid)

$\Delta^{5,8,11,14,17}$-Eicosapentaenoic acid

Figure 16.14   The three 20-carbon fatty acids pictured are the precursors of prostaglandins, leukotrienes, and other biologically active products.

Phospholipase A₂

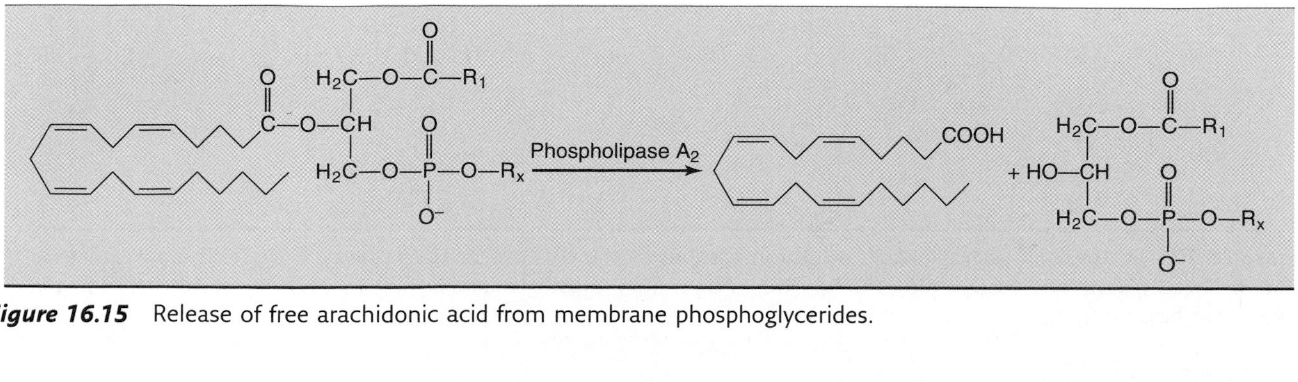

Figure 16.15   Release of free arachidonic acid from membrane phosphoglycerides.

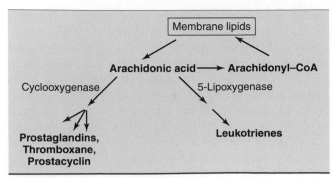

Figure 16.16 Major fates of arachidonic acid. Cyclooxygenase and 5-lipoxygenase are the key enzymes for the synthesis of the biologically active eicosanoids. *CoA,* Coenzyme A.

PROSTAGLANDINS ARE SYNTHESIZED IN ALMOST ALL TISSUES

Prostaglandins and related products are formed by the microsomal **cyclooxygenase complex,** which consists of cyclooxygenase and peroxidase components. Its name indicates that it uses molecular oxygen as an oxidant and that it creates a ring structure in its substrate.

Two isoenzymes of cyclooxygenase are present in the body. **Cyclooxygenase 1 (COX-1)** is a constitutive enzyme that is present in most cells except erythrocytes. **Cyclooxygenase 2 (COX-2)** is an inducible enzyme in white blood cells and in epithelial cells and smooth muscle cells. *It is induced by proinflammatory stimuli.* However, COX-2 is also constitutively expressed in uninflamed tissues such as the vasculature, kidney, heart, spinal cord, brain, and gastric epithelium.

The prostaglandin H that is formed by the cyclooxygenase complex is converted to other products by tissue-specific enzymes (*Fig. 16.17*). *Each cell type makes only one or a few major products.* For example, platelets make thromboxane, and vascular endothelial cells make prostaglandins E and I.

Prostaglandins are named with a capital letter according to the nature of the substituent on the cyclopentane ring and a subscript indicating the number of double bonds outside the ring (*Fig. 16.18*).

The types of prostaglandin, as designated by the capital letter, have different and sometimes antagonistic biological effects. The number of double bonds, on the other hand, affects the potency of the product but not the kind of effect on a particular target tissue.

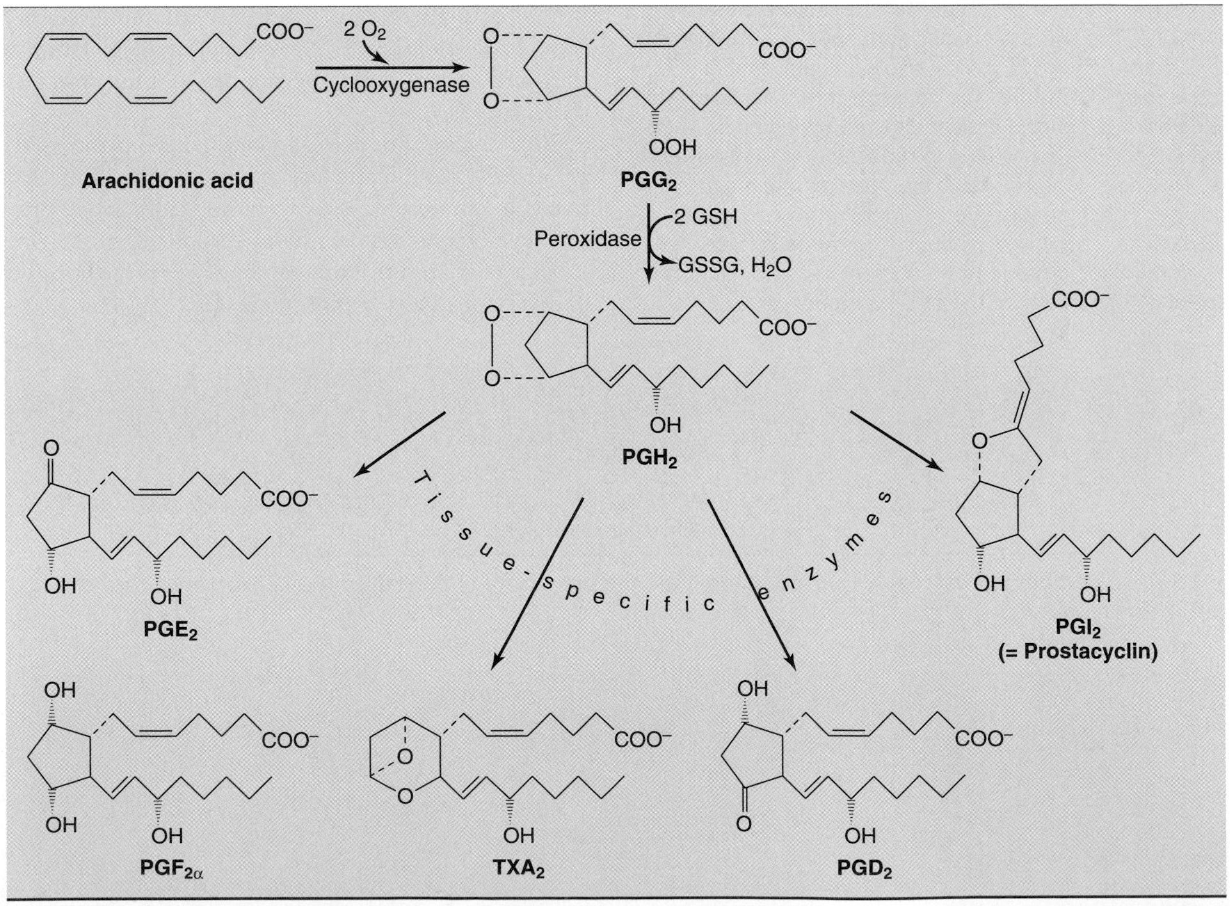

Figure 16.17 Synthesis of prostaglandins and thromboxanes by the cyclooxygenase pathway. *GSH,* Reduced glutathione; *GSSG,* oxidized glutathione; *PGD₂, PGE₂, PGF₂ₐ, PGG₂, PGH₂, PGI₂,* prostaglandins D₂, E₂, F₂ₐ, G₂, H₂, and I₂, respectively; *TXA₂,* thromboxane A₂.

Figure 16.18 Three molecular forms of prostaglandin E (PGE). *PGE₁* is synthesized from eicosatrienoic acid, *PGE₂* from arachidonic acid, and *PGE₃* from eicosapentaenoic acid.

PROSTANOIDS PARTICIPATE IN MANY PHYSIOLOGICAL PROCESSES

Almost every cell in the human body responds to one or more products of the cyclooxygenase pathway. A few of the more interesting actions are mentioned here.

1. *Aggregating platelets release thromboxane A₂ (TXA₂).* This prostaglandin derivative constricts blood vessels and activates platelets. Its actions are short lasting because it is hydrolyzed to an inactive product within 30 to 60 seconds. The actions of TXA_2 on platelets and blood vessels are antagonized by prostaglandin I_2 (PGI_2, or prostacyclin) from endothelial cells. PGI_2 has a half-life of 3 minutes.

2. *Prostaglandin E₂ (PGE₂) and PGI₂ are vasodilators that are formed by endothelial cells.* PGE_1 can be used in infants with pulmonary stenosis to maintain the patency of the ductus arteriosus until surgical correction can be performed. PGI_2 (epoprostenol), which raises cyclic adenosine monophosphate (cAMP) in platelets and vascular smooth muscle, is used for the treatment of pulmonary hypertension.

3. *Prostaglandin E formed by the gastric mucosa stimulates mucus secretion and suppresses gastric acid secretion.* Consequently, it reduces the risk of peptic ulcer. The synthetic PGE_1 analogue **misoprostol** is used for the prevention of gastric ulcer in patients treated with aspirin or other non-steroidal antiinflammatory drugs.

4. *PGE₂ and prostaglandin F₂α (PGF₂α), synthesized in the endometrium, induce uterine contraction.* Their levels in amniotic fluid are low during pregnancy but increase massively at parturition. Together with oxytocin, *they participate in the induction of labor.* Unlike oxytocin, the prostaglandins contract the uterus not only at term of pregnancy but at all times. Therefore *they are used not only for the induction of parturition but also for the induction of abortion.* Outside of pregnancy, the excessive formation of prostaglandins contributes to menstrual cramps.

5. *PGE₂ and TXA₂ are formed by white blood cells as mediators of inflammation.* Together with histamine, bradykinin, leukotrienes, and cytokines, they mediate the cardinal signs of inflammation.

6. *Fever is mediated by the cytokine* **interleukin-1 (IL-1),** a product of activated monocytes and macrophages. IL-1 binds to vascular receptors in the preoptic area of the hypothalamus, where it induces the formation of PGE_2. Diffusing across the blood-brain barrier, PGE_2 causes fever by a direct action on the thermoregulatory center.

LEUKOTRIENES ARE PRODUCED BY THE LIPOXYGENASE PATHWAY

Humans have at least five different molecular forms of lipoxygenase that oxidize arachidonic acid at carbons 5, 12, or 15. Several biologically active products, including the **leukotrienes,** are formed in white blood cells and some other cells (*Fig. 16.19*).

Leukotrienes are powerful constrictors of bronchial and intestinal smooth muscle, and they increase capillary permeability. Unlike the other eicosanoids, *the leukotrienes survive for some hours in the tissue.* Leukotrienes C_4, D_4, and E_4 (LTC_4, LTD_4, and LTE_4), which were originally characterized as the **slow-reacting substance of anaphylaxis,** are responsible for the protracted bronchoconstriction in asthma.

ANTIINFLAMMATORY DRUGS INHIBIT THE SYNTHESIS OF EICOSANOIDS

Two important antiinflammatory drug classes currently are in use. The **glucocorticoids** include cortisol (labeled as "hydrocortisone") and a host of synthetic analogs. *These steroids repress the synthesis of COX-2 and inhibit the action of phospholipase A₂.* The **nonsteroidal antiinflammatory drugs** (**NSAIDs**) include aspirin, indomethacin, and ibuprofen. *The NSAIDs are inhibitors of cyclooxygenase:*

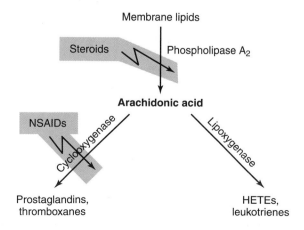

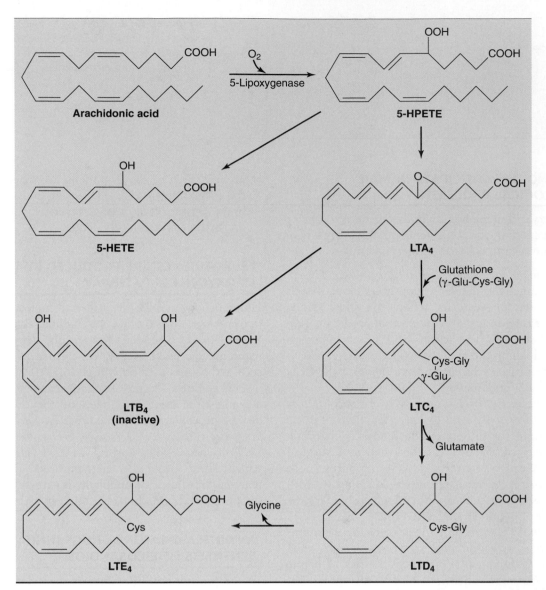

Figure 16.19 Products of 5-lipoxygenase: hydroperoxyeicosatetraenoic acid (*HPETE*), hydroxyeicosatetraenoic acid (*HETE*), and the leukotrienes (*LTA₄, LTB₄, LTC₄, LTD₄, LTE₄*).

By suppressing arachidonic acid release, the steroids suppress the synthesis of all eicosanoids, whereas the NSAIDs inhibit only the cyclooxygenase pathway. Both steroids and NSAIDs are effective in treating arthritis, in which prostaglandins are important mediators of inflammation. In asthma, however, the leukotrienes are the villains. Therefore asthma responds to steroids but not to aspirin and related drugs. Indeed, NSAIDs can make asthma worse. They divert arachidonic acid from prostaglandin synthesis into leukotriene synthesis, and the prostaglandin E that is normally formed in the lungs actually relaxes bronchial smooth muscle. Aspirin prevents the synthesis of this physiological bronchodilator. However, inhibitors of 5-lipoxygenase and drugs that block leukotriene receptors can be effective.

CLINICAL EXAMPLE 16.6: Selective COX-2 Inhibitors

In the stomach, prostaglandin E reduces acid secretion and enhances mucus secretion. Therefore *the suppression of prostaglandin synthesis by aspirin and related drugs can cause gastritis and peptic ulcer.* Selective inhibitors of COX-2 avoid this problem because they suppress prostaglandin synthesis in white blood cells but not in the stomach. Therefore selective COX-2 inhibitors (Vioxx, Celebrex) were developed as antiinflammatory drugs. Although they were effective against inflammation, these drugs had to be withdrawn from the market or their use had to be restricted because of an unexpected increase in the risk of acute myocardial infarction.

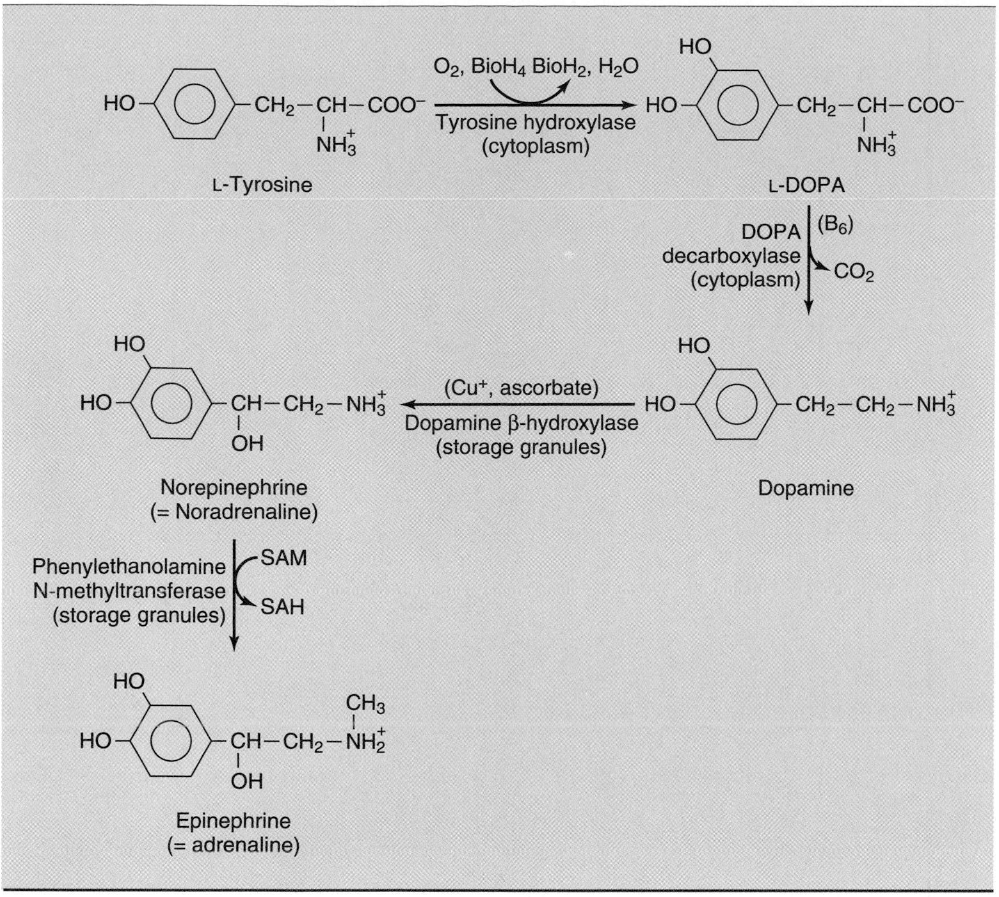

Figure 16.20   Pathway of catecholamine biosynthesis. *SAH*, *S*-adenosyl homocysteine; *SAM*, *S*-adenosyl methionine.

CLINICAL EXAMPLE 16.6: Selective COX-2 Inhibitors—cont'd

The likely explanation is that COX-2 inhibitors block prostacyclin (PGI$_2$) synthesis in endothelial cells and smooth muscle cells of the blood vessels. A reduction in prostacyclin has been shown to accelerate atherosclerotic lesions in injured vessels and to enhance formation of blood clots because prostacyclin normally inhibits platelet aggregation. On the other hand, COX-2 inhibitors, unlike COX-1 inhibitors, do not block the formation of platelet-aggregating thromboxane. A reduction of prostacyclin can also contribute to elevated blood pressure and may have independent detrimental effects on the heart.

CATECHOLAMINES ARE SYNTHESIZED FROM TYROSINE

Several neurotransmitters and hormones are basic products (amines) that are synthesized by the decarboxylation of aromatic amino acids. *These amino acid decarboxylations always depend on pyridoxal phosphate (vitamin B$_6$).* Being water soluble, biogenic amines are stored in membrane-bounded vesicles within the synthesizing cell before they are released by exocytosis.

The **catecholamines** are synthesized from tyrosine (*Fig. 16.20*). The rate-limiting step in this pathway, catalyzed by **tyrosine hydroxylase,** is feedback-inhibited by the amines. The important products are **dopamine, norepinephrine (noradrenaline),** and **epinephrine (adrenaline).** The end product depends on the enzymatic outfit of the cell. For example, the dopamine neurons of the nigrostriatal system in the brain have only tyrosine hydroxylase and DOPA decarboxylase, whereas the adrenal medulla has the enzymes for the complete pathway.

The catecholamines are inactivated by two enzymes (*Fig. 16.21*). **Monoamine oxidase (MAO),** in the outer mitochondrial membrane, inactivates the amines by *oxidative deamination.* The enzyme-bound FAD, which is reduced to FADH$_2$ during the reaction, is regenerated by molecular oxygen with the formation of hydrogen peroxide (H$_2$O$_2$).

Catechol-O-methyltransferase (COMT) inactivates catecholamines by *S-adenosyl methionine (SAM)–dependent methylation* of one of the ring OH groups. These two reactions can occur in either sequence. Dopamine is metabolized to **homovanillic acid,** and norepinephrine and epinephrine are metabolized to

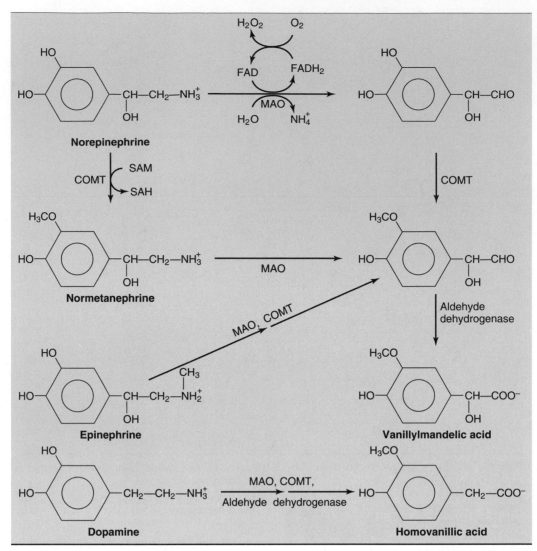

Figure 16.21 Enzymatic inactivation of catecholamines. Besides enzymatic inactivation, which is mostly intracellular, the rapid uptake of catecholamines into the cell is critically important for the termination of their biological actions. *COMT*, Catechol-*O*-methyltransferase; *FAD, FADH₂*, flavin adenine dinucleotide; *MAO*, monoamine oxidase; *SAH*, *S*-adenosyl homocysteine; *SAM*, *S*-adenosyl methionine.

vanillylmandelic acid. These products are excreted in the urine.

INDOLAMINES ARE SYNTHESIZED FROM TRYPTOPHAN

5-Hydroxytryptamine (5-HT), also known as **serotonin**, is synthesized from tryptophan by the enterochromaffin cells of the lungs and digestive tract, platelets, and some neurons in the brain. Its biosynthesis resembles that of the catecholamines. Besides 5-HT, the pineal hormone **melatonin** is the only other indolamine in humans (*Fig. 16.22*).

Serotonin is inactivated by MAO but not by COMT. Humans have two isoenzymes of MAO. **MAO-A** acts on serotonin, and **MAO-B** acts on dopamine. Norepinephrine is inactivated by both.

CLINICAL EXAMPLE 16.7: Diagnosis of Endocrine Tumors

Hormone-secreting tumors arising in the adrenal cortex or sympathetic ganglia are diagnosed as **pheochromocytoma**. They present with hypertension and other autonomic dysfunctions that are caused by the excessive formation of epinephrine, norepinephrine, and, sometimes, dopamine. Overproduction of the hormones is balanced by degradation, and the breakdown products vanillylmandelic acid and homovanillic acid are excreted in the urine. **Carcinoid syndrome** is a similar condition caused by the abnormal proliferation of serotonin-producing endocrine cells in intestine or lungs. In this case the excreted breakdown product is indoleacetic acid. These endocrine tumors are diagnosed by measurements of the breakdown products in the urine.

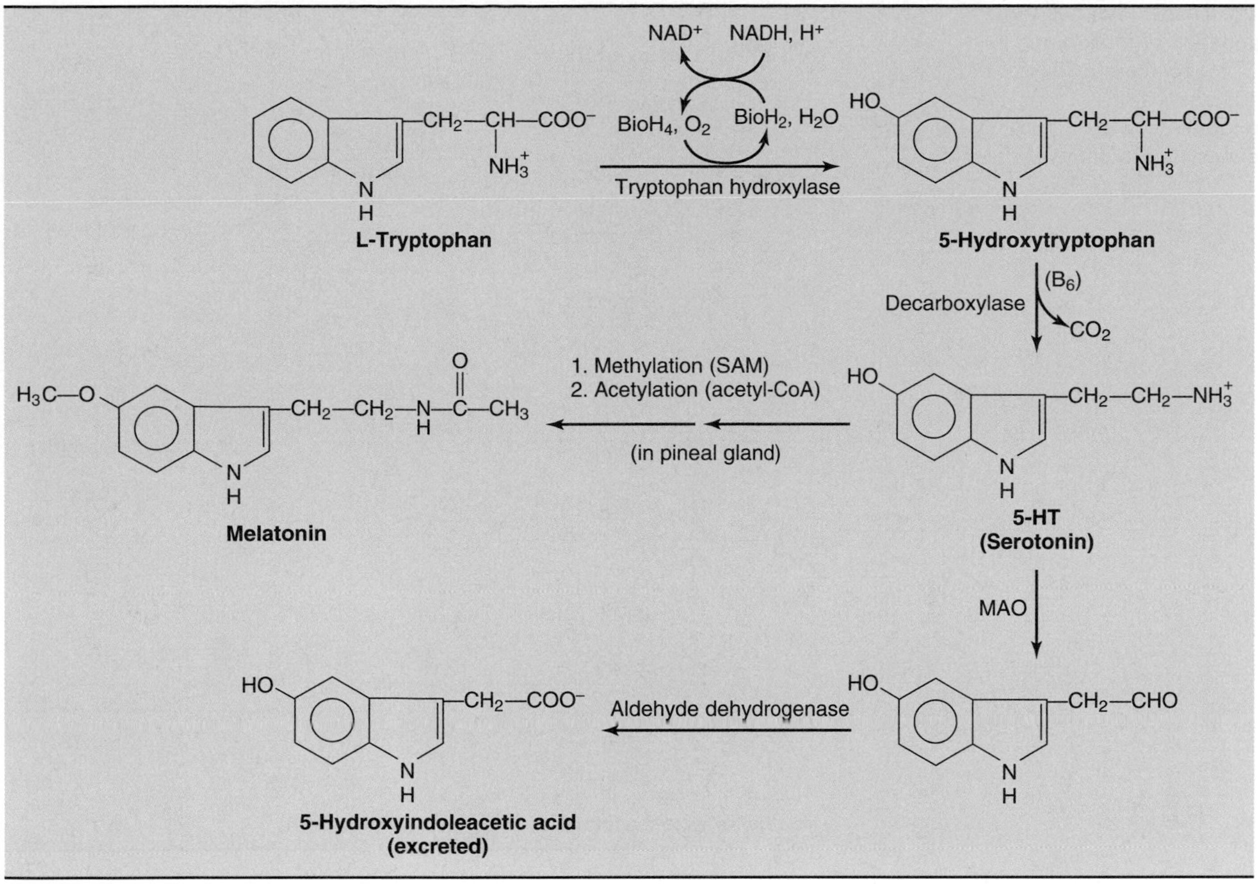

Figure 16.22 Synthesis and degradation of 5-hydroxytryptamine (*5-HT*), or serotonin. *CoA*, Coenzyme A; *SAM*, *S*-adenosyl methionine.

HISTAMINE IS PRODUCED BY MAST CELLS AND BASOPHILS

As a major mediator of allergic responses, *histamine is released by circulating basophils and their sedentary cousins, the mast cells.* Histamine dilates small blood vessels, increases capillary permeability, contracts bronchial and intestinal smooth muscle, stimulates gastric acid secretion and nasal fluid discharge, and regulates the cells of the immune system. Its synthesis and degradation are summarized in *Figure 16.23.*

CLINICAL EXAMPLE 16.8: Pharmacotherapy of Parkinson Disease

Parkinson disease is a movement disorder caused by the degeneration of nigrostriatal dopamine neurons in the brain. The symptoms (tremor, rigor, akinesia) are caused by the deficiency of dopamine action in the corpus striatum.

Direct replacement of the missing neurotransmitter is not possible because dopamine does not cross the blood-brain barrier. However, the dopamine precursor L-DOPA enters the brain on one of the amino acid carriers in the blood-brain barrier. It is taken up by the surviving dopamine neurons, where it is decarboxylated to dopamine. In this way the rate-limiting tyrosine hydroxylase reaction is bypassed. L-DOPA can be combined with carbidopa, a DOPA decarboxylase inhibitor that cannot enter the brain. This prevents the unwanted formation of dopamine outside the brain.

Alternative treatments include dopamine receptor agonists, inhibitors of MAO-B, and inhibitors of catechol-*O*-methyltransferase (COMT).

NEUROTRANSMITTERS ARE RELEASED AT SYNAPSES

Whereas hormones and paracrine messengers broadcast their message, neurotransmitters establish 1:1 communication between two cells. The **presynaptic cell** that synthesizes the neurotransmitter is always a

Figure 16.23 Synthesis and degradation of histamine. *MAO*, Monoamine oxidase; *SAH*, S-adenosyl homocysteine; *SAM*, S-adenosyl methionine.

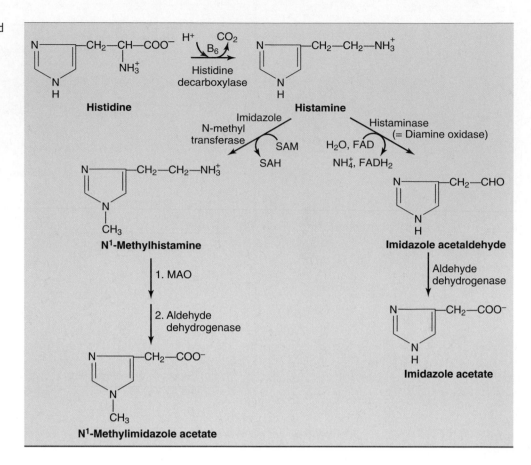

neuron, but the **postsynaptic cell** that responds to the neurotransmitter can be a neuron, a muscle cell, or an epithelial cell in a gland. The site of contact between the two cells is called a **synapse**. The attributes of a "classic" neurotransmitter are as follows:

- It is synthesized in the presynaptic cell.
- It is stored in membrane-bounded vesicles ("synaptic vesicles").
- It is released from the presynaptic cell in response to membrane depolarization.
- It induces a physiological response in the postsynaptic cell, usually by depolarizing or hyperpolarizing its membrane.
- It is rapidly inactivated in the area of the synapse.

ACETYLCHOLINE IS THE NEUROTRANSMITTER OF THE NEUROMUSCULAR JUNCTION

The **neuromuscular junction,** or **motor endplate,** is formed between the terminal of an α-motoneuron and a skeletal muscle fiber (*Fig. 16.24*). Its neurotransmitter **acetylcholine** is formed by the cytoplasmic enzyme **choline acetyltransferase** in the nerve terminal:

where CoA-SH = uncombined coenzyme A. Acetylcholine is packaged in synaptic vesicles (40-nm diameter) in the nerve terminal. When an action potential (reversal of the membrane potential, caused by opening of

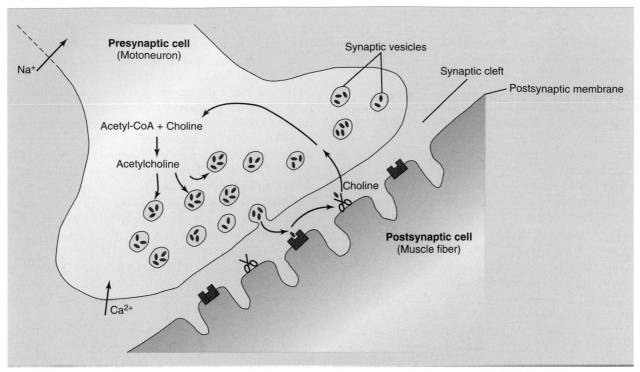

Figure 16.24 Neuromuscular junction: an example of a cholinergic synapse. ⬤, Acetylcholine; ◼, acetylcholine receptor; ✂, acetylcholinesterase; *CoA,* coenzyme A.

voltage gated sodium channels) arrives in the nerve terminal, a voltage-gated calcium channel opens to allow the influx of calcium. Calcium triggers exocytosis of acetylcholine by inducing the fusion of synaptic vesicles with the plasma membrane. *The release of neurotransmitters is always triggered by calcium.*

Within 1 ms, acetylcholine diffuses across the synaptic cleft, a distance of 50 nm. It binds to a receptor in the postsynaptic membrane, but *within a few milliseconds, acetylcholine is degraded by **acetylcholinesterase**, an enzyme in the basal lamina.* The catalytic mechanism of this enzyme resembles that of the serine proteases (see Chapter 4):

This reaction takes place in the synaptic cleft. The breakdown products, choline and acetate, are rapidly taken up into the nerve terminal, where they are used for resynthesis of acetylcholine.

THERE ARE MANY NEUROTRANSMITTERS

Catecholamines, 5-HT, and histamine are used as neurotransmitters by some neurons. Like acetylcholine, these neurotransmitters are stored in synaptic vesicles and are released by a depolarization-induced, calcium-dependent mechanism.

Their synaptic inactivation, however, is different. Unlike acetylcholine, the biogenic amines are not degraded in the synaptic cleft but are removed from their receptors by sodium-dependent, high-affinity uptake back into the nerve terminal. Once back in its home cell, the amine can be repackaged into synaptic vesicles. Alternatively, it is degraded by MAO, the major inactivating enzyme in nervous tissue (*Fig. 16.25*).

Only 1% to 2% of the neurons in the brain use a catecholamine or 5-HT as their neurotransmitter, and perhaps another 2% use acetylcholine. Amino acids are far more popular. **Glutamate** and **aspartate** are the major excitatory neurotransmitters in the central nervous system, and **glycine** is an important inhibitory neurotransmitter in the spinal cord and brainstem. These amino acids are recruited as neurotransmitters simply by being packaged into synaptic vesicles. *Their actions are terminated by sodium-dependent, high-affinity uptake without the need for synthesizing and inactivating enzymes.*

γ-Aminobutyric acid (GABA) is the most important inhibitory neurotransmitter in the brain. It is produced by the decarboxylation of glutamate and used as described in *Figure 16.26, B.*

Small peptides are yet another type of neurotransmitter. Their high-molecular-weight precursors are synthesized at the rough ER in the perikaryon, packaged into vesicles, and transported to the nerve endings. En route, the active transmitter is formed from its precursor protein by proteolytic cleavages. Peptide neurotransmitters are inactivated by enzymes on the surface of neurons and glial cells.

Neurotransmitter systems mediate the actions of many drugs and toxins. Some examples are listed in *Table 16.2.*

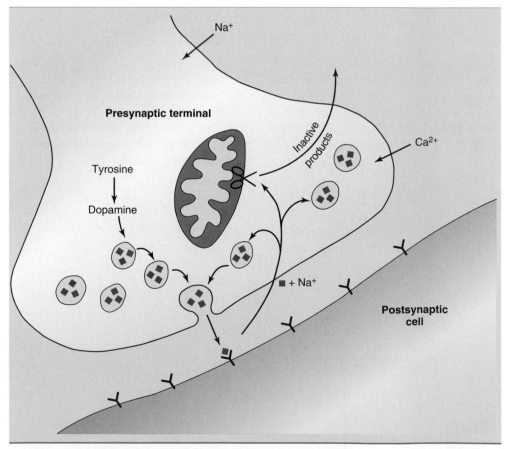

Figure 16.25 Dopaminergic synapse. The transmitter is taken up into the presynaptic nerve terminal by sodium-dependent, high-affinity uptake. Once in the nerve terminal, it is either recycled into the synaptic vesicles or degraded by monoamine oxidase (*MAO*). Y, Postsynaptic receptor; ■, dopamine; ✗, MAO.

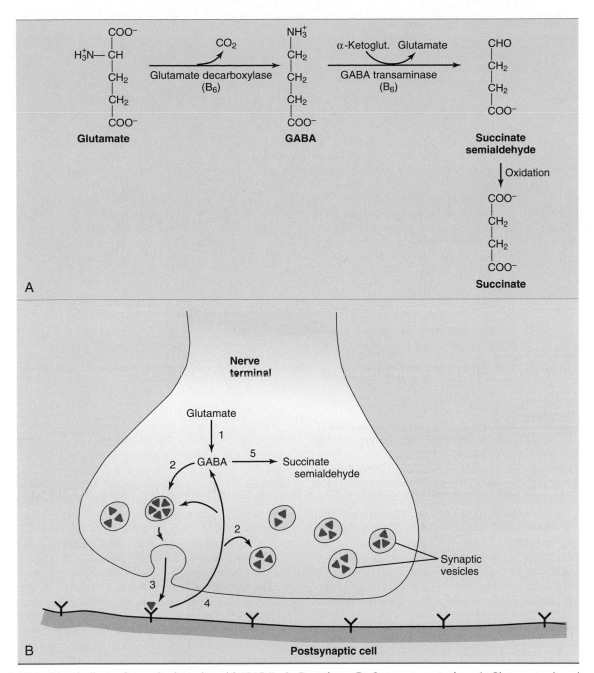

Figure 16.26 Metabolism of γ-aminobutyric acid (*GABA*). **A,** Reactions. **B,** Compartmentation. *1,* Glutamate decarboxylase; *2,* vesicular storage; *3,* release by exocytosis; *4,* sodium-dependent, high-affinity uptake; *5,* GABA transaminase; ▼, γ-aminobutyric acid; Y, postsynaptic receptors.

SUMMARY

Hormones and related extracellular messengers belong to a limited number of structural and biosynthetic classes. **Steroid hormones** are synthesized from cholesterol, and **thyroid hormones** are derived from protein-bound tyrosine. The **biogenic amines,** including catecholamines, serotonin, and histamine, are produced by the decarboxylation of aromatic amino acids. **Protein hormones** are processed through the secretory pathway: ER, Golgi apparatus, and secretory vesicles. Smaller peptide hormones and neurotransmitters are derived from large precursors called "prohormones" by proteolytic cleavages in the organelles of the secretory pathway.

The **eicosanoids** are 20-carbon lipids that are synthesized from polyunsaturated fatty acids. Most are short lived and act only locally in their tissue of origin. They are important mediators of inflammation, and agents that inhibit their synthesis are important antiinflammatory drugs.

Neurotransmitters transmit signals at synapses. Acetylcholine, the biogenic amines, some amino acids, and a variety of peptides are used as neurotransmitters.

Table 16.2 Neurotransmitters as Targets of Drugs and Toxins

Agent	Mechanism of Action	Effects
Drugs		
L-DOPA	Catecholamine precursor	Antiparkinsonian
MAO inhibitors	Inhibit degradation of catecholamines and 5-HT	Antidepressant
Reserpine	Inhibits vesicular storage of catecholamines and 5-HT	Antihypertensive, sedative, depressant
Tricyclics	Inhibit synaptic uptake of norepinephrine and/or 5-HT	Antidepressant
Cocaine	Inhibits synaptic uptake of dopamine, norepinephrine, and 5-HT	Psychostimulant
Amphetamine	Releases nonvesicular (cytoplasmic) dopamine, norepinephrine, and 5-HT	Psychostimulant
Opiates	Agonist action on opiate (endorphin) receptors	Narcotic analgesic
Neuroleptics	Antagonist action on D_2 dopamine receptors	Antipsychotic
Benzodiazepines	Sensitization of GABA-A receptors	Sedative, anxiolytic, anticonvulsant
Bacterial toxins		
Tetanus toxin	Inhibits glycine release in spinal cord	Lockjaw, convulsions
Botulinum toxin	Inhibits acetylcholine release at motor endplate	Flaccid paralysis
Chemical toxins		
Organophosphates	Irreversible inhibition of acetylcholinesterase	Autonomic nervous effects, CNS effects
Curare	Blocks acetylcholine receptors in neuromuscular junction	Flaccid paralysis
Strychnine	Blocks glycine receptors in spinal cord	Convulsions

CNS, Central nervous system; *GABA*, γ-aminobutyric acid; *5-HT*, 5-hydroxytryptamine; *L-DOPA*, L-dihydroxyphenylalanine; *MAO*, monoamine oxidase.

Further Reading

Funk CD: Prostaglandins and leukotrienes: advances in eicosanoid biology, *Science* 294:1871–1875, 2001.

Gross K, Cidlowski JA: Tissue-specific glucocorticoid action: a family affair, *Trends Endocrinol Metab* 19:331–339, 2008.

Grosser T, Yu Y, Fitzgerald GA: Emotion recollected in tranquility: lessons learned from the COX-2 saga, *Annu Rev Med* 61:17–33, 2010.

Hook V, Funkelstein L, Toneff T, et al: Human pituitary contains dual cathepsin L and prohormone convertase processing pathway components involved in converting POMC into the peptide hormones ACTH, α-MSH, and β-endorphin, *Endocrine* 35:429–437, 2009.

Kronenberg HM, Melmed S, Polonsky KS, et al: *Williams textbook of endocrinology*, Philadelphia, WB Saunders, 2007.

Leslie CC: Regulation of arachidonic acid availability for eicosanoid production, *Biochem Cell Biol* 82:1–17, 2004.

Murphy RC, Gijón MA: Biosynthesis and metabolism of leukotrienes, *Biochem J* 405:379–395, 2007.

Rådmark O, Werz O, Steinhilber D, et al: 5-Lipoxygenase: regulation of expression and enzyme activity, *Trends Biochem Sci* 32:332–341, 2007.

Rahman F, Christian HC: Non-classical actions of testosterone: an update, *Trends Endocrinol Metab* 18:371–378, 2008.

Rose SR, Brown RS, Foley T, et al: Update of newborn screening and therapy for congenital hypothyroidism, *Pediatrics* 117:2290–2303, 2006.

Rossi G-P, Sechi LA, Giacchetti G, et al: Primary aldosteronism: cardiovascular, renal and metabolic implications, *Trends Endocrinol Metab* 19:88–90, 2008.

Rouzer CA, Marnett LJ: Cyclooxygenases: structural and functional insights, *J Lipid Res* 50:S29–S34, 2009.

Safe S, Kim K: Non-classical genomic estrogen receptor (ER)/specificity protein and ER/activating protein-1 signaling pathways, *J Mol Endocrinol* 41:263–275, 2008.

Shi L, Mao C, Xu Z, et al: Angiotensin-converting enzymes and drug discovery in cardiovascular diseases, *Drug Discov Today* 15:332–341, 2010.

Smith WL: Nutritionally essential fatty acids and biologically indispensable cyclooxygenases, *Trends Biochem Sci* 33:27–37, 2008.

Visser WE, Friesema ECH, Jansen J, et al: Thyroid hormone transport in and out of cells, *Trends Endocrinol Metab* 19:50–56, 2008.

QUESTIONS

1. **Pheochromocytoma is a tumor of catecholamine-secreting cells that causes dangerous hypertension in patients. In order to prevent these hypertensive episodes, you can try an inhibitor of**

   A. MAO
   B. Tryptophan hydroxylase
   C. COMT
   D. The sodium-dependent norepinephrine carrier in sympathetic nerve terminals
   E. Tyrosine hydroxylase

2. **The pancreatic β-cells secrete not only insulin but also an equimolar amount of**

   A. Glucagon
   B. C-peptide
   C. Renin
   D. Proopiomelanocortin
   E. Enkephalin

3. **The adrenal cortex contains a sizable collection of enzymes for steroid hormone synthesis. Two of these enzymes are required for the synthesis of glucocorticoids but not androgens; therefore, their deficiency leads to an overproduction of adrenal androgens. These two enzymes are**

   A. Cyclooxygenase and 17-hydroxylase
   B. Desmolase and cytochrome P-450
   C. 11β-Hydroxylase and 21-hydroxylase
   D. 17-Hydroxylase and adrenodoxin
   E. 18-Hydroxylase and aromatase

4. **Inhibitors of lipoxygenase can be used for the treatment of asthma because they prevent the formation of**

   A. Prostaglandins
   B. GABA
   C. Thromboxanes
   D. Prostacyclin
   E. Leukotrienes

Chapter 17
INTRACELLULAR MESSENGERS

A key is useless without a matching lock, and a hormone or other extracellular signaling molecule is useless without a matching receptor in its target cell. The receptor is an allosteric protein that changes its conformation when it binds the signaling molecule. Messengers that do not enter the cell activate receptors in the plasma membrane, and many of those that can enter activate receptors in the cytoplasm or nucleus (*Fig. 17.1*).

Receptor binding triggers intracellular signaling cascades with protein-protein interactions and enzymatic reactions. *The phosphorylation of cellular proteins by protein kinases is a recurrent feature of hormonally induced signaling cascades.* These cascades regulate metabolic enzymes, membrane transporters, ion channels, and genes. This chapter describes the most important receptor mechanisms and signaling cascades.

RECEPTOR-HORMONE INTERACTIONS ARE NONCOVALENT, REVERSIBLE, AND SATURABLE

Like the binding of a substrate to its enzyme (see Chapter 4) or an antigen to its antibody (see Chapter 15), *hormone-receptor binding is always noncovalent.* Being noncovalent, it is reversible. The receptor-hormone complex (R·H) can easily dissociate back into free receptor (R) and free hormone (H):

$$R \cdot H \underset{k_{-1}}{\overset{k_1}{\rightleftharpoons}} R + H$$

The **dissociation constant** K_D of the receptor-hormone complex is defined as

$$K_D = \frac{[R] \times [H]}{[R \cdot H]} = \frac{k_1}{k_{-1}}$$

$$\frac{K_D}{[H]} = \frac{[R]}{[R \cdot H]}$$

K_D corresponds to the hormone concentration [H] at which half the receptor molecules are converted to the receptor-hormone complex. It describes the affinity between hormone and receptor.

Hormone binding shows *saturation kinetics* (*Fig. 17.2*). At a hormone concentration far above K_D, almost all receptors are occupied. The physiological response is near maximal and cannot be augmented by adding even more hormone. This is equivalent to zero-order kinetics for enzymes. **Maximal binding** (B_{max}) corresponds to the number of receptor molecules in the cell.

MANY NEUROTRANSMITTER RECEPTORS ARE ION CHANNELS

The job of a neurotransmitter is to change the membrane potential of the postsynaptic cell and to do it quickly. Rather than triggering lengthy signaling cascades, the transmitter should act as directly as possible on the ion channels that determine the membrane potential. *The fastest and most direct mechanism is binding of the neurotransmitter to a ligand-gated ion channel in the plasma membrane.*

The **nicotinic acetylcholine receptor** in the neuromuscular junction is a classic example. This receptor is a channel for the monovalent cations sodium and potassium, with five subunits that each contribute to the channel (*Fig. 17.3*). *The channel is closed in the resting state, opening only when acetylcholine binds.* Opening of the channel causes a rapid influx of sodium down its electrochemical gradient, which depolarizes the membrane.

There is a whole family of ligand-gated ion channels. They all consist of five subunits but differ in their ligand-binding specificities and ionic selectivities. *Most excitatory neurotransmitters open sodium channels, and inhibitory neurotransmitters open chloride or potassium channels.*

The ligand-gated ion channels come in many different variants. For example, the subunits of the nicotinic acetylcholine receptors in the brain are slightly different from those of the receptor in the neuromuscular junction. **Nicotine** stimulates nicotinic receptors in the brain but not in the neuromuscular junction, and the arrow poison **curare** blocks nicotinic receptors in the neuromuscular junction but not in the brain. A drug that activates a receptor is called an **agonist**, and a drug that blocks a receptor is called an **antagonist**. *Like enzymes, receptors are subject to competitive, noncompetitive, and irreversible inhibition by drugs and toxins.*

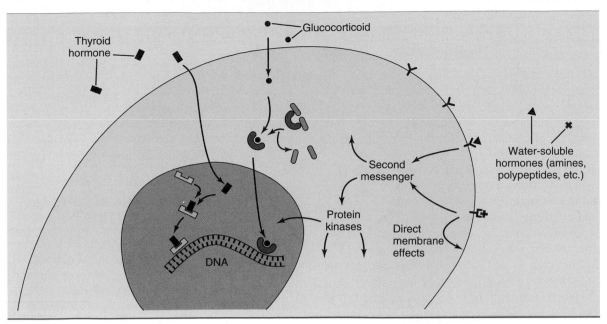

Figure 17.1   Cellular locations of receptors for hormones and other extracellular messengers. ⊏⊐, Thyroid hormone receptor; ☟, glucocorticoid receptor; ☝ and Ⴤ, cell surface receptors.

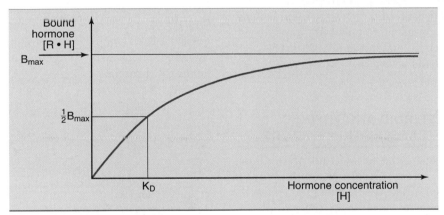

Figure 17.2   Receptor (*R*) binding at various hormone (*H*) concentrations. Maximal binding B_{max} corresponds to the total number of receptors.

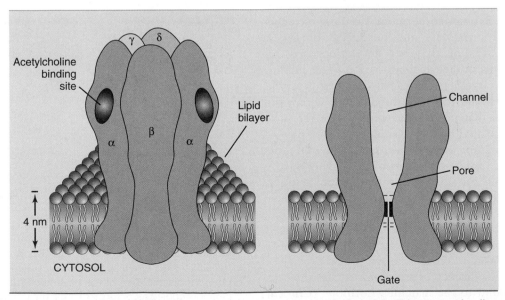

Figure 17.3   Structure of the nicotinic acetylcholine receptor in the neuromuscular junction. This receptor is a ligand-gated channel for small cations (Na^+, K^+). Acetylcholine binds with positive cooperativity to the two α subunits. Each of the five polypeptides traverses the membrane four times, and one of the transmembrane helices in each subunit contributes to the "gate" in the channel.

CLINICAL EXAMPLE 17.1: Androgen Insensitivity Syndrome

The fetal testis produces two important products: androgens (testosterone, dihydrotestosterone), which are required for the development of the male external genitalia, and the protein hormone **müllerian inhibitory factor,** which prevents the formation of the uterus and fallopian tubes.

Inherited defects in the androgen receptor cause androgen insensitivity syndrome, also known as **testicular feminization.** Genetically male individuals with this condition are externally female, and their psychosexual development is feminine. However, they possess undescended testes rather than ovaries, and uterus and fallopian tubes are absent. Although they have male levels of testosterone both during fetal development and in later life, they develop as phenotypic females because the target tissues cannot respond to the male hormones.

This rare condition is inherited as an X-linked recessive trait. Because affected males are infertile and the mutation can be transmitted only by females, the mutations do not persist long in the population. Therefore many patients have a new mutation.

CLINICAL EXAMPLE 17.2: Leprechaunism

Insulin is essential for regulation of the major metabolic pathways, and it participates in normal growth and development. Rarely, a child is born with defective insulin receptors. These infants are born with severe insulin-resistant diabetes, growth retardation, large malformed ears and other physical deformities, and absence of subcutaneous fat. Most die during the first years of life.

SEVEN-TRANSMEMBRANE RECEPTORS ARE COUPLED TO G PROTEINS

Being unable to enter their target cells, water-soluble hormones deliver their message at the cell surface. Their receptors are integral membrane proteins with three functional domains. The *extracellular domain* binds the hormone; one or several *transmembrane α-helices* penetrate the lipid bilayer; and the *intracellular domain* is coupled with an effector mechanism.

Most hormone receptors belong to a family of membrane proteins that crisscross the membrane seven times (*Fig. 17.4*). These receptors do not form a channel and possess no enzymatic activities, but they trigger their signaling cascades by activating a guanine nucleotide-binding **G protein.**

RECEPTORS FOR STEROID AND THYROID HORMONES ARE TRANSCRIPTION FACTORS

Unlike neurotransmitters, the steroid and thyroid hormones can diffuse across membranes and activate receptors in the cytoplasm or the nucleus. For example, the glucocorticoid receptor resides in the cytoplasm, complexed to cytoplasmic proteins that are released when the hormone binds.

The hormone-receptor complex translocates to the nucleus, where it binds to **hormone response elements (HREs)** in the promoters and enhancers of genes. Approximately 1% of all genes have glucocorticoid response elements in their regulatory sites. This implies two levels of targeting: Only cells that possess the receptor can respond to the hormone, and, within the cell, only genes that possess the appropriate response element are regulated by the hormone.

The receptors for steroid hormones, thyroid hormones, retinoic acid, and calcitriol all belong to the same superfamily of hormone-regulated transcription factors. All are zinc finger proteins that bind their response elements in a dimeric form, although the details are variable. For example, unstimulated thyroid hormone receptors are located in the nucleus rather than the cytoplasm.

An inherited deficiency of a receptor makes the cells unable to respond to the matching hormone (*Clinical Examples 17.1* and *17.2*).

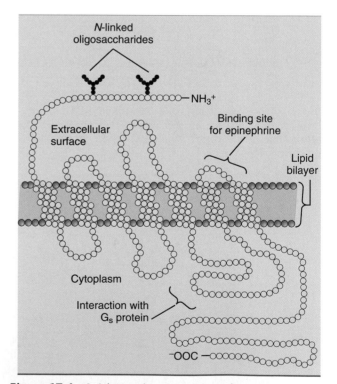

Figure 17.4 β-Adrenergic receptor is an integral membrane protein with seven membrane-spanning α helices. Note that the binding site for β-adrenergic agonists is on the extracellular side, whereas the binding site for the G$_s$ protein is on the cytoplasmic side of the plasma membrane. All G protein–coupled receptors resemble the β-adrenergic receptor in their amino acid sequence and membrane topography.

The G protein is attached to the cytoplasmic surface of the plasma membrane. Its three subunits are designated α (molecular weight [MW] 45,000), β (MW 35,000), and γ (MW 7000). The α subunit has a nucleotide binding site that can accommodate either guanosine diphosphate (GDP) or guanosine triphosphate (GTP). β and γ subunits function as a single unit, but the α subunit is only loosely associated with βγ.

The function of the G protein is described in *Figure 17.5*. The inactive G protein is associated with the unstimulated receptor, with GDP bound to the α subunit. Hormone binding changes the conformation of the receptor and the attached G protein. As a result, the α subunit of the G protein loses its affinity for GDP, which dissociates away and is replaced by GTP.

Once GTP is bound, the G protein leaves the receptor and breaks up into the α-GTP subunit and the βγ complex. Both α-GTP and βγ diffuse along the inner surface of the plasma membrane, where they bind to target proteins known as **effectors**. *The components of the activated G protein are membrane-bound messengers that transmit a signal from the receptor to the effector.* In some cases, α-GTP and βγ can activate their effectors without fully separating from each other.

The α subunit possesses a GTPase activity that is stimulated by its interaction with the effector. As a result, *the α subunit quickly hydrolyzes its bound GTP to GDP and inorganic phosphate.* GDP remains bound to the α subunit, but the α-GDP complex no longer acts on the effector. Rather than transmitting a signal, it returns to the βγ complex. *All G proteins exist in two forms: an active GTP-bound form that acts on the effector, and an inactive GDP-bound form that does not.*

Several molecular forms of α, β, and γ subunits are expressed in different cells. G proteins are classified according to the structure and function of their α subunit. For example, the α-GTP complex of the G_s proteins stimulates adenylate cyclase, and the α-GTP complex of the G_i proteins inhibits adenylate cyclase.

The βγ complex transmits signals as well. The myocardium, for example, responds to acetylcholine from the vagus nerve through a receptor that couples to a G_i protein. The βγ complex of this G_i protein opens a potassium channel in the membrane, thereby hyperpolarizing the membrane and slowing down the heart.

ADENYLATE CYCLASE IS REGULATED BY G PROTEINS

Hormone-activated G proteins carry messages along the plasma membrane but do not travel across the cytoplasm. To send a signal into the interior of the cell, the G protein induces the synthesis of a small, diffusible molecule known as a **second messenger.**

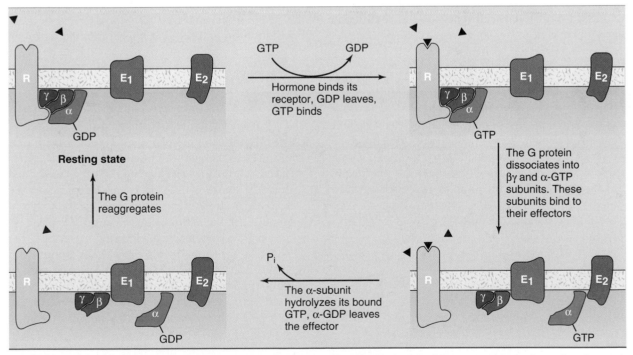

Figure 17.5 Coupling of a hormone receptor (R) to effector proteins (E_1, E_2) in the plasma membrane through a G protein. By an allosteric mechanism, the activation of the receptor causes GDP–GTP exchange and dissociation of the heterotrimeric G protein into βγ and α-GTP subunits. These subunits act allosterically on the effectors. The action on the effector is terminated when the α subunit hydrolyzes its bound GTP. The most important effectors of hormone-regulated G proteins are second messenger–synthesizing enzymes such as adenylate cyclase and phospholipase C, but some calcium and potassium channels also are regulated by this mechanism.

The second messenger **cyclic adenosine monophosphate (cAMP)** is synthesized by **adenylate cyclase** in the plasma membrane:

The rapid hydrolysis of pyrophosphate (PP$_i$) by cellular pyrophosphatases makes this reaction irreversible. Adenylate cyclases are integral membrane proteins that are stimulated by the α_s subunit of the stimulatory G proteins (G$_s$ proteins). Humans have nine isoenzymes of adenylate cyclase that are encoded by different genes, are expressed in different cell types, and have different regulatory properties.

cAMP is degraded by **phosphodiesterases:**

There are 11 families of phosphodiesterases for the inactivation of cAMP and the related second messenger cyclic guanosine monophosphate (cGMP), with at least 100 different molecular forms. Most are inhibited by **methylxanthines,** including caffeine, theophylline, and aminophylline. These drugs potentiate the effects of cAMP. After drinking a cup of coffee, for example, the level of plasma free fatty acids rises because fat breakdown in adipose tissue is stimulated by cAMP.

CLINICAL EXAMPLE 17.3: Cholera

Cholera is a severe form of diarrhea that kills its victims through rapid dehydration. The offending bacterium, *Vibrio cholerae*, remains confined to the intestinal lumen but produces a secreted protein toxin. One of the toxin's subunits enters the intestinal mucosal cells. Using the ubiquitous coenzyme NAD as a substrate, it acts as an enzyme that covalently modifies the α subunit of the G$_s$ protein:

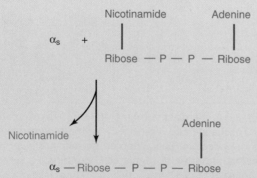

The modified α subunit can still activate adenylate cyclase, but it can no longer hydrolyze its bound GTP. The G protein cannot switch itself off, and adenylate cyclase is stimulated permanently. The cell is flooded with cAMP, which causes the excessive secretion of water and electrolytes.

Some strains of *Escherichia coli* cause the common traveler's diarrhea by raising the cAMP level with a similar toxin, although other strains do the same by raising cGMP. The best symptomatic treatment of traveler's diarrhea is opium taken by mouth. Opiate receptors couple to the G$_i$ protein (***Table 17.1***), thereby antagonizing the out-of-control G$_s$ protein.

Table 17.1   Roles of Cyclic Adenosine Monophosphate (cAMP) in Different Tissues

Tissue/Cell Type	Agents Increasing cAMP	Agents Decreasing cAMP	Effects of Elevated cAMP
Liver	Glucagon, epinephrine	Insulin*	Glycogen degradation, gluconeogenesis
Skeletal muscle	Epinephrine	—	Glycogen degradation, glycolysis
Adipose tissue	Epinephrine	Insulin*	Lipolysis
Renal tubular epithelium	Antidiuretic hormone	—	Water reabsorption
Intestinal mucosa	Vasoactive intestinal polypeptide, adenosine, epinephrine	Endorphins (peptides that activate opiate receptors)	Water and electrolyte secretion
Vascular smooth muscle	Epinephrine (β receptor)	Epinephrine (α_2 receptor)	Relaxation, growth inhibition
Bronchial smooth muscle	Epinephrine (β receptor)	—	Relaxation
Platelets	Prostacyclin, prostaglandin E	ADP	Maintenance of inactive state
Adrenal cortex	ACTH	—	Hormone secretion
Melanocytes	MSH	Melatonin	Melanin synthesis
Thyroid gland	TSH	—	Hormone secretion

*Insulin does not act through a G protein; it decreases cAMP levels by alternative routes.
ACTH, Adrenocorticotropic hormone; *MSH,* melanocyte-stimulating hormone; *TSH,* thyroid-stimulating hormone.

HORMONES CAN BOTH ACTIVATE AND INHIBIT THE cAMP CASCADE

*The most important target of cAMP is **protein kinase A**.* In the absence of cAMP, two catalytic subunits of this enzyme form an inactive complex with two regulatory subunits. When the cAMP level rises, the two regulatory subunits bind up to four cAMP molecules, and the active catalytic subunits are released:

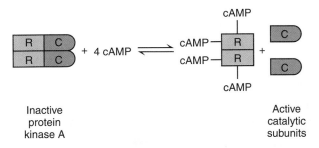

Inactive protein kinase A   Active catalytic subunits

The catalytic subunits phosphorylate proteins on serine and threonine side chains. The enzyme phosphorylates only a small proportion of the cellular proteins, including several metabolic enzymes and nuclear transcription factors. In addition, many of the actions of protein kinase A are localized to specific intracellular sites because a portion of the enzyme is already bound to A-kinase anchoring proteins (AKAPs), which place the enzyme near its substrate proteins.

The cAMP cascade amplifies the hormonal signal (***Fig. 17.6***). For example, the binding of a single epinephrine molecule to a β-adrenergic receptor activates up to 20 G_s proteins. Each α_s-GTP subunit activates adenylate cyclase long enough to cause the synthesis of hundreds of cAMP molecules. Although only four cAMP molecules are needed to activate two catalytic subunits of protein kinase A, each active subunit phosphorylates hundreds or thousands of proteins before it returns to the regulatory subunits.

Some hormones do not stimulate but rather inhibit adenylate cyclase (see ***Table 17.1***). In most cases inhibition is mediated by the α_i subunit of an **inhibitory G protein (G_i)**. Most cells possess both G_s-linked and G_i-linked hormone receptors, and *the activity of adenylate cyclase depends on the balance between stimulatory and inhibitory hormones* (***Fig. 17.7***).

Many hormones and neurotransmitters can act through different receptors and second messengers. For example, epinephrine (adrenaline) can raise the cAMP level by activating **β-adrenergic receptors**, or it can reduce cAMP by activating **α_2-adrenergic receptors**. A third receptor type, the **α_1-adrenergic receptor**, raises the calcium level by activating the IP_3 second messenger system (see section "Phospholipase C generates two second messengers"). Therefore *the effect of epinephrine depends on the type of receptor that is present on the cell.* Acetylcholine acts not only on nicotinic receptors, which are ligand-gated ion channels, but also on several subtypes of **muscarinic receptors**, which are linked to G proteins and either lower the cAMP level or raise the levels of IP_3 and calcium.

CLINICAL EXAMPLE 17.4: Whooping Cough

Whooping cough is an acute inflammation of the upper respiratory tract caused by *Bordetella pertussis,* a denizen of the respiratory epithelium. Pathogenic strains of this bacterium produce a secreted protein toxin that is similar to cholera toxin but which modifies the α_i subunit rather than the α_s subunit. In this case, the covalently modified α_i subunit is unable to inhibit adenylate cyclase. *By inhibiting the inhibition of adenylate cyclase, pertussis toxin leads to excessive cAMP formation.*

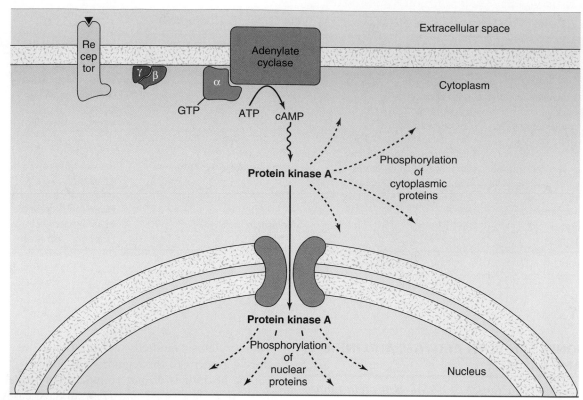

Figure 17.6 Cyclic AMP (cAMP) cascade. Receptor and adenylate cyclase are coupled by the stimulatory G protein (G$_s$), which consists of the α_s, β, and γ subunits. Almost all known cAMP effects in humans are mediated by protein kinase A. This protein kinase phosphorylates a variety of proteins in the cytoplasm and the nucleus. *ATP*, Adenosine triphosphate; *GTP*, guanosine triphosphate.

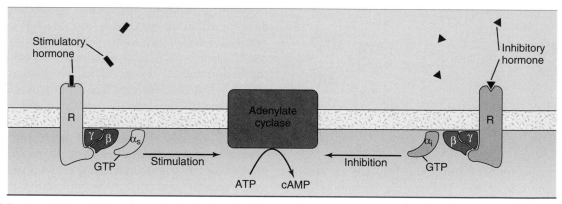

Figure 17.7 Regulation of adenylate cyclase by the α subunits of the stimulatory and inhibitory G proteins. Some isoforms of adenylate cyclase are affected by $\beta\gamma$ complexes of the G proteins as well. *cAMP*, Cyclic adenosine monophosphate; *R*, receptor.

CLINICAL EXAMPLE 17.5: Toxic Thyroid Nodules

Most cases of hyperthyroidism ("thyrotoxicosis") are caused by Graves disease (see Chapter 16). Benign thyroid adenomas that overproduce the hormones ("toxic nodules") are a less common cause of thyrotoxicosis. These tumors are derived from a single cell that proliferates abnormally as a consequence of somatic mutations.

Many thyroid adenomas have a mutant thyroid-stimulating hormone (TSH) receptor that is in the active conformation at all times, even in the absence of TSH. Other adenomas have a normal TSH receptor, but a point mutation makes the α subunit of the G$_s$ protein unable to hydrolyze its bound GTP. In both cases the cell's cAMP system, which ordinarily is controlled by TSH, is in overdrive even in the absence of TSH. This results in overproduction of the hormones and abnormal cell proliferation with tumor formation.

CLINICAL EXAMPLE 17.6: Pseudohypoparathyroidism

The function of parathyroid hormone (PTH) is the minute-to-minute maintenance of a sufficient plasma calcium level. PTH deficiency, or **hypoparathyroidism,** causes hypocalcemia, with involuntary muscle twitching (tetany) and other abnormalities. Patients with **pseudohypoparathyroidism** have signs of PTH deficiency even though their PTH level is elevated. Their problem is PTH resistance.

The usual cause of pseudohypoparathyroidism is an abnormal G$_s$ protein that couples poorly between the PTH receptor and adenylate cyclase. Many patients with this disorder have mild skeletal deformities, a condition known as **Albright hereditary osteodystrophy.** This condition is caused by a heterozygous gene defect inherited from the mother. The gene is paternally imprinted by DNA methylation (see Chapter 7); therefore, most of the encoded protein is produced from the maternally inherited gene.

These patients also have short stature and developmental delay. These abnormalities are not caused by PTH resistance but by poor responsiveness to other hormones that stimulate adenylate cyclase, such as TSH and the gonadotropins.

CYTOPLASMIC CALCIUM IS AN IMPORTANT INTRACELLULAR SIGNAL

The calcium concentration is 1.25 mmol/L in the extracellular fluid but only 0.2 μmol/L in the cytoplasm. The most elementary reason for maintaining this enormous concentration gradient is that phosphate is the principal inorganic anion in the cytoplasm. Phosphate forms insoluble salts with calcium, and if the calcium concentration were as high in the cytoplasm as in the extracellular fluid, the cell would soon be filled with obnoxious calcium phosphate crystals.

Therefore the cell goes out of its way to keep the cytoplasmic calcium concentration low. Calcium is pumped out of the cell by both an ATP-dependent calcium pump and a sodium/calcium antiporter in the plasma membrane. In addition, it is pumped from the cytoplasm into the endoplasmic reticulum (ER) by the ATP-dependent calcium pump. Therefore the calcium concentration is about as high in the ER as in the extracellular fluid.

External signals can trigger a transient rise of the cytoplasmic calcium concentration in several ways.

1. *An extracellular messenger opens a ligand-gated calcium channel in the plasma membrane.* The only important example is the N-methyl-D-aspartate (NMDA) type of glutamate receptor in the brain.
2. *A stimulus depolarizes the plasma membrane, thereby opening voltage-gated calcium channels.* One example is the release of neurotransmitters from nerve terminals in response to opening of a voltage-gated calcium channel (see Chapter 16). In smooth muscle cells, voltage-gated calcium channels open when the membrane becomes depolarized by the action of an excitatory neurotransmitter. These channels are the targets of **calcium channel blockers.** These drugs are used for treatment of hypertension, vasospastic disorders, angina pectoris, and cardiac arrhythmias.
3. *A hormone-stimulated protein kinase phosphorylates a calcium channel in the plasma membrane.* For example, epinephrine and norepinephrine activate the cAMP cascade in the myocardium by an action on β-adrenergic receptors. The cAMP-activated protein kinase A phosphorylates a voltage-gated calcium channel in the plasma membrane, thereby raising calcium influx during contraction.
4. *A hormone induces release of calcium from the ER.* This mechanism is discussed in the following.

PHOSPHOLIPASE C GENERATES TWO SECOND MESSENGERS

Most calcium-elevating hormones trigger the release of calcium from the ER. The hormone activates a seven-transmembrane receptor that is coupled to a G protein of the G$_q$ family. G$_q$ proteins do not act on adenylate cyclase. Rather they activate a **phospholipase C,** a type of enzyme that cleaves the bond between glycerol and phosphate in position 3 of phosphoglycerides.

The hormone-stimulated phospholipase C cleaves phosphatidylinositol and related lipids in the inner leaflet of the plasma membrane. Phosphatidylinositol 4,5-bisphosphate (PIP$_2$) is the most important substrate because its cleavage forms the second messengers **1,2-diacylglycerol** and **inositol 1,4,5-trisphosphate (IP$_3$)** (*Fig. 17.8*).

1,2-Diacylglycerol remains membrane bound but diffuses laterally in the inner leaflet of the lipid bilayer. In the presence of calcium and phosphatidylserine, it activates several proteins, including the membrane-associated enzyme **protein kinase C** (*Fig. 17.9*). Like protein kinase A, protein kinase C phosphorylates serine and threonine side chains in proteins. Although some proteins can be phosphorylated by both, the substrate specificities of the two kinases are quite different.

Protein kinase C promotes the proliferation of many cells. **Phorbol esters,** which are naturally present in croton oil, act as tumor promoters by activating protein kinase C.

Being small and water soluble, IP$_3$ can diffuse across the cytoplasm. *It raises cytoplasmic calcium by opening a calcium channel in the ER membrane.* IP$_3$ is inactivated by successive dephosphorylations, either directly or after an initial phosphorylation to inositol 1,3,4,5-tetrakisphosphate.

Calcium induces its effects by binding to specific regulatory proteins. **Troponin C** has already been described as a calcium sensor on the thin filaments of striated muscle (see Chapter 13). The structurally related **calmodulin**

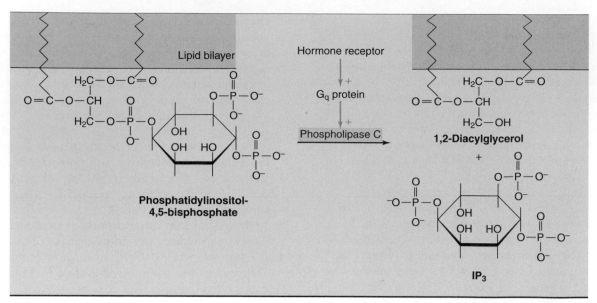

Figure 17.8 Formation of the second messengers 1,2-diacylglycerol and inositol 1,4,5-trisphosphate (*IP₃*) from phosphatidylinositol-4,5-bisphosphate. *Green arrows* represent allosteric stimulation.

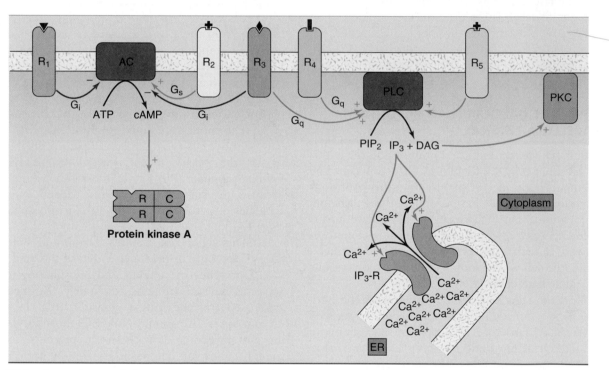

Figure 17.9 G protein–coupled receptors (R_1, R_2, and so forth) and their second messenger systems. Note that more than one hormone receptor can couple to an effector in the plasma membrane (⬤). The effector produces the second messenger, and the second messenger stimulates intracellular targets (▢). Note also that some receptors can couple to more than one G protein (G_i and G_q in the case of R_3) and thereby act on different effectors. *AC*, Adenylate cyclase; *cAMP*, cyclic adenosine monophosphate; *DAG*, 1,2-diacylglycerol; *IP₃*, inositol 1,4,5-trisphosphate; *IP₃-R*, IP₃ receptor (an IP₃-regulated calcium channel in the endoplasmic reticulum [*ER*]); *PIP₂*, phosphatidylinositol-4,5-bisphosphate; *PKC*, protein kinase C; *PLC*, phosphatidylinositol-specific phospholipase C.

(MW, 17000) is present in all nucleated cells. At a Ca^{2+} concentration range from 10^{-7} mol to 10^{-6} mol, *calmodulin forms a calcium complex that activates many enzymes.* The Ca^{2+}-calmodulin–regulated enzymes include a family of protein kinases that phosphorylate serine and threonine side chains but with substrate specificities different from those of protein kinases A and C.

BOTH cAMP AND CALCIUM REGULATE GENE TRANSCRIPTION

The catalytic subunits of the cAMP-dependent protein kinase A can translocate to the nucleus, where they phosphorylate transcription factors including the **cAMP response element-binding (CREB) protein.** The dimeric

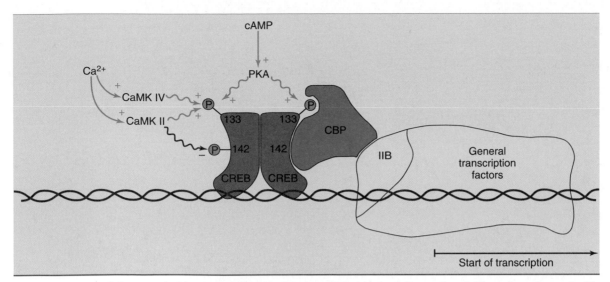

Figure 17.10 Actions of the protein kinase A catalytic subunit (*PKA*) and of calcium-calmodulin–activated protein kinases (*CaMK II, CaMK IV*) on the cyclic AMP (*cAMP*) response element-binding (*CREB*) protein, which mediates cAMP effects on transcription. The phosphorylation of Ser[133] is thought to induce transcription through a CREB-binding protein (*CBP*) that binds both to phosphorylated CREB and to transcription factor IIB in the transcriptional initiation complex. Phosphorylation of Ser[142] is thought to prevent this interaction. *Straight arrow* indicates allosteric stimulation; *green wavy arrow* indicates activating phosphorylation; *red wavy arrow* indicates inhibitory phosphorylation.

forms of these transcription factors bind to the **cAMP response element**, a palindromic sequence (TGACGTCA) in the promoters and enhancers of cAMP-regulated genes. *The CREB protein stimulates transcription only after the phosphorylation of a single serine residue (Ser[133]) by protein kinase A* (**Fig. 17.10**).

The calcium-dependent calmodulin kinase II (CaMK II) phosphorylates a different serine residue (Ser[142]) in CREB, but this phosphorylation prevents transcriptional activation. Both CaMK II and CaMK IV, another Ca[2+]-calmodulin–dependent protein kinase, can also phosphorylate Ser[133] and thereby activate transcription. As a result, *calcium can act either synergistically or antagonistically with cAMP in the regulation of gene expression*, depending on the Ca[2+]-calmodulin–regulated protein kinases that are present in the cell.

MUSCLE CONTRACTION AND EXOCYTOSIS ARE TRIGGERED BY CALCIUM

Muscle contraction is always calcium dependent. The calcium-sensing protein is troponin C in striated muscle and calmodulin in smooth muscle (*Fig. 17.11*). The Ca[2+]-calmodulin complex activates the enzyme **myosin light chain kinase**, which causes contraction by phosphorylating a pair of light chains on the globular head of myosin.

cAMP decreases the calcium concentration in most types of smooth muscle, either by reducing IP₃-stimulated calcium release from the ER or by activating a potassium channel that hyperpolarizes the plasma membrane and thereby prevents membrane depolarization and opening of voltage-gated calcium channels. Therefore *most types of smooth muscle are contracted by agents that raise cytoplasmic calcium and are* *relaxed by agents that raise cytoplasmic cAMP* (*Tables 17.1* and *17.2*).

In addition, *the release of water-soluble products by exocytosis is always triggered by calcium.* Examples include the release of neurotransmitters from nerve terminals, zymogens from the pancreas, insulin from pancreatic β-cells, and histamine from mast cells (see *Table 17.2*).

CLINICAL EXAMPLE 17.7: Treatment of Asthma

Asthma is characterized by recurrent attacks of bronchospasm leading to obstruction of the bronchial tree. Bronchial smooth muscle is contracted by calcium-elevating agents, including histamine (through H₁ receptors) and acetylcholine (through muscarinic receptors). It is relaxed by epinephrine, which raises cAMP levels through β-adrenergic receptors. Therefore asthma can be treated with epinephrine, synthetic β-adrenergic agonists (e.g., salbutamol), and the phosphodiesterase inhibitors theophylline and aminophylline.

RECEPTOR FOR ATRIAL NATRIURETIC FACTOR IS A MEMBRANE-BOUND GUANYLATE CYCLASE

Synthesis and degradation of the second messenger **cyclic guanosine monophosphate (cGMP)** are analogous to the corresponding steps in cAMP metabolism:

$$GTP \xrightarrow[\text{Guanylate cyclase}]{PP_i} cGMP \xrightarrow[\text{Phosphodiesterase}]{H_2O} GMP$$

Unlike the adenylate cyclases, guanylate cyclases are not activated by hormone-coupled G proteins. The two families of guanylate cyclases are membrane-bound

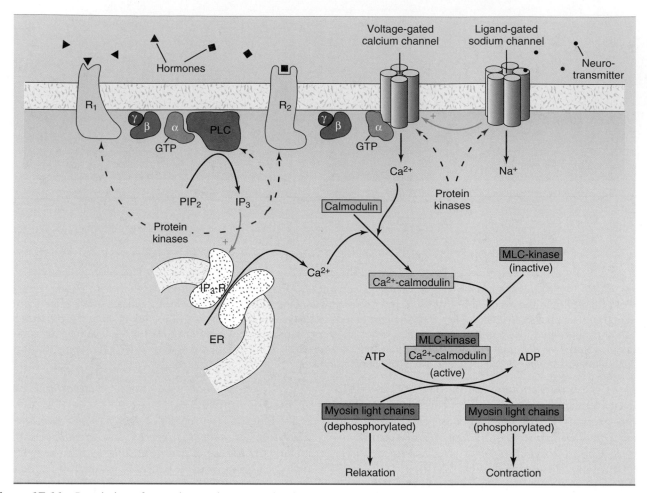

Figure 17.11 Regulation of smooth muscle contraction by calcium. Calcium enters the cytoplasm either from the extracellular space through voltage-gated calcium channels or through the inositol 1,4,5-trisphosphate (*IP₃*)–operated channel in the ER (*IP₃-R*). Voltage-gated calcium channels are regulated indirectly by neurotransmitters that act on ligand-gated ion channels. However, they also are regulated by hormone-operated G proteins, and they can be phosphorylated by protein kinases that are themselves under the control of second messengers. *ER*, Endoplasmic reticulum; *MLC-kinase*, myosin light chain kinase; *PIP₂*, phosphatidylinositol 4,5-bisphosphate; *PLC*, phospholipase C; *R₁* and *R₂*, G-protein–linked hormone receptors.

Table 17.2 Effects of Elevated Cytoplasmic Calcium Levels in Different Tissues

Tissue/Cell Type	Agents Inducing Release from Endoplasmic Reticulum	Effects
Pancreatic acinar cells	Cholecystokinin, acetylcholine	Zymogen secretion
Intestinal mucosa	Acetylcholine	Water and electrolyte secretion
Platelets	Thromboxane, collagen, thrombin, platelet-activating factor, ADP	Shape change, degranulation
Endothelial cells	Histamine, bradykinin, ATP, acetylcholine, thrombin	Nitric oxide synthesis
Vascular smooth muscle cells	Epinephrine (α₁ receptor), angiotensin II, vasopressin	Contraction
Bronchial smooth muscle cells	Histamine, leukotrienes	Contraction
Thyroid gland	TSH	Hormone synthesis and release
Corpus luteum	LHRH	Hormone synthesis
Liver	Epinephrine (α₁ receptor)	Glycogen degradation

LHRH, Luteinizing hormone–releasing hormone; *TSH*, thyroid-stimulating hormone.

enzymes, which are activated directly by extracellular ligands, and soluble cytoplasmic enzymes, which respond to small diffusible molecules.

Vascular smooth muscle cells have both types of guanylate cyclase (*Fig. 17.12*). The membrane-bound enzyme is a receptor for **atrial natriuretic factor (ANF)**. This peptide hormone (28 amino acids) is released from the atrium of the heart in response to elevated blood pressure. It increases sodium excretion by the kidneys, inhibits renin release from the juxtaglomerular cells and aldosterone release from the adrenal cortex, and relaxes vascular smooth muscle.

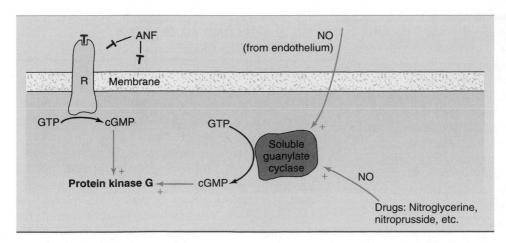

Figure 17.12 Formation of cyclic guanosine monophosphate (*cGMP*) in vascular smooth muscle cells. These cells have two guanylate cyclases. The membrane-bound enzyme is the receptor for atrial natriuretic factor (*ANF*), and the soluble enzyme is activated by the "endothelium-derived relaxing factor" nitric oxide (*NO*). *Straight green arrows* indicate allosteric stimulation. *R*, atrial natriuretic factor receptor.

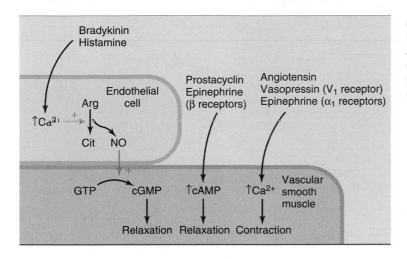

Figure 17.13 Roles of endothelium and vascular smooth muscle in the regulation of vascular tone. Agents that raise the calcium level in endothelial cells relax vascular smooth muscle because they stimulate the synthesis of nitric oxide (*NO*). *cAMP*, Cyclic AMP; *cGMP*, cyclic GMP.

The ANF receptor has an extracellular ligand-binding domain, a single transmembrane helix, and an intracellular guanylate cyclase domain. *The guanylate cyclase domain is active only when ANF is bound to the extracellular domain.*

Like cAMP, *cGMP induces its effects by activating a protein kinase.* This kinase is conveniently named **protein kinase G.** The cyclic nucleotides are not entirely specific for their respective protein kinases. To some extent cAMP can dilate vascular smooth muscle by activating protein kinase G, and high levels of cGMP in the intestinal mucosa can cause fluid secretion and diarrhea by an action on protein kinase A.

NITRIC OXIDE STIMULATES A SOLUBLE GUANYLATE CYCLASE

Although some vascular beds are relaxed by ANF, the major guanylate cyclase of vascular smooth muscle is a soluble, cytoplasmic enzyme that is activated by **nitric oxide (NO).** Before its chemical identity was known, NO had been described as the "endothelium-derived relaxing factor." NO is synthesized by a Ca^{2+}-calmodulin–activated **nitric oxide synthase** in endothelial cells. Being small and lipid soluble, it diffuses rapidly to the underlying smooth

muscle cells, in which it activates the soluble guanylate cyclase. NO is chemically unstable and decomposes within a few seconds, without the need for degrading enzymes.

Vascular smooth muscle is contracted by elevated cytoplasmic calcium and relaxed by cAMP and cGMP. Some vasodilators act by stimulating cAMP synthesis in vascular smooth muscle. Others act indirectly, by raising the calcium level in endothelial cells and thereby inducing the synthesis of the vasodilator NO. Vasoconstrictors act by raising the calcium level in vascular smooth muscle cells (*Fig. 17.13*).

Nitroglycerin is a fast-acting vasodilator that is used to treat acute attacks of angina pectoris:

Nitroglycerine

It is effective because it is rapidly metabolized to produce NO.

CLINICAL EXAMPLE 17.8: Treatment of Erectile Dysfunction

The blood vessels in the corpora cavernosa of the penis are expected to dilate profoundly in response to parasympathetic nerve stimulation. NO is the most important mediator. In this tissue, NO is formed mainly in the nerve terminals and only to a lesser extent in the vascular endothelium. As in other vascular beds, however, it acts by stimulating the soluble guanylate cyclase in vascular smooth muscle.

Erectile dysfunction (formerly known as impotence) is treated with **sildenafil (Viagra)** and related drugs that inhibit phosphodiesterase-5. This cGMP-specific phosphodiesterase is responsible for the degradation of cGMP in the vascular smooth muscle cells of the penis.

cGMP IS A SECOND MESSENGER IN RETINAL ROD CELLS

The retinal rod cells register light and transmit the information to the next cell in the neural signaling chain. The receptive part of the cell is its outer segment (actually a vastly modified cilium) that is filled with flattened membrane stacks (*Fig. 17.14*).

Embedded in these membranes is the light-absorbing protein **rhodopsin.** Ordinary proteins do not absorb visible light, but rhodopsin contains the light-absorbing prosthetic group **retinal.** Visible light isomerizes the 11-*cis* double bond in retinal into the *trans* configuration, leading to a substantial steric change not only in retinal but in the whole rhodopsin molecule:

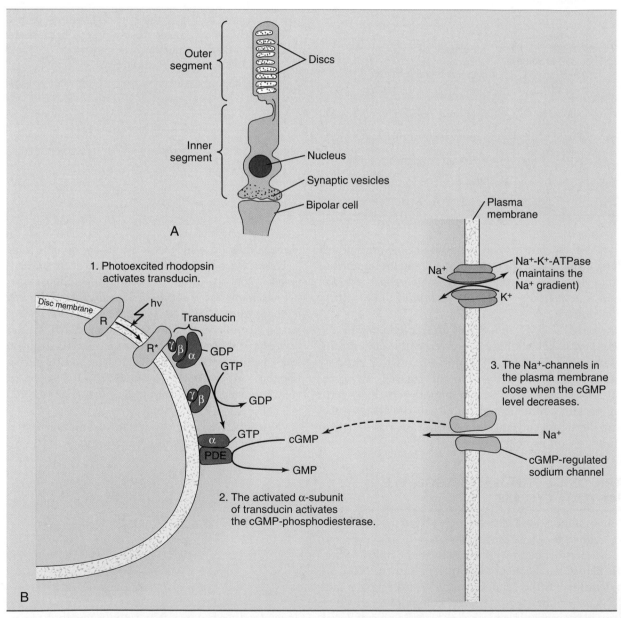

Figure 17.14 Signal transduction in the retinal rod cell. **A,** Structure of the retinal rod cell. **B,** Visual cascade. *cGMP*, Cyclic GMP; *hv*, visible light; *PDE*, cGMP phosphodiesterase; *R*, rhodopsin; *R**, photoexcited rhodopsin.

11-*cis* retinal in
unexcited rhodopsin

All-*trans* retinal in
photoexcited rhodopsin

All-*trans* retinal   +   Opsin

This photoisomerization switches rhodopsin to an activated, "photoexcited" conformation (R*). The labile aldimine bond between all-*trans* retinal and the apoprotein in R* hydrolyzes, and all-*trans* retinal dissociates from the apoprotein.

Although it responds to light rather than a hormone, rhodopsin is a seven-transmembrane protein that functions as a G-protein–coupled receptor. When activated by light, it switches the G-protein **transducin** into the active, GTP-bound form.

In the dark, the membrane of the rod cell is half depolarized because a sodium channel in the plasma membrane is kept in a half-open state by a tightly bound molecule of cGMP. *The light-activated transducin stimulates a phosphodiesterase.* cGMP is hydrolyzed, and the sodium channel loses its bound cGMP. Closure of the sodium channel hyperpolarizes the membrane, and the cell stops releasing its neurotransmitter.

This cascade amplifies the stimulus enormously. A single photoexcited rhodopsin molecule activates about 500 transducin molecules, each transducin-activated phosphodiesterase molecule hydrolyzes about 1000 cGMP molecules per second, and removal of cGMP from a single sodium channel prevents the influx of thousands of sodium ions. Therefore a single photon hyperpolarizes the cell by about 1 mV.

RECEPTORS FOR INSULIN AND GROWTH FACTORS ARE TYROSINE-SPECIFIC PROTEIN KINASES

Growth factors in the widest sense are soluble proteins that regulate growth, mitosis, differentiation, migration, and programmed cell death. They help in determining cell fate during embryonic and fetal development, and they regulate cell turnover and regeneration throughout life. Although growth factors induce most of their effects at the level of gene transcription, their receptors are in the plasma membrane.

The intracellular domain of most growth factor receptors is a ligand-activated protein kinase (**Fig. 17.15**). Unlike most other protein kinases, which phosphorylate their substrates on serine and threonine side chains, *the activated growth factor receptors attach phosphate groups to tyrosine side chains.* The substrate specificity of these receptor tyrosine kinases is unusual. After ligand binding, *the receptors aggregate in the membrane and phosphorylate each other.* This is called "autophosphorylation."

Tyrosine protein kinase receptors autophosphorylate on multiple tyrosine side chains, sometimes more than a dozen. Autophosphorylation has two effects: *It stimulates receptor kinase activity toward other substrates,* and *it creates docking sites for signaling proteins.* Most of these proteins bind to tyrosine-phosphorylated sites through a specialized **SH2 domain** (SH for src homology). Because each protein tyrosine kinase receptor has a unique combination of autophosphorylation sites, *each receptor interacts with a unique set of SH2 containing proteins.* Binding to the autophosphorylated receptor can have several consequences:

1. *Soluble cytoplasmic proteins are recruited to the plasma membrane.* Some are enzymes that are brought in contact with their membrane-bound substrates, and others are allosteric links in signaling cascades.
2. *Receptor binding induces allosteric changes in the bound molecules.* For example, some enzymes are allosterically activated by binding to the autophosphorylated receptor.
3. *Some of the bound proteins become tyrosine phosphorylated by the receptor.* This changes their biological properties.

The insulin receptor is similar to the growth factor receptors (**Fig. 17.16**). It phosphorylates two insulin receptor substrates (**IRS-1** and **IRS-2**) on about 20 tyrosine side chains. Signaling proteins become activated by binding to the phosphotyrosines of the IRS proteins.

GROWTH FACTORS AND INSULIN TRIGGER MULTIPLE SIGNALING CASCADES

Growth factors and insulin have a common evolutionary origin, but *in vertebrates, growth factors stimulate mainly growth and mitosis, whereas insulin stimulates*

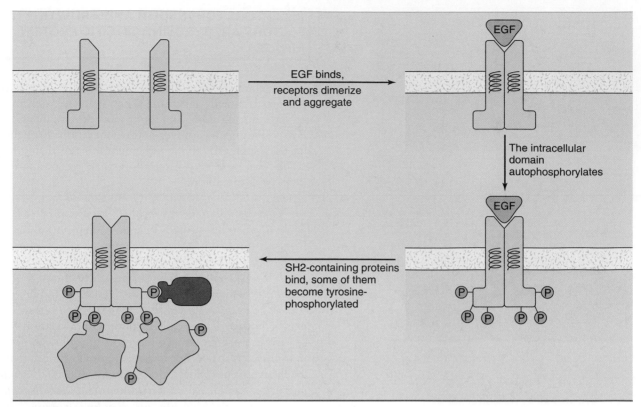

Figure 17.15 Receptor for epidermal growth factor (*EGF*). Ligand binding induces dimerization or oligomerization of the receptor, followed by autophosphorylation on tyrosine side chains. Most growth factors act by this general mechanism. Their actions are terminated by tyrosine-specific protein phosphatases that dephosphorylate the receptor and its substrates.

mainly the utilization of nutrients. Nevertheless, there is extensive overlap in the signaling cascades of the two types of hormones.

Figure 17.17 shows how growth factors can stimulate the IP$_3$ second messenger system. The key enzyme in this cascade, phospholipase C, comes in several isoforms. One group of isoforms, called **phospholipase Cβ,** is activated by the α subunits of G$_q$ proteins (see *Figs. 17.9* and *17.11*). Another type, **phospholipase Cγ,** associates with growth factor receptors and becomes activated by tyrosine phosphorylation.

Figure 17.18 shows another cascade. The activated tyrosine kinase receptor initiates a bucket brigade of allosteric protein-protein interactions to convert the membrane-bound G protein **Ras** into the active GTP-bound form. Like the heterotrimeric G proteins that are coupled to seven-transmembrane receptors, the Ras protein cycles between an inactive GDP-bound form and an active GTP-bound form. However, Ras consists of a single subunit.

In yet another pathway (*Fig. 17.19*), the autophosphorylated receptor recruits the enzyme phosphoinositide 3-kinase (PI3K) to the membrane. PI3K is allosterically activated by binding to the autophosphorylated growth factor receptor or to tyrosine-phosphorylated IRS-1. It also can be activated by Ras-GTP. PI3K phosphorylates inositol lipids in the plasma membrane in position 3. For example, it converts phosphatidylinositol 4,5-bisphosphate (PIP$_2$) into phosphatidylinositol 3,4,5-trisphosphate (PIP$_3$).

The 3-phosphorylated inositol lipids recruit a set of proteins to the membrane that includes **protein kinase B,** also known as **Akt,** together with two protein kinases that activate protein kinase B by phosphorylations of a serine and a threonine side chain. Once activated by these phosphorylations, *protein kinase B detaches from the membrane and phosphorylates a large number of proteins in cytoplasm and nucleus.*

Humans have three isoforms of protein kinase B: one mediating the growth-promoting and antiapoptotic effects of growth factors, one mediating insulin effects, and one of unknown function. These kinases phosphorylate their substrates on serine and threonine side chains.

SOME RECEPTORS RECRUIT TYROSINE-SPECIFIC PROTEIN KINASES TO THE MEMBRANE

Cytokines, including the interleukins and interferons, are secreted by white blood cells during inflammation to coordinate the immune response. Their receptors

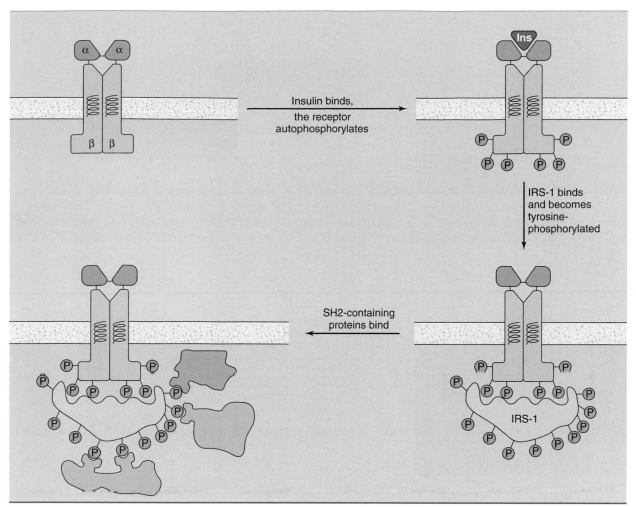

Figure 17.16 Insulin receptor. Unlike the growth factor receptors, which are monomers in the unstimulated state, the insulin receptor is a disulfide-bonded tetramer. Also, the insulin receptor does not bind SH2-containing signaling proteins itself but rather recruits insulin receptor substrate 1 (*IRS-1*) for this purpose.

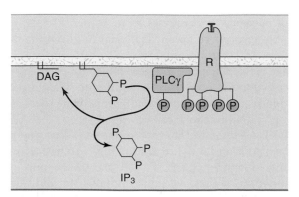

Figure 17.17 Activation of phospholipase Cγ (*PLCγ*) by growth factor receptors (*R*). PLCγ is activated by binding to the autophosphorylated receptor and by tyrosine phosphorylation. *DAG*, 1,2-Diacylglycerol; *IP₃*, inositol 1,4,5-trisphosphate.

have no enzymatic activity, but the ligand-activated receptor binds and thereby activates a **Janus kinase** (also called **JAK**, for "just another kinase"). Several JAKs associate with different receptors. *The receptor-bound kinases phosphorylate both each other and the receptor on tyrosine side chains* (**Fig. 17.20**).

Next, *the tyrosine-phosphorylated receptor attracts a protein of the* **signal transducer and activator of transcription (STAT)** *family*. Several STATs associate selectively with different receptors by means of an SH2 domain. The STAT becomes phosphorylated by the receptor-bound JAK and then moves to the nucleus, where it binds to response elements in promoters and enhancers to regulate transcription.

In addition to the cytokine receptors, the receptors for growth hormone, prolactin, and erythropoietin (*Clinical Example 17.9*) recruit JAKs and STATs. Some of the protein tyrosine kinase receptors use STATs, although they do not require a JAK for phosphorylation of the STAT.

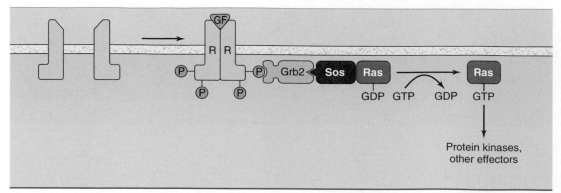

Figure 17.18 Activation of the Ras protein by growth factors (*GF*). The sequence of events is as follows: dimerization or oligomerization of the stimulated growth factor receptor (*R*) → receptor autophosphorylation → binding of an SH2-containing adapter protein (*Grb2*) → recruitment of a nucleotide exchange factor (*Sos*) to the plasma membrane → activation of Ras.

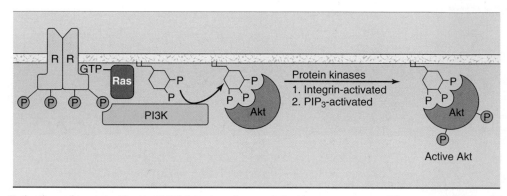

Figure 17.19 Activation of protein kinase B (*Akt*) by tyrosine protein kinase receptors. The autophosphorylated receptor (*R*) recruits the SH2 protein phosphoinositide 3-kinase (*PI3K*). This enzyme can also be recruited by Ras-GTP. The 3-phosphorylated inositol lipids formed by PI3K recruit Akt. After activating phosphorylations on serine and threonine, Akt phosphorylates serine and threonine side chains in its substrates. *PIP₃*, Phosphatidylinositol 3,4,5-trisphosphate.

CLINICAL EXAMPLE 17.9: Polycythemia Vera

Polycythemia is an abnormal increase in the number of circulating erythrocytes, which in most cases is caused by chronic oxygen deficiency. However, in patients with **polycythemia vera** the polycythemia has no obvious external cause and is of neoplastic origin. In essence, an abnormal, somatically mutated erythropoietic stem cell has formed a clone that overproduces erythrocytes.

Using high-throughput sequencing of granulocyte DNA, a somatic missense mutation (val→phe in position 617) in the gene for the tyrosine protein kinase JAK-2 was identified in 121 of 164 patients. The mutated kinase is constitutively active even in the absence of the kidney-derived hormone **erythropoietin**, which is the physiological ligand for the receptor with which JAK-2 associates.

THE T-CELL RECEPTOR RECRUITS CYTOSOLIC TYROSINE PROTEIN KINASES

In the presence of cytokines from helper T cells, lymphocytes respond to an unusual class of growth factors: antigens. B cells proliferate and differentiate into plasma cells when an antigen binds to their surface immunoglobulin, and T cells proliferate when an antigen binds to their functional equivalent of surface immunoglobulin, the **T-cell receptor.**

The T-cell receptor has two antigen-binding polypeptides called α and β that end in highly variable antigen-binding domains. Each T cell expresses only one combination of these variable domains. In addition to the α and β chains, the receptor contains a dimer of two ζ chains, as well as the **CD3** complex, which consists of a γ chain, a δ chain, and two ε chains (*Fig. 17.21*).

Antigen binding induces a conformational change that exposes the cytoplasmic tails of the γ, δ, ε, and ζ chains to the action of a tyrosine-specific protein

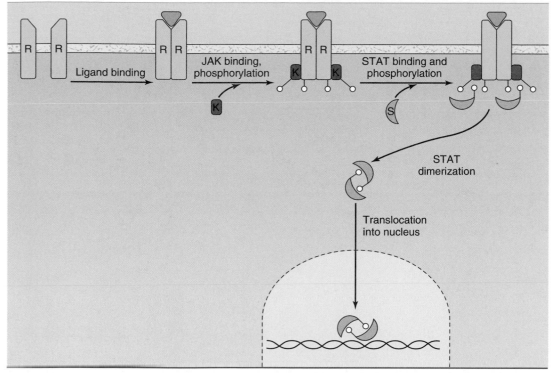

Figure 17.20   Signaling through cytokine receptors. The ligand-activated receptor (*R*) attracts a Janus (*JAK*) kinase (*K*). This kinase tyrosine phosphorylates both itself and the receptor. A signal transducer and activator of transcription (*STAT*) protein (S) binds to the tyrosine-phosphorylated receptor-kinase complex. After being phosphorylated by the Janus kinase, the STATs form active dimers that translocate into the nucleus to regulate transcription. ⓸, Phosphotyrosine groups.

kinase of the **Src** family (named after avian sarcoma, a virus induced cancer in chickens). These protein kinases are attached to the inner surface of the plasma membrane by a covalently bound myristoyl group. Besides Src itself, there are eight different Src-related protein kinases in different cells. Two of them, Lck and Fyn, are the major kinases phosphorylating the T-cell receptor.

Once the tyrosines are phosphorylated by the Src family kinases, a second type of tyrosine protein kinase, **zeta-associated protein 70 (ZAP-70)**, anchors itself to the tyrosine-phosphorylated receptor and phosphorylates target proteins. One of the target proteins, phospholipase Cγ, induces mitosis through 1,2-diacylglycerol, IP$_3$, and calcium.

An inherited deficiency of ZAP-70 has been identified as a cause of severe combined immunodeficiency in some patients. Although signaling through the surface immunoglobulin of B cells does not require ZAP-70, B cells are crippled as well because their activation requires activated helper T cells in addition to antigen.

MANY RECEPTORS BECOME DESENSITIZED AFTER OVERSTIMULATION

Many cells lose their responsiveness when they are exposed to high concentrations of a hormone for several minutes, hours, or days. For G-protein–coupled receptors, this **desensitization** is initiated by *phosphorylation of the receptor after agonist exposure.* For example, the β-adrenergic receptor is desensitized by two protein kinases: protein kinase A, which is activated by the β-adrenergic receptor through cAMP, and a **β-adrenergic receptor kinase (BARK)**, which phosphorylates the stimulated receptor but not the unstimulated receptor. These phosphorylations impair the activation of the G$_s$ protein by the activated receptor.

The phosphorylated receptor either becomes reactivated by a protein phosphatase, or it becomes deactivated entirely by binding of the cytoplasmic protein arrestin, which triggers endocytosis of the receptor (*Fig. 17.22*). The receptors either are stored in the membranes of intracellular vesicles or are sent to the lysosomes for degradation. *When receptors are degraded, desensitization can be reversed only by the synthesis of new receptors.*

In some cases, the receptor-bound arrestin protein itself can initiate additional signal transduction cascades that carry out characteristic actions of the hormone in the cell.

In addition to G-protein–coupled receptors, many tyrosine kinase receptors are endocytosed in response to overstimulation. For example, overeating leads to excessive insulin release. The overstimulated insulin receptors are prone to endocytosis, and some of the endocytosed receptors are destroyed in lysosomes.

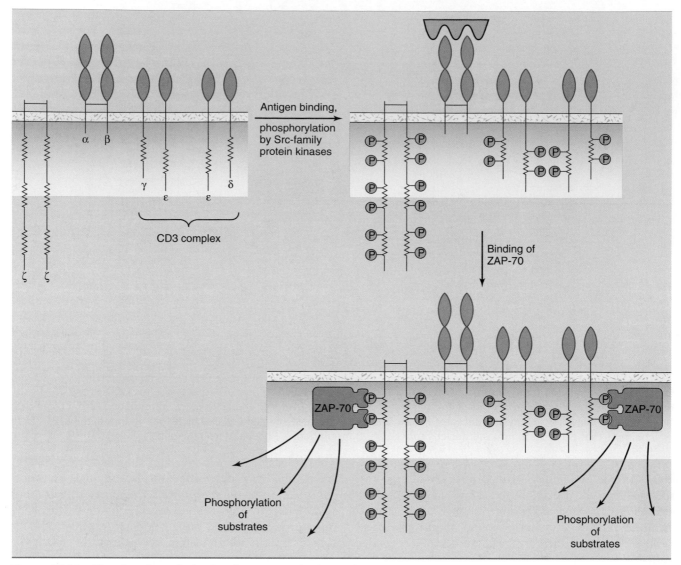

Figure 17.21 Signaling through the T-cell receptor. The intracellular tails of the γ, δ, ε, and ζ chains possess antigen-recognition activation motifs (ARAMs; ‑www‑) that become tyrosine phosphorylated by tyrosine protein kinases of the Src family. The extracellular portions of the α, β, γ, and δ chains contain immunoglobulin-like domains, but only the α and β chains have variable domains for antigen recognition. T cells can respond specifically to an antigen on the surface of a presenting cell. Like many other signal transducing proteins, zeta-associated protein 70 (*ZAP-70*) has SH2 domains (𝕏) that bind to tyrosine-phosphorylated sites.

Figure 17.22 Desensitization of the β-adrenergic receptor (*R*). Phosphorylation by protein kinase A prevents interaction of the receptor with the G_s protein. Alternatively, the ligand-activated receptor is phosphorylated by a specialized β-adrenergic receptor kinase (*BARK*). The cytoplasmic protein arrestin binds to the phosphorylated receptor, preventing activation of the G_s protein and triggering receptor endocytosis. *PKA*, Protein kinase A.

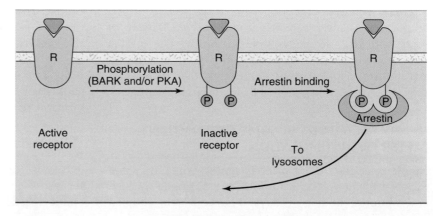

Some overeaters can balance this loss by making more insulin receptors, but those who cannot are at risk for type 2 diabetes. Many obese type 2 diabetics have a reduced number of insulin receptors, although defects in the downstream signaling cascades appear to be more important than reduced receptor number as a cause for their insulin resistance. Weight loss can nevertheless increase the number of insulin receptors in obese type 2 diabetics, restore a normal insulin response, and reduce the level of circulating insulin.

SUMMARY

Binding to a cellular receptor protein is the first step in the action of an extracellular messenger on its target cell. Receptors are allosteric proteins that bind their ligand with high affinity and selectivity. The receptors for steroid hormones, thyroid hormones, calcitriol, and retinoic acid are ligand-regulated transcription factors, but water-soluble agents bind to receptors on the cell surface.

Many neurotransmitters open a ligand-gated ion channel in the plasma membrane by direct binding to the channel, but water-soluble hormones trigger lengthy signaling cascades. Most hormone receptors activate a G protein that triggers the synthesis of a second messenger. cAMP, cGMP, IP$_3$ (acting through Ca^{2+}), and 1,2-diacylglycerol are important second messengers. The second messengers activate protein kinases, including kinases A (cAMP-activated), C (Ca^{2+}-diacylglycerol-activated), and G (cGMP-activated), and the calcium-calmodulin–dependent protein kinases.

The receptors for insulin and many growth factors are tyrosine-specific protein kinases. They autophosphorylate in response to ligand binding and can activate other proteins by recruiting them to the membrane, activating them allosterically, or phosphorylating them.

Further Reading

Assinder SJ, Dong Q, Kovacevic Z, et al: The TGF-β, PI3K/Akt and PTEN pathways: established and proposed biochemical integration in prostate cancer, *Biochem J* 417:411–421, 2009.

Bai Y, Sanderson MJ: Airway smooth muscle relaxation results from a reduction in the frequency of Ca^{2+} oscillations induced by a cAMP-mediated inhibition of the IP$_3$ receptor, *Respir Res* 7:34, 2006.

Bastepe M, Jüppner H: GNAS locus and pseudohypoparathyroidism, *Horm Res* 63:65–74, 2005.

Biel M: Cyclic nucleotide-regulated cation channels, *J Biol Chem* 284:9017–9021, 2009.

Carrasco S, Mérida I: Diacylglycerol, when simplicity becomes complex, *Trends Biochem Sci* 32:27–36, 2007.

Clapham DE: Calcium signaling, *Cell* 131:1047–1058, 2007.

Conti M, Beavo J: Biochemistry and physiology of cyclic nucleotide phosphodiesterases: essential components in cyclic nucleotide signaling, *Annu Rev Biochem* 76:481–511, 2007.

Cooper DMF: Regulation and organization of adenylyl cyclases and cAMP, *Biochem J* 375:517–529, 2003.

Dessauer CW: Adenylyl cyclase-A-kinase anchoring protein complexes: the next dimension in cAMP signaling, *Mol Pharmacol* 76:935–941, 2009.

Di Paolo G, De Camilli P: Phosphoinositides in cell regulation and membrane dynamics, *Nature* 443:651–657, 2006.

Eszlinger M, Jaeschke H, Paschke R: Insights from molecular pathways: potential pharmacologic targets of benign thyroid nodules, *Curr Opin Endocrinol Diabetes Obes* 14:393–397, 2007.

Fishman MC, Porter JA: A new grammar for drug discovery, *Nature* 437:491–493, 2005.

Gáboric Z, Hunyadi L: Intracellular trafficking of hormone receptors, *Trends Endocrinol Metab* 15:286–293, 2004.

Garbers DL, Chrisman TD, Wiegn P, et al: Membrane guanylyl cyclase receptors: an update, *Trends Endocrinol Metab* 17:251–258, 2006.

Houslay MD, Baillie GS, Maurice DH: cAMP-specific phosphodiesterase-4 enzymes in the cardiovascular system: a molecular toolbox for generating compartmentalized cAMP signaling, *Circ Res* 100:950–966, 2007.

Huang J, Manning BD: A complex interplay between Akt, TSC2 and the two mTOR complexes, *Biochem Soc Trans* 37:217–222, 2009.

Lefkowitz RJ, Shenoy SK: Transduction of receptor signals by β-arrestins, *Science* 308:512–517, 2005.

Levine R, Wadleigh M, Cools J, et al: Activating mutation in the tyrosine kinase JAK2 in polycythemia vera, essential thrombocythemia, and myeloid metaplasia with myelofibrosis, *Cancer Cell* 7:387–397, 2005.

Manning BD, Cantley LC: AKT/PKB signaling: navigating downstream, *Cell* 129:1261–1274, 2007.

Pestka S: The interferons: 50 years after their discovery, there is much more to learn, *J Biol Chem* 282:20047–20051, 2007.

Schindler C, Levy DE, Decker T: JAK-STAT signaling: from interferons to cytokines, *J Biol Chem* 282:20059–20063, 2007.

Shabsigh R, Anastasiadis AG: Erectile dysfunction, *Annu Rev Med* 54:153–168, 2003.

Thirone ACP, Huang C, Klip A: Tissue-specific roles of IRS proteins in insulin signaling and glucose transport, *Trends Endocrinol Metab* 17:70–76, 2006.

Umar S, van der Laarse A: Nitric oxide and nitric oxide synthase isoforms in the normal, hypertrophic, and failing heart, *Mol Cell Biochem* 333:191–201, 2010.

QUESTIONS

1. **Vascular smooth muscle contracts in response to increased cytoplasmic calcium. Nevertheless, many natural agents that stimulate the IP$_3$/calcium system (including acetylcholine, histamine, and bradykinin) are potent vasodilators. Why?**

   A. In the vascular smooth muscle cell, calcium rapidly equilibrates across the plasma membrane.
   B. The calcium-calmodulin complex blocks voltage-gated calcium channels in vascular smooth muscle.
   C. Calcium is transferred from endothelial cells to vascular smooth muscle through gap junctions.
   D. The calcium-calmodulin complex stimulates NO synthase in endothelial cells.
   E. The calcium-calmodulin complex inhibits adenylate cyclase in vascular smooth muscle cells.

2. **Activation of the IP$_3$/calcium system leads to growth stimulation in many cells, including cancer cells. In order to inhibit this second messenger system, you could try to develop a drug that**

   A. Inhibits the dephosphorylation of IP$_3$
   B. Stimulates protein kinase C
   C. Reacts chemically with the α subunits of the G$_q$ proteins, thereby making them unable to activate phospholipase C
   D. Inhibits the GTPase activity of the G$_q$ proteins
   E. Inhibits the active transport of calcium in the plasma membrane

3. **cAMP regulates the transcription of many genes. What is the major mechanism for this action?**

   A. It induces the phosphorylation of transcription factors.
   B. It binds directly to cAMP response elements in promoters and enhancers.
   C. It mediates this effect by increasing the calcium concentration in the cytoplasm and the nucleus.
   D. It binds directly to nuclear transcription factors.
   E. It induces the phosphorylation of STAT proteins, thus enabling them to translocate into the nucleus.

4. **Most growth factor receptors are able to phosphorylate tyrosine side chains of proteins. Although the substrates of the activated receptors differ, one protein always becomes tyrosine phosphorylated. This protein is**

   A. Adenylate cyclase
   B. Inositol triphosphate
   C. Protein kinase C
   D. Protein kinase A
   E. The receptor itself

5. **A drug that inhibits the hydrolysis of 3-phosphorylated inositol lipids (e.g., phosphatidylinositol 3,4,5-trisphosphate) is likely to increase the cell's responsiveness to some of the effects of**

   A. Glucocorticoids
   B. Hormones acting through G$_s$ protein-coupled receptors
   C. Hormones acting through G$_i$ protein-coupled receptors
   D. Insulin
   E. NO

Chapter 18

CELLULAR GROWTH CONTROL AND CANCER

The human body is produced from the fertilized ovum in a succession of mitotic cell divisions. Each mitotic cycle consists of an orderly sequence of events, including growth, DNA replication, and cell division.

As they go through repeated rounds of cell division, the totipotent cells of the embryo metamorphose into the differentiated cells of the mature body: blood cells, neurons, muscle cells, and so forth. Cell growth, mitotic rate, and cell differentiation are controlled by external stimuli, including nutrients, hormones, growth factors, and contacts with neighboring cells and the extracellular matrix.

Derangements in the controls on the cell's proliferation, differentiation, and survival cause cancer. This chapter describes the elements of cell cycle control and their abnormalities in cancer.

THE CELL CYCLE IS CONTROLLED AT TWO CHECKPOINTS

Under the microscope, only two phases of the cell cycle can be distinguished in dividing cells: **interphase** and **mitosis** (*Fig. 18.1*). Mitosis, which lasts between 1 and 4 hours, is the stage of cell division. All of the rest is interphase. Chromosomes are visible as distinct entities only during mitosis, when the DNA is packaged for relocation into the daughter cells. During interphase, there is only dispersed chromatin all over the nucleus.

Interphase is subdivided into three phases. **G_1 phase** (G for gap) is the regular, diploid state of the cell. G_1 is followed by **S phase** (S for synthesis), during which the DNA is replicated, and finally by **G_2**. *S phase can be identified by feeding the cells with radiolabeled thymidine.* Cells in S phase, which lasts about 6 hours, incorporate a large amount of the thymidine into DNA (but not RNA). Outside S phase, only a small amount of DNA synthesis takes place during DNA repair.

The cell makes three important all-or-none decisions during the cell cycle. At the **G_1 checkpoint** in late G_1, it decides about *entry into S phase.* DNA replication should be initiated only when the cell is ready to progress through the complete cell cycle and only after any DNA damage that may have been sustained has

been thoroughly repaired. *The overall rate of cell proliferation is controlled by G_1.*

At the **G_2 checkpoint** in late G_2, the cell decides about *entry into mitosis.* Mitosis should begin only after the completion of DNA replication and only if the replicated chromosomes are structurally intact.

The **spindle assembly checkpoint,** finally, ensures that the cell proceeds from mitotic metaphase to anaphase only if the mitotic spindle is intact and all chromosomes are attached to the spindle fibers.

Nondividing cells are said to be in **G_0**. Some nondividing cells, including neurons and skeletal muscle fibers, are in G_0 forever. Others, including fibroblasts, hepatocytes, and lymphocytes, are usually in G_0 but can be coaxed into the cell cycle by growth factors or, in the case of lymphocytes, by antigen along with cytokines from helper T cells.

CELLS CAN BE GROWN IN CULTURE

The cell cycle is most easily studied in cultured cells. Leukocytes, fibroblasts, and many other cells (but not neurons) can be induced to grow and divide in culture. Typical features of these cultured cells include the following:

1. *Cell proliferation is mitogen dependent.* Normal cells in the human body enter the cell cycle only when told to do so by soluble mitogens.
2. *Cell growth is anchorage dependent.* Cells in the body are attached to the extracellular matrix, and they proliferate only as long as these attachments are maintained. Cultured cells other than white blood cells need a solid or semisolid surface to substitute for the extracellular matrix.
3. *Cell growth is contact inhibited.* In the body, cells stop dividing when they are surrounded by other cells in the tissue. In the test tube, they stop dividing as soon as a continuous cell layer has been formed.
4. *Cells are mortal.* For example, cultured fibroblasts divide between 25 and 50 times until they turn senile and die. Fibroblasts from a baby have a higher life expectancy in culture than do those from a senior citizen.

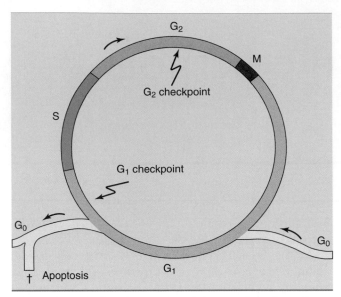

Figure 18.1 Cell cycle. G_1, S, and G_2 constitute interphase. DNA is replicated during synthesis (S) phase; the chromosomes segregate during mitosis (M). Nondividing cells are in G_0 phase.

These limitations apply only to normal cells. Cancer cells are mitogen independent and anchorage independent, are not inhibited by contact with neighboring cells, and are immortal.

CYCLINS PLAY KEY ROLES IN CELL CYCLE CONTROL

Cell cycle progression depends on the phosphorylation of multiple proteins by the **cyclin-dependent kinases (Cdks)** in the nucleus and their regulatory subunits, the **cyclins**. The Cdks are present more or less at all times, but most of the cyclins come and go with the phases of the cell cycle (*Fig. 18.2*).

Only cyclin D is not controlled by the cell cycle; it is controlled by mitogens. It rises when a cell in G_1 is exposed to mitogens. By activating **Cdk4** and **Cdk6,** cyclin D induces the synthesis of **cyclin E,** an activator of **Cdk2.** Cyclin E and Cdk2 push the cell through the G_1 checkpoint. Next comes **cyclin A,** which activates Cdk1 (formerly called Cdc2) and Cdk2. It brings the cell through S phase and remains active through G_2.

Finally **cyclin B,** working with Cdk1, accumulates during G_2 and early mitosis. It condenses the chromosomes by phosphorylating chromosomal scaffold proteins and histone H1, and it breaks down the nuclear envelope by phosphorylating and thereby dismantling the lamin network under the inner nuclear membrane. At the spindle assembly checkpoint in mitosis, a ubiquitin ligase complex is formed that destroys cyclin B along with cyclin A and some other proteins of early mitosis suddenly during the metaphase-anaphase transition.

The Cdks are controlled primarily by cyclins, but also by stimulatory and inhibitory phosphorylations and by **Cdk inhibitors** that are formed under the influence of antimitotic agents.

RETINOBLASTOMA PROTEIN GUARDS THE G_1 CHECKPOINT

Progression through the cell cycle and DNA synthesis require the transcription factor E2F, which regulates more than 500 genes. It activates the transcription of genes for cyclins D1 (there are three closely related D cyclins), E, A, and B, Cdk1, thymidylate synthetase, dihydrofolate reductase, DNA polymerase α, topoisomerase II, the clamp protein PCNA (see Chapter 7), and the

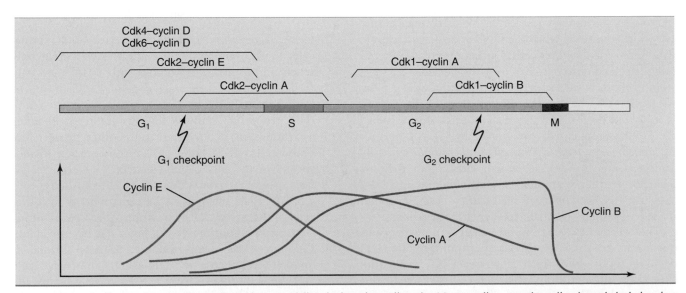

Figure 18.2 Cyclins and cyclin-dependent kinases (*Cdks*) during the cell cycle. Most cyclins are short lived, and their levels fluctuate with the stages of the cell cycle. The cyclin-dependent kinases and cyclin D, on the other hand, are present throughout the cell cycle. G_1, S, G_2, and M are the stages of the cell cycle (see *Fig. 18.1*).

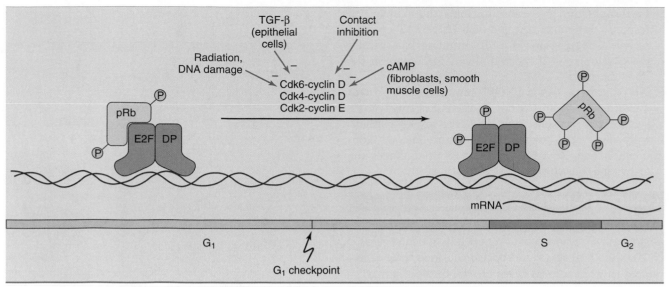

Figure 18.3 Function of the retinoblastoma protein (*pRb*) in the control of the G$_1$ checkpoint. Phosphorylation of pRb by cyclin-dependent protein kinases (*Cdks*) releases the transcription factor E2F/DP from inhibitory control, thus enabling the transcription of genes for cell cycle progression. Growth-inhibiting stimuli prevent pRb phosphorylation indirectly by increasing the activity of cyclin/Cdk inhibitors. *cAMP*, Cyclic AMP; *mRNA*, messenger RNA; *P*, phosphate groups; *TGF-β*, transforming growth factor β.

proto-oncogenes *MYC* and *MYCL1* (which code for the transcription factors c-Myc and N-Myc, respectively).

In quiescent cells, E2F is prevented from activating the transcription of these genes by the **retinoblastoma protein (pRb)**, which is encoded by the *RB1* gene (*Fig. 18.3*). Throughout G$_0$ and early G$_1$, pRb is tightly bound to E2F. It prevents gene expression by masking the transcriptional activation domain of E2F and by recruiting a histone deacetylase. At the G$_1$ checkpoint, however, both pRb and E2F become phosphorylated by the kinase complexes of cyclins D and E. The phosphorylated pRb falls off the transcription factor, and the genes can be transcribed.

These events are all or none because they are subject to *positive feedback*. Once the activity of the cyclin D-Cdk complexes has passed a threshold, the cyclin genes become derepressed. Even more cyclin-Cdk is formed, pushing the cell through the G$_1$ checkpoint.

CELL PROLIFERATION IS TRIGGERED BY MITOGENS

During embryonic development, cell proliferation is tightly linked to cell differentiation. Undifferentiated stem cells divide frequently, but once the cell has morphed into a specialized cell type, it withdraws from the cell cycle. For some cells, including neurons and skeletal muscle fibers, the withdrawal into G$_0$ is final. However, other cells, including hepatocytes and fibroblasts, behave like Sleeping Beauty. They can be restored to reproductive life by external agents. The prince's kiss that causes these cells to abandon G$_0$ and reenter the cell cycle is delivered by agents called **mitogens.**

Mitogenic stimuli can be provided by the extracellular matrix. The integrins in focal adhesions (see Chapter 13) not only mediate adhesion to extracellular matrix components but also provide an assembly point for signaling molecules. Cell-matrix contacts tend to be mitogenic, but cell-cell contacts usually are antimitogenic.

Soluble **growth factors** allow the cell to respond to signals from more distant sources. The term is used loosely to refer to proteins that stimulate cell growth (growth factors in the strict sense), cell proliferation (mitogens), or cell survival (survival factors). Examples of growth factors include the following:

1. **Platelet-derived growth factor** (PDGF) is present in the α-granules of platelets from which it is released during platelet activation. Acting on fibroblasts, smooth muscle cells, and other cells, *PDGF participates in wound healing.* The discovery of PDGF followed the observation that added serum but not plasma stimulates the proliferation of cultured cells. The serum effect could be traced to PDGF, which is released from activated platelets during blood clotting.
2. **Epidermal growth factor** (EGF) stimulates the proliferation of epithelial cells and some other cells. It acts primarily in its tissues of origin.
3. **Fibroblast growth factors** (FGFs) are a family of at least 22 proteins that act on four different tyrosine kinase receptors. They stimulate not only fibroblasts but also many other cells.
4. **Insulin-like growth factor 1** (IGF-1) is released from the liver in response to growth hormone. Pygmies are short because they have a reduced number of growth hormone receptors in the liver and therefore a reduced level of circulating IGF-1.

5. **Erythropoietin** is released from the kidney in response to hypoxia. Acting on a JAK-STAT coupled receptor (see Chapter 17), it stimulates specifically the development of red blood cell precursors in the bone marrow.

6. **Nerve growth factor (NGF)** stimulates the growth and differentiation (but not mitosis) of postganglionic sympathetic neurons. Being released by sympathetically innervated tissues during embryonic development, it acts as a chemoattractant that guides the growing axons to their proper destinations.

CLINICAL EXAMPLE 18.1: Achondroplasia

Achondroplasia is an autosomal dominant form of short-limbed dwarfism with a population incidence of 1:10,000. Because achondroplastic dwarves have a low reproductive rate, most cases are the result of a new mutation. The mutation occurs in a mutational hotspot in the gene for **fibroblast growth factor receptor 3 (FGFR3)** and leads to a glycine→arginine substitution next to a transmembrane helix. This missense mutation causes a slight shift in the transmembrane helix that leads to constitutive activation of the receptor's tyrosine kinase activity.

   This constitutively active receptor causes aberrant development of chondrocytes in the epiphyseal plates of long bones, leading to abnormally short bones. Milder mutations in the *FGFR3* gene lead to mildly reduced stature, diagnosed as **hypochondroplasia.** Mutations that lead to greater receptor activation than the achondroplasia mutation cause **thanatophoric dysplasia,** with growth abnormalities that are serious enough to cause death shortly after birth. Homozygosity for the achondroplasia mutation leads to a fatal condition similar to thanatophoric dysplasia.

MITOGENS REGULATE GENE EXPRESSION

Mitogens push cells through the G_1 checkpoint. Figure 18.4 shows two mitogenic signaling cascades that are triggered by autophosphorylated growth factor receptors and activate the nuclear cyclin D-Cdk complexes.

   One of these cascades signals through **phosphoinositide 3-kinase (PI3K)** and **protein kinase B (PKB, or Akt)** (see Chapter 17). PKB phosphorylates and thereby inhibits another protein kinase, **glycogen synthase kinase 3 (GSK3).** GSK3 inhibits the expression of cyclin D1 by phosphorylating transcriptional regulators bound to the promoter of the cyclin D1 gene. *By inhibiting these inhibitory phosphorylations, PKB stimulates the expression of the cyclin D1 gene.*

   The other mitogenic cascade shown in *Figure 18.4* is the **mitogen-activated protein (MAP) kinase cascade.** It starts with activation of the small G protein **Ras** at the cytoplasmic surface of the plasma membrane (see Chapter 17). Three isoforms of Ras occur in human tissues.

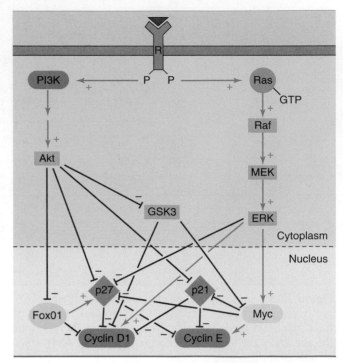

Figure 18.4 Two mitogenic signaling cascades. On the left side, the activated growth factor receptor *R* activates phosphoinositide 3-kinase (*PI3K*). By producing 3-phosphorylated inositol lipids, PI3K assists in the activation of protein kinase B (*Akt*). Akt inhibits glycogen synthase kinase-3 (*GSK3*) by phosphorylation. The right side shows the mitogen-activated protein (MAP) kinase pathway. Ras is a small monomeric G protein; Akt, GSK3, Raf, MEK, and ERK are protein kinases; p21 and p27 are cyclin-Cdk inhibitors; FoxO1 (Forkhead box-O) and Myc are transcription factors.

   Activated Ras recruits the serine-threonine protein kinase **Raf** to the plasma membrane, where it becomes activated by phosphorylation. Some isoenzymes of protein kinase C can activate Ras-bound Raf.

   Raf phosphorylates and thereby activates the protein kinases **MEK1** and **MEK2** (MAPK/ERK kinases). The MEKs phosphorylate the serine-threonine kinases **ERK1** and **ERK2** (extracellular signal-regulated kinases) on threonine and tyrosine residues in the sequence Thr-Glu-Tyr. The ERKs are also known as **MAP kinases.**

   The activated MAP kinases phosphorylate proteins in both the cytoplasm and the nucleus. They regulate transcription factors by phosphorylation, both directly and indirectly by phosphorylating nuclear protein kinases. The products of some of the activated genes, including the proto-oncogene *MYC*, are themselves regulators of transcription. In addition to the cyclins, cyclin-Cdk inhibitors including p21 and p27 are regulated both by phosphorylation and at the transcriptional level.

   Negative controls on mitogenic signaling include the *dephosphorylation of proteins by protein phosphatases* at all levels, from the autophosphorylated growth factor receptors to the phosphorylated transcription factors. Another negative control is the *hydrolysis of its bound GTP by the Ras protein.* The GTPase activity of Ras is stimulated by regulatory proteins, including **neurofibromin** (*Clinical Example 18.2*).

CLINICAL EXAMPLE 18.2: Neurofibromatosis Type 1

Neurofibromatosis type 1 is a dominantly inherited condition (incidence 1:4000) that presents at birth with light brown spots on the skin (café au lait spots). Benign but disfiguring nerve sheath tumors (neurofibromas) develop along the peripheral nerves throughout life. Some patients develop rhabdomyosarcoma or neuroblastoma during childhood, and malignant peripheral nerve sheath tumors can arise at any age.

The mutation inactivates the protein **neurofibromin**, which stimulates the GTPase activity of Ras and thereby reduces signaling through Ras and the MAP kinase pathway. In the tumors that form in this condition, the second, originally intact copy of the neurofibromin gene is disabled by a somatic mutation. Therefore the tumor cells (but not the normal somatic cells in the patient) have greatly elevated signaling through this pathway.

CELLS CAN COMMIT SUICIDE

When a cell dies by **necrosis,** the environment gets polluted with proteases and other damaging and inflammation-inducing proteins that leak out of the dying cells. Programmed cell death by **apoptosis,** by contrast, is a clean process in which the dying cell presents itself to macrophages with its membrane intact.

Apoptosis is a normal part of early human development. In adults it remains important as a response to cellular damage, viral infections, somatic mutations, hormonal influences, or lack of extracellular survival factors. *Apoptosis eliminates many virus-infected and genetically altered cells.* These cells must be prevented from evolving into cancer cells.

Apoptotic stimuli destroy the cell by recruiting proteases of the **caspase** family. Caspases are present in the cell as inactive precursors (procaspases) that have to be activated by a proteolytic cascade.

Initiator procaspases are activated by death-promoting stimuli. Once activated, their main function is the activation of **executioner procaspases** that destroy target proteins in the cell. Cleavage of nuclear lamins destroys the nuclear envelope; degradation of a DNase inhibitor unleashes a DNase that cleaves DNA in the spacers between nucleosomes; and cleavage of cytoskeletal and cell adhesion proteins causes the cell to curl up and detach from neighboring cells. This facilitates the removal of the dying cell by macrophages. There are two apoptotic pathways:

1. The **extrinsic pathway** is triggered by external agents that activate **death receptors** on the cell surface (*Fig. 18.5*). These receptors contain a **death domain** in their cytoplasmic portion. Once activated by an extracellular signal, for example, **tumor necrosis**

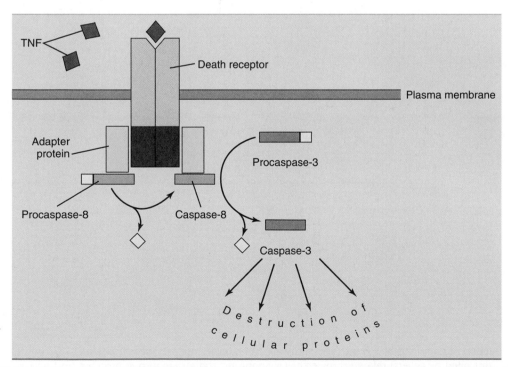

Figure 18.5 The extrinsic pathway of apoptosis consists of a receptor (*pink*) with a death domain (*red*). Adapter proteins that bind to the death domain of the activated receptor recruit procaspase-8 or -10. Tumor necrosis factor (*TNF*) is a well-studied extracellular trigger of apoptosis.

factor (**TNF**) or the **Fas ligand,** the death domain binds the precursor of an initiator caspase (either **Casp-8** or **Casp-10**) through adapter proteins. *Binding to this complex activates the bound procaspases allosterically, enabling them to cleave each other into the active caspases.* The activated initiator caspases proceed to activate **Casp-3** and other executioner caspases.

2. The **intrinsic pathway** is triggered by stimuli that arise within the cell. *Apoptotic stimuli trigger the release of cytochrome c from the intermembrane space of the mitochondria.* In the cytoplasm, cytochrome *c* associates with the scaffold protein apoptotic protease

activating factor 1 (**Apaf1**) and the precursor of the initiator caspase **Casp-9.** The procaspase-9 molecules in this "apoptosome" activate each other to form active Casp-9, which then proceeds to activate the effector caspase **Casp-3** (*Fig. 18.6*).

The intrinsic pathway depends on proteins that bind to the outer mitochondrial membrane to control the release of cytochrome *c*. In unimpaired cells, **Bcl-2** and related proteins prevent cytochrome *c* release and apoptosis. This effect can be overcome by **Bax** and related proteins. Other proapoptotic proteins participate in this process by binding and inactivating Bcl-2 and its relatives.

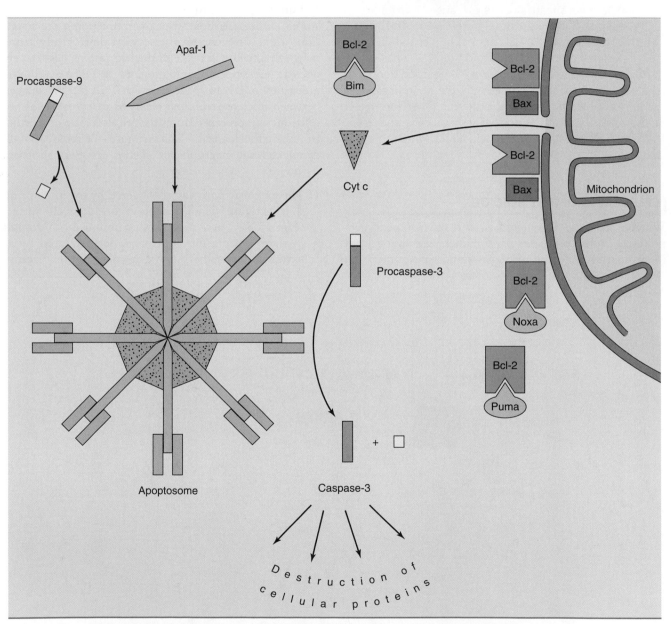

Figure 18.6 Induction of apoptosis by the intrinsic pathway. The intermembrane space contains cytochrome *c*. Its release into the cytoplasm is controlled by several related families of proapoptotic and antiapoptotic proteins (*red/pink* and *green,* respectively). Antiapoptotic Bcl-2 competes with proapoptotic Bax, whereas proteins with such names as Puma, Noxa, and Bim help Bax by tying up Bcl-2. In the cytoplasm, an "apoptosome" is constructed from the scaffold protein Apaf-1, procaspase-9, and cytochrome *c.* Procaspase-9 activates itself in the apoptosome, and caspase-9 activates procaspase-3.

CANCERS ARE MONOCLONAL IN ORIGIN

Because they are genetically identical and depend on one another for transmission of their genes into the next generation, the cells of the human body behave unselfishly toward one another. Each cell grows and divides only to the extent that it furthers the greater good of the body, and some cells even die dutifully—by apoptosis—once their task has been fulfilled.

Cancer cells, however, have the cellular equivalent of antisocial personality disorder. A cancer cell arises when a somatic mutation creates a "selfish gene" that causes the cell to proliferate without regard for the greater good of the organism. This single abnormal cell grows into a cell mass called a **neoplasm** or **tumor.** *Most tumors are monoclonal in origin.* This means that all tumor cells are derived from a single abnormal ancestor. **Benign tumors** limit their growth without doing much harm, but **malignant tumors,** commonly called **cancer,** kill the organism. Cancer causes more than 20% of all deaths in industrialized countries. *Figure 18.7* shows the incidence of various kinds of cancer in the United States.

Malignant cells retain morphological and biochemical features typical for their cells of origin. Some tumors of epithelial origin, for example, known as **carcinomas,** still produce keratins; some connective tissue tumors, known as **sarcomas,** still produce constituents of the extracellular matrix; and some endocrine tumors still secrete hormones. However, these specialized features tend to get lost when cancers become more malignant. Characteristic differences between cancer cells and the normal cells from which they are derived include the following:

1. *Cancer cells have an abnormally high mitotic rate.* The percentage of mitotic cells (**mitotic index**) is determined diagnostically to estimate the malignant potential of a tumor.

2. *Cancer cells lose many specialized functions and become more similar to stem cells.* The cells in epithelial cancers (carcinomas), for example, lose the normal squamous, cuboidal, or columnar shape of their normal progenitors and come to resemble embryonic cells.

3. *Cancer cells show disordered growth.* They have no respect for anatomical boundaries but grow as a chaotic mass, spreading and sprawling in all directions. The dedifferentiation and disordered growth of cancerous cells are called **anaplasia.** The degree of anaplasia predicts the malignant behavior of the tumor and the patient's survival chances.

4. *Cancer cells can colonize distant tissues.* They can break loose from the primary tumor to be disseminated by lymph or blood, and they take root in distant tissues to form secondary growths called **metastases.**

5. *Cancer cells are genetically unstable.* Most cancers have aberrations in chromosome number, major deletions and translocations, gene amplifications, and even extrachromosomal genetic elements. They keep mutating because their ability to prevent and repair DNA damage is defective.

6. *Cancer cells can grow in the absence of mitogens.* Their mitogenic signaling cascades are switched on permanently, even in the absence of mitogens.

7. *Cancer cells are immortal.* Although many cancer cells succumb to haphazard mutations, they escape the normal process of senescence. Most cancer cells have also lost the ability for apoptosis in response to growth factor deprivation, DNA damage, and other environmental insults.

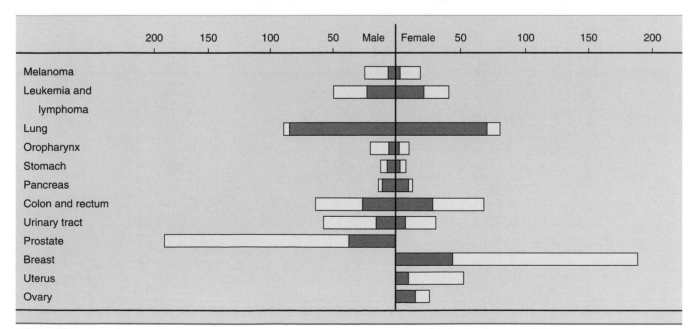

Figure 18.7   Incidence of new cancer cases in the United States in 1998 *(complete bars)* and the annual death rate *(dark-colored portions),* in thousands per year. Basal cell carcinomas and squamous cell carcinomas of the skin are not included. These skin cancers have a very high incidence, but most are readily cured by resection of the tumor.

CANCER IS CAUSED BY ACTIVATION OF GROWTH-PROMOTING GENES AND INACTIVATION OF GROWTH-INHIBITING GENES

Some gene products, including growth factors, growth factor receptors, components of mitogenic signaling cascades, and the G_1 cyclins, promote cell proliferation. Others, including cyclin-Cdk inhibitors and pRb, are inhibitory. Therefore two types of mutation can favor mitosis (*Fig. 18.8*):

1. *A gene that codes for a promitotic protein becomes abnormally activated.* The normal promitotic gene is called a **proto-oncogene,** and its mutationally activated form is called an **oncogene** (from Greek ὄγκος for "mass"). Mutation in a regulatory site and gene amplification can cause overproduction of a structurally normal gene product. In other cases, a point mutation creates a structurally abnormal "superactive" gene product. Many signaling proteins are normally restrained by a regulatory domain. Loss of this domain through a nonsense mutation, frameshift mutation, or partial gene deletion can produce a truncated protein that no longer responds to negative controls. There are even cases in which a proto-oncogene becomes translocated to a site where it is overexpressed under the influence of the enhancers or promoters of other genes or in which an abnormal protein is created by the fusion of two genes (*Fig. 18.9*).

2. *A gene that codes for a growth-inhibiting protein becomes inactivated.* The normal gene that prevents cancerous growth is called a **tumor suppressor gene.** Oncogene activation changes the cell's growth habits even when only one copy of a proto-oncogene becomes activated, but both copies of a tumor suppressor gene have to be inactivated to cause abnormal growth. From the cell's point of view, *oncogene activations are expressed as dominant traits, whereas inactivations of tumor suppressor genes are expressed as recessive traits.*

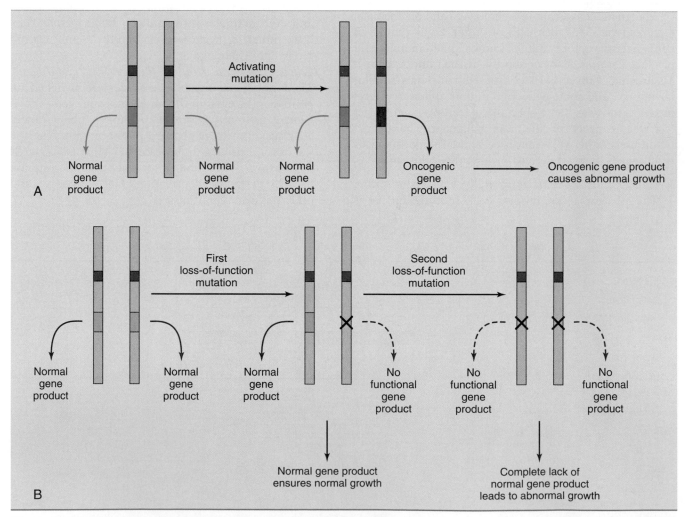

Figure 18.8 Difference between an oncogene and a tumor suppressor gene. **A,** Products of cellular proto-oncogenes (■) are growth-stimulating proteins. A single activating mutation ("gain-of-function" mutation) is sufficient to produce abnormal cell growth. **B,** Products of tumor suppressor genes (■) are growth-inhibiting proteins. Two inactivating mutations ("loss-of-function" mutations) are necessary to produce abnormal cell growth.

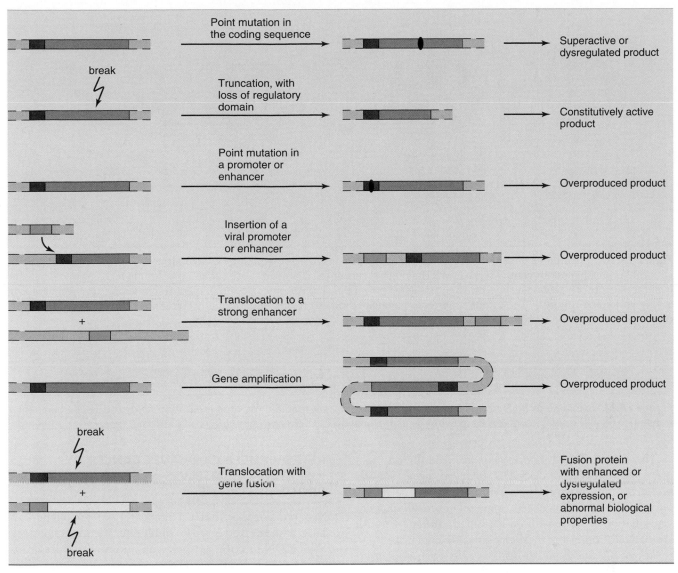

Figure 18.9 Oncogenic activation of a cellular proto-oncogene.

A single mutation is rarely sufficient to convert a cell to malignancy. Common cancers contain a whole assortment of activated oncogenes and inactivated tumor suppressor genes.

Inactivation of tumor suppressor genes is even more important than activation of cellular proto-oncogenes in most spontaneous cancers. This can be demonstrated in cultured cells (*Fig. 18.10*). When a cancer cell is fused with a normal cell, the resulting hybrid cell grows like a normal cell because the intact tumor suppressor gene from the normal cell produces the tumor-suppressing protein. If malignant transformation were caused by dominantly acting oncogenes, the hybrid cells would grow like cancer cells.

SOME RETROVIRUSES CONTAIN AN ONCOGENE

As early as 1910, Peyton Rous established the transmissible nature of a rare connective tissue tumor in chickens. Much later the transmissible agent, now known

as the **Rous sarcoma virus,** was identified as a retrovirus.

Like all retroviruses, Rous sarcoma virus has a small RNA genome with three major genes: *gag, pol,* and *env.* A fourth gene, v-*src* (v for viral, *src* for sarcoma), is not required for viral replication. v-*src* is a **viral oncogene** that causes abnormal proliferation of the virus-infected cells (*Fig. 18.11*). It gets inserted into the host cell DNA along with the rest of the viral genome and is expressed at a high rate under the direction of the viral promoter and enhancer in the long terminal repeats.

The v-*src* oncogene is closely related to a normal cellular gene. Both the normal *SRC* proto-oncogene and the v-*src* oncogene code for a nonreceptor tyrosine protein kinase that is loosely bound to cellular membranes. The normal Src kinase is controlled by growth factor receptors and by proteins in focal adhesions. It stimulates mitosis by phosphorylating many of the same proteins that are phosphorylated by activated growth factor receptors.

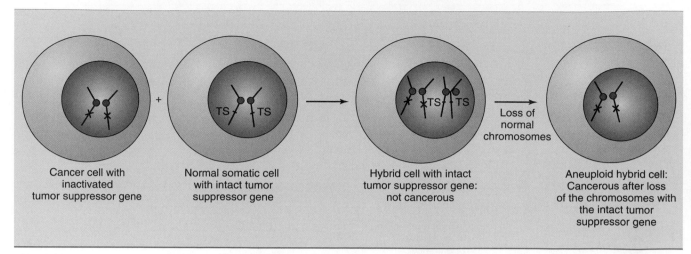

Figure 18.10 Importance of tumor suppressor genes, as demonstrated by somatic cell hybridization. Only the chromosome with the tumor suppressor gene (*TS*) is shown. The original cancer cell is able to cause tumors in immunodeficient mice, but the hybrid cell is not. The hybrid cell becomes tumorigenic only if the chromosomes with the intact tumor suppressor gene are lost during prolonged culturing. The tumor suppressor gene slows down growth. Therefore any cultured cell that loses the chromosomes with the tumor suppressor gene can outgrow the "normal" hybrid cells.

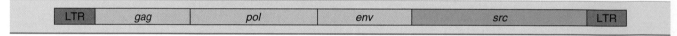

Figure 18.11 Genome of Rous sarcoma virus. *gag, pol,* and *env* are required for virus replication, and *src* causes malignant transformation. The total length of the provirus is approximately 11,000 base pairs. *LTR,* Long terminal repeat.

The virus acquired its oncogene accidentally during a previous infectious cycle. *This hijacked gene, slightly mutated and grossly overexpressed, turns the virus-infected cell into a cancer cell.* Some other retroviral oncogenes besides v-*src* have been identified (*Table 18.1*). All are derived from normal cellular proto-oncogenes.

Retroviral oncogenes transform cells only after insertion into the cellular genome. Rous sarcoma virus is fully infective, but the other oncogenic retroviruses have lost some of the essential retroviral genes during acquisition of their oncogene. They can reproduce only in a cell that is also infected by a second, intact retrovirus that supplies the missing gene products.

RETROVIRUSES CAN CAUSE CANCER BY INSERTING THEMSELVES NEXT TO A CELLULAR PROTO-ONCOGENE

Even retroviruses that do not carry an oncogene can cause cancer. Retroviruses integrate a complementary DNA (cDNA) copy of their genome more or less randomly in the host cell DNA. On occasion, the virus inserts itself next to a cellular proto-oncogene. This can boost the transcription of the proto-oncogene in two ways (*Fig. 18.12*):

1. In **promoter insertion,** the retroviral cDNA is lodged immediately upstream of the proto-oncogene. This

Table 18.1 Examples of Retroviral Oncogenes

Oncogene	Protein Product	Tumor (Species)
sis	Truncated version of platelet-derived growth factor (PDGF)	Simian sarcoma (monkey)
erb-B	Epidermal growth factor (EGF) receptor	Erythroblastosis (chicken)
src	Nonreceptor tyrosine kinase	Sarcoma (chicken)
abl	Nonreceptor tyrosine kinase	Leukemia (mouse), sarcoma (cat)
H-ras } *K-ras* }	Ras protein (a G protein)	Sarcoma, erythroleukemia (rat)
raf	Raf protein (a serine/threonine protein kinase)	Sarcoma (chicken, mouse)
myc	Transcription factor of the helix-loop-helix family	Sarcoma, myelocytoma (chicken)
erb-A	Thyroid hormone receptor	Erythroblastosis (chicken)
fos } *jun* }	DNA-binding proteins, components of the heterodimeric transcription factor AP 1 (activator protein 1)	Sarcoma (mouse, chicken), erythroblastosis (chicken)

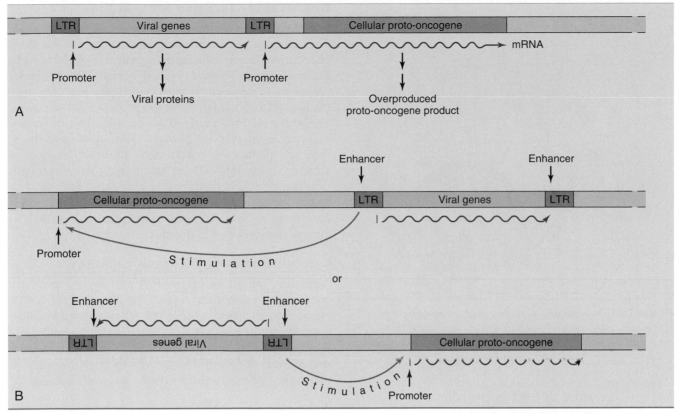

Figure 18.12 Activation of a cellular proto-oncogene by an integrated retrovirus. The two long terminal repeats (*LTRs*) of the provirus are identical. Note that the proto-oncogene is not damaged during retroviral integration, but its rate of transcription is increased. **A,** Promoter insertion. The promoter in the downstream LTR is used for transcription of the proto-oncogene. Messenger RNA. **B,** Enhancer insertion. The viral enhancer stimulates transcription from the normal promoter even if it is inserted downstream of the proto-oncogene or if it is inserted with opposite polarity.

can lead to transcription of the proto-oncogene from the promoter in the downstream long terminal repeat of the virus, at an abnormally high rate and without the usual negative controls.

2. In **enhancer insertion,** the enhancer in the long terminal repeats of the inserted retrovirus stimulates the transcription of a neighboring proto-oncogene. Because enhancers can act over distances of more than 10,000 base pairs, this mechanism works even if the virus is inserted some distance away from the transcriptional start site.

MANY ONCOGENES CODE FOR COMPONENTS OF MITOGENIC SIGNALING CASCADES

Abnormal cell proliferation results when a somatic mutation activates a protein in a mitogenic signaling cascade, keeping it active even in the absence of mitogens. *These mutations are responsible for the mitogen independence of cancers.* Many oncogenes code for components of mitogenic cascades, described as follows.

Growth Factors

Growth factors are uncommon as oncogene products. Only one viral oncogene, the **simian sarcoma** (*sis*) oncogene, is known to code for a growth factor. However, *some spontaneous cancers secrete growth factors that stimulate the tumor cells through an autocrine loop* (**Fig. 18.13**). For example, normal melanocytes respond to fibroblast growth factor (FGF) although they do not produce it, but many malignant melanomas stimulate their own growth by producing FGF.

Receptor Tyrosine Kinases

Receptor tyrosine kinases are overexpressed or structurally altered in many malignant tumors. The *erb-B* oncogene of the avian erythroblastosis virus codes for a truncated version of the epidermal growth factor (EGF) receptor that has lost the extracellular ligand-binding domain (**Fig. 18.14**). The tyrosine protein kinase domain is intact but is no longer controlled by the ligand. It phosphorylates substrates at all times, even in the absence of EGF.

The *neu* oncogene, which is found in some spontaneous neuroblastomas, codes for an aberrant growth

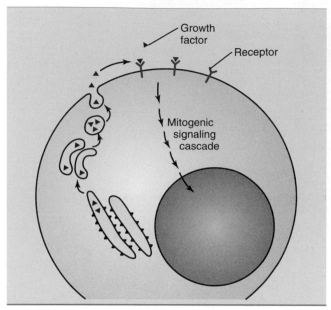

Figure 18.13 Autocrine stimulation of a neoplastic cell. Some tumor cells express both a growth factor and the corresponding receptor, thereby stimulating their own growth.

factor receptor that differs from its normal counterpart by only a single amino acid substitution at one end of the transmembrane helix. This point mutation keeps the protein kinase active at all times, even in the absence of the ligand.

Besides structurally abnormal receptors, overexpressed receptors are common in cancers. Many squamous cell carcinomas and glioblastomas, for example, have an overexpressed or amplified gene for the EGF receptor.

Nonreceptor Tyrosine Protein Kinases

Nonreceptor tyrosine protein kinases include the **Src** protein. The normal Src protein kinase is inhibited by tyrosine phosphorylation. In normal cells, more than 90% of Src is in the inactive, tyrosine-phosphorylated form. The inhibitory phosphate is removed by protein phosphatases only after binding of Src to growth factor receptors or focal adhesions.

Some structurally altered oncogenic forms of Src are mutated at the tyrosine phosphorylation site and therefore are permanently activated. In other cancers, a structurally normal cellular *SRC* gene is overexpressed. Because Src relays mitogenic stimuli from both growth factor receptors and focal adhesions, *SRC* mutations contribute to both mitogen independence and anchorage independence of malignant growth.

Cytoplasmic Serine/Threonine Kinases

Activating mutations of the *RAF1* proto-oncogene are encountered in some tumors. The Raf protein kinase encoded by this gene (see *Fig. 18.4*) is regulated by phosphorylations at multiple sites, some activating and some inhibitory. Oncogenic forms of Raf frequently have point mutations that destroy negative phosphorylation sites, or they have lost part or all of their regulatory domain.

G Proteins

Oncogenic forms of one or another of the *RAS* genes are found in about 30% of all spontaneous cancers, including 30% to 50% of lung and colon cancers and 90% of pancreatic cancers. Most oncogenic forms of Ras have amino acid substitutions that disrupt the protein's GTPase activity or make it unresponsive to GTPase-activating proteins. *These oncogenic Ras proteins have lost their "off" switch and remain in the active state at all times.*

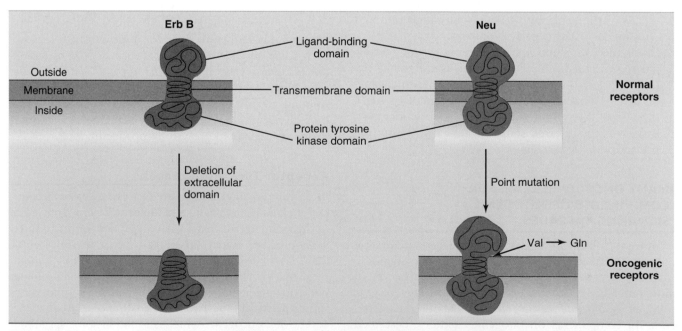

Figure 18.14 Abnormal growth factor receptors as oncogene products. The intracellular protein tyrosine kinase domains of the abnormal receptors are constitutively active, even in the absence of the ligand.

CLINICAL EXAMPLE 18.3: Chronic Myelogenous Leukemia

In most patients with chronic myelogenous leukemia, the malignant cells are distinguished from normal white blood cells by the presence of the **Philadelphia chromosome**, created by a translocation between the long arms of chromosomes 9 and 22. The chromosomal break points are in two genes, *ABL1* and *BCR*, and the translocation creates a fusion gene that starts with a small piece of *BCR* and continues with the major portion of *ABL1*.

ABL1 encodes a nonreceptor tyrosine protein kinase that is located in the nucleus and participates in the regulation of cell proliferation. The fusion protein still has this protein kinase activity but is overexpressed under the control of the *BCR* promoter. This deregulated protein kinase causes abnormal cell proliferation.

Gleevec has been designed specifically as an inhibitor of the Bcr-Abl protein kinase. It is a highly effective drug, although many patients with later stages of the disease develop resistance. The reason for the resistance is that, as the disease progresses, the leukemic cells evolve defects in cell cycle control and a high mutation rate. This increases the likelihood of further mutations in the *BCR-ABL1* gene that make the encoded protein resistant to Gleevec.

Nuclear Transcription Factors

Many cellular oncogenes code for transcriptional regulators. The *MYC* genes, including *MYC* (c-*myc*), *MYCN* (N-*myc*), and *MYCL1* (L-*myc*), are among the most common targets of mitogenic signaling chains from growth factor receptors and focal adhesions (see *Fig. 18.4*). They are among the most commonly mutated genes in cancers.

MYC genes are amplified in many malignant tumors, leading to overproduction of structurally normal gene products. *MYC* is amplified in a great variety of tumors, including many breast, colon, and stomach cancers, small cell lung cancers, and glioblastomas. *MYCN* is amplified in some neuroblastomas, retinoblastomas, and small cell lung carcinomas. *MYCL1* is amplified in some small cell lung carcinomas.

Most of these amplifications occur late during tumor progression and are associated with an aggressively malignant phenotype. The isolated overexpression of a *MYC* gene in an otherwise normal cell can lead to abnormal proliferation but is also likely to cause apoptosis. Therefore *MYC* overexpression is most dangerous in aberrant cells that have lost the capacity for apoptosis.

In **Burkitt lymphoma**, the *MYC* gene on chromosome 8 is translocated into the locus for immunoglobulin κ chains (on chromosome 2), λ chains (chromosome 22), or heavy chains (chromosome 14). *The translocation places the MYC gene into a transcriptionally active spot of the genome, where it is overexpressed under the influence of local enhancers.*

CANCER SUSCEPTIBILITY SYNDROMES ARE CAUSED BY INHERITED MUTATIONS IN TUMOR SUPPRESSOR GENES

Not all cancer-promoting mutations occur in somatic cells. Individuals with a dominantly inherited **cancer susceptibility syndrome** are born with a heterozygous mutation in a tumor repressor gene. *Clinical Example 18.4* describes the prototype for this class of diseases, and *Clinical Examples 9.2, 18.2, 18.5, 18.7, and 18.8* further illustrate this principle. Affected individuals are otherwise healthy, but *when a cell loses the single intact copy of the tumor suppressor gene through a somatic mutation, the cell is at risk of becoming cancerous*. Although the inheritance of the cancer susceptibility is dominant for the patient, for the cell the mutation behaves as a recessive trait because *only cells that have lost both copies of the tumor suppressor gene become cancerous*.

CLINICAL EXAMPLE 18.4: Retinoblastoma

Retinoblastoma is a rare cancer of immature retinal cells (retinoblasts) that afflicts 1:20,000 children during the first 5 years of life. *The major mutation in this cancer is the homozygous inactivation of the retinoblastoma gene (RB1) in the cancer cells*, leading to a defective G_1 checkpoint (see *Fig. 18.3*).

Only the homozygous inactivation of *RB1* in an immature retinal cell causes a tumor. Cells with a single intact copy of the gene are normal. Therefore *two mutations in* RB1 *are required for malignant transformation* (see *Fig. 18.15*).

Sixty percent of patients have the sporadic form of the disease, which presents as a single tumor without family history. The other 40% have the familial form, which is heritable as an autosomal dominant trait and frequently presents with more than one primary tumor. *Patients with the familial form are heterozygous for an inactivating* RB1 *mutation*. Heterozygotes have a 90% chance of getting at least one malignant eye tumor.

In the sporadic form of the disease, *two* mutations in *RB1* have to occur in the retinoblast to eliminate both copies of *RB1* and make the cell cancerous. Only *one* mutation is sufficient for patients who are heterozygous for an inherited mutation. There is a strong chance that this occurs in more than one retinoblast; therefore, the tumors in the inherited disease often are multifocal.

Patients who survive familial retinoblastoma in childhood have an increased risk of osteosarcoma (bone cancer) and perhaps other cancers in later life. Somatic mutations of the *RB1* gene are also seen in many spontaneous cancers other than retinoblastoma, including most small cell lung carcinomas and one third of breast and bladder cancers.

This somatic mutation can be an independent small mutation, but more often it is a large deletion, loss of the normal chromosome, or replacement of the normal gene by the defective one through homologous recombination in mitosis (*Fig. 18.16*). These events lead to loss of heterozygosity both for the tumor suppressor gene and for genetic markers (microsatellite polymorphisms, single-nucleotide polymorphisms) close to it. Loss of heterozygosity in cancer cells is used for mapping of tumor suppressor genes.

Figure 18.15 Homozygous inactivation of the *Rb* gene (■) in the spontaneous and inherited forms of retinoblastoma. **A,** Spontaneous tumor. Two inactivating mutations ("hits") are required for malignant transformation. **B,** Inherited tumor. The first mutation is already present in the germ line. A single somatic mutation in a retinoblast is sufficient for malignant transformation.

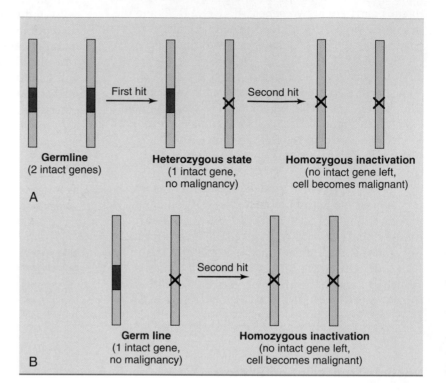

Figure 18.16 Mechanisms for the "second hit" in retinoblastoma (see *Fig. 18.15*) and other cancers. The mechanisms shown in **B, C,** and **D** lead to loss of heterozygosity both for the gene itself and for nearby genetic markers. **D** (somatic recombination in mitosis) is the most common mechanism for tumor suppressor genes that are located far away from the centromere.

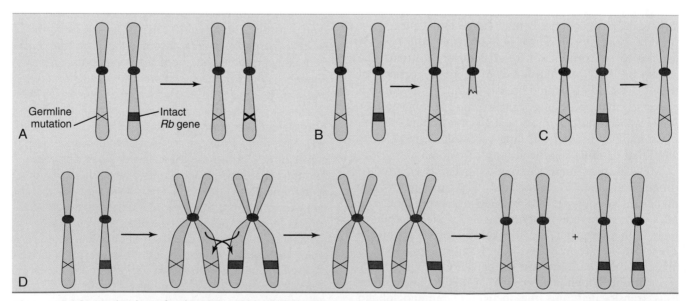

MANY TUMOR SUPPRESSOR GENES ARE KNOWN

Table 18.2 lists some of the more important tumor suppressor genes. The products of these genes include the following:

1. *Negative regulators of the G_1 checkpoint.* The most important examples are pRb and the Cdk inhibitor INK4a.
2. *Proteins that respond to DNA damage.* Proteins that induce senescence or apoptosis in response to DNA damage or oncogene activation are among the most commonly mutated tumor suppressor genes in spontaneous cancers.
3. *Negative regulators of mitogenic or antiapoptotic signaling cascades.* The lipid phosphatase PTEN, which hydrolyzes phosphatidylinositol 3,4,5-trisphosphate, is inactivated in many cancers. Other negative regulators of mitogenic cascades include neurofibromin (see *Clinical Example 18.2*), hamartin-tuberin (*Clinical Example 18.5*), and APC (see *Clinical Example 18.7*).
4. *Cell adhesion molecules.* The loss of E-cadherin, for example, is associated with loss of contact inhibition during the transition from benign tumors to invasive cancer. In many cancers, the E-cadherin gene is not lost by somatic mutation, but it is silenced by DNA methylation.

For many tumor suppressor genes, germline mutations that lead to a dominantly inherited cancer susceptibility syndrome are known. These syndromes are rare, accounting for 4% to 8% of all breast and colon cancers and even fewer of other common cancers.

CLINICAL EXAMPLE 18.5: Tuberous Sclerosis

This dominantly inherited disease (incidence at birth 1:10,000) is characterized by tumorlike growths called "hamartomas," which consist of more than one cell type. Although abnormal growths are found in many organs, the most consequential lesions are in the brain. They lead to epilepsy in 80% of patients and mental deficiency in 50%.

The disease is caused by mutations in either the **TSC1** gene or the **TSC2** gene, which code for the proteins **hamartin** and **tuberin**, respectively. The mutations are heterozygous in normal cells but are homozygous (or hemizygous) in at least one of the tumor-forming cell types.

Hamartin and tuberin form a complex that inhibits the protein kinase **mTOR** (mammalian target of rapamycin) indirectly, through the G protein Rheb (*Fig. 18.17*). mTOR phosphorylates and activates **S6 kinase**, which in turn phosphorylates the ribosomal protein S6. mTOR also phosphorylates the protein **4E-BP1**, which binds to the translational initiation factor 4E. Both effects increase the rate of ribosomal

Continued

Table 18.2 Examples of Tumor Suppressor Genes

Gene	Location*	Encoded Protein	Inherited Disease[†]	Inactivation or Lack of Expression in Spontaneous Tumors
WT1	11p	Transcription factor	Wilms tumor	Some leukemias
NF1	17q	Neurofibromin, a Ras-GTPase activating protein	Neurofibromatosis type 1	Some tumors of neural crest origin
NF2	5q	Cytoskeleton/membrane protein mediating contact inhibition	Neurofibromatosis type 2	Rare
APC	5q	Required for degradation of β-catenin	Adenomatous polyposis coli (APC)	Most colon cancers
CDH1	16q	E-cadherin, a cell adhesion molecule	Hereditary diffuse gastric cancer	Many epithelial cancers
CDKN2A[‡]	9p	INK4a, an inhibitor of Cdk4	Some familial melanomas	Some esophageal and pancreatic cancers
BRCA1	17q	DNA repair	Familial breast and ovarian cancer	Some sporadic breast cancers
BRCA2	13q	Homologous repair of DNA double-strand breaks	Familial breast and ovarian cancer	20%-40% of spontaneous breast cancers
NME1	17q	Transcription factor and protein kinase	?	Many metastatic cancers
VHL	3p	Ubiquitin ligase	von Hippel–Lindau disease	Many renal cell carcinomas
ATM	11q	Protein kinase	Ataxia-telangiectasia	Rare
SMAD4	18q	DNA-binding signal transducer	Juvenile polyposis	Colon and pancreatic cancers
PTEN	10q	Lipid phosphatase	Cowden disease	30%-50% of spontaneous cancers
TSC1	9q	Inhibitor of mTOR	Tuberous sclerosis	Rare
TSC2	16p	Inhibitor of mTOR	Tuberous sclerosis	Rare

*p, Short arm of chromosome; q, long arm.
[†]These diseases are inherited as autosomal dominant traits.
[‡]This gene also encodes Arf, and most mutations affect both gene products.

protein synthesis, including synthesis of the oncogenic proteins cyclin D1 and Myc.

The hamartin-tuberin complex is subject to inhibitory phosphorylations by Akt (protein kinase B) and the MAP kinases ERK1 and ERK2. Thereby it links the major mitogenic signaling cascades to mTOR. Mutations that inactivate hamartin or tuberin lead to overactivity of mTOR and abnormal growth.

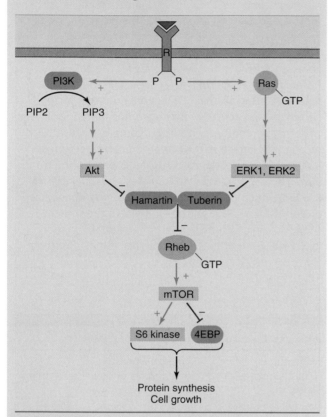

Figure 18.17 Stimulation of ribosomal protein synthesis by growth factor–induced cascades that signal through the tuberous sclerosis (hamartin-tuberin) complex and the protein kinase *mTOR* (mammalian target of rapamycin). Inherited defects in hamartin-tuberin lead to tuberous sclerosis. *4EBP,* Binding protein for translational initiation factor 4E; *PI3K,* phosphoinositide 3-kinase; *PIP₂,* phosphatidylinositol bisphosphate; *PIP₃,* phosphatidylinositol trisphosphate; *R,* growth factor receptor. Ras and Rheb are G proteins. Akt (protein kinase B), ERK1 and ERK2 ("MAP kinases"), mTOR, and S6 kinase are protein kinases.

COMPONENTS OF THE CELL CYCLE MACHINERY ARE ABNORMAL IN MOST CANCERS

The mechanisms of cell cycle control are exceedingly complex, and they vary according to the cell type. For example, there are three different isoforms of cyclin D (D1, D2, and D3) and two proteins related to pRb, p107 and p130, that bind to transcription factors of the E2F type. There are six genes for E2F and two for its dimerization partner DP. With alternative splicing and use of alternative promoters in some of the genes, the actual number of gene products is even greater.

Among the components of the G₁ checkpoint, pRb is abnormal or missing in many spontaneous cancers (**Fig. 18.18** and **Table 18.3**).

Phosphorylation of pRb is controlled by cyclins. *Cyclin D1 is overexpressed in many cancers.* Amplifications of its gene have been found in 43% of squamous cell carcinomas of the head and neck, 34% of esophageal cancers, and 10% of small cell lung cancers and liver cancers. More than 50% of breast cancers overexpress cyclin D1, although in most cases the gene is not amplified. Cdk4, the most important catalytic partner of the D cyclins, also is overexpressed or structurally abnormal in some cancers.

The cyclin-dependent kinases are controlled by Cdk inhibitors. **p21** is induced by p53 (see following) in response to DNA damage. The related inhibitor **p27** is induced by contact inhibition and other growth-inhibiting stimuli from outside the cell but inhibited by mitogen-induced phosphorylations (see **Fig. 18.4**). The complexes of cyclin D with Cdk4 and Cdk6 are inhibited by a whole family of Cdk inhibitors that includes inhibitor of kinase 4a (INK4a), INK4b, INK4c, and INK4d.

Of the Cdk inhibitors, the p53-induced p21 protein is rarely affected in cancers (but see **Clinical Example 18.6**). p27 is underproduced or mislocalized in many cancers, and *mutations that inactivate INK4a are very common.* Fifty-five percent of gliomas and mesotheliomas, 50% of biliary tract cancers, 40% of nasopharyngeal carcinomas, and 30% of esophageal cancers and acute lymphocytic leukemias, as well as many sarcomas and bladder and ovarian cancers, have lost functional INK4a. Some cases of familial melanoma are caused by inactivating germline mutations in the INK4a gene.

Tumors that overexpress cyclin D1 or are deficient in INK4a usually retain pRb, whereas those with pRb loss express cyclin D1 and INK4a normally. Therefore it seems that control of the G₁ checkpoint is defective in most and possibly all cancers, but the molecular defect is variable.

Cyclin-Cdk complexes, Cdk inhibitors, and pRb work mainly through the E2F transcription factors. Therefore overexpression of E2F in tumor cells might be expected. However, E2F mutations actually are rare in human cancers. Cultured cells that are transfected with overexpressed E2F genes do increase their mitotic rate, but this is followed by apoptosis. It is quite possible that activating E2F mutations are not seen in cancers because such mutations lead to apoptosis.

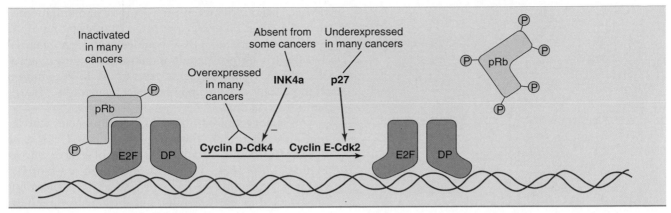

Figure 18.18   Abnormalities of the G_1 checkpoint in human cancers. See text for details. *pRb*, Retinoblastoma protein.

Table 18.3   Cell Cycle Regulators in Cancer

Protein	Normal Function	Abnormalities in Cancer Cells
Cyclin D1	Major G_1 cyclin; responds to mitogens	Overexpressed in many cancers
Cyclin D2 Cyclin D3 }	G_1 cyclins	None known
Cyclin E	Entry into S phase	None known
Cyclin A	Entry into S phase and progression toward mitosis	Rarely overexpressed in cancers
Cdk4	Major catalytic partner of the D cyclins	Amplification in sarcomas and gliomas; activating mutations in some melanomas
p27	Inhibitor of cyclin-Cdk2 complexes	Underexpressed or mislocalized in many cancers
INK4a	Inhibitor of Cdk4, induced by growth-inhibiting stimuli	Deleted or mutated in many cancers
INK4b INK4c } INK4d	Similar to INK4a	None known
pRb	Negative regulator of E2F	Mutated or deleted in many cancers
p107, p130	Similar to pRb	None known
E2F	Transcription factors; regulated by pRb, p107, and p130	None known

CLINICAL EXAMPLE 18.6: Tamoxifen in Breast Cancer

Tamoxifen is an estrogen-related drug with both agonist and antagonist effects on estrogen receptors. Acting as an estrogen antagonist, it inhibits the growth of most hormone-responsive breast cancers. In some cases, however, a breast cancer not only loses the growth-suppressive response to tamoxifen after prolonged treatment but actually becomes stimulated by the drug.

Molecular analysis showed that the response switches from inhibition to stimulation when a cancer cell clone arises that has lost the Cdk inhibitor p21 as a result of somatic mutations. This finding suggests that the antiproliferative effect of tamoxifen is mediated by p21. Growth stimulation appears to be mediated by increased phosphorylation of the estrogen receptor, which enhances estrogen effects on the tumor.

DNA DAMAGE CAUSES EITHER GROWTH ARREST OR APOPTOSIS

When DNA is damaged, the cell practices triage. Cells with good DNA proceed through the cell cycle; those with remediable damage are prevented from DNA replication until the damage is repaired; and irreversibly damaged cells are eliminated by senescence and/or apoptosis.

Responses to DNA damage are coordinated by the nuclear phosphoprotein **p53** (molecular weight 53,000 D), which is encoded by the *TP53* (tumor protein 53) gene. *p53 is a transcription factor that drives the expression of genes for growth arrest, DNA repair, senescence, and apoptosis.* It is present in low concentrations at all times, with a half-life of less than 1 hour in unstressed cells. The reason for its fast turnover is its rapid ubiquitination by the E3 ubiquitin ligase **Mdm2**, which sends p53 to the proteasome (*Fig. 18.19*).

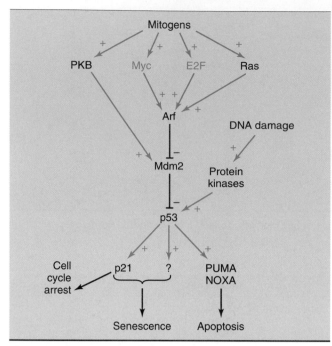

Figure 18.19 Regulation of p53 by DNA damage and activated oncogenes, and its effects on cell fate. Mdm2 inhibits p53 and induces its degradation, and Mdm2 is inhibited by the tumor suppressor protein Arf. Note that many oncogene products (Myc, Ras, E2F) can activate p53 through Arf and Mdm2. This tends to suppress cancer because it leads to apoptosis of oncogenically mutated cells. However, protein kinase B (PKB) inhibits p53 by phosphorylating Mdm2, thereby promoting the entry of Mdm2 into the nucleus.

DNA damage activates several protein kinases. For example, DNA double-strand breaks activate the **"ataxia-telangiectasia mutated" (ATM)** protein kinase (see Chapter 9, *Clinical Example 9.5*). ATM is only one of several damage-activated protein kinases that phosphorylate p53 at up to 12 sites.

These phosphorylations make p53 a poor substrate for MDM2 and allow it to accumulate in the nucleus. In addition to DNA damage, oxidative stress, hypoxia, inhibition of transcription or translation, and telomere erosion can activate p53. These stimuli induce phosphorylations and acetylations of p53.

Oncogene activation stabilizes p53 through the tumor suppressor protein ARF, which inhibits Mdm2. For example, overexpression of the oncogenes *E2F* and *MYC* leads to apoptosis of otherwise normal cells. There is evidence that this is the most important pathway for the antitumor effect of p53.

*Even mild elevations of p53 induce cell cycle arrest by inducing synthesis of the Cdk inhibitor **p21*** (MW 21,000 D), which inhibits the cyclin-Cdk complexes that phosphorylate pRb. Prolonged p21 induction contributes to replicative senescence of the cell.

More substantial elevations of p53 induce the synthesis of proapoptotic proteins, thereby tilting the delicate balance between proapoptotic and antiapoptotic proteins in favor of apoptosis. By preventing DNA replication until all DNA damage has been repaired and by driving irreversibly damaged cells into apoptosis, *p53 has antimutagenic properties.* In recognition of these achievements, p53 has been named the "guardian of the genome."

p53 is not required for normal development. Knockout mice that lack both copies of the *TP53* gene develop normally, although they die of cancer during midlife (*Table 18.4*). Transgenic mice with substantially elevated expression of p53 are resistant to cancer but are afflicted by early senility, but those with three normally regulated copies of *TP53* are cancer resistant without paying the price of accelerated aging.

MOST SPONTANEOUS CANCERS ARE DEFECTIVE IN *p53* ACTION

Mutations in TP53 *have been identified in 50% to 60% of all spontaneous human cancers,* including 70% of colorectal cancers, 50% of lung cancers, and 40% of breast cancers. 70% to 80% of the cancer-associated *TP53* mutations are missense mutations. The mutant forms of the p53 protein are conformationally changed and fail to activate gene transcription.

Are *TP53* mutations carcinogenic because they prevent cell cycle arrest or because they prevent apoptosis? p53-mediated cell cycle arrest depends on the Cdk inhibitor p21. If p21 activation by p53 prevents tumors, mutational inactivation of p21 is expected to cause tumors. Actually, however, such mutations are rare in malignant tumors. Therefore apoptosis appears to be more important than cell cycle arrest for the cancer-preventing effect of p53. This is important for cancer treatment because *tumor cells without functional p53 fail to go into apoptosis after treatment with radiation or DNA-damaging chemicals.*

CLINICAL EXAMPLE 18.7: Li-Fraumeni Syndrome

About 1:30,000 people are born with a heterozygous mutation in the *TP53* gene that is serious enough to cause grossly enhanced cancer susceptibility. This condition, known as **Li-Fraumeni syndrome**, presents with sarcomas, breast cancer, leukemias, brain tumors, and adrenocortical carcinomas. Fifty percent develop invasive cancers by age 30 years and 90% by age 70 years. These cancers develop when the second copy of *TP53* is knocked out by a somatic mutation, making the cell unable to synthesize any functional p53 protein. This is the same two-hit model described for retinoblastoma in *Clinical Example 18.4*.

Many cancer cells that have intact p53 overexpress Mdm2. The *MDM2* gene is a proto-oncogene that is amplified in approximately 30% of all soft tissue

Table 18.4 Abnormalities in Knockout Mice Homozygously Deficient in Cell Cycle Regulators

Protein	Viability of Mice	Tumors
Regulators of G₁ Checkpoint		
Cyclin D1	Viable, but small size and behavioral abnormalities	None
pRb	Death at gestational day 14	—
p27*	Viable, but increased body size and female sterility	Pituitary tumors
INK4a*	Viable	Tumors by age 6 months
E2F1†	Viable, but T-cell hyperplasia	None
Components of DNA Damage Response		
p53	Viable, few abnormalities	Tumors by age 3 months
p21*	Normal	None
Mdm2	Embryos dying at implantation‡	—
Mitogenic Signal Transducers		
N-Ras	Viable, T-cell defects	None
K-Ras	Embryonic lethal	—
Src	Viable, but osteoclast malfunction (osteopetrosis)	None
Myc	Early death	—

*CDK inhibitors.
†Isoform of E2F that is regulated by pRb but not by p107 and p130.
‡Mice lacking both Mdm2 and p53 are viable.

sarcomas as well as in some glial tumors. Although these tumor cells possess structurally normal p53, they show the abnormalities of p53-deficient cells.

THE PI3K/PROTEIN KINASE B PATHWAY IS ACTIVATED IN MANY CANCERS

Many oncogene products, including Myc, Ras, and E2F, can activate p53 (see ***Fig. 18.19***). Therefore in the presence of intact p53, the mutationally activated oncogenes are likely to induce cell cycle arrest, senescence, or apoptosis. Only protein kinase B (PKB, or Akt) suppresses p53 by phosphorylating and thereby activating Mdm2.

The PKB cascade transmits a survival signal that prevents apoptosis by multiple mechanisms. It regulates the synthesis of proapoptotic and antiapoptotic proteins by phosphorylating several transcription factors, including nuclear factor kappa-B (NFκB) and transcription factors of the forkhead family (***Fig. 18.20***). It also phosphorylates and thereby inactivates the proapoptotic protein Bad and the initiator caspase Casp-9.

The genes for PI3K and PKB are amplified in some cancers. The most common alteration, however, is the mutational inactivation of **PTEN**. This lipid phosphatase dampens the signaling cascade by hydrolyzing the phosphatidylinositol 3,4,5-trisphosphate that is generated by PI3K (***Fig. 18.21***). Without PTEN, levels of this lipid remain permanently elevated and PKB remains active at all times. Apoptosis is suppressed, whereas cell cycle progression is stimulated. Between 30% and 50% of spontaneous cancers have lost PTEN through somatic mutations.

The PTEN gene is itself an important target of p53. Its transcription is stimulated by p53, and the resulting inhibition of the PI3K/PKB pathway contributes to p53-induced apoptosis.

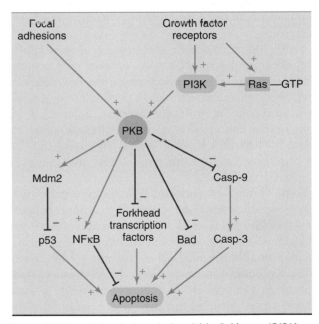

Figure 18.20 Role of phosphoinositide 3-kinase (*PI3K*) and protein kinase B (*PKB*) in the prevention of apoptosis. This signaling pathway prevents apoptosis by multiple mechanisms that involve nuclear transcription factors (p53, NFκB, forkhead proteins), the protease caspase-9, and the proapoptotic protein Bad, which acts as a Bcl-2 antagonist in the intrinsic pathway of apoptosis.

THE PRODUCTS OF SOME VIRAL ONCOGENES NEUTRALIZE THE PRODUCTS OF CELLULAR TUMOR SUPPRESSOR GENES

Retrovirus-induced cancers are extremely rare in humans, but DNA viruses are risk factors for some common cancers. Some DNA viruses promote cancer simply by causing chronic tissue damage and a stimulation of

Figure 18.21 The phosphatase *PTEN* removes a phosphate from phosphatidylinositol 3,4,5-trisphosphate (*PIP₃*) in the plasma membrane, thereby inactivating this second messenger. PTEN is inactivated in many cancers, and the resulting overactivity of protein kinase B prevents apoptosis. *PIP₂*, Phosphatidylinositol 4,5-bisphosphate.

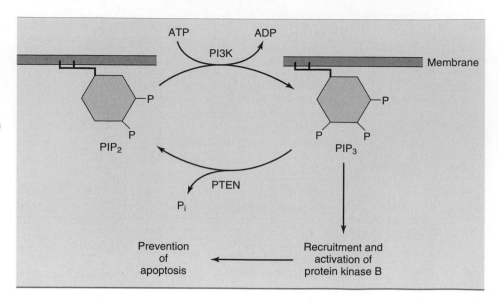

cell division in the surviving cells. This increases the pool of mitotic cells that can potentially acquire oncogenic mutations.

Unlike the retroviruses, *DNA viruses do not habitually integrate their DNA into the host cell genome.* Integration into a host cell chromosome is a rare accident, but when it occurs, it can activate a cellular proto-oncogene by promoter insertion, enhancer insertion, or disruption of a tumor suppressor gene. For example, **hepatitis B virus** carries no oncogene, but the cancers induced by this virus almost always contain integrated viral DNA.

Some strains of the **human papillomavirus** (wart virus), which infects the cells of squamous epithelia in the skin and mucous membranes, have their own oncogenes. This virus is a genetic pauper, with a small circular double-stranded DNA genome of 8000 base pairs that codes for about half a dozen proteins. Viral replication requires DNA polymerases, helicases, and other host cell proteins that are present only in dividing cells.

Therefore the virus can reproduce only by forcing its host to reproduce while avoiding apoptosis. It achieves these two aims through the products of its two oncogenes, *E6* and *E7*. *The viral oncogene products inactivate the products of the major cellular tumor suppressor genes.* E6 binds tightly to p53, and E7 binds to pRb (**Fig. 18.22**). These complexes are destroyed by the proteasome. Untroubled by suicidal thoughts, the virus-infected cell now can sail through the cell cycle, replicating the viral DNA along with its own. Unlike the retroviral oncogenes, the oncogenes of the papillomavirus and other DNA viruses are not related to normal cellular proto-oncogenes.

Ordinarily the papillomavirus produces a common wart, with abnormally proliferating epithelial cells that contain viral DNA as plasmidlike entities. The abnormal growth is benign, and eventually the infected cells either die or lose their virus. In rare cases, however, snippets of viral DNA containing *E6* and/or *E7* become integrated into a host cell chromosome. *These cells cannot lose the viral DNA, and they are at risk for malignant transformation by additional somatic mutations.*

The papillomavirus plays a sinister role in cancer of the uterine cervix. Ninety-three percent of cervical cancers worldwide contain the viral *E6* and/or *E7* genes integrated into their genome. The papillomavirus can be transmitted by sexual intercourse; therefore, cervical cancer can be considered a "sexually transmitted cancer." The viral oncogenes are found not only in cervical cancers but also in more than 50% of other anogenital cancers, many nonmelanoma skin cancers, and some cancers of the oral cavity.

INTESTINAL POLYPS ARE PREMALIGNANT LESIONS

Even cancers that are derived from the same cell type vary greatly in their clinical behavior, depending on their unique combinations of mutations and epigenetic changes. Cancers also change their character over time. For example, a benign mole can turn into a malignant melanoma; a slowly progressive chronic leukemia that had been present for years can suddenly transform into an acute disease ("blast crisis") that kills the patient within weeks; and a long-standing, indolent astrocytoma or oligodendroglioma can mutate into a highly aggressive, rapidly fatal glioblastoma.

These are examples of **tumor progression.** Tumor progression is evolution in the fast track. New variants are formed continuously by mutation, and more malignant

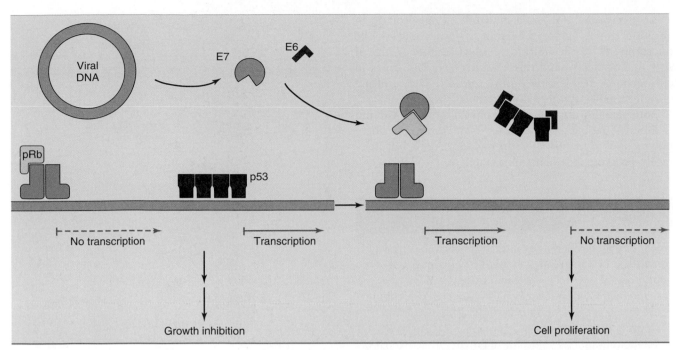

Figure 18.22   Molecular mechanism by which human papillomavirus stimulates the growth of infected cells. The viral *E6* and *E7* proteins bind to the p53 protein and the retinoblastoma protein (*pRb*), respectively, tying them up in inactive complexes. The resulting changes in gene transcription lead to increased cell proliferation and an increased rate of somatic mutations. In ordinary warts, the viral DNA exists as a plasmid-like episome, but in most cervical cancers, the viral *E6* and/or *E7* genes are integrated in the host cell DNA. Although the product of the *E6* gene acts like the product of the cellular *mdm2* gene (see *Fig. 18.19*), the two proteins are not structurally related.

clones with higher mitotic rate, greater invasiveness, or greater resistance to apoptosis take over the ecosystem from less malignant clones. Like all other life forms, neoplastic cells are subject to darwinian selection: *Fast-reproducing variants replace slower-reproducing variants.* This process is accelerated by the genetic instability and high mutation rate that are typical for most cancers.

Colorectal cancers develop from benign polyps. Homozygous inactivation of the **APC** (adenomatous polyposis coli) tumor suppressor gene is sufficient for the formation of a benign polyp. *The product of the APC gene is a negative regulator in the **Wnt** signaling pathway* (**Fig. 18.23**). Normally, a signaling protein from the mitogenic Wnt signaling pathway prevents the destruction of the multifunctional protein **β-catenin**, which is otherwise a constituent of adherens junctions (see Chapter 13). This allows the β-catenin to escape into the nucleus, where it stimulates transcription from the genes for cyclin D1, the Myc protein, and other mitogenic proteins.

Normally, any β-catenin that strays away from its adherens junction is scavenged by a protein complex that contains the APC protein along with a protein kinase. Phosphorylation of β-catenin in this complex marks it for ubiquitination and destruction by the proteasome. *Mutational inactivation of the APC gene prevents the destruction of β-catenin, and the accumulating β-catenin stimulates gene expression permanently.*

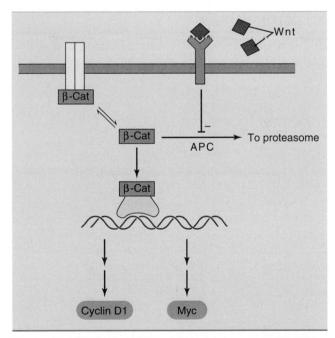

Figure 18.23   Role of the tumor suppressor protein *APC* (adenomatous polyposis coli) in the Wnt signaling cascade. APC is required for the breakdown of β-catenin by the proteasome system. The Wnt pathway prevents the breakdown of β-catenin (*β-Cat*). This allows β-catenin to reach the nucleus, where it stimulates the expression of promitotic genes. Without functional APC, β-catenin cannot be degraded even in the absence of Wnt signaling. Therefore the Wnt pathway is switched on at all times.

Like β-catenin, APC is a multifunctional protein. In addition to scavenging β-catenin, it interacts with the microtubules of the mitotic spindle. Mutant forms of APC fail to do so, and this leads to frequent errors in chromosome segregation during mitosis. The resulting chromosomal instability favors tumor progression.

Some small polyps have normal APC, but β-catenin is mutated to make it resistant to degradation. These polyps look like those with missing APC, but they rarely progress to a malignant state.

CLINICAL EXAMPLE 18.8: Adenomatous Polyposis Coli

Most people develop a few intestinal polyps as they get older, but in dominantly inherited **adenomatous polyposis coli (APC),** the colonic mucosa becomes studded with thousands of polyps. Affected patients have a heterozygous loss of *APC* in all their cells, and inactivation of the single remaining *APC* gene by a somatic mutation is sufficient to create a polyp. Most of these polyps remain benign, but there is an 80% chance that at least one of them eventually will turn malignant. APC accounts for approximately 2% of all colon cancers.

SEVERAL MUTATIONS CONTRIBUTE TO COLON CANCER

Intestinal polyps can evolve into colorectal cancer in a typical sequence of mutational events:

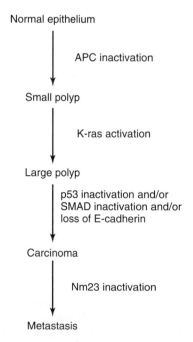

Activating mutations of the **KRAS** proto-oncogene (which codes for the K-Ras protein) are not seen in small polyps but occur in 40% of large polyps and carcinomas.

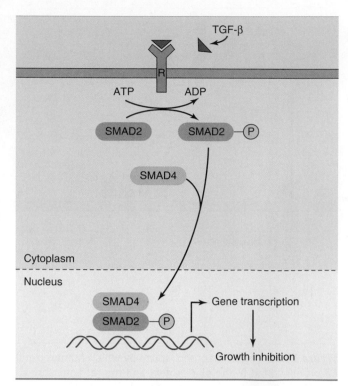

Figure 18.24 Signaling by transforming growth factor β (*TGF-β*), which inhibits the proliferation of cells in the colon mucosa. The TGF-β receptor (*R*) is a ligand-activated serine/threonine protein kinase. Inactivations of this pathway are common in colon cancer and some other cancers.

Loss of a tumor suppressor gene, either **TP53, CDH1 (which codes for E-cadherin),** or **SMAD4,** appears to mark the transition from a benign polyp to a true carcinoma. E-cadherin is a cell adhesion protein that is involved in the contact inhibition of cell growth. SMAD proteins are signal transducers and transcriptional regulators in yet another signaling pathway that is triggered by the antimitotic protein **transforming growth factor β (TGF-β)** (*Fig. 18.24*). The receptor for TGF-β is also mutationally inactivated in about 30% of spontaneous colon cancers.

Little is known about the genetic changes that predispose cancer cells to metastasis. The **NME1** (nonmetastatic-1) gene has frequently been found mutated in metastases but not the primary tumor. The encoded nm23 protein is a signal transducer that, in its unmutated form, prevents metastasis by poorly known mechanisms.

Some molecular markers are useful for the prognosis of cancer. For example, deletion of the long arm of chromosome 18 in the tumor cells signals a loss of the *SMAD4* gene and is associated with decreased survival in patients with colorectal cancer. Reduced or absent expression of the *NME1* gene indicates a high metastatic potential, not only in colorectal cancers but also in many other malignancies.

SUMMARY

Cell cycle progression is coordinated by the cyclin-dependent kinases (Cdks) and their regulatory subunits, the cyclins. The Cdk complexes of cyclins D and E bring the cell through the G_1 checkpoint by phosphorylating and thereby inactivating pRb; cyclin A is most important in S phase; and cyclin B initiates mitosis.

Cells can commit suicide, or apoptosis, under adverse conditions. Apoptosis can be triggered by external stimuli through the extrinsic ("death receptor") pathway and by internal stimuli through the intrinsic ("mitochondrial") pathway.

Growth, differentiation, proliferation, and survival of cells are regulated by extracellular signals. Focal adhesions favor survival and mitosis and are responsible for the anchorage dependence of cell proliferation; contacts with neighboring cells lead to contact inhibition; and soluble extracellular signaling proteins can both stimulate and inhibit growth, mitosis, and apoptosis.

The PI3K/PKB and MAP kinase cascades are the prototypical mitogenic signaling pathways. Both lead to phosphorylation of nuclear transcription factors, thereby regulating the expression of genes for cell cycle progression, differentiation, and apoptosis.

Although some viruses can contribute to cancer, somatic mutations are the most important cause of spontaneous cancers. Oncogenes are mitogenic or antiapoptotic genes that are abnormally activated in cancer cells, and tumor suppressor genes are antiproliferative or proapoptotic genes that are inactivated in cancers. In cancer susceptibility syndromes, inherited defects of tumor suppressor genes contribute to the development of cancer. Cancers tend to become more malignant over time because the cancer cells are subject to frequent mutations and to darwinian selection acting on the mutant cells.

Further Reading

Abukhdeir AM, Vitolo MI, Argani P, et al: Tamoxifen-stimulated growth of breast cancer due to p21 loss, *Proc Natl Acad Sci U S A* 105:288–293, 2008.

Adrain C, Martin SJ: Double knockout blow for caspases, *Science* 311:785–786, 2006.

Aylon Y, Oren M: Living with p53, dying of p53, *Cell* 130:597–600, 2007.

Bozzola M, Travaglino P, Marzilliano N, et al: The shortness of pygmies is associated with severe under-expression of the growth hormone receptor, *Mol Genet Metab* 98:310–313, 2009.

Bracken AP, Ciro M, Cocito A, et al: E2F target genes: unraveling the biology, *Trends Biochem Sci* 29:409–417, 2004.

Broemer M, Meier P: Ubiquitin-mediated regulation of apoptosis, *Trends Cell Biol* 19:130–140, 2009.

Chu IM, Hengst L, Slingerland JM: The Cdk inhibitor p27 in human cancer: prognostic potential and relevance to anticancer therapy, *Nat Rev Cancer* 8:253–267, 2008.

Clarke PR, Allan LA: Cell-cycle control in the face of damage—a matter of life or death, *Trends Cell Biol* 19:89–98, 2009.

Clevers H: Wnt/β-catenin signaling in development and disease, *Cell* 127:469–479, 2006.

Conboy CM, Spyrou C, Thorne NP, et al: Cell cycle genes are the evolutionarily conserved targets of the E2F4 transcription factor, *PLoS ONE* 2(10):e1061, 2007.

Denayer E, de Ravel T, Legius E: Clinical and molecular aspects of RAS related disorders, *J Med Genet* 45:695–703, 2008.

Efeyan A, Garcia-Cao I, Herranz D, et al: Policing of oncogene activity by p53, *Nature* 443:159, 2006.

Engelman JA, Chen L, Tan X, Crosby K, et al: Effective use of PI3K and MEK inhibitors to treat mutant *Kras* G12D and *PIK3CA* H1047R murine lung cancers, *Nat Med* 14:1351–1361, 2008.

Faivre S, Kroemer G, Raymond E: Current development of mTOR inhibitors as anticancer agents, *Nat Rev Drug Discov* 5:671–688, 2006.

Ferner RE: Neurofibromatosis 1, *Eur J Hum Genet* 15:131–138, 2007.

Firestein R, Bass AJ, Kim SY, et al: CDK8 is a colorectal cancer oncogene that regulates β-catenin activity, *Nature* 455:547–551, 2008.

Guicciardi ME, Gores GJ: Life and death by death receptors, *FASEB J* 23:1625–1637, 2009.

Hill R, Wu H: PTEN, stem cells, and cancer stem cells, *J Biol Chem* 284:11755–11759, 2009.

Hirsch E, Braccini L, Ciraolo E, et al: Twice upon a time: PI3K's secret double life exposed, *Trends Biochem Sci* 34:244–248, 2009.

Huang CH, Mandelker D, Schmidt-Kittler O, et al: The structure of a human p110α/p85α complex elucidates the effects of oncogenic PI3Kα mutations, *Science* 318:1744–1748, 2007.

Huang J, Manning BD: The TSC1-TSC2 complex: a molecular switchboard controlling cell growth, *Biochem J* 412:179–190, 2008.

Ikushima H, Miyazono K: TGFβ signaling: a complex web in cancer progression, *Nat Rev Cancer* 10:415–424, 2010.

Inoki K, Guan K-L: Tuberous sclerosis complex, implication from a rare genetic disease to common cancer treatment, *Hum Mol Genet* 18:R94–R100, 2009.

Joerger AC, Fersht AR: Structural biology of the tumor suppressor p53, *Annu Rev Biochem* 77:557–582, 2008.

Kruse J-P, Gu W: Modes of p53 regulation, *Cell* 137:609–622, 2009.

Lupberger J, Hildt E: Hepatitis B virus induced oncogenesis, *World J Gastroenterol* 13:74–81, 2007.

Malumbres M, Barbacid M: Cell cycle kinases in cancer, *Curr Opin Genet Dev* 17:60–65, 2007.

Murphy LO, Blenis J: MAPK signal specificity: the right place at the right time, *Trends Biochem Sci* 31:268–275, 2006.

Nagata S, Hanayama R, Kawane K: Autoimmunity and the clearance of dead cells, *Cell* 140:619–630, 2010.

Pleasance ED, Stephens PJ, O'Meara S, et al: A small-cell lung cancer genome with complex signatures of tobacco exposure, *Nature* 463:184–190, 2010.

Pleasance ED, Cheetham RK, Stephens PJ, et al: A comprehensive catalogue of somatic mutations from a human cancer genome, *Nature* 463:191–196, 2010.

Raaijmakers JH, Bos JL: Specificity in ras and rap signaling, *J Biol Chem* 284:10995–10999, 2009.

Roos WP, Kaina B: DNA damage-induced cell death by apoptosis, *Trends Mol Med* 12:440–450, 2006.

Salmena L, Carracedo A, Pandolfi PP: Tenets of PTEN tumor suppression, *Cell* 133:403–414, 2008.

Soucek L, Evan GI: The ups and downs of Myc biology, *Curr Opin Genet Dev* 20:91–95, 2010.

Vassilev LT: MDM2 inhibitors for cancer therapy, *Trends Mol Med* 13:23–31, 2007.

Vervoorts J, Lüscher-Firzlaff J, Lüscher B: The ins and outs of MYC regulation by posttranslational mechanisms, *J Biol Chem* 281:34725–34729, 2006.

Vogt PK, Kang S, Elslinger M-A, et al: Cancer-specific mutations in phosphatidylinositol 3-kinase, *Trends Biochem Sci* 32:342–349, 2007.

Vousden KH, Prives C: Blinded by the light: the growing complexity of p53, *Cell* 137:413–431, 2009.

Winder T, Lenz H-J: Vascular endothelial growth factor and epidermal growth factor signaling pathways as therapeutic targets for colorectal cancer, *Gastroenterology* 138:2163–2176, 2010.

Wong K-K, Engelman JA, Cantley LC: Targeting the PI3K pathway in cancer, *Curr Opin Genet Dev* 20:87–90, 2010.

Yates JRW: Tuberous sclerosis, *Eur J Hum Genet* 14:1065–1073, 2006.

QUESTIONS

1. An activating mutation in the *ras* gene will most likely

A. Prevent the autophosphorylation of growth factor receptors

B. Inhibit the release of calcium from the endoplasmic reticulum

C. Increase the activity of the MAP kinases

D. Activate the Src protein kinase

E. Reduce the nuclear concentration of cyclin D

2. What type of structural/functional change would be most likely in an oncogenically activated variant of the Ras protein?

A. Inability to interact with the Raf-1 protein kinase

B. Reduced GTPase activity

C. A point mutation in a transmembrane helix

D. Resistance to the phosphatase PTEN

E. An increased ability to tyrosine-phosphorylate proteins

3. Most of the cyclins are induced and repressed periodically during the cell cycle. One cyclin, however, is controlled primarily by mitogens rather than the cell cycle machinery. This mitogen-sensing cyclin is

A. Cyclin A

B. Cyclin B

C. Cyclin C

D. Cyclin D

E. Cyclin E

4. pRb is a major control element of the cell cycle. It normally becomes

A. Transcriptionally induced at the G_1 checkpoint

B. Dephosphorylated at the G_1 checkpoint

C. Phosphorylated at the G_1 checkpoint

D. Phosphorylated at the G_2 checkpoint

E. Transcriptionally induced at the G_2 checkpoint

5. The homozygous loss of a cell cycle regulator or signaling molecule can contribute to malignant transformation. This is most likely for the homozygous loss of

A. The Cdk4 protein kinase

B. Cyclin E

C. E-cadherin

D. A MAP kinase

E. The transcription factor E2F

6. The oncogenes of the human papillomavirus

A. Bind to the host cell DNA, stimulating the transcription of antiapoptotic genes

B. Inactivate the retinoblastoma and p53 proteins

C. Activate growth factor receptors in the absence of the normal ligand

D. Activate cyclin-dependent kinases by direct binding to the catalytic subunit

E. Are protein kinases that phosphorylate many of the same proteins as the MAP kinases

7. The entry into mitosis is accompanied by the phosphorylation of histone H1, chromosomal scaffold proteins, and nuclear lamins. The protein kinase that is responsible for these phosphorylations is activated by

A. The p53 protein

B. Cyclin D

C. The Ras protein

D. The ERK protein kinases through phosphorylation

E. Cyclin B

8. Mutations in the p53 gene are the most common aberrations in spontaneous human cancers. The normal p53 protein affects the cell cycle by

A. Inducing cell cycle arrest and apoptosis in response to DNA damage

B. Inducing the phosphorylation of pRb in response to mitogens

C. Directly inhibiting Cdk inhibitors in response to cell-cell contact and other growth-inhibiting stimuli

D. Increasing the activity of cyclin-dependent protein kinases by inducing their phosphorylation

E. Binding and thereby inactivating the products of many proapoptotic genes

9. **The loss of the lipid phosphatase PTEN is likely to**

A. Increase the activity of the Ras protein

B. Make the cell more vulnerable to apoptosis-inducing stimuli

C. Raise the cellular levels of p53

D. Activate PKB (Akt)

E. Lead to the dephosphorylation of pRb

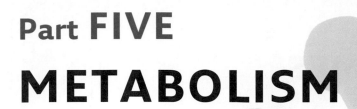

Part FIVE

METABOLISM

Chapter 19
DIGESTIVE ENZYMES

Most dietary nutrients come in the form of large polymeric structures that cannot be absorbed in the intact state. They have to be hydrolyzed by enzymes in the gastrointestinal (GI) tract, and the breakdown products, including monosaccharides, amino acids, and fatty acids, are absorbed. *The whole process of digestion consists of hydrolytic cleavage reactions.*

Approximately 30 g of digestive enzymes is secreted per day. Because each enzyme has a fairly narrow substrate specificity and hydrolyzes only certain bonds, several enzymes have to cooperate in the digestion of complex nutrients (*Table 19.1*).

SALIVA CONTAINS α-AMYLASE AND LYSOZYME

The main function of saliva is not the digestion of nutrients but the conversion of food into a homogeneous mass during mastication. The only noteworthy enzymes in saliva are **α-amylase** and **lysozyme.** Both are **endoglycosidases** that cleave internal glycosidic bonds in a polysaccharide substrate. **Exoglycosidases,** in contrast, cleave glycosidic bonds at the ends.

α-Amylase cleaves α-1,4-glycosidic bonds in starch. Starch occurs in two forms. **Amylose** is a linear polymer of glucose, linked by α-1,4-glycosidic bonds. **Amylopectin,** which usually forms the larger part of the starch in plants, is a branched molecule with α-1,6-glycosidic bonds at the branch points.

α-Amylase does not act on disaccharides and trisaccharides, and it does not cleave α-1,6 bonds. Therefore it produces **maltose, maltotriose,** and **α-limit dextrins** rather than free glucose (*Fig. 19-1*). Maltose is a disaccharide, and maltotriose is a trisaccharide of glucose residues in α-1,4-glycosidic linkage. α-Limit dextrins are oligosaccharides containing an α-1,6-glycosidic bond.

Table 19.1 Dietary Nutrients and Their Fates in the Gastrointestinal Tract

Nutrient	Products Generated	Enzymes	Sites of Digestion
Starch, glycogen	Glucose	α-Amylase, disaccharidases, oligosaccharidases	Saliva, intestinal lumen, brush border
Maltose	Glucose	Glucoamylase, sucrase	
Sucrose	Glucose + fructose	Sucrase	Brush border
Lactose	Glucose + galactose	Lactase	
Proteins	Amino acids, dipeptides, tripeptides	Pepsin, pancreatic enzymes, brush border enzymes	Stomach, intestinal lumen, brush border
Triglycerides	Fatty acids, 2-monoacylglycerol	Pancreatic lipase	Intestinal lumen
Nucleic acids	Nucleosides, bases	DNAses, RNAses	Intestinal lumen
"Fiber": cellulose, lignin, hemicelluloses	Acetate, propionate, lactate, H_2, CH_4, CO_2		Only very limited fermentation by colon bacteria

DNAse, Deoxyribonuclease; *RNAse,* ribonuclease.

Figure 19.1 Pattern of starch digestion by α-amylase. This enzyme acts strictly as an endoglycosidase. It is unable to cleave the bonds in maltose, maltotriose, and the α-limit dextrins. *Arrows* indicate cleavage sites.

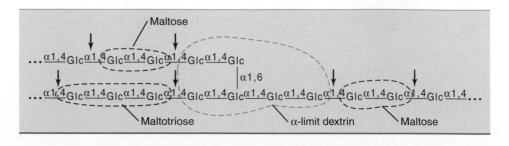

The salivary α-amylase is active at the normal salivary pH of 6.5 to 7.0 but is rapidly denatured in the acidic environment of the stomach. Therefore it makes only a minor contribution to starch digestion. Its main function is to keep the teeth clean by dissolving starchy bits of food that remain lodged between the teeth after a meal. Cancer patients whose salivary glands have been destroyed by radiation therapy develop rapid tooth decay.

The other salivary endoglycosidase, **lysozyme,** hydrolyzes β-1,4-glycosidic bonds in the bacterial cell wall polysaccharide **peptidoglycan** (*Fig. 19.2*). *Lysozyme kills some types of bacteria.* However, other bacteria are resistant because their peptidoglycan is protected from the enzyme by other cell wall components or, in the case of gram-negative bacteria, by an overlying outer membrane. The members of the normal bacterial flora in the mouth (including those that cause bad breath) are resistant to lysozyme. However, many bacteria from other ecosystems are killed by lysozyme, and animals make use of this effect by licking their wounds. They use their saliva as an antiseptic.

PROTEIN AND FAT DIGESTION START IN THE STOMACH

With a pH close to 2.0, the stomach is a forbidding place. The proton gradient between gastric juice and the blood—an almost million-fold concentration difference—is the steepest ion gradient anywhere in the body. The gastric acid has three major functions:

1. *It kills most microorganisms.* Because solid foods remain in the stomach far longer than do fluids, pathogens are more likely to establish an intestinal infection when they are ingested in water or other fluids than in solid food. People with achlorhydria (lack of gastric acid) and those who have had a gastrectomy (surgical removal of the stomach) have an increased risk of intestinal infections.

2. *It denatures dietary proteins.* This helps with protein digestion because it makes the peptide bonds more accessible for proteases.

3. *It is required for the action of pepsin.* Pepsin is a protease with an unusually low optimum pH of 2.0. It is considered an **endopeptidase,** but it also cleaves peptide bonds at the ends of the polypeptide. Pepsin cleaves only some peptide bonds, with a preference for bonds formed by the amino groups of large hydrophobic amino acids. Therefore it produces a mix of oligopeptides with some free amino acids. This mix is known as **peptone.** Protein digestion has to be completed by other enzymes in the small intestine (*Table 19.2*).

In addition to protein, 10% to 20% of dietary fat is digested by an acid-tolerant gastric lipase in the stomach. Neither gastric acid nor the gastric enzymes are essential for life, and patients can live reasonably normal lives after total gastrectomy.

THE PANCREAS IS A FACTORY FOR DIGESTIVE ENZYMES

Pancreatic juice supplies a cocktail of enzymes for the digestion of nearly all major nutrients. α-**Amylase** is

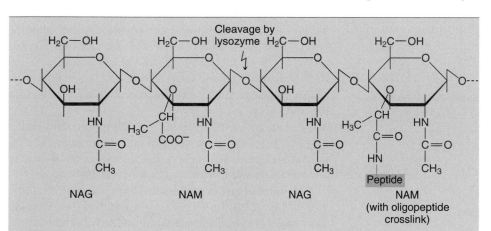

Figure 19.2 Structure of peptidoglycan, the substrate of lysozyme. NAG, *N*-acetylglucosamine; NAM, *N*-acetylmuramic acid.

Table 19.2 Enzymes of Protein Digestion

Enzyme	Source	Type	Catalytic Mechanism	Cleavage Specificity
Pepsin	Stomach	Endopeptidase	Carboxyl protease	NH side of hydrophobic amino acids
Trypsin	Pancreas	Endopeptidase	Serine protease	CO side of basic amino acids
Chymotrypsin	Pancreas	Endopeptidase	Serine protease	CO side of hydrophobic amino acids
Elastase	Pancreas	Endopeptidase	Serine protease	CO side of small amino acids
Carboxypeptidase A	Pancreas	Carboxypeptidase	Metalloprotease (Zn^{2+})	Hydrophobic amino acids at C-terminus
Carboxypeptidase B	Pancreas	Carboxypeptidase	Metalloprotease (Zn^{2+})	Basic amino acids at C-terminus

secreted in large amounts. This enzyme is different from the salivary α-amylase, which has a slightly different structure and is encoded by a separate gene. Closely related enzymes that catalyze the same reaction but differ in molecular structure, physical properties, and reaction kinetics are called **isoenzymes.**

For protein digestion, the pancreas supplies the endopeptidases (and exopeptidases) **trypsin, chymotrypsin,** and **elastase.** All three are serine proteases (see Chapter 4), but with different cleavage specificities (see *Table 19.2*). Their action is complemented by exopeptidases. **Carboxypeptidase A** cleaves nonpolar amino acids from the carboxyl end of peptides, and **carboxypeptidase B** cleaves basic amino acids. Other pancreatic enzymes include **pancreatic lipase,** various **phospholipases,** and **nucleases.**

FAT DIGESTION REQUIRES BILE SALTS

Triglycerides (also known as "fat") are almost totally insoluble in water. They form large fat droplets that provide only a small surface area for enzymatic attack, and the first task in fat digestion is to disperse the fat into smaller particles with a larger surface/volume ratio.

During mastication, fat is emulsified with the help of dietary phospholipids and proteins. In the stomach, this process continues with the help of fatty acids, monoglycerides, and diglycerides formed by the gastric lipase.

In the small intestine, **pancreatic lipase** and **colipase** bind to the surface of the emulsion droplets. The colipase maintains the activity of the lipase in the presence of bile salts. Pancreatic lipase hydrolyzes dietary triglycerides to free fatty acids and 2-monoacylglycerol (2-monoglyceride):

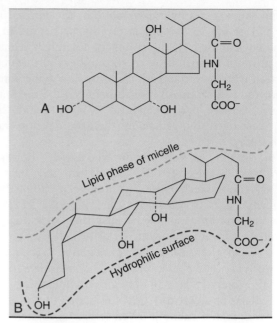

Figure 19.3 Structure of glycocholate, the most abundant bile salt in humans. The protonated forms of the bile salts are called "bile acids." **A,** Structure. **B,** Stereochemistry. Note that the molecule has a hydrophilic surface and a hydrophobic surface.

Unlike the triglycerides, *the products of fat digestion are slightly soluble in water.* Their efficient absorption requires **mixed micelles,** which are formed with the help of **bile salts** (deprotonated bile acids) (*Fig. 19.3*). Between 20 and 50 g of bile salts reaches the intestine every day.

The mixed micelles look like little shreds of lipid bilayer. The products of fat digestion form the two layers of the bilayer, and the bile salt covers the hydrophobic edges. *Mixed micelles ferry the lipids through the unstirred layer overlying the intestinal mucosa.* Being slightly water soluble, fatty acids and 2-monoglyceride diffuse from the micelles to the microvilli for uptake into the mucosal cells (*Fig. 19.4*).

Bile salts are also needed for the absorption of other dietary lipids, including cholesterol and the fat-soluble vitamins. In general, *lipids with the lowest water solubility are most dependent on bile salts for their absorption.*

Fat malabsorption can result from pancreatic failure, lack of bile salts due to biliary obstruction, or extensive intestinal diseases. Pancreatic failure leads to bulky, fatty, floating stools that contain undigested triglycerides. This condition is called **steatorrhea.** Deficiencies of fat-soluble vitamins can occur because the vitamins are excreted in the stools along with the fat rather than being absorbed. A lack of bile salts has similar consequences, but in this case most of the "fat" in the stools consists of unabsorbed fatty acids, monoglycerides, and diglycerides.

Fat malabsorption can be treated with oral supplements of pancreatic enzymes in patients with pancreatic failure and with bile salts in patients with biliary obstruction.

Triglyceride

Pancreatic lipase (+ colipase)

2-Monoacylglycerol   Fatty acids

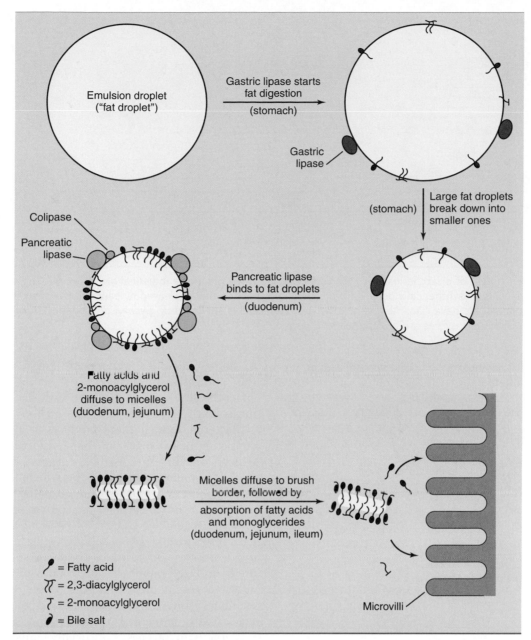

Figure 19.4 Sequence of events in fat digestion. A small amount of fat is hydrolyzed by gastric lipase in the stomach, but pancreatic lipase is the major enzyme of fat digestion. Bile salts containing micelles are required for efficient absorption of fatty acids, monoglycerides, and other dietary lipids.

SOME DIGESTIVE ENZYMES ARE ANCHORED TO THE SURFACE OF THE MICROVILLI

The crypts of Lieberkühn in the small intestine secrete between 1 and 2 L of a watery fluid every day, but this secretion is almost devoid of digestive enzymes. However, there are enzymes attached to the luminal surface of the mucosal cells. This surface, known as the intestinal **brush border,** measures more than 200 m^2 because of the extensive folding of the villi and the innumerable microvilli. The brush border enzymes are firmly anchored to the surface of the microvilli, with their catalytic domains protruding into the intestinal lumen (*Fig. 19.5*).

Several **peptidases** (proteases) are present on the brush border, including aminopeptidases, endopeptidases, carboxypeptidases, and dipeptidases that act on the small oligopeptides formed by pepsin and the pancreatic enzymes. Nevertheless, a sizable portion of the dietary protein is absorbed not in the form of free amino acids but as dipeptides and tripeptides. These are further hydrolyzed to free amino acids by cytoplasmic enzymes in the mucosal cells.

Disaccharidases and **oligosaccharidases** (*Table 19.3*) hydrolyze sucrose and lactose, as well as the maltose, maltotriose, and α-limit dextrins that are formed by the action of α-amylase on starch.

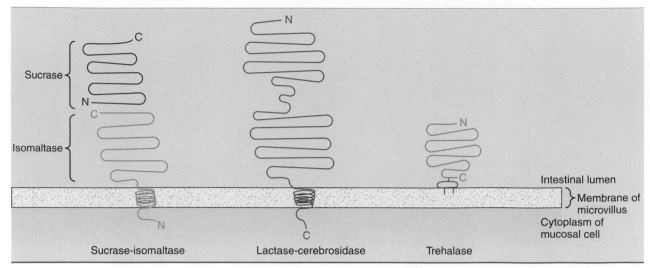

Figure 19.5 Anchoring of disaccharidases to the surface of the microvilli in the intestinal brush border. The sucrase-isomaltase complex is biosynthetically derived from a single polypeptide that is cleaved by pancreatic proteases. Isomaltase and lactase/cerebrosidase have transmembrane α-helices. Trehalase is anchored by glycosyl phosphatidylinositol (see *Fig. 12.11*). All of these enzymes are glycoproteins.

Table 19.3 Disaccharidases and Oligosaccharidases of the Intestinal Brush Border

Enzyme	Cleavage Specificity
Glucoamylase	Maltose, maltotriose; acts as exoglycosidase on α-1,4 bonds at the nonreducing end of starch and starch-derived oligosaccharides
Sucrase	Sucrose, maltose, maltotriose
Isomaltase	α-1,6 Bonds in isomaltose and α-limit dextrins
Lactase*	Lactose; also cellobiose†
Cerebrosidase*	Glucocerebroside, galactocerebroside
Trehalase	Trehalose‡

*The lactase and cerebrosidase activities reside in two different globular domains of the same polypeptide (see Fig. 19.5).
†Cellobiose is a disaccharide of two glucose residues in β-1,4-glycosidic linkage.
‡Trehalose is a disaccharide of two glucose residues in α,α′-1,1-glycosidic linkage; it is common only in mushrooms and insects.

POORLY DIGESTIBLE NUTRIENTS CAUSE FLATULENCE

In comparison with other animals, humans have a substandard digestive system. Although 95% of dietary fat and variable proportions of other dietary lipids are utilized, the efficiency of starch digestion is only 70% to 90% depending on the dietary source. Protein digestion is variable. Keratins and some plant proteins are incompletely digested, and between 5 to 20 g of protein is excreted in the stools every day. This includes both undigested dietary protein and protein from digestive enzymes and desquamated mucosal cells.

Many plant polymers, including cellulose, hemicelluloses, inulin, pectin, lignin, and suberin, are resistant to human digestive enzymes. A small percentage of this undigestible "dietary fiber" is hydrolyzed and anaerobically fermented by the lush bacterial flora of the colon.

Bacterial fermentation produces a flammable gas consisting of **hydrogen, methane,** and **carbon dioxide,** which contributes to global warming because of its methane content. Other products include the organic acids **acetate, propionate, butyrate,** and **lactate.** Most of this is absorbed through the colonic mucosa.

Some vegetables contain oligosaccharides in which galactose forms an α-1,6-glycosidic bond. These α-galactosides are resistant to digestive enzymes but are hydrolyzed rapidly by intestinal bacteria. Raffinose and stachyose in beans and peas are the most notorious examples (*Fig. 19.6*). The released oligosaccharides are rapidly fermented to acids and gas by colon bacteria, with harmless but socially embarrassing flatulence. The acids can cause abdominal discomfort through their acidity and diarrhea through their osmotic activity.

Lactose is another carbohydrate that is not always well digested (see *Clinical Example 19.1*).

MANY DIGESTIVE ENZYMES ARE RELEASED AS INACTIVE PRECURSORS

Among the digestive enzymes, *proteases and phospholipases are dangerous.* They must be kept chained and muzzled until they reach the lumen of the GI tract, lest they attack proteins and membrane lipids in the cells of their birth.

To prevent self-digestion, the dangerous enzymes (but not lipases and glycosidases) are synthesized and

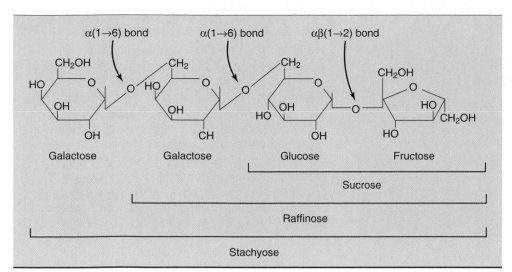

Figure 19.6 Structures of raffinose and stachyose. The α-1,6 bonds formed by galactose are undigestible but are hydrolyzed by bacterial α-galactosidases, leading to excessive bacterial growth and flatulence.

secreted as inactive precursors called **zymogens.** The zymogens are synthesized at the rough endoplasmic reticulum, stored in secretory vesicles, released by exocytosis, and activated by selective proteolytic cleavage in the lumen of the GI tract.

CLINICAL EXAMPLE 19.1: Lactose Intolerance

Lactose ("milk sugar") is abundant only in milk and milk products. Accordingly, the activity of intestinal lactase is maximal in infants. Some people maintain abundant lactase throughout life and can digest almost any amount of lactose. In other individuals, lactase declines to only 5% to 10% of the original level, resulting in **lactose intolerance,** which consists of flatulence and other intestinal symptoms after the consumption of more than 200 to 500 ml of milk.

Lactose intolerance is not an important clinical problem because most people have enough common sense to adjust their milk consumption to their digestive capacity. Lactose-free milk products and lactase in pill and capsule forms are commercially available. The latter products contain lactases of microbial origin.

In most parts of the world, a majority of the population is lactose intolerant. Persistent lactase prevails only in Europeans and in some desert nomads of Arabia and Africa (*Table 19.4*).

In Europe, lactase persistence is caused by a point mutation in an enhancer 13,910 base pairs upstream of the start of the lactase gene. This genetic variant became common only after the introduction of cattle raising and milking; it has not been found in fossil DNA from Europeans dated to between 5000 and 5800 years BC. It appears that lactase persistence was selected because in Neolithic Europe, those who

Table 19.4 Approximate Prevalence of Lactase Restriction (Nonpersistent Lactase) in Various Populations

Population/Country	Percent with Low Lactose-Digesting Capacity
Sweden	1
Britain	6
Germany	15
Greece	53
Morocco	78
Tuareg (Niger)	13
Fulani (Nigeria, Senegal)	0–22
Ibo, Yoruba (Nigeria)	89
Saudi Arabia: Bedouins	23
Saudi Arabia: Other Arabs	56
India (different areas)	27–67
Thailand	98
China	93–100
North American Indians	63–95

could digest the milk of their animals were slightly more likely to survive and reproduce than were those who could not. Thus a Roman anthropologist reported about the Germans: "They do not eat much cereal food, but live chiefly on milk and meat...." (Caesar, *Gallic War,* 4.1).

Biochemically, lactose intolerance can be demonstrated in two ways. In the **lactose tolerance test,** the blood glucose level is determined before and after ingestion of 50 g of lactose. A rise in blood glucose of less than 20 mg/100 ml signals a delay in the absorption of lactose-derived glucose and galactose. Alternatively, the hydrogen content of breath can be determined before and after an oral lactose load. Increased hydrogen signals the fermentation of undigested lactose by colon bacteria.

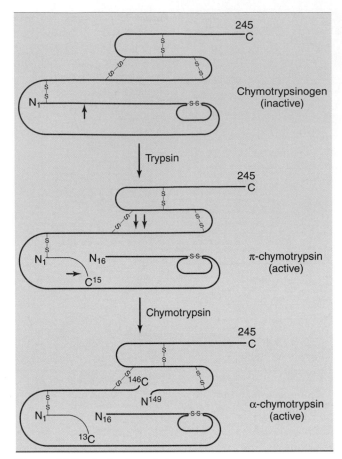

Figure 19.7 Activation of chymotrypsinogen to chymotrypsin. These reactions take place in the duodenum. Although π-chymotrypsin is fully active, α-chymotrypsin is the predominant form in the small intestine.

Pepsinogen, which is secreted from the chief cells of the stomach, activates itself to pepsin by cleavage of a 44–amino acid peptide from its amino terminus. This reaction requires a pH less than 5 and therefore takes place only in the lumen of the stomach. Even after this activating reaction, *pepsin is essentially inactive at pH values close to 7.0.*

The pancreatic zymogens include **trypsinogen, chymotrypsinogen** (*Fig. 19.7*), **proelastase, procarboxypeptidases,** and **prophospholipases.** *All of these zymogens are activated by trypsin in the intestinal lumen.* Trypsinogen itself is activated by either trypsin or the duodenal enzyme **enteropeptidase.**

The pancreas protects itself not only by synthesizing the dangerous enzymes as inactive zymogens but also by a **trypsin inhibitor,** a small (6-kD) polypeptide that binds very tightly (but noncovalently) to trypsin. It is present in the cytoplasm of the acinar cells and in the ductal system, in which it inactivates any trypsin that is accidentally activated within the organ.

CLINICAL EXAMPLE 19.2: Acute Pancreatitis

The accidental activation of zymogens within the pancreatic duct system leads to **acute pancreatitis,** a life-threatening condition in which the pancreas digests itself. The enzymes even spill over into the abdominal cavity, where the pancreatic lipase finds ample substrate in the intraabdominal adipose tissue.

The cause of acute pancreatitis remains unknown in most cases. It is associated with alcoholism, and a gallstone blocking the ampulla of Vater can be demonstrated in some cases. Acute pancreatitis is diagnosed by determining the presence of lipase or amylase in the blood (see Chapter 15).

SUMMARY

Digestive enzymes are hydrolases that degrade macromolecular nutrients into their constituent monomers. Because the digestive enzymes have fairly narrow cleavage specificities, many enzymes have to cooperate for the complete digestion of nutrients.

Proteins are digested by pepsin in the stomach and by the pancreatic enzymes trypsin, chymotrypsin, elastase, carboxypeptidase A, and carboxypeptidase B in the lumen of the small intestine. Their digestion is completed by peptidases on the surface of the intestinal mucosal cells. Starch is digested to maltose, maltotriose, and α-limit dextrins by the pancreatic α-amylase. Together with sucrose and lactose, these products are hydrolyzed by brush border enzymes. Dietary triglycerides are digested to free fatty acids and 2-monoacylglycerol by pancreatic lipase, and these breakdown products are absorbed with the help of bile salts.

Digestive enzymes are products of the "secretory pathway." Proteases and phospholipases are generally synthesized as inactive zymogens, which are activated by partial proteolysis in the lumen of the GI tract.

Further Reading

Aloulou A, Carrière F: Gastric lipase: an extremophilic interfacial enzyme with medical applications, *Cell Mol Life Sci* 65:851–854, 2008.

Armand M: Lipases and lipolysis in the human digestive tract: where do we stand? *Curr Opin Clin Nutr Metabol Care* 10:156–164, 2007.

Burger J, Kirchner M, Bramanti B, et al: Absence of the lactase-persistence-associated allele in early Neolithic Europeans, *Proc Natl Acad Sci U S A* 104:3736–3741, 2007.

Ingram CJE, Mulcare CA, Itan Y, et al: Lactose digestion and the evolutionary genetics of lactase persistence, *Hum Genet* 124:579–591, 2009.

Perry GH, Dominy NJ, Claw KG, et al: Diet and the evolution of human amylase gene copy number variation, *Nat Genet* 39:1256–1260, 2007.

Singh H, Ye A, Horne D: Structuring food emulsions in the gastrointestinal tract to modify lipid digestion, *Progr Lipid Res* 48:92–100, 2009.

QUESTIONS

1. **A Chinese student at a U.S. medical school complains to the school physician that he suffers from bouts of flatulence and diarrhea shortly after each breakfast. His usual breakfast consists of two candy bars, a small bag of peanuts, and three glasses of fresh milk. He never had digestive problems in his home country, where his diet consisted only of vegetables, meat, and rice. He has most likely a low level of**

   A. Pepsin
   B. Pancreatic lipase
   C. Lactase
   D. Trypsin
   E. α-Amylase

2. **Patients who had a pancreatectomy (surgical removal of the pancreas) should take supplements of digestive enzymes with each meal. These enzyme supplements need *not* contain**

   A. α-Amylase
   B. Proteases
   C. Lipase
   D. Disaccharidases

Chapter 20
INTRODUCTION TO METABOLIC PATHWAYS

The metabolic activities of cells are dictated by two major concerns:

1. *The cell has to synthesize its macromolecules.* Proteins have to be synthesized from amino acids; complex carbohydrates from monosaccharides; membrane lipids from fatty acids and other building blocks; and nucleic acids from nucleotides. These biosynthetic processes are called **anabolic.** They require metabolic energy, usually in the form of adenosine triphosphate (ATP).
2. *The cell has to generate metabolic energy.* Nutrients must be oxidized to supply energy in the form of ATP for biosynthesis, active membrane transport, cell motility, and muscle contraction. Degradative processes are called **catabolic.** Most ATP is produced during the end-oxidation of metabolic intermediates to CO_2 and H_2O in the mitochondria (pathway ⑤ in *Fig. 20.1*).

Therefore an unsuspecting nutrient molecule entering a cell has two alternative fates: either it becomes incorporated into a cellular macromolecule or it is oxidized for the generation of ATP.

The biosynthesis of cellular macromolecules has to be balanced by their degradation (pathway ② in *Fig. 20.1*). Under **steady-state** conditions, the rates of synthesis and degradation are balanced and the amount of the macromolecule remains constant. Different nutrients can also be interconverted through metabolic intermediates. For example, most amino acids can be converted to glucose, and glucose can be converted to amino acids and fatty acids (pathways ③ and ④ in *Fig. 20.1*).

ALTERNATIVE SUBSTRATES CAN BE OXIDIZED IN THE BODY

Several nutrients can be used as a source of metabolic energy. During their oxidation to carbon dioxide and water, carbohydrates yield about 4 kcal/g, triglycerides 9.3 kcal/g, proteins between 4.0 and 4.5 kcal/g, and alcohol 7.1 kcal/g. Molecular oxygen is consumed during oxidative metabolism, and carbon dioxide is produced:

$$C_6H_{12}O_6 + 6\,O_2 \rightarrow 6\,CO_2 + 6\,H_2O$$
Glucose

$$C_{51}H_{98}O_6 + 72\tfrac{1}{2}\,O_2 \rightarrow 51\,CO_2 + 49\,H_2O$$
Tripalmitate, a triglyceride

The stoichiometry of O_2 consumption and CO_2 production is described by the **respiratory quotient (RQ):**

$$RQ = \frac{CO_2\ (produced)}{O_2\ (consumed)}$$

The RQ for the oxidation of carbohydrates is 1.0; for fat, about 0.7; and for protein, about 0.8.

Most cells have a choice among alternative substrates, including glucose, fatty acids, and amino acids.

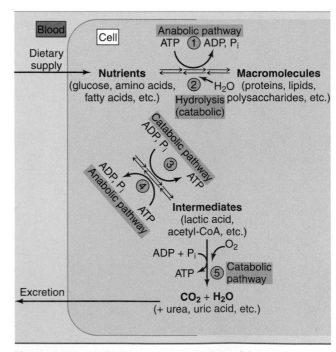

Figure 20.1 Major types of metabolic activity in the cell. *ADP,* Adenosine diphosphate; *ATP,* adenosine triphosphate; *CoA,* coenzyme A; *P_i,* inorganic phosphate.

Others are more specialized. A few cell types, such as neurons and red blood cells, depend mainly or exclusively on glucose for their energy needs.

METABOLIC PROCESSES ARE COMPARTMENTALIZED

In the cell, metabolic processes are compartmentalized. Each organelle has its own enzymatic outfit and metabolic activities (*Fig. 20.2*).

1. The **cytoplasm** contains biosynthetic pathways and some nonoxidative catabolic pathways, and it is the place where glycogen and fat are stored as energy reserves.
2. The **endoplasmic reticulum (ER)** and **Golgi apparatus** are concerned with the synthesis and processing of proteins and membrane lipids.

3. **Lysosomes** are filled with hydrolytic enzymes for the degradation of macromolecules. They hydrolyze endocytosed materials and some cellular macromolecules.
4. **Peroxisomes** are specialized organelles for some oxidative reactions.
5. **Mitochondria** generate more than 90% of the cell's ATP by oxidative phosphorylation.

FREE ENERGY CHANGES IN METABOLIC PATHWAYS ARE ADDITIVE

Complex metabolic transactions, such as the synthesis of glucose from lactate and the oxidation of lactate to carbon dioxide and water, cannot occur in a single step. They require a whole sequence of reactions that form a **metabolic pathway**. *The direction in which the pathway proceeds depends on the sum of the free energy changes of the individual reactions.* Consider the simple pathway:

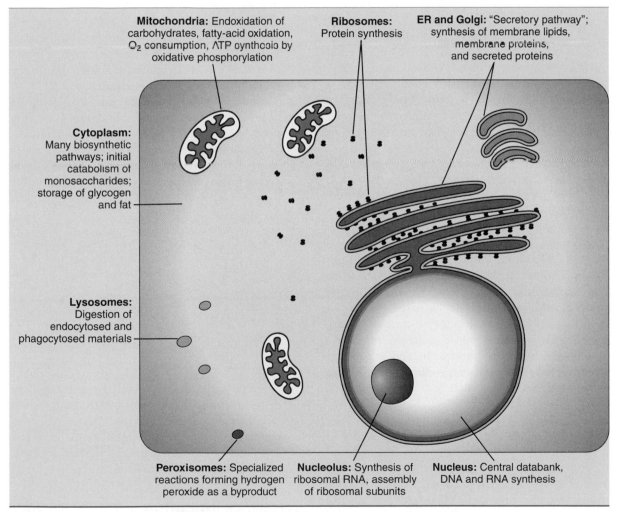

Figure 20.2   Metabolic functions of the major organelles. *ATP*, Adenosine triphosphate; *DNA*, deoxyribonucleic acid; *ER*, endoplasmic reticulum; *RNA*, ribonucleic acid.

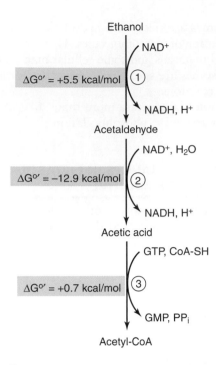

Ethanol

$\Delta G^{0'} = +5.5$ kcal/mol (1)

NAD$^+$

NADH, H$^+$

Acetaldehyde

$\Delta G^{0'} = -12.9$ kcal/mol (2)

NAD$^+$, H$_2$O

NADH, H$^+$

Acetic acid

$\Delta G^{0'} = +0.7$ kcal/mol (3)

GTP, CoA-SH

GMP, PP$_i$

Acetyl-CoA

where $\Delta G^{0'}$ = standard free energy change, and PP$_i$ = inorganic pyrophosphate. Two of the three reactions have an unfavorable equilibrium with a positive $\Delta G^{0'}$. Nevertheless, the sum of the free energy changes is negative at -6.7 kcal/mol. Therefore, under standard conditions, the pathway will turn ethanol into acetyl coenzyme A (acetyl-CoA) rather than turn acetyl-CoA into ethanol.

However, the actual free energy change is quite different from the standard free energy change. For example, reaction (1) has a very unfavorable equilibrium. With equal concentrations of NAD$^+$ and NADH, there would be only one molecule of acetaldehyde at equilibrium for every 10,000 molecules of ethanol (see Chapter 4)! However, under aerobic conditions, [NAD$^+$] is always far higher than [NADH]. When NAD$^+$ is 100 times more abundant than NADH, one molecule of acetaldehyde is expected to be in equilibrium with 100 molecules of ethanol. Therefore this seemingly "irreversible" reaction actually is reversible under cellular conditions. Indeed, it proceeds in the right direction because its product, acetaldehyde, is rapidly mopped up by the next enzyme in the pathway.

Reaction (3) appears freely reversible with its $\Delta G^{0'}$ of +0.7 kcal/mol. In the cell, however, the GTP concentration is about 100 times higher than the GMP concentration, and the level of PP$_i$ is extremely low because this product is rapidly cleaved to inorganic phosphate by various pyrophosphatases. Therefore the reaction actually proceeds only in the direction of acetyl-CoA formation.

The terms **freely reversible** and **(physiologically) irreversible** are used to indicate whether or not a reaction can proceed in both directions under ordinary cellular conditions.

MOST METABOLIC PATHWAYS ARE REGULATED

The cells of the human body have to adjust their metabolic activities to both their own survival needs and the physiological needs of the body. Therefore they have to respond to their own energy status, the availability of nutrients, and hormones. Of the more important hormones,

- **Insulin** is released after a carbohydrate-rich meal and stimulates the utilization of dietary nutrients.
- **Glucagon** is released during fasting and maintains an adequate blood glucose level during fasting.
- **Epinephrine** and **norepinephrine** are released during acute stress and stimulate the mobilization of stored nutrients (fat, glycogen).
- **Cortisol** is released during more prolonged stress, when it promotes glucose synthesis and fat breakdown.

These internal and external signals regulate metabolic pathways by three mechanisms:

1. *The amount of the enzyme is adjusted by changes in its rate of synthesis or degradation.* The lactose operon of the bacterium *Escherichia coli* (see Chapter 6) is the classic example of regulated enzyme synthesis. Human metabolic enzymes have lifespans ranging from 1 hour to several days. Therefore regulation of enzyme levels is a long-term type of regulation.

2. *Some enzymes are modified covalently, usually by phosphorylation of amino acid side chains.* Either the phosphorylated or the dephosphorylated enzyme is the catalytically active form. This regulatory mechanism requires a **protein kinase** (phosphorylating enzyme) and a **protein phosphatase** (dephosphorylating enzyme):

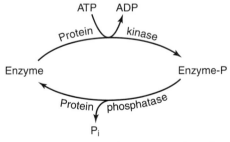

ATP   ADP

Protein   kinase

Enzyme   Enzyme-P

Protein   phosphatase

P$_i$

The protein kinases and protein phosphatases are regulated by nutrients, metabolites, or hormones.

3. *Some enzymes are regulated by allosteric effectors.* In most cases, the allosteric effector is a substrate, intermediate, or product of the pathway. In some regulated enzymes, the equilibrium between active and inactive conformations is affected by both phosphorylation and allosteric effectors.

FEEDBACK INHIBITION AND FEEDFORWARD STIMULATION ARE THE MOST IMPORTANT REGULATORY PRINCIPLES

Consider a biosynthetic pathway in which an important product such as heme, cholesterol, or a purine is synthesized from a simple precursor:

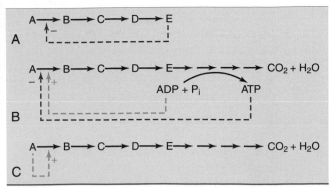

Figure 20.3 Regulation of metabolic pathways. The indicated regulatory influences (⊸, stimulation; ⇢, inhibition) may work through changes in enzyme concentration (regulation of enzyme synthesis or degradation), by direct allosteric effects, or by effects on protein kinases and protein phosphatases that regulate the phosphorylation state of the enzyme. **A,** Anabolic pathway: feedback inhibition. **B,** Catabolic pathway: regulation by ATP and ADP. P_i, Inorganic phosphate. **C,** Catabolic pathway: regulation by feedforward stimulation.

$$\text{Substrate A} \xrightarrow{(1)} \text{B} \xrightarrow{(2)} \text{C} \xrightarrow{(3)} \text{D} \xrightarrow{(4)} \text{Product E}$$

This pathway should be active when the end product E is needed, but it should be switched off when there is enough product E in the cell already. In fact, *most biosynthetic pathways are inhibited by high concentrations of their end product.* This is called **feedback inhibition** (*Fig. 20.3, A*).

Not all enzymes in a pathway are regulated. Short-term regulation, in particular, affects only one or a few enzymes in the pathway. But which enzyme is most suitable for regulation?

1. A regulated enzyme must be present in lower activity than the other enzymes in the pathway. It has to catalyze the rate-limiting step.
2. It should serve an essential function in only one metabolic pathway.
3. It should catalyze the first irreversible reaction in the pathway. This reaction is called the **committed step.** Regulation of the committed step ensures that only the substrate of the pathway accumulates when the regulated enzyme is inhibited. If a later reaction were regulated, metabolic intermediates would accumulate and possibly cause toxic effects. For example, inhibition of the last enzyme in pathway A in *Figure 20.3* would cause accumulation of intermediate D and, possibly, C and B as well.

In energy-producing catabolic pathways (see *Fig. 20.3, B*), the important product is ATP. Therefore *ATP is used as a feedback inhibitor.* When ATP is scarce, the catabolic pathways are stimulated; when it is abundant, they are inhibited. The ATP level is inversely related to the

concentrations of ADP and AMP, and *ADP and/or AMP act opposite to ATP in the regulation of many catabolic pathways.*

In **feedforward stimulation,** a substrate stimulates the pathway by which it is utilized (see *Fig. 20.3, C*). Induction of the *lac* operon of *E. coli* by lactose (see Chapter 6) is an example of feedforward stimulation.

INHERITED ENZYME DEFICIENCIES CAUSE METABOLIC DISEASES

Inborn errors of metabolism are caused by inherited enzyme deficiencies. The immediate effects of the enzyme deficiency are always *accumulation of the substrate* and *deficiency of the product.*

If a biosynthetic pathway is affected (*Fig. 20.4, A*), *clinical signs and symptoms can be caused by the lack of the end product.* A classic example is **oculocutaneous albinism.** In this benign condition, the dark pigment melanin is not formed because one of the steps in melanin synthesis is blocked. In some other metabolic disorders, however, it is not the lack of the end product but the accumulation of a toxic metabolic intermediate that causes problems.

The deficiency of an enzyme in a major catabolic, ATP-producing pathway will cause serious problems for the cells that depend on that pathway for generation of their metabolic energy. More commonly, an enzyme deficiency affects only the catabolism of a specialized substrate such as fructose or galactose (see Chapter 22) or the amino acid phenylalanine (see Chapter 26). In these cases, ATP can still be synthesized from other substrates, but *the accumulation of the nutrient or its immediate metabolites can cause problems* (see *Fig. 20.4, B*). Some of these diseases can be treated simply by avoiding the offending nutrient.

In **storage diseases,** intracellular degradation of a macromolecule by hydrolytic enzymes (pathway ② in *Fig. 20.1*) is blocked, and problems arise through the *abnormal accumulation ("storage") of the nondegradable macromolecule* (see *Fig. 20.4, C*). The mucopolysaccharidoses (see Chapter 14), glycogen storage diseases (see Chapter 22), and lipid storage diseases (see Chapter 24) are the most prominent examples. Many but not all storage diseases are caused by the deficiency of a lysosomal enzyme.

Many metabolic enzymes come in the form of tissue-specific **isoenzymes** that are encoded by different genes. Therefore *many inherited enzyme deficiencies are expressed only in some tissues but not others.*

Hundreds of enzyme deficiencies have been recognized in inherited metabolic diseases. Most of them are rare, with frequencies of less than 1:10,000 in the population. These diseases are expressed as recessive traits. This means that heterozygotes, who still have half of the normal enzyme activity, are healthy. Only the complete loss of the enzyme in homozygotes causes the disease.

Figure 20.4 Consequences of an enzyme deficiency. **A,** Anabolic pathway. Metabolite C accumulates, and the product is deficient. Clinical signs and symptoms can be caused by either deficiency of the product or accumulation of C. **B,** Catabolic pathway. A nutrient or one of its metabolites accumulates. Unless the pathway is essential for ATP synthesis (e.g., glycolysis, tricarboxylic acid cycle), the clinical signs are caused not by ATP deficiency but by the accumulation of the nutrient and/or its metabolites. **C,** Degradation of a macromolecule. The undegraded molecule C accumulates, mostly within the cells. The result is a storage disease. P_i, inorganic phosphate.

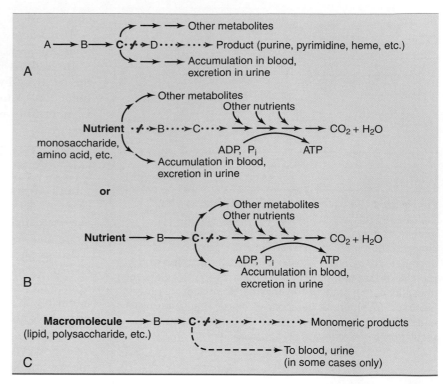

VITAMIN DEFICIENCIES, TOXINS, AND ENDOCRINE DISORDERS CAN DISRUPT METABOLIC PATHWAYS

Many **toxins** are inhibitors of metabolic enzymes. For example, the metal lead causes accumulation of toxic intermediates by inhibiting enzymes of heme biosynthesis, and cyanide blocks cell respiration by inhibiting the mitochondrial cytochrome oxidase.

Vitamin deficiencies can affect metabolic pathways because many metabolic enzymes require a coenzyme, and many coenzymes are made from a vitamin (see Chapter 29). Most vitamin-derived coenzymes, including NAD, flavin adenine dinucleotide (FAD), and CoA, participate in multiple metabolic pathways. All of these pathways are impaired when the vitamin is deficient.

Endocrine disorders are the most complex metabolic diseases because each hormone controls a whole set of metabolic pathways. In diabetes mellitus, for example, insufficient insulin action disrupts most of the major pathways in carbohydrate and fat metabolism.

SUMMARY

Anabolic, or biosynthetic, pathways produce complex biosynthetic products from simple precursors. The energy necessary for biosynthesis is generated during catabolic processes, particularly by the oxidation of nutrients in the mitochondria.

Enzymes in metabolic pathways are regulated by nutrients, metabolites, and hormones. These signals regulate important enzymes in three ways: by adjustments of enzyme synthesis or degradation, by covalent modifications, or by means of reversible binding of allosteric effectors. In feedback inhibition, the regulated enzyme is inhibited by a product of the pathway; in feedforward stimulation, it is stimulated by a substrate.

QUESTIONS

1. **The generation of metabolic energy from glucose requires a pathway known as glycolysis. What would be the most appropriate mechanism of regulation for this pathway?**

   A. Inhibition of the first irreversible step by glucose
   B. Inhibition of the first irreversible step by ADP
   C. Inhibition of the last irreversible step by ADP
   D. Inhibition of the first irreversible step by ATP
   E. Inhibition of the first irreversible step by carbon dioxide and water

2. **Under physiological conditions, the "reversibility" of a metabolic reaction is affected by all of the following *except***

   A. Concentrations of the substrates and products
   B. Concentration of the enzyme
   C. The energy charge if ATP and ADP participate in the reaction
   D. The standard free energy change of the reaction
   E. The pH if protons are formed or consumed in the reaction

Chapter 21

GLYCOLYSIS, TRICARBOXYLIC ACID CYCLE, AND OXIDATIVE PHOSPHORYLATION

For the generation of metabolic energy, *all major nutrients are degraded to* **acetyl coenzyme A (acetyl-CoA)**. These include carbohydrates, fat, protein, and alcohol (*Fig. 21.1*). Acetyl-CoA is also called "activated acetic acid" because it consists of an acetyl (acetic acid) group that is bound to coenzyme A by an energy-rich thioester bond.

In the mitochondria, the two carbons of the acetyl group become oxidized to CO_2 in the **tricarboxylic acid (TCA) cycle** (also called the citric acid cycle or Krebs cycle), whereas hydrogen (consisting of electron and proton) is transferred from the substrate to the coenzymes *nicotinamide adenine dinucleotide* (NAD^+) and *flavin adenine dinucleotide* (FAD). Finally, the electrons are transferred from the reduced coenzymes NADH and $FADH_2$ to the respiratory chain to react with molecular oxygen. The reoxidation of the reduced coenzymes produces the bulk of the cellular ATP in the process of **oxidative phosphorylation.**

This chapter shows how glucose is oxidized and how this process produces energy in the form of ATP. Glucose is not only the most abundant monosaccharide in food but is also produced from other monosaccharides, by the breakdown of the storage polysaccharide glycogen, and from amino acids and other noncarbohydrate substrates (*Fig. 21.2*).

GLUCOSE UPTAKE INTO THE CELLS IS REGULATED

Glucose is not sufficiently lipid soluble to enter cells by passive diffusion across the plasma membrane. Dietary glucose enters the intestinal mucosal cells mainly by sodium cotransport, but the uptake of glucose from blood or interstitial fluid into cells occurs by facilitated diffusion.

Table 21.1 summarizes the most important facilitated-diffusion glucose carriers. *One of these carriers, GLUT4,*

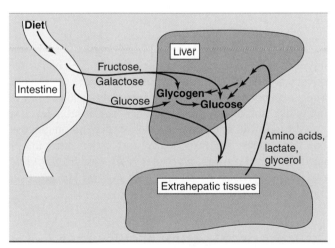

Figure 21.2 Role of glucose as the principal transported carbohydrate in the human body. Note the important role of the liver in glucose metabolism.

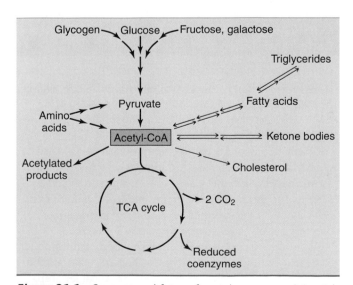

Figure 21.1 Sources and fates of acetyl coenzyme A (*acetyl-CoA*).

Table 21.1 Most Important Glucose Transporters

Transporter	Expressed in	Function
GLUT1	Most tissues	Basal glucose uptake
GLUT2	Liver, intestine, pancreatic β-cells	High-capacity glucose uptake
GLUT3	Brain	Neuronal glucose uptake
GLUT4	Muscle, adipose tissue, heart	Insulin-dependent glucose uptake
GLUT5	Intestine	Fructose transport

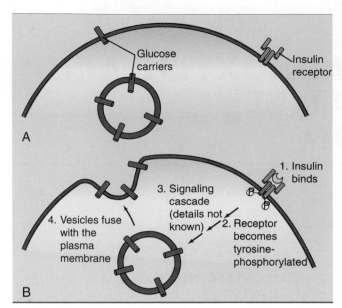

Figure 21.3 Effect of insulin on the glucose carriers in adipocytes. A similar mechanism is thought to operate in skeletal muscle. **A,** In the resting state, most glucose carriers are present in the membrane of intracellular vesicles. **B,** After insulin binding and receptor autophosphorylation, the carrier-containing vesicles fuse with the plasma membrane. This leads to an increased V_{max} of glucose transport across the plasma membrane.

is insulin dependent. Its deposition in the plasma membrane is enhanced by insulin (**Fig. 21.3**). The consequence is that muscle and adipose tissue take up glucose after a carbohydrate-rich meal, when the insulin level is high, but not during fasting, when the insulin level is low. Muscle and adipose tissue do not depend on glucose but can subsist on fatty acids and other nutrients if needed. *During fasting, glucose is redirected from muscle and adipose tissue to tissues that depend on glucose, including brain and erythrocytes.*

GLUCOSE DEGRADATION BEGINS IN THE CYTOPLASM AND ENDS IN THE MITOCHONDRIA

The steps in glucose oxidation are summarized in **Figure 21.4**. The initial reaction sequence, known as **glycolysis,** is cytoplasmic. It turns one molecule of glucose (six carbons) into two molecules of the three-carbon compound **pyruvate.** All cells of the body are capable of glycolysis.

Under aerobic conditions, pyruvate is transported into the mitochondrion, where it is turned into the two-carbon compound **acetyl-CoA.** Acetyl-CoA then enters the **TCA cycle** by reacting with the four-carbon compound oxaloacetate to form the six-carbon compound citrate. Citrate is converted back to oxaloacetate in the remaining reactions of the TCA cycle.

In these pathways, *the hydrogen of the substrate is transferred to the coenzymes NAD^+ and FAD* (see Chapter 5). The reduced coenzymes donate electrons to the **respiratory chain** of the inner mitochondrial membrane, which in turn donates them to molecular oxygen. *The reoxidation of the reduced coenzymes is highly exergonic.* It is the energy source for ATP synthesis by **oxidative phosphorylation.** The TCA cycle and oxidative phosphorylation take place in all cells that contain mitochondria.

GLYCOLYSIS BEGINS WITH ATP-DEPENDENT PHOSPHORYLATIONS

After entering the cell, glucose is phosphorylated to glucose-6-phosphate by **hexokinase** (**Fig. 21.5**). *The hexokinase reaction is irreversible* for two reasons: Its $\Delta G^{0'}$ is strongly negative (-4.0 kcal/mol) because an energy-rich phosphoanhydride bond in ATP is cleaved while a "low-energy" phosphate ester bond is formed (**Table 21.2**), and the ATP concentration in a healthy cell is always far higher than the ADP concentration.

The hexokinase reaction is always the first step in glucose metabolism, whether glucose is being used for glycolysis or for other metabolic pathways. Glucose-6-phosphate cannot leave the cell on a membrane carrier as glucose can. Indeed, *phosphorylated intermediates in general do not cross the plasma membrane.*

In glycolysis, glucose-6-phosphate is in equilibrium with fructose-6-phosphate through the reversible **phosphohexose isomerase** reaction. Fructose-6-phosphate is then phosphorylated to fructose-1,6-bisphosphate by **phosphofructokinase** (PFK). This is the first irreversible reaction specific for glycolysis. It is its **committed step.**

The reactions from glucose to fructose-1,6-bisphosphate require two high-energy phosphate bonds in ATP. This initial investment has to be recovered in later reactions of the pathway.

CLINICAL EXAMPLE 21.1: Prevention of Dental Caries with Fluoride

Dental caries are caused by *Streptococcus mutans*. This bacterium takes advantage of an abundant sugar supply by converting sugars into lactic acid. The lactic acid erodes the acid-sensitive calcium phosphates in the tooth enamel, causing cavities.

Both the bacterial and the human varieties of the glycolytic enzyme enolase are inhibited by fluoride ions, a common ingredient of toothpaste. Actually, *fluoride protects the teeth by two mechanisms: It strengthens the teeth by being incorporated in dentin and enamel, and it prevents glycolytic lactic acid formation by bacteria.*

As an inhibitor of human enolase, sodium fluoride is routinely added to blood samples that are used for the determination of blood glucose in the clinical laboratory to prevent the breakdown of glucose by blood cells.

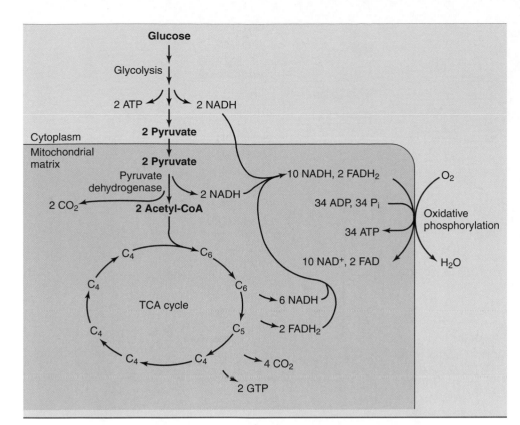

Figure 21.4 Steps in glucose oxidation. The catabolic pathways convert the carbon of the substrate to carbon dioxide. The hydrogen initially is transferred to the coenzymes NAD^+ and *FAD*. The reduced coenzymes then are reoxidized by the respiratory chain. Most of the *ATP* is produced by oxidative phosphorylation, which couples the oxidation of the reduced coenzymes to ATP synthesis.

MOST GLYCOLYTIC INTERMEDIATES HAVE THREE CARBONS

The six-carbon intermediate fructose-1,6-bisphosphate is cleaved into two triose phosphates by the enzyme **aldolase**. Carbons 1, 2, and 3 of the sugar form dihydroxyacetone phosphate, and carbons 4, 5, and 6 form glyceraldehyde-3-phosphate. The triose phosphates are interconverted in the reversible **triose phosphate isomerase** reaction.

Aldolase and triose phosphate isomerase establish an equilibrium between fructose-1,6-bisphosphate, dihydroxyacetone phosphate, and glyceraldehyde-3-phosphate. Although only glyceraldehyde-3-phosphate proceeds through the remaining glycolytic reactions, triose phosphate isomerase ensures that all six glucose-derived carbons can proceed through the pathway.

Glyceraldehyde-3-phosphate is converted to the energy-rich intermediate 1,3-bisphosphoglycerate by **glyceraldehyde-3-phosphate dehydrogenase**. The enzyme couples the exergonic oxidation of the aldehyde group in the substrate with the endergonic formation of an energy-rich bond between the newly created carboxyl group and inorganic phosphate. The reaction also forms a substrate for oxidative phosphorylation by reducing NAD^+ to NADH.

Simple hydrolysis of the mixed anhydride bond in 1,3-bisphosphoglycerate would release 11.8 kcal/mol

in the form of heat. Rather than wasting this energy by hydrolyzing the bond, the enzyme **phosphoglycerate kinase** transfers the phosphate to ADP, forming ATP. This strategy of forming an energy-rich intermediate that is then used for ATP synthesis is called **substrate-level phosphorylation**.

3-Phosphoglycerate is isomerized to 2-phosphoglycerate by **phosphoglycerate mutase**. "Mutase" is an old-fashioned name for isomerases that shift the position of a phosphate group in the molecule. 2-Phosphoglycerate, in turn, is dehydrated to phosphoenolpyruvate (PEP) by **enolase**.

The last enzyme of glycolysis, **pyruvate kinase**, makes substrate-level phosphorylation by transferring the phosphate group of PEP to ADP. Although ATP is synthesized, this reaction is highly exergonic with a standard free energy change ($\Delta G^{0'}$) of −7.5 kcal/mol. This implies a free energy content of 14.8 kcal/mol for the phosphate ester bond in PEP. Why is this phosphate ester so unusually energy rich? The initial transfer of phosphate from PEP to ADP is indeed endergonic. However, the enolpyruvate formed in this reaction rearranges almost immediately to pyruvate. This highly exergonic reaction removes enolpyruvate from the equilibrium (*Fig. 21.6*).

Overall, the reactions of glycolysis produce a net yield of *two ATP molecules and two NADH molecules* for each molecule of glucose (*Table 21.3*).

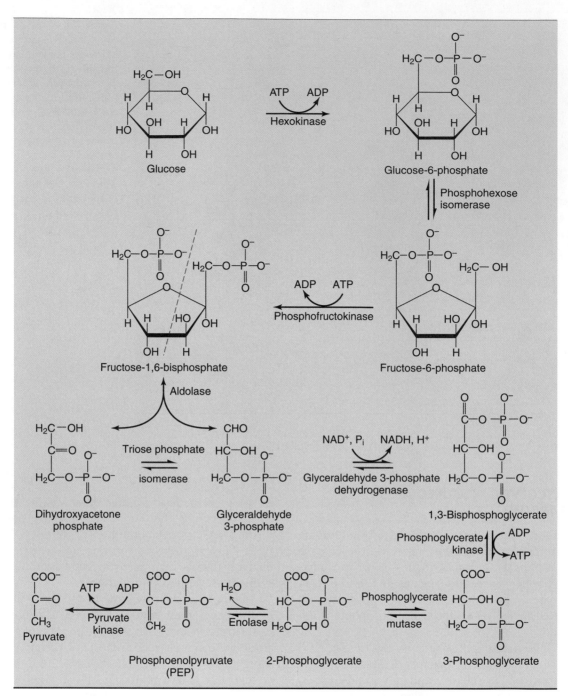

Figure 21.5 Reactions of glycolysis, the major catabolic pathway for glucose. It is active in the cytoplasm of all cells in the human body.

Only the hexokinase, PFK, and pyruvate kinase reactions are "irreversible." The aldolase and triose phosphate isomerase reactions have very unfavorable equilibria (see *Table 21.2*). Nevertheless they can proceed because fructose-1,6-bisphosphate is formed in the irreversible PFK reaction and glyceraldehyde-3-phosphate is rapidly consumed in the next reactions of the pathway. The actual equilibrium of the glyceraldehyde-3-phosphate dehydrogenase reaction is far more favorable than suggested by its $\Delta G^{0'}$ value of +1.5 kcal/mol because NAD$^+$ is far more abundant than NADH in the aerobic cell.

CLINICAL EXAMPLE 21.2: Pyruvate Kinase Deficiency

A complete deficiency of any glycolytic enzyme would be fatal, at least if it affects cells such as neurons or erythrocytes that depend on glucose as an energy source. Anaerobic glycolysis is the only energy source for erythrocytes, and partial deficiencies of glycolytic enzymes in red blood cells are seen as rare causes of chronic hemolytic anemia.

CLINICAL EXAMPLE 21.2: Pyruvate Kinase Deficiency—cont'd

Recessively inherited **pyruvate kinase deficiency** has a frequency of 1:20,000 in the white population. The erythrocytes of affected individuals have between 5% and 25% of the normal pyruvate kinase activity, and the severity of the hemolytic anemia depends on the residual enzyme activity. Enzyme activity less than 5% of normal causes fetal death, and activity greater than 25% of normal is asymptomatic.

The affected isoenzyme is present only in erythrocytes. Therefore glycolysis is unimpaired in other tissues.

PHOSPHOFRUCTOKINASE IS THE MOST IMPORTANT REGULATED ENZYME OF GLYCOLYSIS

Most tissues glycolyze heavily after a carbohydrate meal but switch to fatty acid oxidation during fasting. The *long-term control* of glycolysis, particularly in the liver, is affected by changes in the amounts of some key glycolytic enzymes, triggered by nutrients and hormones. In general, *insulin and glucose increase the levels of glycolytic enzymes, whereas glucagon and fatty acids have the opposite effect.*

Of the important hormones, *insulin rises in response to elevated blood glucose after a meal.* It stimulates glucose consumption in many tissues, both by glycolysis and by other pathways. *Glucagon rises in response to low blood glucose during fasting.* It reduces glucose consumption and stimulates glucose production by the liver.

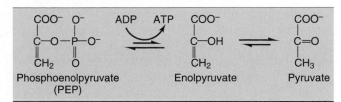

Figure 21.6 Pyruvate kinase reaction. Pyruvate shows keto-enol tautomerism, the keto form being energetically far more stable than the enol form.

Table 21.3 Products Formed during Conversion of One Molecule of Glucose to Two Molecules of Pyruvate in Aerobic Glycolysis*

Enzyme	Product (Molecules)
Hexokinase	−1 ATP
Phosphofructokinase	−1 ATP
Glyceraldehyde-3-phosphate dehydrogenase	+2 NADH
Phosphoglycerate kinase	+2 ATP
Pyruvate kinase	+2 ATP
	2 ATP + 2 NADH

*Note that all reactions beyond the aldolase reaction occur twice for each glucose molecule.

The *short-term control* of glycolysis depends mainly on the allosteric enzyme PFK, which catalyzes the committed step of glycolysis. PFK is

- inhibited by ATP and stimulated by AMP and ADP
- inhibited by low pH
- inhibited by citrate
- stimulated by insulin and inhibited by glucagon (in the liver)

Table 21.2 Standard Free Energy Changes of Glycolytic Reactions

Reaction	Enzyme	$\Delta G^{0'}$ (kcal/mol)
Glucose $\xrightarrow{\text{ATP} \ \text{ADP}}$ Glucose-6-phosphate	Hexokinase	−4.0
Glucose-6-phosphate ⇌ Fructose-6-phosphate	Phosphohexose isomerase	+0.4
Fructose-6-phosphate $\xrightarrow{\text{ATP} \ \text{ADP}}$ Fructose-1,6-bisphosphate	Phosphofructokinase	−3.4
Fructose-1,6-bisphosphate ⇌ Dihydroxyacetone phosphate + Glyceraldehyde-3-phosphate	Aldolase	+5.7
Dihydroxyacetone phosphate ⇌ Glyceraldehyde-3-phosphate	Triose phosphate isomerase	+1.8
Glyceraldehyde-3-phosphate $\xrightarrow{\text{NAD}^+, \text{P}_i \ \text{NADH, H}^+}$ 1,3-bisphosphoglycerate	Glyceraldehyde-3-phosphate dehydrogenase	+1.5
1,3-Bisphosphoglycerate $\xrightarrow{\text{ADP} \ \text{ATP}}$ 3-Phosphoglycerate	Phosphoglycerate kinase	−4.5
3-Phosphoglycerate ⇌ 2-Phosphoglycerate	Phosphoglycerate mutase	+1.1
2-Phosphoglycerate $\xrightarrow{\text{H}_2\text{O}}$ Phosphoenolpyruvate (PEP)	Enolase	+0.4
Phosphoenolpyruvate $\xrightarrow{\text{ADP} \ \text{ATP}}$ Pyruvate	Pyruvate kinase	−7.5

$\Delta G^{0'}$, Standard free energy change; P_i, inorganic phosphate.

The response to adenine nucleotides ensures that *glycolytic activity increases when more ATP is needed* (e.g., in contracting muscle). Citrate is a mitochondrial metabolite that signals an abundance of energy and metabolic intermediates, and *low pH dampens glycolytic activity when pyruvic and lactic acid, the end products of glycolysis, accumulate to dangerous levels.*

Additional control sites are insulin-dependent glucose uptake into the cell by the GLUT4 transporter in muscle and adipose tissue as well as the other irreversible enzymes of glycolysis, hexokinase and pyruvate kinase. In most tissues (but not the liver), *hexokinase is competitively inhibited by its own product, glucose-6-phosphate.* This prevents the accumulation of glucose-6-phosphate when the supply of glucose exceeds the capacity of the metabolizing pathways. Glucose-6-phosphate must not be allowed to accumulate because it would tie up the cell's phosphate and thereby impair ATP synthesis. Pyruvate kinase, finally, is inhibited by ATP in many tissues, including the liver.

LACTATE IS PRODUCED UNDER ANAEROBIC CONDITIONS

Glycolysis produces ATP without consuming oxygen. Does this mean that we can live without oxygen by turning glucose into pyruvate? Not quite. The immediate problem is that glycolysis turns NAD^+ into NADH. Without a mechanism to regenerate NAD^+, glycolysis would soon grind to a screeching halt for lack of NAD^+.

The solution to this problem is simple (***Fig. 21.7***). The enzyme **lactate dehydrogenase (LDH)** regenerates NAD^+ by transferring the hydrogen of NADH to the keto group of pyruvate:

$$Pyruvate + NADH + H^+ \rightarrow Lactate + NAD^+$$

$$\Delta G^{0'} = -6.0 \text{ kcal/mol}$$

The equilibrium of the LDH reaction favors lactate, but the reaction is physiologically reversible because NAD^+ is far more abundant than NADH under aerobic conditions. In fact, *lactate is a metabolic dead end.* The LDH reaction is the only way to channel lactate back into the metabolic pathways.

The overall balance of lactate formation by anaerobic glycolysis is

$$Glucose + 2 ADP + 2P_i \rightarrow 2 \text{ Lactate} + 2 \text{ ATP} + 2H^+$$

Thus it is possible to make ATP in the absence of oxygen. *Carbohydrates are the only metabolic substrates that can produce ATP under anaerobic conditions.* A major limitation of anaerobic glycolysis is that the protons that are formed along with the lactate anion can create a serious pH problem.

Another limitation is that the two ATP molecules formed in glycolysis capture only 14.6 kcal of useful energy, whereas the complete oxidation of glucose produces approximately 270 kcal (see ***Table 21.7***). Therefore anaerobic glycolysis is useful only under certain circumstances, for example:

1. *Mature erythrocytes* have no mitochondria. They can afford an anaerobic lifestyle because their energy requirement is so modest that it can be met by the anaerobic glycolysis of 15 to 20 g of glucose per day.
2. *Skeletal muscle* has to increase its ATP production more than 20-fold during bouts of vigorous contraction. For example, during a 100-m sprint, the oxygen supply becomes a limiting factor. To keep going, the muscles turn blood glucose and their own stored glycogen into lactic acid. The lactate concentration in the blood rises 5-fold to 10-fold in this situation.
3. *Ischemic tissues* use anaerobic glycolysis for crisis management. This allows them to survive for some time on the ATP generated by glycolysis. However, the accumulating lactic acid contributes to cell death (see ***Clinical Example 21.9***).

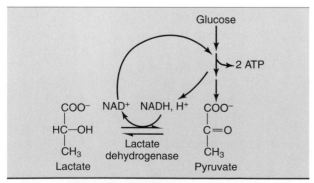

Figure 21.7 Anaerobic glycolysis. Lactate dehydrogenase regenerates NAD^+ for the glyceraldehyde-3-phosphate dehydrogenase reaction. The conversion of glucose to lactic acid can proceed smoothly with a net synthesis of two *ATP* molecules.

CLINICAL EXAMPLE 21.3: Lactic Acidosis

The overproduction or underutilization of lactic acid leads to **lactic acidosis.** The most common cause is *impairment of oxidative metabolism* by respiratory failure, insufficient oxygen transport, or toxins that prevent oxidative phosphorylation. As in tissue ischemia, PFK is stimulated by low energy charge, and large amounts of lactate are formed by glycolysis. Without oxygen, the mitochondria cannot oxidize NADH to NAD^+. As a result, *the accumulating NADH makes the LDH reaction irreversible in the direction of lactate formation.*

Some other causes of lactic acidosis are listed in *Table 21.4.* In alcohol intoxication, for example, the rapid formation of NADH during alcohol oxidation increases the [NADH]/[NAD^+] ratio. This makes the liver unable to oxidize lactate, and lactate is released into the blood.

CLINICAL EXAMPLE 21.3: Lactic Acidosis—cont'd

Table 21.4   Conditions Resulting in Lactic Acidosis

Condition	Mechanism
Physical exercise	Anaerobic glycolysis in muscle
Severe lung disease	
High altitude	Impaired respiration
Drowning	
Severe anemia	
Carbon monoxide poisoning	Impaired oxygen delivery
Sickling crisis	
Cyanide poisoning	Inhibition of oxidative phosphorylation
Alcohol intoxication	Elevated [NADH]/[NAD⁺] ratio
von Gierke disease	Impaired gluconeogenesis
Pyruvate dehydrogenase deficiency	Impaired pyruvate oxidation
Leukemia	Anaerobic glycolysis by neoplastic cells
Metastatic carcinoma	

PYRUVATE IS DECARBOXYLATED TO ACETYL-CoA IN THE MITOCHONDRIA

Under aerobic conditions, pyruvate is oxidized in the mitochondria. It diffuses through the pores in the outer mitochondrial membrane and is transported across the inner mitochondrial membrane into the mitochondrial matrix, where it is oxidatively decarboxylated to acetyl-CoA:

$$\text{Pyruvate} + \text{NAD}^+ + \text{CoA-SH}$$
$$\rightarrow \text{Acetyl-CoA} + \text{NADH} + \text{CO}_2$$

where CoA-SH = uncombined CoA. This irreversible reaction is catalyzed by **pyruvate dehydrogenase,** a multienzyme complex with three components:

1. *Pyruvate dehydrogenase component* (E_1), which contains **thiamin pyrophosphate** as a prosthetic group

2. *Dihydrolipoyl transacetylase component* (E_2), which contains **lipoic acid** covalently bound to a lysine side chain

3. *Dihydrolipoyl dehydrogenase component* (E_3), an FAD-containing flavoprotein

In addition to the tightly bound prosthetic groups, the cosubstrates NAD⁺ and CoA are required for the reaction.

The structures of thiamin pyrophosphate (TPP) and lipoic acid are shown in ***Figure 21.8***. TPP acts as a carrier of pyruvate and of the hydroxyethyl group that is formed by pyruvate decarboxylation. Lipoic acid participates as a redox system and carrier of the acetyl group. The reaction sequence is shown in ***Figure 21.9***.

With the exception of lipoic acid, the coenzymes of pyruvate dehydrogenase require vitamins for their synthesis: pantothenic acid (CoA), niacin (NAD), riboflavin (FAD), and thiamin (TPP). A deficiency of any of these vitamins can impair the pyruvate dehydrogenase reaction. In thiamin deficiency (**beriberi**), for example, the blood levels of pyruvate, lactate, and alanine are elevated after a carbohydrate-rich meal. Pyruvate accumulates because its major reaction is blocked, and most of it is either reduced to lactate or transaminated to alanine.

THE TCA CYCLE PRODUCES TWO MOLECULES OF CARBON DIOXIDE FOR EACH ACETYL RESIDUE

The **TCA cycle,** also known as the **citric acid cycle** or **Krebs cycle,** is the final common pathway for the oxidation of all major nutrients. It takes place in the mitochondrial matrix, and *it is active in all cells that possess mitochondria.*

In the first reaction, the acetyl group of acetyl-CoA reacts with the four-carbon compound oxaloacetate to form the six-carbon compound citrate. This irreversible reaction (***Table 21.5***) is catalyzed by **citrate synthase.** The remaining reactions regenerate oxaloacetate from citrate, with two carbons released as carbon dioxide (***Fig. 21.12***).

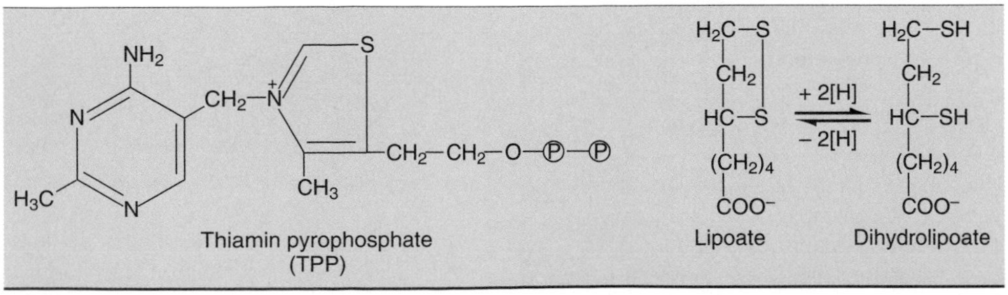

Figure 21.8   Structures of thiamin pyrophosphate (*TPP*) and lipoic acid. In the pyruvate dehydrogenase complex, TPP is bound noncovalently to the apoprotein, whereas lipoic acid is bound covalently by an amide bond with a lysine side chain.

Figure 21.9 Pyruvate dehydrogenase reaction.

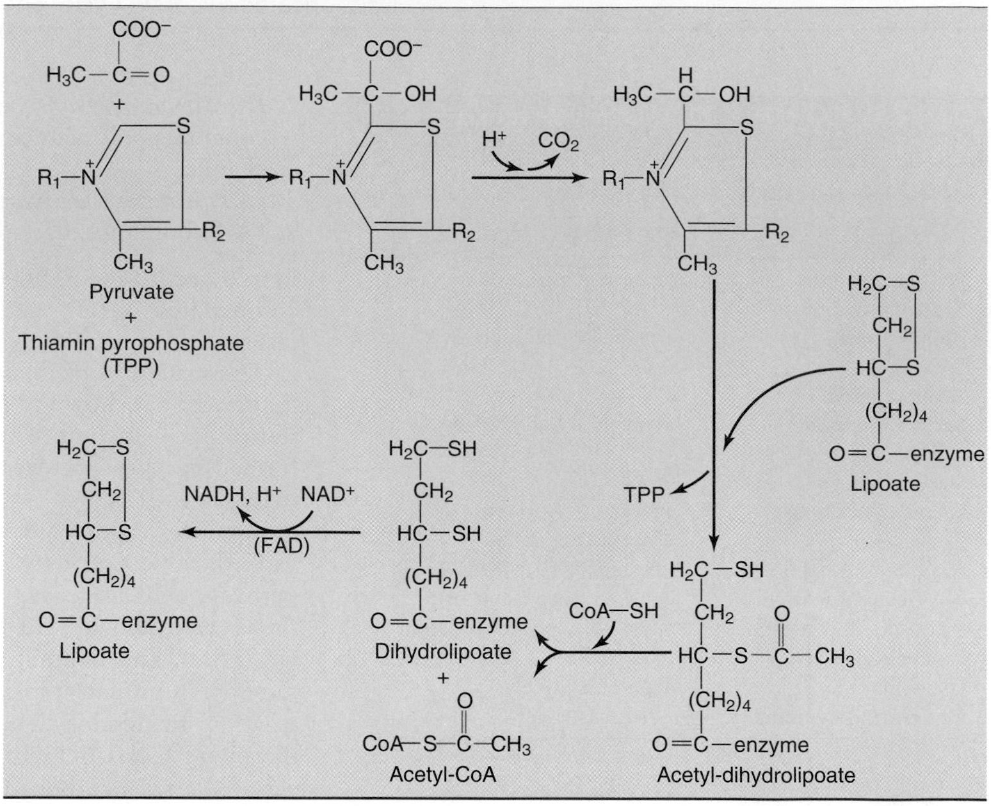

CLINICAL EXAMPLE 21.4: Arsenic Poisoning

Arsenic occurs in two forms that are toxic by different mechanisms. **Arsenate** is a structural analog of phosphate that competes with phosphate in many biochemical reactions. However, *the bonds that arsenate forms with phosphate and carboxyl groups are unstable and hydrolyze spontaneously*. **Figure 21.10** shows how it uncouples substrate-level phosphorylation in glycolysis. The term "uncoupling" implies that *the pathway can proceed, but without ATP synthesis*.

Arsenite is even more toxic than arsenate. It poisons pyruvate dehydrogenase and other lipoic acid containing enzymes by binding to the sulfhydryl groups in dihydrolipoic acid (*Fig. 21.11*). A similar reaction of arsenite with closely spaced sulfhydryl groups in immature keratin leads to its incorporation in hair and fingernails. Its determination in hair is used forensically in cases of alleged arsenic poisoning.

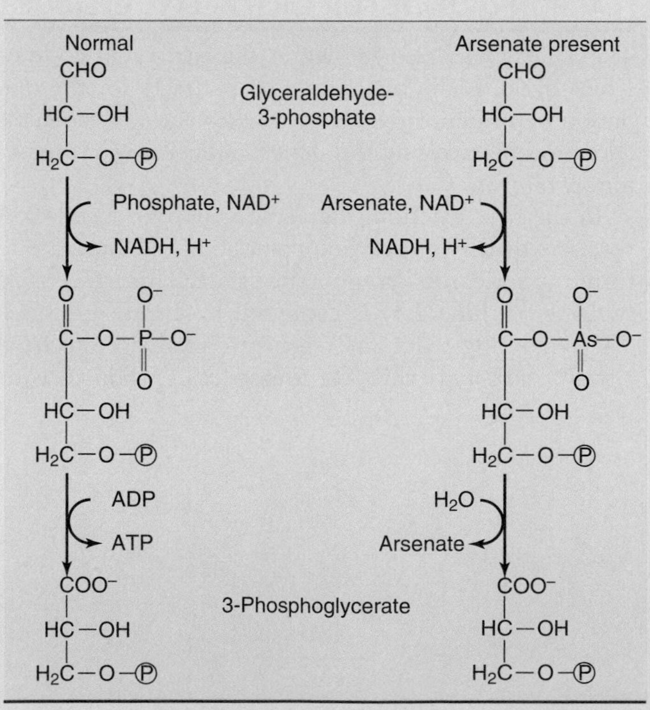

Figure 21.10 Uncoupling of substrate-level phosphorylation in glycolysis by arsenate. An unstable mixed anhydride is formed between arsenate and 3-phosphoglycerate. This anhydride hydrolyzes spontaneously. The pathway can proceed because the product of this hydrolysis, 3-phosphoglycerate, is a normal glycolytic intermediate.

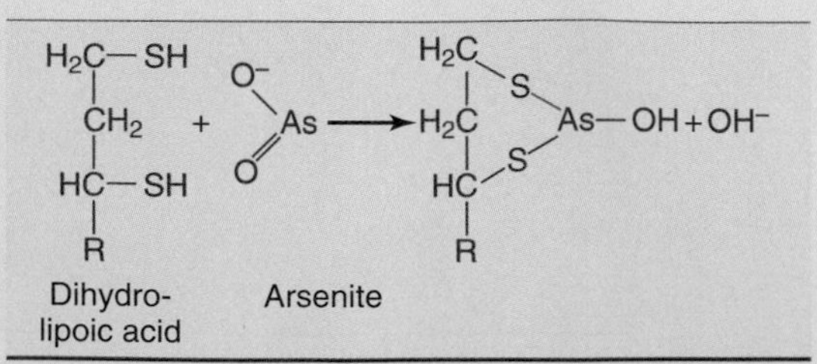

Figure 21.11 Reaction of arsenite with dihydrolipoic acid.

CLINICAL EXAMPLE 21.5: Pyruvate Dehydrogenase Deficiency

Inherited partial deficiencies of pyruvate dehydrogenase cause *lactic acidosis* and *central nervous system dysfunction.* Clinical expression and prognosis depend on the residual enzyme activity. Severe deficiencies (<40% of normal) cause mental deficiency, microcephaly, optical atrophy, and severe motor dysfunction starting in infancy. Less severe cases present with slowly progressive spinocerebellar ataxia (motor incoordination).

The brain is most severely affected because it depends on carbohydrate oxidation, being unable to oxidize alternative fuels. Pyruvate dehydrogenase deficiency impairs only carbohydrate oxidation, but not the oxidation of other nutrients. Treatment can be attempted by placing the patient on a low-carbohydrate diet. Megadoses of thiamin or other required vitamins also can be tried.

Table 21.5 Standard Free Energy Changes ($\Delta G^{0'}$) of Pyruvate Dehydrogenase Reaction and Tricarboxylic Acid Cycle Reactions

Enzyme	$\Delta G^{0'}$ (kcal/mol)	Products
Pyruvate dehydrogenase	−8.0	CO_2, NADH
Citrate synthase	−8.5	
Aconitase	+1.6	
Isocitrate dehydrogenase	−2.0	CO_2, NADH
α-Ketoglutarate dehydrogenase	−8.0	CO_2, NADH
Succinyl-CoA synthetase	−0.7	GTP
Succinate dehydrogenase	≈0	$FADH_2$
Fumarase	−0.9	
Malate dehydrogenase	+7.1	NADH

Citrate is isomerized to isocitrate by **aconitase.** The enzyme first dehydrates citrate to aconitate and then hydrates aconitate to isocitrate (*Fig. 21.13*). At equilibrium, the composition is 90% citrate, 3% aconitate, and 7% isocitrate.

Fluoroacetate has occasionally been used as a rat poison but is interesting for terrorists as well. It is metabolically converted to fluorocitrate by the same enzymes that otherwise metabolize acetate (*Fig. 21.14*). The resulting fluorocitrate is a potent inhibitor of aconitase.

Isocitrate is oxidatively decarboxylated to α-ketoglutarate (2-oxoglutarate) by isocitrate dehydrogenase. Oxalosuccinate is an enzyme-bound intermediate in

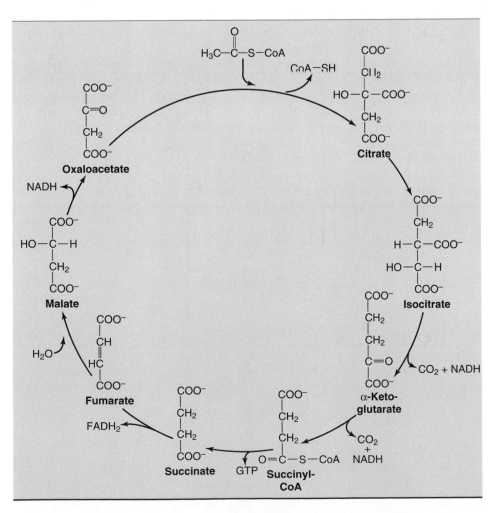

Figure 21.12 Tricarboxylic acid (*TCA*) cycle.

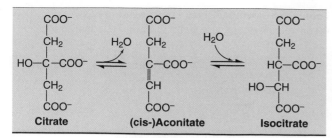

Figure 21.13 Aconitase reaction.

this reaction (*Fig. 21.15*). The isocitrate dehydrogenase of the TCA cycle is an NAD-linked enzyme.

The next enzyme of the cycle, α-**ketoglutarate dehydrogenase**, resembles pyruvate dehydrogenase in structure, reaction mechanism, and coenzyme requirements. However, it works on α-ketoglutarate rather than pyruvate and produces succinyl-CoA rather than acetyl-CoA.

In the reversible **succinyl-CoA synthetase** (also known as **succinyl thiokinase**) reaction, the hydrolysis of the energy-rich thioester bond in succinyl-CoA is coupled to the synthesis of GTP. This is yet another example of substrate-level phosphorylation, in which a high-energy bond in a metabolic intermediate is used for the synthesis of an energy-rich nucleotide. GTP is equivalent to ATP, with which it is in equilibrium through the nucleoside diphosphate kinase reaction:

$$GTP + ADP \rightleftharpoons GDP + ATP$$

Succinate is a four-carbon dicarboxylic acid. In the remaining reactions, two hydrogen atoms of succinate are replaced by oxygen to complete the cycle with the formation of oxaloacetate.

The enzyme **succinate dehydrogenase** (**SDH**) forms fumarate by transferring two hydrogen atoms from succinate to its prosthetic group FAD and from $FADH_2$ to the respiratory chain. Unlike the other TCA cycle enzymes, which are soluble in the mitochondrial matrix,

SDH is an integral protein of the inner mitochondrial membrane.

Why does SDH use enzyme-bound FAD rather than soluble NAD^+ to abstract hydrogen from its substrate? The reason is that FAD has the higher affinity for hydrogen. If NAD^+ were used, the reaction would be irreversible in the direction of succinate formation, but with FAD it is freely reversible.

Fumarate is hydrated to l-malate by **fumarase**, and malate is oxidized to oxaloacetate in the NAD^+-dependent **malate dehydrogenase** reaction. Like LDH, malate dehydrogenase equilibrates an α-hydroxy acid with its corresponding α-keto acid, and, as in the LDH reaction, the equilibrium favors the hydroxy acid (see *Table 21.5*). The reaction can nevertheless proceed toward oxaloacetate because the $[NAD^+]/[NADH]$ ratio in the mitochondrion is very high under aerobic conditions and because oxaloacetate is consumed in the irreversible citrate synthase reaction.

REDUCED COENZYMES ARE THE MOST IMPORTANT PRODUCTS OF THE TCA CYCLE

The important products of the TCA cycle are shown in *Figure 21.12* and *Table 21.5*. To balance the two carbons of acetyl-CoA that enter the cycle, each turn of the cycle releases two carbons as carbon dioxide. The hydrogen in the substrate does not form water, but it is transferred to the coenzymes NAD^+ and FAD. *Three molecules of NADH and one molecule of $FADH_2$ are formed in each turn of the cycle.* Along with the NADH from glycolysis and pyruvate dehydrogenase, these reduced coenzymes go to the respiratory chain, in which they are reoxidized by molecular oxygen.

The energy yield is about 3 ATP for NADH oxidation and 2 ATP for $FADH_2$ oxidation. Therefore the overall energy yield from the oxidation of one acetyl residue is 12 high-energy phosphate bonds: one from

Figure 21.14 Metabolic activation of fluoroacetate to fluorocitrate. Fluorocitrate is an inhibitor of aconitase.

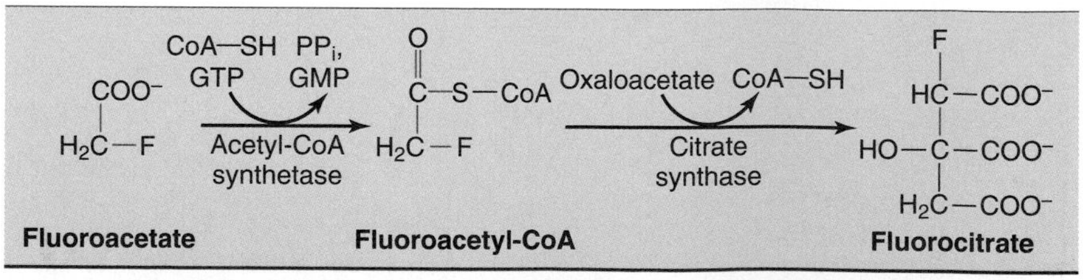

Figure 21.15 Isocitrate dehydrogenase reaction.

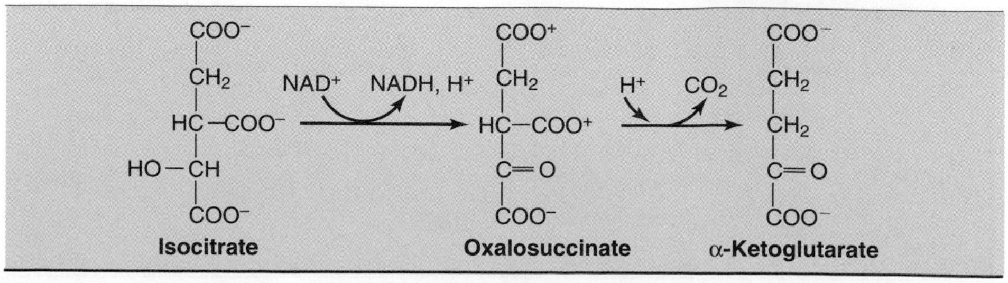

substrate-level phosphorylation and 11 by the reoxidation of the reduced coenzymes.

OXIDATIVE PATHWAYS ARE REGULATED BY ENERGY CHARGE AND [NADH]/[NAD⁺] RATIO

The oxidative pathways produce NADH directly and ATP indirectly through the oxidation of NADH. Accordingly, most of the regulated enzymes in these pathways are inhibited by an elevated [ATP]/[ADP] ratio and an elevated [NADH]/[NAD⁺] ratio. This ensures that a constant ATP level is maintained at all times and that NADH production matches the rate of NADH oxidation in the respiratory chain. There is also direct feedback inhibition of the irreversible reactions to prevent an undesirable accumulation of metabolic intermediates (*Fig. 21.16*).

Pyruvate dehydrogenase, which is outside the TCA cycle, is important because *it channels carbohydrate-derived carbons irreversibly into acetyl-CoA*. It is inhibited by its products NADH and acetyl-CoA and stimulated by AMP. It is also inactivated by the phosphorylation of a single serine side chain and reactivated by dephosphorylation.

The protein kinase that phosphorylates the enzyme complex is allosterically activated by the same factors that inhibit pyruvate dehydrogenase allosterically: high energy charge, high [NADH]/[NAD⁺] ratio, and high [acetyl-CoA]/[CoA] ratio. It is also inhibited by pyruvate. The action of the protein kinase is opposed by an insulin-stimulated protein phosphatase.

In the TCA cycle, **citrate synthase** is inhibited by ATP. However, more important is the availability of oxaloacetate. Citrate inhibits the reaction by competing with oxaloacetate for the active site of the enzyme.

Isocitrate dehydrogenase is inhibited by high energy charge and high [NADH]/[NAD⁺] ratio. Citrate accumulates along with isocitrate when isocitrate dehydrogenase is inhibited. It can leave the mitochondrion to act as an allosteric effector in the cytoplasmic pathways of glycolysis, gluconeogenesis (see Chapter 22), and fatty acid biosynthesis (see Chapter 23). Therefore elevations of mitochondrial energy charge and [NADH]/[NAD⁺] ratio can control these cytoplasmic pathways by inhibiting isocitrate dehydrogenase.

α-Ketoglutarate dehydrogenase, like pyruvate dehydrogenase, is inhibited by its own products (succinyl-CoA and NADH) and by high energy charge, but unlike pyruvate dehydrogenase it is not regulated by phosphorylation.

Except in anoxia, the mitochondrial [NAD⁺]/[NADH] ratio is so high that NAD⁺ is not a limiting factor as a substrate for the dehydrogenase reactions. However, the equilibrium of the NAD⁺-dependent malate dehydrogenase reaction is so unfavorable (see *Table 21.5*) that an elevated [NADH]/[NAD⁺] ratio seriously impairs the formation of oxaloacetate. As a result, citrate synthase suffers from a shortage of its substrate oxaloacetate.

TCA CYCLE PROVIDES AN IMPORTANT POOL OF METABOLIC INTERMEDIATES

The TCA cycle is not only the final common pathway for the oxidation of metabolic fuels. It is also a source of precursors for biosynthetic reactions (*Fig. 21.17*). Most of these reactions are tissue specific. For example, the synthesis of glucose from oxaloacetate occurs only in liver and kidneys, and the synthesis of heme from succinyl-CoA is most active in bone marrow and liver.

The removal of TCA cycle intermediates for biosynthesis can create a shortage of oxaloacetate as a substrate for the citrate synthase reaction. Therefore *biosynthetic reactions that consume TCA cycle intermediates must be balanced by reactions that produce them.* This latter type of reaction is called **anaplerotic** (from Greek words meaning "to fill up").

The three α-keto acids pyruvate, α-ketoglutarate, and oxaloacetate are structurally related to the amino acids alanine, glutamate, and aspartate (*Fig. 21.18*). When the amino acids are in demand, they can be synthesized from the α-keto acids. Under most conditions, however, excess dietary amino acids are metabolized to their corresponding α-keto acids. Most of the 20 amino acids are degraded to TCA cycle intermediates.

Another important anaplerotic reaction is the synthesis of oxaloacetate from pyruvate by **pyruvate carboxylase**.

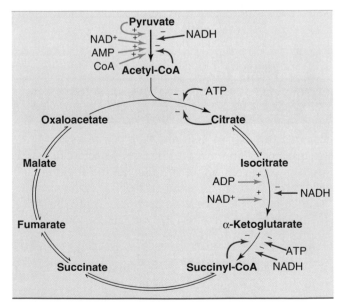

Figure 21.16 Regulatory effects on pyruvate dehydrogenase and the tricarboxylic acid cycle. Note the importance of energy charge and [NADH]/[NAD⁺] ratio. Also note the product inhibition of the irreversible reactions. →, Stimulation; ⊣, inhibition.

Figure 21.17 Some reactions of tricarboxylic acid cycle intermediates.

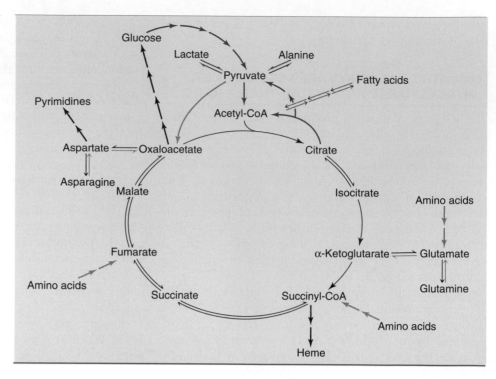

Figure 21.18 α-Keto acids and their corresponding α-amino acids.

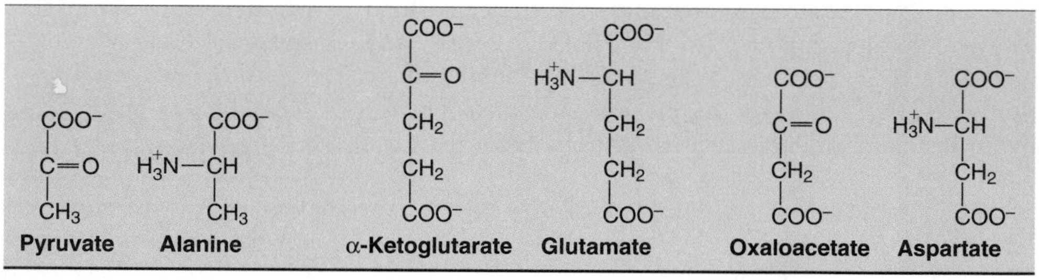

This *ATP-dependent carboxylation* introduces a carboxyl group from inorganic bicarbonate. The reaction requires enzyme-bound **biotin,** and it proceeds in two steps (*Fig. 21.19*). First, CO_2 binds to a nitrogen atom in biotin to produce **carboxy-biotin.** This endergonic reaction ($\Delta G^{0'} = +4.7$ kcal/mol) is fueled by the hydrolysis of ATP to ADP + phosphate ($\Delta G^{0'} = -7.3$ kcal/mol), resulting in an overall free energy change of -2.6 kcal/mol ($4.7 - 7.3$ kcal/mol). In the next step, the "activated carboxyl group" of carboxy-biotin is transferred to pyruvate, forming oxaloacetate.

Pyruvate carboxylase is a strictly mitochondrial enzyme. It requires manganese or magnesium for its activity, and acetyl-CoA is a positive allosteric effector. When the citrate synthase reaction is impaired by a lack of oxaloacetate, acetyl-CoA accumulates in the mitochondrion and activates pyruvate carboxylase.

CLINICAL EXAMPLE 21.6: Pyruvate Carboxylase Deficiency

Pyruvate carboxylase deficiency is a rare recessively inherited condition characterized by elevated blood levels of pyruvate, lactate and alanine, metabolic acidosis, hypoglycemia, and neurological dysfunction. Near-complete deficiency leads to early death, but in the mildest form there is only mild lactic acidosis with normal psychomotor development.

Pyruvate accumulates because pyruvate carboxylase is a major consumer of pyruvate, and accumulating pyruvate is converted to lactate and alanine. Hypoglycemia is caused by the inability to convert pyruvate to glucose in the gluconeogenic pathway (*Fig. 21.17*). Neurological deficits and mental retardation are attributed mainly to dysfunction of the TCA cycle, which suffers from insufficient oxaloacetate.

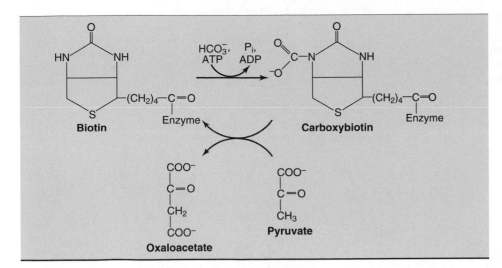

Figure 21.19 Pyruvate carboxylase reaction. This general mechanism applies to all biotin- and ATP-dependent carboxylations.

ANTIPORTERS TRANSPORT METABOLITES ACROSS THE INNER MITOCHONDRIAL MEMBRANE

The outer mitochondrial membrane is riddled with pores that allow the passage of small water-soluble molecules, but transport across the inner mitochondrial membrane requires specific carriers. Most of the important substrates, intermediates, and products of the TCA cycle, with the exceptions of acetyl-CoA, oxaloacetate, fumarate, NAD^+, and NADH, have carriers in the inner mitochondrial membrane. Other transported molecules include ATP and ADP (but not the other nucleotides), pyruvate, phosphate, and the amino acids alanine, aspartate, and glutamate.

The mitochondrial translocases (***Fig. 21.20***) are antiporters. They do not hydrolyze ATP, but energy is consumed whenever actively maintained ion gradients or the membrane potential are dissipated. For example, the transport of hydroxyl ions out of the mitochondrion by the phosphate carrier dissipates an actively maintained proton gradient, and ATP/ADP exchange weakens the membrane potential because ADP has about three negative charges at physiological pH, whereas ATP has about four.

NADH can donate an electron to the respiratory chain only from the mitochondrial matrix, not from the cytoplasm. This creates a problem for the use of the cytoplasmic NADH produced in glycolysis because neither NADH nor NAD^+ is transported across the inner mitochondrial membrane. Therefore two shuttle systems are used: the **glycerol phosphate shuttle** and the **malate-aspartate shuttle** (***Fig. 21.21***).

The glycerol phosphate shuttle transfers the hydrogen first to dihydroxyacetone phosphate, forming glycerol phosphate, and then to the FAD prosthetic group of the mitochondrial glycerol phosphate dehydrogenase, an integral protein of the inner mitochondrial membrane. Like SDH, this enzyme regenerates its FAD by the direct transfer of electrons to the respiratory chain, *producing two ATP molecules.*

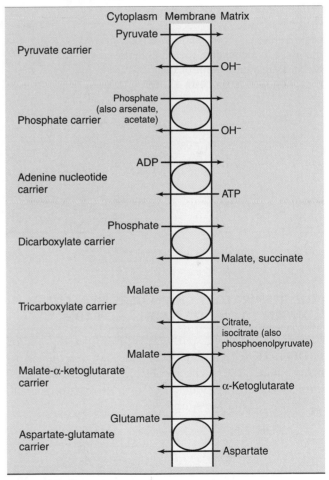

Figure 21.20 Translocases that transport metabolites across the inner mitochondrial membrane. *ADP,* Adenosine diphosphate; *ATP,* adenosine triphosphate.

The malate-aspartate shuttle transfers hydrogen from cytoplasmic NADH to oxaloacetate, forming malate. Malate is transported into the mitochondrion, where it donates its hydrogen to NAD^+, forming NADH. This NADH is oxidized by the respiratory chain, *producing three ATP molecules.*

Figure 21.21 Two ways of transferring electrons from cytoplasmic NADH to the respiratory chain. **A,** Glycerol phosphate shuttle. Mitochondrial glycerol phosphate dehydrogenase is an integral protein of the inner mitochondrial membrane that reacts with glycerol phosphate on the cytoplasmic surface. Therefore glycerol phosphate need not cross the membrane. The FAD prosthetic group of the enzyme is regenerated by transfer of its hydrogen to ubiquinone (Q), a component of the respiratory chain. **B,** Malate-aspartate shuttle. Cytoplasmic NADH transfers its hydrogen to oxaloacetate, forming malate. Malate is transported across the inner mitochondrial membrane, and donates hydrogen to NAD^+ in the malate dehydrogenase reaction of the tricarboxylic acid cycle. Because oxaloacetate is not transported across the inner mitochondrial membrane, its carbons are shuttled out of the mitochondrion in the form of aspartate.

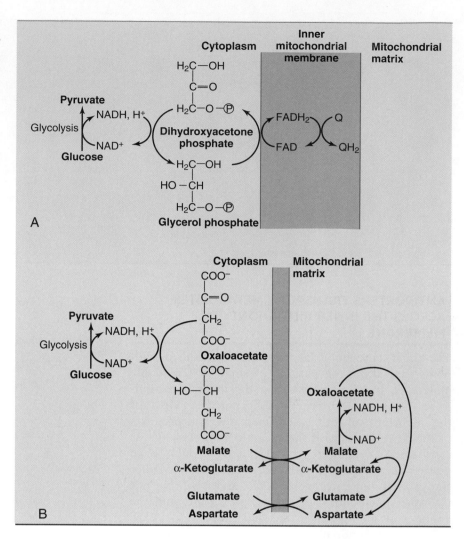

THE RESPIRATORY CHAIN USES MOLECULAR OXYGEN TO OXIDIZE NADH AND FADH$_2$

All major catabolic pathways form NADH and/or FADH$_2$. These reduced coenzymes are reoxidized to NAD$^+$ and FAD by the **respiratory chain** in the inner mitochondrial membrane. The overall reactions in the respiratory chain are simple enough:

$$NADH + H^+ + \tfrac{1}{2} O_2 \rightarrow NAD^+ + H_2O$$

$$FADH_2 + \tfrac{1}{2} O_2 \rightarrow FAD + H_2O$$

The free energy changes, however, are enormous. The oxidation of NADH + H$^+$ releases 52.6 kcal/mol under standard conditions. This corresponds to the free energy content of seven phosphoanhydride bonds in ATP! Oxidation of the FADH$_2$ in mitochondrial flavoproteins yields approximately 40 kcal/mol.

In **oxidative phosphorylation,** some of this energy is harvested as ATP. First, *the oxidations are broken down into sequential reactions with smaller free energy changes.* In these reactions, the components of the

respiratory chain accept and donate electrons, either with or without accompanying protons. A simple hydrogen transport chain looks somewhat like this:

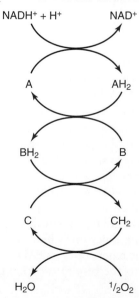

The individual reactions in this chain are as follows:

1. $NADH + H^+ + A \rightarrow NAD^+ + AH_2$
2. $AH_2 + B \rightarrow A + BH_2$
3. $BH_2 + C \rightarrow B + CH_2$
4. $CH_2 + \frac{1}{2} O_2 \rightarrow C + H_2O$

These four reactions add up to the overall reaction:

$$NADH + H^+ + \frac{1}{2} O_2 \rightarrow NAD^+ + H_2O$$

Electron carriers can react with "hydrogen" carriers because a hydrogen atom consists of an electron and a proton. Protons are readily exchanged with the solvent during redox reactions. For example:

$$FADH_2 + 2Fe^{3+} \rightarrow FAD + 2Fe^{2+} + 2H^+$$

Fe^{2+}, in turn, can donate an electron to a hydrogen carrier:

$$2Fe^{2+} + \frac{1}{2} O_2 + 2H^+ \rightarrow 2Fe^{3+} + H_2O$$

STANDARD REDUCTION POTENTIAL DESCRIBES THE TENDENCY TO DONATE ELECTRONS

Redox reactions are electron transfers by definition. This implies the participation of two substrates: a reduced substrate, or **reductant,** which donates electrons (e^-) and becomes oxidized during the reaction, and an oxidized substrate, or **oxidant,** which accepts electrons and becomes reduced.

A substance that can exist in oxidized and reduced forms is called a **redox couple.** $FAD/FADH_2$, Fe^{3+}/Fe^{2+}, and $\frac{1}{2} O_2/H_2O$ are redox couples. During a redox reaction, each redox couple undergoes a "half-reaction." For example:

$$FAD + 2H^+ + 2e^- \rightleftharpoons FADH_2$$

$$Fe^{3+} + e^- \rightleftharpoons Fe^{2+}$$

$$\frac{1}{2} O_2 + 2H^+ + 2e^- \rightleftharpoons H_2O$$

The reduction potential, also called the redox potential, is a measure of the tendency of a redox couple to donate electrons. It can be determined experimentally by allowing the two half-reactions of a redox reaction to proceed in separate compartments and measuring the resulting electron motive force in volts.

The (biological) **standard reduction potential** $E^{o'}$, also called the **standard redox potential,** is determined under standard conditions, with a temperature of 25°C and reactant concentrations of 1 mol/L, but with the proton concentration fixed at 10^{-7} mol/L (pH = 7.0). These are the same "biological" standard conditions that are used for the definition of standard free energy changes.

A low $E^{o'}$ means that the reduced form of the redox couple has a strong tendency to donate electrons, or a

Table 21.6 Standard Reduction Potentials of Some Biologically Important Redox Couples

Oxidant/Reductant	$E^{o'}$ (V)
Acetate/acetaldehyde	−0.60
$2 H^+/H_2$	−0.42*
$NAD^+/NADH + H^+$	−0.32
$NADP^+/NADPH + H^+$	−0.32
Lipoate/dihydrolipoate	−0.29
Acetoacetate/β-hydroxybutyrate	−0.27
Glutathione oxidized/reduced	−0.23
Acetaldehyde/ethanol	−0.20
Pyruvate/lactate	−0.19
Oxaloacetate/malate	−0.17
Fumarate/succinate	+0.03
Cytochrome b Fe^{3+}/Fe^{2+}	+0.08
Dehydroascorbate/ascorbate	+0.08
Ubiquinone/ubiquinol	+0.10
Cytochrome c Fe^{3+}/Fe^{2+}	+0.22
Fe^{3+}/Fe^{2+}	+0.77†
$\frac{1}{2} O_2/H_2O$	+0.82

*The reduction potential of the hydrogen electrode is set at zero for "chemical" standard conditions, with a proton concentration of 1M. The shift into the negative range is caused by the far lower proton concentration under "biological" standard conditions (at pH = 7.0).
†Standard reduction potential of inorganic iron. The reduction potentials of the iron in heme proteins and iron-sulfur proteins may be markedly different.

great "reducing power." Therefore *electrons are transferred from the redox couple with the lower reduction potential to the redox couple with the higher reduction potential.* **Table 21.6** shows the standard reduction potentials of some redox couples.

Under standard conditions, the equilibrium of a redox reaction is determined by the difference between the standard reduction potentials of the participating redox couples ($\Delta E^{o'}$):

$$\Delta E^{o'} = E^{o'}_{oxidant} - E^{o'}_{reductant}$$

For the reaction

$$NADH + H^+ + \frac{1}{2} O_2 \rightarrow NAD^+ + H_2O$$

the standard reduction potentials are

$$NAD^+/NADH + H^+ : E^{o'} = -0.32\ V$$

$$\frac{1}{2} O_2 + 2H^+/H_2O : E^{o'} = +0.82\ V$$

Therefore

$$\Delta E^{0'} = E^{0'}_{1/2 O_2 + 2H^+/H_2O} - E^{0'}_{NAD^+/NADH + H^+}$$
$$= 0.82\ volt - (-0.32\ volt)$$
$$= +1.14\ volt$$

As in the case of free energy changes, the actual driving force of the reaction under nonstandard conditions (ΔE) also depends on the relative reactant concentrations. There is a simple relationship between $\Delta G^{0'}$ and $\Delta E^{o'}$:

$$\Delta G^{0'} = -n \times F \times \Delta E^{o'}$$

where n = the number of electrons transferred, and F = the Faraday constant ($23.06\ kcal \times V^{-1} \times mol^{-1}$).

A positive $\Delta E^{o'}$, like a negative $\Delta G^{0'}$, signifies an exergonic reaction. In the previous example of NADH oxidation by molecular oxygen, $\Delta G^{0'}$ can be calculated as

$$\begin{aligned} \Delta G^{0'} &= -n \times F \times \Delta E^{o'} \\ &= -2 \times 23.06 \times 1.14 \\ &= -52.6\ kcal/mol \end{aligned}$$

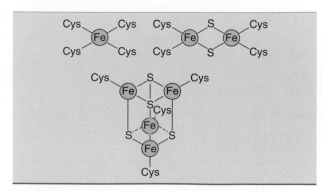

Figure 21.23 Iron-sulfur complexes in proteins. The iron in these complexes can change its oxidation state reversibly between the ferrous (Fe^{2+}) and ferric (Fe^{3+}) forms.

THE RESPIRATORY CHAIN CONTAINS FLAVOPROTEINS, IRON-SULFUR PROTEINS, CYTOCHROMES, UBIQUINONE, AND PROTEIN-BOUND COPPER

Because none of the functional groups in "ordinary" proteins can transfer hydrogen or electrons easily, the components of the respiratory chain have to use metal ions and coenzymes.

The **flavoproteins** contain protein-bound FAD or flavin mononucleotide (FMN), which can transfer two electrons sequentially (***Fig. 21.22***). For example, single-electron transfers occur when the flavin coenzyme exchanges an electron with iron. The standard reduction potentials of FAD and FMN are intermediate between NAD^+/NADH and the cytochromes. Therefore *the flavoproteins accept electrons (+ protons) from NADH and donate the electrons to the cytochromes.*

The **iron-sulfur proteins,** also known as **nonheme iron proteins,** contain iron complexed to cysteine side chains. *This iron transfers electrons by switching between the ferrous (Fe^{2+}) and ferric (Fe^{3+}) states.* Many iron-sulfur proteins contain inorganic sulfide as well (***Fig. 21.23***). Both the iron-sulfur proteins and the flavoproteins of the respiratory chain are integral membrane proteins.

The **cytochromes** contain iron in the form of an iron-porphyrin, usually the heme group. In contrast to hemoglobin and myoglobin, in which the iron is always in the ferrous state, *the heme iron of the cytochromes switches back and forth between Fe^{2+} and Fe^{3+}.* Also,

in most cytochromes (but not cytochrome a/a_3), the heme iron is bound to two amino acid side chains rather than one. This prevents the binding of molecular oxygen, carbon monoxide, and other potential ligands.

Cytochromes a and a_3 contain **heme a,** which has a hydrophobic isoprenoid chain covalently attached to one of its vinyl groups. With the exception of cytochrome c, the cytochromes of the respiratory chain are integral membrane proteins.

Ubiquinone, also known as **coenzyme Q,** is a mobile hydrogen carrier that is not permanently associated with an apoprotein. A long hydrocarbon tail, consisting of 10 isoprene (branched five-carbon) units, makes it strongly hydrophobic and confines it to the lipid bilayer of the inner mitochondrial membrane. Like the flavin coenzymes, ubiquinone carries two hydrogen atoms but can act in one-electron transfers by forming a somewhat stable intermediate (***Fig. 21.24***).

Protein-bound **copper** participates in the last reaction of the respiratory chain, the transfer of electrons to molecular oxygen. It switches between the Cu^{1+} and Cu^{2+} forms during these electron transfers.

THE RESPIRATORY CHAIN CONTAINS LARGE MULTIPROTEIN COMPLEXES

Four members of the respiratory chain are diffusible: NADH, ubiquinone, cytochrome c, and molecular oxygen. NADH is in the mitochondrial matrix, ubiquinone is mobile in the lipid bilayer, and cytochrome c is loosely

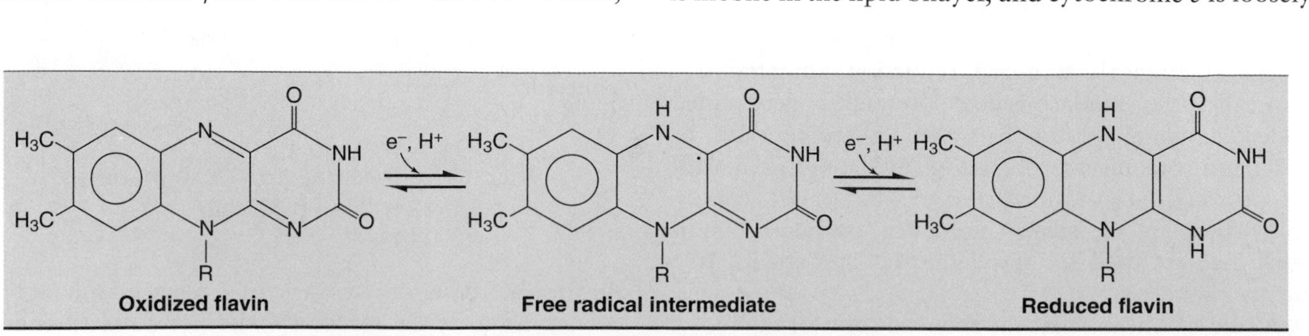

Figure 21.22 Structures of oxidized and reduced flavin coenzymes. e^-, Electron.

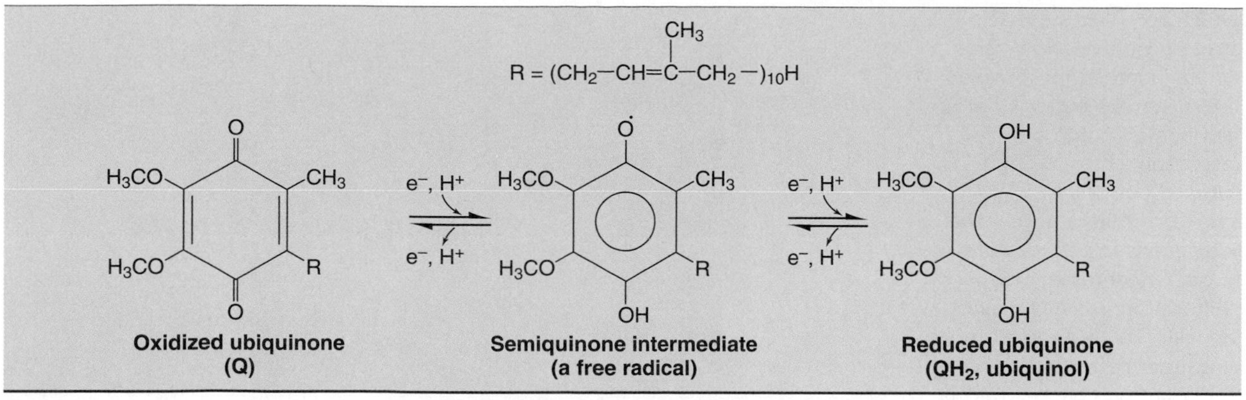

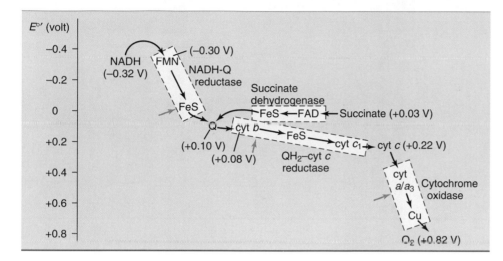

Figure 21.24   Structure of ubiquinone (coenzyme Q). e^-, Electron.

Figure 21.25   Respiratory chain. *Shaded structures* are multiprotein complexes in the inner mitochondrial membrane. NADH and succinate are in the matrix space, ubiquinone (Q) is in the lipid bilayer of the membrane, and cytochrome *c* is a peripheral membrane protein on the outer surface of the inner mitochondrial membrane. The standard redox potentials are shown for some components. *Orange arrows* indicate sites of proton pumping ("phosphorylation sites"). *cyt,* Cytochrome; *FAD,* flavin adenine dinucleotide; *FeS,* iron-sulfur protein; *FMN,* flavin mononucleotide; *Q,* ubiquinone.

bound to the outer surface of the inner mitochondrial membrane. Molecular oxygen, freely diffusible across membranes, receives electrons and protons on the matrix side of the inner mitochondrial membrane.

The other components are organized in large protein complexes that are arranged asymmetrically in the membrane (*Fig. 21.25*):

1. **NADH-Q reductase,** also called **NADH dehydrogenase** or **complex I,** transfers electrons from NADH to ubiquinone. It contains FMN and several iron-sulfur centers. Electrons are transferred from NADH to FMN, then through a succession of iron-sulfur centers to ubiquinone.

2. **QH₂-cytochrome *c* reductase,** also called **cytochrome reductase** or **complex III,** transfers electrons from ubiquinone to cytochrome *c*. It contains cytochrome *b*, an iron-sulfur protein, and cytochrome c_1.

3. **Cytochrome oxidase (complex IV)** contains two heme *a* groups (heme *a* and heme a_3) located next to a copper ion. O_2 is tightly held between heme a_3 and copper, to be released only after its complete

reduction to H_2O by the sequential transfer of four electrons. Cytochrome oxidase has a very high affinity for molecular oxygen. This ensures a near-maximal rate of oxidative phosphorylation even at very low oxygen partial pressure.

4. **Mitochondrial flavoproteins,** including SDH (**complex II**) and the mitochondrial glycerol phosphate dehydrogenase, bypass the NADH-Q reductase complex. They transfer their electrons directly to ubiquinone.

THE RESPIRATORY CHAIN CREATES A PROTON GRADIENT

Oxidative phosphorylation proceeds in two steps (*Fig. 21.26*):

1. *Protons are pumped out of the mitochondrion.* Proton pumping is driven by the redox reactions in the respiratory chain.

2. *Protons are admitted back into the mitochondrion through a proton channel.* This entropically favored process drives ATP synthesis.

Figure 21.26 Two steps in oxidative phosphorylation. The inner mitochondrial membrane acts like a storage battery that is charged by the proton pumps of the respiratory chain. **A,** Protons are pumped out of the mitochondrial matrix during the redox reactions in the respiratory chain. *cyt,* Cytochrome; *FeS,* iron-sulfur protein; *FMN,* flavin mononucleotide. **B,** Protons move back into the matrix space through a proton channel that is coupled to an ATP-synthesizing enzyme (F_1F_o-ATP synthase). ATP synthesis is fueled by the flow of protons down their electrochemical gradient.

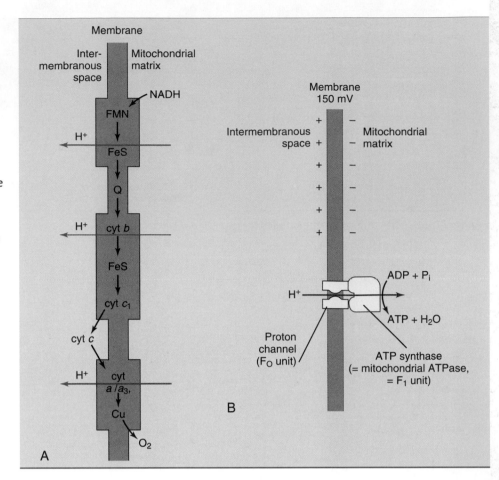

Protons are pumped in each of the three protein complexes (see **Figs. 21.25** and **21.26**). Approximately four protons are pumped by the NADH-Q reductase complex and another four by the QH_2-cytochrome *c* reductase complex. Cytochrome oxidase removes four protons from the mitochondrial matrix, translocating two to the intermembranous space and consuming the other two in the reduction of O_2.

The passage of a pair of electrons through these "phosphorylation sites" leads to the synthesis of approximately one ATP molecule per phosphorylation site. There are three phosphorylation sites for the oxidation of NADH and two for the oxidation of $FADH_2$. Therefore the **P/O ratio,** defined as the number of high-energy phosphate bonds formed for each oxygen atom (or each pair of electrons) consumed, is conventionally stated as 3 for NADH and 2 for $FADH_2$. However, under "real-world" conditions the ratio seems to be a bit lower.

The respiratory chain creates a proton gradient of about one pH unit, inside alkaline. It also helps to maintain a membrane potential of 100 to 200 mV, inside negative. Concentration gradient and electrical membrane potential add up to a steep electrochemical gradient for protons.

To maintain this gradient, the inner mitochondrial membrane must be impermeable to protons and also to other ions (which would dissipate the membrane potential). This is the reason why most translocases of the inner mitochondrial membrane make electroneutral exchanges, thereby minimizing the effects of substrate transport on the membrane potential (see **Fig. 21.20**).

THE PROTON GRADIENT DRIVES ATP SYNTHESIS

The proton gradient fuels **mitochondrial ATP synthase,** also known as **F_1F_o-ATP synthase.** The F_1 unit (F_1 = coupling factor 1) of the enzyme is a protein complex of subunit structure $\alpha_3\beta_3\gamma\delta\epsilon$ and a molecular weight of 380 kD. It is visible under the electron microscope as small buttons on the inner surface of the inner mitochondrial membrane. The F_1 unit is **attached to the F_o unit** (F_o = oligomycin-sensitive factor), an integral membrane protein with the subunit structure a,b_2,c_1. The *c* subunits form a circular array, and the proton channel is formed by the interface between the *a* and *c* subunits.

The ATP synthase works like a rotary motor (**Fig. 21.27**). The F_1 unit has three catalytic sites on a circular array of three α subunits and three β subunits.

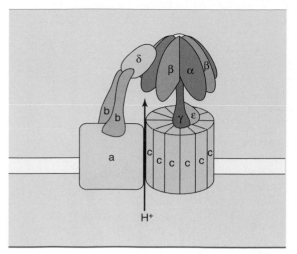

Figure 21.27 Structure of the F_1F_o-ATP synthase. The *a*, *b*, δ, α, and β subunits are stationary. The ring of *c* subunits with the attached γ and ε subunits rotates when protons move through the channel. The rotation of γ induces sequential changes in the conformation of the catalytic $α_3β_3$ "button." These conformational changes drive ATP synthesis.

This array is kept stationary by the *b* and δ subunits, which attach it firmly to the *a* subunit in the membrane. The centrally located γ subunit is tightly anchored to the ring of *c* subunits in the membrane.

The ring of c subunits rotates during proton flow. The movement of a single proton through the channel seems to be sufficient to ratchet one *c* subunit out of its interaction with the stationary *a* subunit while the next *c* subunit ratchets in. This amounts to a rotation of 30 degrees. The attached γ subunit rotates with the

ring of *c* subunits, forming a "rotor stalk" in the axis of the F_1 unit.

Each of the three catalytic sites on the $α_3β_3$ array goes through a sequence of conformational changes that are driven by the rotation of the γ subunit (*Fig. 21.28*). In the **L (loose) conformation,** the β subunit binds ADP + phosphate. The rotating γ subunit then switches it to the **T (tight) conformation** while ATP is synthesized. This conformation binds ATP with very high affinity. This tight binding stabilizes ATP thermodynamically and makes its synthesis possible. To release the ATP, the catalytic site has to be switched from the T conformation to the **O (open) conformation,** which has low affinity for ATP.

Proton flow is tightly coupled to ATP synthesis. *ATP is synthesized only when protons flow, and protons can flow only when ATP is synthesized.* A 360-degree rotation of the motor produces three molecules of ATP while 12 protons are translocated. Thus four protons are required for the synthesis of one ATP molecule.

In the absence of a sufficient proton gradient, the ATP synthase does not synthesize but rather hydrolyzes ATP, as shown in the experiment of *Figure 21.29.* Therefore the term **mitochondrial ATPase** is sometimes applied to the ATP-synthesizing complex.

THE EFFICIENCY OF GLUCOSE OXIDATION IS CLOSE TO 40%

We can now examine the efficiency of ATP synthesis from the oxidation of glucose, assuming an ATP yield of three molecules for each NADH and two for each

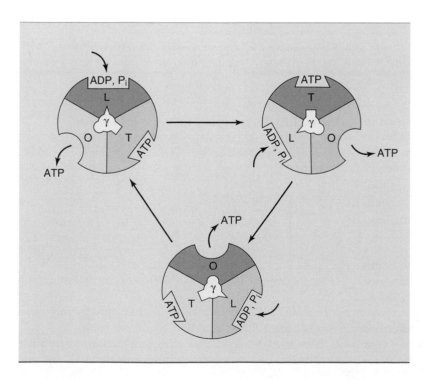

Figure 21.28 Sequence of reactions in the synthesis of ATP by F_1F_o-ATP synthase in the inner mitochondrial membrane. The conformational transitions between the tight (T), open (O), and loose (L) conformations are driven by the rotating γ subunit.

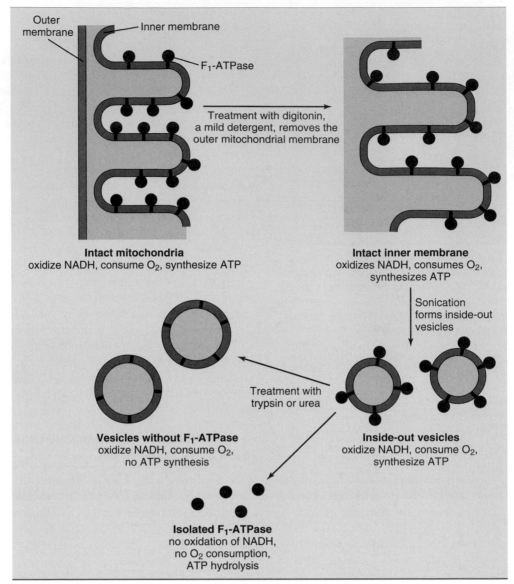

Figure 21.29 Isolation of the F_1-ATPase. Note that the isolated ATP synthase does not synthesize but rather hydrolyzes ATP. Therefore this enzyme is often called the "mitochondrial ATPase" or "F_1-ATPase." An intact membrane with a steep proton gradient is an absolute requirement for ATP synthesis.

$FADH_2$ oxidized in the respiratory chain. As shown in *Table 21.7*, 36 to 38 high-energy phosphate bonds are generated, far more than the two ATP generated in anaerobic glycolysis. Assuming a production of 37 ATP and a free energy of hydrolysis of 7.3 kcal/mol for a phosphoanhydride bond in ATP, the energy yield from glucose oxidation is therefore

$$37 \times 7.3 = 270.1 \text{ kcal/mol}$$

The total heat released by glucose oxidation in the bomb calorimeter is 686 kcal/mol. Therefore the efficiency of ATP synthesis during glucose oxidation is 270.1/686 = 0.394 = 39.4%. The balance is released as heat.

Even with ATP synthesis, the overall equilibrium of the oxidative pathways is so overwhelmingly in favor of substrate oxidation that *the cells are able to maintain*

Table 21.7 Energy Yield from Glucose Oxidation

Pathway	Yield (Molecules)		
Glycolysis			2 ATP
	2 NADH	→	4 or 6 ATP*
Pyruvate dehydrogenase	2 NADH	→	6 ATP
Tricarboxylic acid cycle	2 GTP	→	2 ATP
	6 NADH	→	18 ATP
	2 FADH2	→	4 ATP
			36 or 38 ATP

*The energy yield from cytoplasmic NADH depends on the shuttle system used.

a high [ATP]/[ADP] ratio. In resting muscle, this ratio approaches 100:1.

Nevertheless, oxidative phosphorylation is not quite as efficient as it looks. Approximately 20% of the energy in the proton gradient is dissipated by the phosphate carrier and the ATP/ADP exchanger in the membrane, reducing the true ATP yield to about 30 ATP molecules per molecule of glucose.

Oxidative phosphorylation would be more efficient if ATP were synthesized on the outer rather than inner surface of the inner mitochondrial membrane, obviating the need for wasteful membrane carriers. The reason for this suboptimal design is that the ancestors of current human mitochondria were free-living bacteria that had to synthesize their ATP inside the cell. This fundamental design has never been changed since the enslavement of the mitochondria by the eukaryotic cell.

OXIDATIVE PHOSPHORYLATION IS LIMITED BY THE SUPPLY OF ADP

Electron flow in the respiratory chain and ATP synthesis are tightly coupled. *ATP cannot be synthesized without electron flow, and electrons cannot flow without ATP synthesis.* Unless the proton gradient is dissipated through the F_1F_0-ATP synthase, it will build up to such proportions that the redox reactions in the respiratory chain grind to a halt, being unable to pump against the overwhelming gradient.

There is no "rate-limiting step" in oxidative phosphorylation, but its rate depends on substrate availability. Possible limiting factors include

- NADH
- Oxygen
- ADP
- Phosphate
- The capacity of the respiratory chain itself when all substrates are freely available (its V_{max})

Phosphate and (except in starvation) NADH are rarely in short supply. *Usually, ADP is the rate-limiting substrate.* With increased metabolic activity, as in contracting muscle, oxidative phosphorylation increases initially in proportion to the rising ADP concentration until either the oxygen supply or the capacity of the respiratory chain becomes limiting.

An increased rate of oxidative phosphorylation consumes NADH and raises the mitochondrial $[NAD^+]/[NADH]$ ratio. Together with the low energy charge that raised the rate of oxidative phosphorylation in the first place, the high $[NAD^+]/[NADH]$ ratio stimulates pyruvate dehydrogenase and the regulated enzymes of the TCA cycle. Nutrient degradation and NADH production in the catabolic pathways are thereby adjusted to NADH consumption in the respiratory chain.

CLINICAL EXAMPLE 21.7: Acute Cyanide Poisoning

Cyanide (CN^-) blocks the electron transport chain by binding to the ferric (Fe^{3+}) iron in cytochrome oxidase. It is not especially potent, with an LD_{50} of approximately 1 mg/kg in humans, but its acid form hydrocyanic acid (HCN, historically called "prussic acid") is highly diffusible and can cause death almost instantly.

Cyanide poisoning causes hyperventilation, not because of hypoxia but because of massive lactic acidosis. Being unable to synthesize ATP by oxidative phosphorylation, *all tissues switch to anaerobic glycolysis and release lactic acid into the blood.* Acidosis is a powerful stimulus for the respiratory center in the brain. Consciousness is lost fast, and death after a fatal dose can ensue in minutes.

HCN's rapid action makes it a popular poison for suicide, but its bitter almond smell makes it less suitable for homicide. Because of its rapid and painless action, cyanide was used in Nazi gas chambers during the holocaust and for the execution of criminals in the United States.

Treatment of acute poisoning is aimed at the removal of cyanide from cytochrome oxidase. Injected sodium nitrite and inhaled amyl nitrite are used to oxidize some of the hemoglobin to methemoglobin. Cyanide binds with high affinity to the ferric iron in methemoglobin, and this removes it from the ferric iron in cytochrome oxidase.

Ordinarily, cyanide from dietary sources is detoxified by the enzyme **rhodanase** in the liver, which reacts cyanide with thiosulfate to form harmless thiocyanate:

$$N\equiv C^- + {}^-S - \underset{\underset{O}{\parallel}}{\overset{\overset{O}{\parallel}}{S}} - O^- \longrightarrow N\equiv C - S^- + \underset{\underset{O}{\parallel}}{\overset{\overset{O^-}{\mid}}{S}} - O^-$$

Cyanide   Thiosulfate   Thiocyanate   Sulfite

Thiosulfate is used along with nitrites for the emergency treatment of cyanide poisoning.

OXIDATIVE PHOSPHORYLATION IS INHIBITED BY MANY POISONS

Electron flow through the respiratory chain can be blocked by *site-specific inhibitors* (*Table 21.8*). **Rotenone,** obtained from the roots of some tropical plants, inhibits electron flow from the iron-sulfur complexes in the NADH-Q reductase complex to ubiquinone. It is a very effective poison for fish, which take it up through their gills. Humans can eat the poisoned fish with impunity because rotenone is absorbed poorly by the intestine. Rotenone is also in favor as a "natural" insecticide.

In addition to rotenone, some **barbiturates** inhibit electron flow through the NADH-Q reductase complex. This action is unrelated to their sedative-hypnotic properties, which are mediated by an effect on a γ-aminobutyric acid (GABA)–operated chloride channel in the brain.

Antimycin A, an antibiotic produced by a streptomycete, blocks electron flow through the QH_2-cytochrome *c* reductase complex.

In the cytochrome oxidase complex, several inhibitors bind to the heme iron in cytochrome a/a_3, whose sixth coordination position is otherwise reserved for oxygen. **Cyanide** and **azide** bind to the ferric form of the iron, and **carbon monoxide** binds to the ferrous form. Whereas carbon monoxide binds more tightly to hemoglobin than to cytochrome oxidase, the other poisons induce their effects by inhibiting electron flow.

Uncouplers of oxidative phosphorylation prevent ATP synthesis despite continuing electron flow. Most uncouplers disrupt the proton gradient across the inner mitochondrial membrane. **2,4-Dinitrophenol** and **pentachlorophenol** (*Fig. 21.30*) are weak, lipid-soluble organic acids that dissipate the proton gradient by

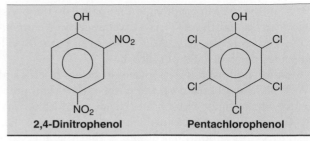

Figure 21.30 Structures of 2,4-dinitrophenol and pentachlorophenol. These weakly acidic substances can diffuse across the inner mitochondrial membrane even in the negatively charged deprotonated form. They uncouple oxidative phosphorylation by transporting protons across the membrane.

ferrying protons across the inner mitochondrial membrane. ATP synthesis is impaired, but electron flow accelerates because ADP rises and the respiratory chain no longer has to pump protons against a steep gradient.

Even some endogenous products, including free fatty acids and bilirubin, act as uncouplers at high concentrations. Bilirubin can cause brain damage in infants with severe hyperbilirubinemia (see Chapter 27), possibly by uncoupling oxidative phosphorylation.

Valinomycin is a transport antibiotic that makes the inner mitochondrial membrane permeable for potassium. This dissipates the membrane potential, which is an essential component of the proton-motive force.

Oligomycin is an antibiotic that prevents ATP synthesis by blocking the proton channel in the F_1F_o-ATP synthase. A steep proton gradient builds up and inhibits electron flow through the respiratory chain.

The plant product **atractyloside** blocks the ATP/ADP antiporter in the inner mitochondrial membrane. The resulting lack of ADP in the mitochondrial matrix stops both ATP synthesis and electron flow.

Table 21.8 Inhibitors of Oxidative Phosphorylation

Inhibitor	Mechanism
Inhibitors of Electron Flow	
Rotenone, Amytal	Inhibits NADH-Q reductase
Antimycin A	Inhibits QH_2-cytochrome *c* reductase
Cyanide, azide, hydrogen sulfide, carbon monoxide	Inhibits cytochrome oxidase
Oligomycin	Inhibits the F_o proton channel
Uncouplers	
2,4-Dinitrophenol, pentachlorophenol	Transports protons across the inner mitochondrial membrane
Valinomycin	Transports potassium across the inner mitochondrial membrane
Arsenate	Substitutes for phosphate during ATP synthesis
Atractyloside	Inhibits ATP-ADP translocation

ADP, Adenosine diphosphate; *ATP,* adenosine triphosphate; *NADH,* reduced form of nicotinamide adenine dinucleotide.

CLINICAL EXAMPLE 21.8: Use of 2,4-Dinitrophenol for Weight Loss

Uncouplers of oxidative phosphorylation reduce the efficiency of ATP synthesis. This is compensated for by increased electron flow in the respiratory chain and increased nutrient oxidation. *The result is massive heat production with only marginally reduced ATP synthesis.* Indeed, death after a lethal dose appears to be caused by rampant hyperthermia rather than ATP depletion.

The prototypical uncoupler, 2,4-dinitrophenol, had been used in diet pills during the 1930s but was banned in the United States in 1938 after its toxicity had been recognized. Today it is again available through Internet outlets and is used by some bodybuilders and athletes in an attempt to lose body fat fast. Its therapeutic index is rather narrow, though. The dose recommended (by some) for weight loss is 5 to 8 mg/kg/day, but a single dose of 20 to 50 mg/kg can be lethal.

CLINICAL EXAMPLE 21.9: Ischemia

Local obstruction of the blood supply is called **ischemia**. Tissue necrosis due to ischemia is called **infarction**. Gangrene, acute myocardial infarction, and thromboembolic stroke are examples of infarction.

The immediate cause of infarction is the inability of the ischemic tissue to produce sufficient ATP by oxidative phosphorylation. The average ATP molecule has a lifespan of only 1 to 5 minutes, and most cells will be depleted of ATP within minutes when its synthesis is blocked. Ischemic anoxia causes cell death within a few minutes (neurons), half an hour to 2 hours (myocardium, liver, kidney), or several hours (fibroblasts, epidermis, skeletal muscle). Cells in the hair follicles are so resistant to anoxia that a beard keeps growing for 2 to 3 days after death.

Insufficient ATP makes the cells unable to maintain ion gradients across the plasma membrane and the organelle membranes (*Fig. 21.31*). This leads both to aberrant activation of intracellular signaling cascades (especially by calcium) and to membrane damage by osmotic stress. Cellular proteins leak out of the cell, and hydrolytic enzymes leak out of the lysosomes.

The shortfall of ATP stimulates glycolysis at the level of phosphofructokinase, with lactic acid formed as the end product. Although ATP from anaerobic glycolysis can tide the cell over for some time, the accumulating lactic acid acidifies the tissue, thereby activating lysosomal enzymes and contributing to cell death. In animal experiments, tissues that are perfused with oxygen-free blood survive far longer than tissues whose blood supply has been interrupted. A likely reason is that the accumulation of lactic acid contributes to cell death in ischemic tissues.

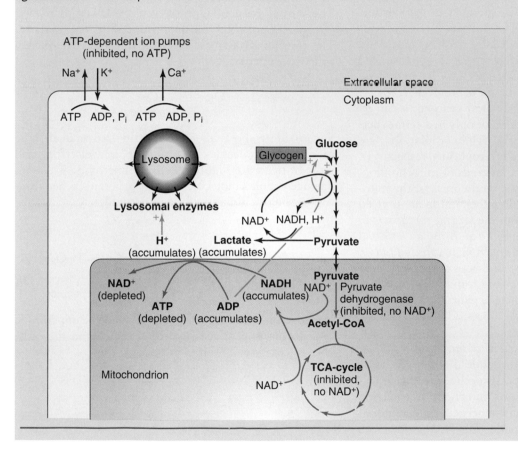

Figure 21.31 Metabolic consequences of hypoxia. Decreased energy charge and [NAD$^+$]/[NADH] ratio are the initial results of oxygen deficiency. The mitochondrial oxidative pathways are arrested for lack of NAD$^+$. The regulated enzymes of glycolysis and glycogen degradation (phosphofructokinase and glycogen phosphorylase) are stimulated by low energy charge. Lactic acid accumulates and acidifies the cell. Membranes are damaged by the increased acidity and by osmotic imbalances that result from the failure of ATP-dependent ion pumps. Lysosomal enzymes, which are active at low pH, initiate autolysis.

BROWN ADIPOSE TISSUE CONTAINS AN UNCOUPLING PROTEIN

Ordinarily, the oxidative pathways are designed to maximize ATP production while minimizing heat production. During cold stress, however, heat is a valuable product. For this contingency, many mammals, including human infants, have a small amount of brown adipose tissue, mainly in the neck and upper back. Unlike white adipose tissue, brown adipose tissue contains large numbers of mitochondria whose cytochromes are responsible for its brown color.

The mitochondria of brown adipose tissue contain an uncoupling protein (**UCP1**, or **thermogenin**) in their inner membrane, which forms a proton channel. Ordinarily, the channel is kept closed by physiological concentrations of purine nucleotides.

Like white adipose tissue, brown adipose tissue is innervated by the sympathetic nervous system. Norepinephrine, released during cold stress, activates the cAMP system through a β-adrenergic receptor. The cAMP cascade activates the lipase that hydrolyzes the stored triglyceride. Fat hydrolysis forms free fatty acids, which are both catabolic substrates and activators of thermogenin, causing massive heat production.

MUTATIONS IN MITOCHONDRIAL DNA CAN CAUSE DISEASE

The mitochondrial genome (see Chapter 7) consists of 16,569 base pairs that encode 13 polypeptides, 22 transfer RNA (tRNAs), and the two RNAs (12S and 16S) of the mitochondrial ribosomes. The mitochondria-encoded polypeptides include 7 (of 42) subunits of NADH-Q reductase, 1 subunit (of 11) of QH_2-cytochrome c reductase, 3 (of 13) subunits of cytochrome oxidase, and 2 subunits of ATP synthase. All other mitochondrial proteins are encoded by nuclear genes and synthesized by cytoplasmic ribosomes.

Therefore *mitochondrial diseases can be caused by mutations in either nuclear or mitochondrial DNA.* If the mutation is in the mitochondrial genome, it can be present either in all mitochondria or only in a certain percentage of the mitochondria. These situations are described as **homoplasmy** and **heteroplasmy,** respectively. Most cells have hundreds to thousands of mitochondria, and each mitochondrion has several copies of the mitochondrial genome. Because all mitochondria are derived from the ovum and none from the sperm, *mutations in mitochondrial DNA are transmitted from an affected mother to all her children but not from an affected father.*

Mitochondrial diseases affect tissues that have a high energy demand and rely heavily on oxidative metabolism. Typical presentations include neurological deficits, abnormalities of red muscle fibers, cardiomyopathy, and/or retinal degeneration.

Mitochondrial DNA has a higher mutation rate than nuclear DNA. Therefore mitochondrial mutations accumulate, and the oxidative capacity declines, with advancing age. The gradual decline of mitochondrial function with age explains why many inherited mitochondrial mutations become symptomatic only at an advanced age, when the combined effects of the inherited mutation and of acquired somatic mutations depress oxidative phosphorylation below a critical threshold (*Clinical Example 21.10*).

CLINICAL EXAMPLE 21.10: Leber Hereditary Optic Neuropathy

Leber hereditary optic neuropathy (LHON) is characterized by the sudden onset of blindness in young adults, caused by degeneration of the optic nerve. The most common mutation in patients with this disease is a single-base substitution that replaces an arginine residue in one of the subunits of NADH-Q reductase with histidine. Other patients have different point mutations in genes for subunits of NADH-Q reductase, QH_2-cytochrome c reductase, or cytochrome oxidase.

All of these mutations impair electron flow through the respiratory chain and reduce ATP synthesis. They lead to blindness because the optic nerve has a high energy demand and depends almost entirely on oxidative phosphorylation for its ATP supply.

REACTIVE OXYGEN DERIVATIVES ARE FORMED DURING OXIDATIVE METABOLISM

The reduction of one molecule of oxygen to two molecules of water requires four electrons and four protons. The partial reduction of oxygen by fewer than four electrons is possible, but the products are very reactive. The transfer of a single electron to molecular oxygen produces **superoxide:**

$$O_2 + e^- \rightarrow O_2^{-}$$
Superoxide

Superoxide is both an anion and a **free radical.** Free radicals are molecules with an unpaired electron, and most of them are highly reactive. Superoxide itself can damage cellular molecules, and it generates other reactive species including **hydrogen peroxide:**

$$O_2^{-} \underset{}{\overset{H^+}{\rightleftharpoons}} HO_2^{\bullet} \xrightarrow{HO_2^{\bullet} \quad O_2} H_2O_2$$

Superoxide radical — Hydroperoxide radical — Hydrogen peroxide

Hydrogen peroxide is less reactive than the superoxide radical, but it produces **hydroxyl radicals** in the presence of catalytic amounts of ferrous iron:

$$H_2O_2 + Fe^{2+} + H^+ \longrightarrow HO^{\bullet} + H_2O + Fe^{3+}$$

Hydrogen peroxide — Hydroxyl radical

The hydroxyl radical is the most reactive of all oxygen-derived free radicals. It behaves like the most indiscriminate suicide terrorist because it reacts with almost any organic molecule it collides with, destroying both itself and the molecule in the reaction.

The superoxide radical is thought to be formed in small quantity by many oxygenases including cytochrome oxidase, but the major source is most likely the haphazard leakage of electrons from the respiratory chain and other electron transport chains to molecular oxygen (see *Clinical Example 21.11*).

Hydrogen peroxide is formed not only from the superoxide radical but also as a normal product of many flavoproteins. Unlike NAD and NADP, FAD and FMN are tightly bound prosthetic groups. After being reduced in a dehydrogenase reaction, the flavin coenzyme cannot simply diffuse away to donate its hydrogen in a different enzymatic reaction. Flavoproteins of the inner mitochondrial membrane, including SDH and the mitochondrial glycerol phosphate dehydrogenase, donate their hydrogen to ubiquinone (coenzyme Q):

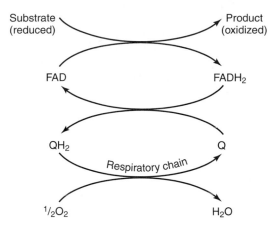

Flavoproteins in other locations transfer their hydrogen directly to molecular oxygen, forming hydrogen peroxide:

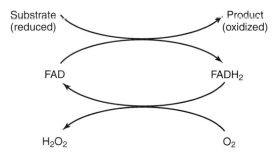

Several enzymes have evolved to destroy reactive oxygen derivatives. **Superoxide dismutase** eliminates the superoxide radical by accelerating the formation of hydrogen peroxide from the superoxide radical:

$$2\ O_2^{\cdot -} + 2\ H^+ \xrightarrow[\text{dismustase}]{\text{Superoxide}} H_2O_2 + O_2$$

It is present in the cytoplasm and mitochondria of all cells. The mitochondrial enzyme is activated by manganese, and the cytoplasmic enzyme contains copper and zinc. *Superoxide dismutase is required for aerobic life.* It is present in all aerobic organisms but not in obligate anaerobes.

The heme-containing enzyme **catalase** destroys hydrogen peroxide:

$$2\ H_2O_2 \xrightarrow{\text{Catalase}} 2\ H_2O + O_2$$

It is present in blood and tissues, accounting for 40% of the total protein in peroxisomes. Because of catalase, hydrogen peroxide bubbles when it is applied to wounds.

Peroxidases destroy hydrogen peroxide by reacting it with an organic substrate. The most important of them, **glutathione peroxidase,** uses the sulfhydryl-containing tripeptide glutathione (see Chapter 22):

$$2\ \text{Glutathione-SH} + H_2O_2 \rightarrow \begin{array}{c}\text{Glutathione-S}\\ |\\ \text{Glutathione-S}\end{array} + 2\ H_2O$$

Many metabolites, vitamins, and phytochemicals can eliminate dangerous free radicals. Water-soluble antioxidants, including bilirubin, uric acid, and ascorbate, patrol the aqueous compartments, while the fat-soluble vitamins A and E do police duty in the membranes. *These molecules form stable free radicals that are sufficiently reactive to react readily with other free radicals but not sufficiently reactive to damage normal constituents of the cell.* Ubiquinone and the flavin coenzymes are examples of molecules that form stable free radicals (see *Figs. 21.22* and *21.24*). Ubiquinone is available in health food stores as an antioxidant and free radical scavenger.

However, because free radical scavengers themselves form free radicals, there is always the possibility that the scavenger can cause some collateral damage while it is eliminating the more dangerous free radicals.

Reactive oxygen derivatives can initiate the nonenzymatic oxidation of polyunsaturated fatty acid residues in membrane lipids and triglycerides (see Chapter 23), and they contribute to somatic mutations. The mitochondria, in particular, are badly polluted with reactive oxygen species. This is a likely reason for the high mutation rate of mitochondrial DNA.

CLINICAL EXAMPLE 21.11: Oxygen Toxicity

Experimental animals die in an atmosphere of pure oxygen. The likely reason is that much of the superoxide that is formed during oxidative metabolism is formed by the accidental transfer of an electron from a redox catalyst to molecular oxygen in solution. This process is expected to be directly proportional to the oxygen concentration in the solution.

Human tissues contain proteins that bind oxygen with rather high affinity, including hemoglobin and myoglobin. Cytochrome oxidase contributes to the maintenance of a low oxygen concentration because of its very high oxygen affinity. These proteins ensure that the concentration of free, unbound oxygen in the cell is very low.

Oxygen toxicity becomes a problem whenever pure oxygen is administered for medical or other reasons. For example, divers know to avoid oxygen concentrations greater than 36% to prevent the risk of oxygen toxicity. Another situation is oxygen treatment of newborns. Premature infants have developed retrolental fibroplasia with resulting blindness after oxygen treatment.

SUMMARY

Glycolysis converts the six carbons of glucose into two molecules of the three-carbon compound pyruvate. Under aerobic conditions, pyruvate enters the mitochondrion, where it is oxidatively decarboxylated to the two-carbon acetyl group in acetyl-CoA. Acetyl-CoA is formed not only from carbohydrates but also from fatty acids and amino acids.

The TCA cycle converts the acetyl group into carbon dioxide and reduced coenzymes. Its first reaction forms citrate from oxaloacetate and acetyl-CoA, and the remaining reactions of the cycle regenerate the oxaloacetate. Each round of the cycle produces two molecules of carbon dioxide, one of GTP, three of NADH, and one of $FADH_2$.

The reduced coenzymes are reoxidized by molecular oxygen in the respiratory chain. These reactions create a proton gradient across the inner mitochondrial membrane that fuels ATP synthesis by the mitochondrial ATP synthase. The efficiency of ATP synthesis during glucose oxidation is close to 40%. Oxidative phosphorylation is the principal energy source for most tissues, and inhibitors of oxidative phosphorylation can be rapidly fatal.

Oxidative phosphorylation is controlled by the availability of ADP for ATP synthesis, while most of the regulated enzymes in the oxidative pathways are stimulated by low energy charge and a high $[NAD^+]/[NADH]$ ratio. These mechanisms maintain a high ATP/ADP ratio in the cell.

Under anaerobic conditions, the pyruvate formed in glycolysis is reduced to lactate by LDH. Anaerobic glycolysis produces only two molecules of ATP for each glucose molecule. It can tide the cell over during brief periods of hypoxia, but only cells with very low energy needs can subsist permanently on anaerobic glycolysis.

Further Reading

Belenky P, Bogan KL, Brenner C: NAD^+ metabolism in health and disease, *Trends Biochem Sci* 32:12–19, 2007.

Cameron JM, Maj M, Levandovskiy V, Barnett CP, et al: Pyruvate dehydrogenase phosphatase 1 (PDP1) null mutation produces a lethal infantile phenotype, *Hum Genet* 125:319–326, 2009.

Choe E, Min DB: Chemistry and reactions of reactive oxygen species in foods, *Crit Rev Food Sci Nutr* 46:1–22, 2006.

Elliott HR, Samuels DC, Eden JA, et al: Pathogenic mitochondrial DNA mutations are common in the general population, *Am J Hum Genet* 83:254–260, 2008.

Halliwell B: Oxidative stress and neurodegeneration: where are we now? *J Neurochem* 97:1634–1658, 2006.

Halliwell B: Phagocyte-derived reactive species: salvation or suicide? *Trends Biochem Sci* 31:509–515, 2006.

Harper M-E, Green K, Brand MD: The efficiency of cellular energy transduction and its implications for obesity, *Annu Rev Nutr* 28:13–33, 2008.

Imlay JA: Cellular defenses against superoxide and hydrogen peroxide, *Annu Rev Biochem* 77:755–776, 2008.

Jitrapakdee S, St Maurice M, Rayment I, et al: Structure, mechanism and regulation of pyruvate carboxylase, *Biochem J* 413:369–387, 2008.

Kellett GL, Brot-Laroche E, Mace OJ, et al: Sugar absorption in the intestine: the role of GLUT2, *Annu Rev Nutr* 28:35–54, 2008.

Leney SE, Tavaré JM: The molecular basis of insulin-stimulated glucose uptake: signaling, trafficking and potential drug targets, *J Endocrinol* 203:1–18, 2009.

Platanias LC: Biological responses to arsenic compounds, *J Biol Chem* 284:18583–18587, 2009.

Pollak N, Dölle C, Ziegler M: The power to reduce: pyridine nucleotides—small molecules with a multitude of functions, *Biochem J* 402:205–218, 2007.

Porter RK: Uncoupling protein 1: a short-circuit in the chemiosmotic process, *J Bioenerget Biomembr* 40:457–461, 2008.

Von Ballmoos C, Wiedenmann A, Dimroth P: Essentials for ATP synthesis by F_1F_o ATP synthases, *Annu Rev Biochem* 78:649–672, 2009.

Yu-Wai-Man P, Griffiths PG, Hudson G, et al: Inherited mitochondrial optic neuropathies, *J Med Genet* 46:145–158, 2009.

Zanella A, Fermo E, Bianchi P, et al: Red cell pyruvate kinase deficiency: molecular and clinical aspects, *Br J Haematol* 130:11–25, 2005.

QUESTIONS

1. **Some enzymes of the TCA cycle are physiologically regulated. The most common regulatory effect on these enzymes is**

   A. Inhibition by ATP
   B. Inhibition by ADP
   C. Inhibition by NAD^+
   D. Stimulation by citrate
   E. Inhibition by acetyl-CoA

2. **Some individuals are born with a partial deficiency of pyruvate dehydrogenase in all tissues. What tissue suffers most from this abnormality?**

   A. Liver tissue
   B. Muscle tissue
   C. Erythrocytes
   D. Adipose tissue
   E. Brain tissue

3. **What biochemical changes take place in brain cells shortly after decapitation?**

   A. The rate of glycolysis is reduced
   B. TCA cycle activity is increased
   C. The [lactate]/[pyruvate] concentration ratio is increased
   D. All electron carriers in the respiratory chain are converted to the oxidized state
   E. The potassium concentration in the cells increases, and the sodium concentration decreases

4. **Assume that the concentration of one of the glycolytic enzymes is reduced to 50% of normal as a result of a heterozygous mutation. The reduced activity of which enzyme would decrease overall glycolytic activity to the greatest extent?**

   A. Hexokinase
   B. PFK
   C. Aldolase
   D. Enolase
   E. Pyruvate kinase

5. **Assume that the NADH-Q reductase complex is inhibited by the fish poison rotenone. A likely result of this inhibition will be**

   A. The mitochondria can no longer oxidize succinate to fumarate
   B. Most or all of the mitochondrial NAD will be in the oxidized state
   C. Most or all of the mitochondrial ubiquinone will be in the oxidized state
   D. The proton gradient across the inner mitochondrial membrane will be very steep
   E. PFK will be inhibited

6. **Following the advice of her biochemistry professor, an overweight medical student goes on a sawdust diet (it fills the stomach but cannot be digested). She should make sure that the sawdust is not from wood that has been treated with the uncoupler pentachlorophenol. Pentachlorophenol would cause**

   A. Weight gain
   B. Reduced oxygen consumption (while she is still alive)
   C. Reduced TCA cycle activity
   D. Hyperthermia
   E. An increased [NADH]/[NAD$^+$] concentration ratio

7. **Muscle contraction causes an *immediate* increase in the rate of oxidative phosphorylation because it**

   A. Decreases the pH
   B. Increases the NAD$^+$ concentration
   C. Increases the activity of PFK
   D. Decreases the activity of pyruvate dehydrogenase
   E. Increases the ADP concentration

Chapter 22
CARBOHYDRATE METABOLISM

In addition to the catabolism of glucose (see Chapter 21), carbohydrate metabolism has several other functions:

1. *The maintenance of an adequate blood glucose level.* Brain and erythrocytes require glucose at all times. The liver has to provide this glucose in the fasting state, both by the degradation of stored glycogen and by synthesis from noncarbohydrates.
2. *The utilization of dietary monosaccharides other than glucose.* Fructose and galactose, in particular, have to be channeled into the major metabolic pathways of glucose.
3. *The provision of specialized monosaccharides as biosynthetic precursors:* ribose for the synthesis of nucleotides and nucleic acids, and amino sugars and acidic sugar derivatives for the synthesis of glycolipids, glycoproteins, and proteoglycans.

AN ADEQUATE BLOOD GLUCOSE LEVEL MUST BE MAINTAINED AT ALL TIMES

Some cells and tissues, including brain and erythrocytes, depend on glucose because they cannot oxidize alternative fuels. The brain alone consumes nearly 120 g of glucose per day. Therefore the body maintains a blood glucose level of 4.0 to 5.5 mmol/L (70–100 mg/dl) at all times. Dietary carbohydrates provide glucose for a few hours after a meal. During these hours, the blood glucose concentration can rise as high as 8.5 mmol/L (150 mg/dl). In the fasting state, however, the liver has to produce glucose by two pathways:

1. *Glycogen degradation* is fast and cheap. It requires no metabolic energy, but the glycogen reserves of the liver rarely exceed 100 g and therefore are depleted within 24 hours. Only liver glycogen, but not the glycogen of muscle and other tissues, can be used to maintain the blood glucose level.
2. *Gluconeogenesis* produces glucose from amino acids, lactic acid, and glycerol. Liver and kidney both have a complete gluconeogenic pathway, but the liver is the major gluconeogenic organ because of its larger size. Gluconeogenesis is the only source of glucose during prolonged fasting.

GLUCONEOGENESIS BYPASSES THE THREE IRREVERSIBLE REACTIONS OF GLYCOLYSIS

The easiest strategy for glucose synthesis would be to reverse glycolysis by making glucose from pyruvate and lactate. To do so, however, *the gluconeogenic pathway has to bypass the three irreversible reactions of glycolysis: those catalyzed by hexokinase, phosphofructokinase (PFK), and pyruvate kinase* (*Fig. 22.1*).

The pyruvate kinase reaction of glycolysis is irreversible despite ATP synthesis. Reversing this reaction by going back from pyruvate to phosphoenolpyruvate (PEP) requires 14.8 kcal/mol, or at least two high-energy phosphate bonds.

This feat is accomplished in a sequence of two reactions (*Fig. 22.2*). First, pyruvate is carboxylated to oxaloacetate by **pyruvate carboxylase**. This ATP-dependent carboxylation reaction was described as an anaplerotic reaction of the tricarboxylic acid (TCA) cycle in Chapter 21. The second reaction, catalyzed by **PEP-carboxykinase**, converts oxaloacetate into PEP. It requires GTP, which supplies the phosphate group in PEP. The two reactions combined have a standard free energy change ($\Delta G^{0'}$) of +0.2 kcal/mol, but in the cell they proceed only from pyruvate to PEP because of the high cellular concentration ratios of [ATP]/[ADP], [GTP]/[GDP], and [pyruvate]/[PEP].

Whereas pyruvate carboxylase is strictly mitochondrial, PEP-carboxykinase is both mitochondrial and cytoplasmic. PEP is transported across the inner mitochondrial membrane, whereas oxaloacetate is shuttled into the cytoplasm after being reduced to malate or transaminated to aspartate (see *Fig. 21.21*).

The remaining irreversible reactions of glycolysis, catalyzed by PFK and hexokinase, are bypassed by the hydrolytic removal of phosphate. **Fructose-1,6-bisphosphatase** hydrolyzes the phosphate from carbon 1 of fructose-1,6-bisphosphate (*Fig. 22.3*), and **glucose-6-phosphatase** removes the phosphate from glucose-6-phosphate. Both reactions are irreversible. Unlike the other gluconeogenic enzymes, which are cytoplasmic (except pyruvate carboxylase), glucose-6-phosphatase resides on the inner surface of the endoplasmic reticulum membrane.

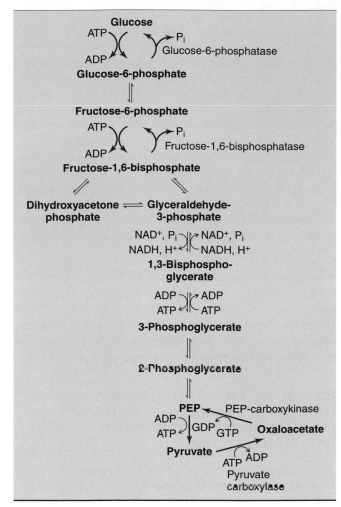

Figure 22.1 Reactions of glycolysis and gluconeogenesis. *NAD,* Nicotinamide adenine dinucleotide; *PEP,* phosphoenolpyruvate; *P_i,* inorganic phosphate.

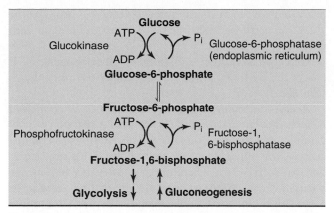

Figure 22.3 Second and third bypasses of gluconeogenesis.

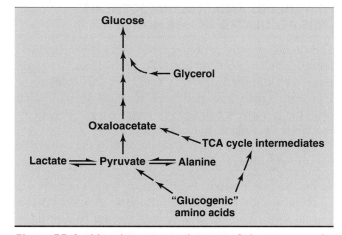

Figure 22.4 Most important substrates of gluconeogenesis. Although acetyl-coenzyme A enters the tricarboxylic acid (*TCA*) cycle, it is not a substrate of gluconeogenesis because the citrate synthase reaction does not involve the net synthesis of a TCA cycle intermediate.

Gluconeogenesis requires *six phosphoanhydride bonds* for the synthesis of one glucose molecule from two molecules of pyruvate or lactate. Pyruvate carboxylase consumes two ATP molecules, PEP-carboxykinase consumes two GTP molecules, and phosphoglycerate kinase consumes two ATP molecules in the reversal of substrate-level phosphorylation.

FATTY ACIDS CANNOT BE CONVERTED INTO GLUCOSE

Lactate and **alanine** are convenient substrates of gluconeogenesis because they are readily converted to pyruvate by lactate dehydrogenase and by transamination, respectively (*Fig. 22.4*). **Oxaloacetate** is not only a gluconeogenic intermediate but also a member of the TCA cycle. This is important because most amino acids are

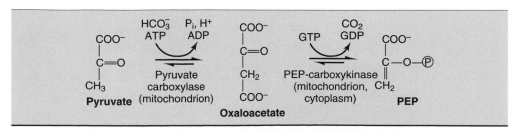

Figure 22.2 First bypass of gluconeogenesis, from pyruvate to phosphoenolpyruvate (*PEP*).

degraded to TCA cycle intermediates. Through the TCA cycle, these *"glucogenic" amino acids* feed into gluconeogenesis.

Glycerol is another substrate of gluconeogenesis. It enters the pathway at the level of the triose phosphates (*Fig. 22.5*).

Acetyl-coenzyme A (acetyl-CoA) cannot be converted to glucose. The pyruvate dehydrogenase reaction is irreversible, and there are no alternative reactions to channel acetyl-CoA into gluconeogenesis. Fatty acids are degraded to acetyl-CoA. Therefore *the fatty acids that are released from adipose tissue during fasting cannot be turned into glucose.* Gluconeogenesis depends on amino acids and, to a lesser extent, on lactic acid and glycerol.

GLYCOLYSIS AND GLUCONEOGENESIS ARE REGULATED BY HORMONES

Simultaneous activity of glycolysis and gluconeogenesis would achieve nothing but ATP hydrolysis. To minimize such a **futile cycle,** it is mandatory to control the irreversible reactions at all three bypasses to ensure that only the glycolytic reactions or only the gluconeogenic reactions take place, but not both.

The following hormones participate in the control of hepatic glycolysis and gluconeogenesis:

1. **Insulin** is released from pancreatic β-cells in response to increased blood glucose level after a carbohydrate-rich meal. The insulin level can rise up to 10-fold in this situation. Insulin regulates gene expression, and it reduces the cyclic AMP (cAMP) level in the liver by activating a cAMP-degrading phosphodiesterase. By stimulating the glucose-*consuming* pathways and inhibiting the glucose-*producing* pathways in the liver, *insulin lowers the blood glucose level.*
2. **Glucagon** is a polypeptide hormone from the α-cells of the endocrine pancreas. It is released in response

to hypoglycemia (decreased blood glucose level); therefore, its plasma level is higher in the fasting state than after a carbohydrate meal. By stimulating the glucose-producing pathways and inhibiting the glucose-consuming pathways in the liver, *glucagon raises the blood glucose level.* Glucagon achieves these effects by raising the cAMP level.
3. **Epinephrine** and **norepinephrine** are stress hormones that are released during physical exertion, cold exposure, and emotional turmoil. Their task is to provide fuel for contracting muscles. In the liver, *they favor gluconeogenesis over glycolysis* by inducing a modest rise of cAMP.
4. **Glucocorticoids** are released during sustained stress. *They stimulate gluconeogenesis by inducing the synthesis of gluconeogenic enzymes.*

The hormones regulate the synthesis of the distinctive glycolytic and gluconeogenic enzymes at the level of transcription (*Fig. 22.6, A*). Because this involves the synthesis of new enzyme protein and most of the enzymes have lifespans of a few days in the cell, *regulation of enzyme synthesis works on a time scale of days rather than minutes.*

GLYCOLYSIS AND GLUCONEOGENESIS ARE FINE TUNED BY ALLOSTERIC EFFECTORS AND HORMONE-INDUCED ENZYME PHOSPHORYLATIONS

The short-term control of glycolysis and gluconeogenesis is shown in *Figure 22.6, B.*

The glycolytic enzyme **pyruvate kinase** is the most important regulated enzyme in the PEP-pyruvate cycle. It is allosterically inhibited by ATP and alanine and activated by fructose-1,6-bisphosphate. The concentration of fructose-1,6-bisphosphate is high when PFK is activated and fructose-1,6-bisphosphatase is inhibited. Its effect on pyruvate kinase is an example of *feedforward*

Figure 22.5 Glycerol enters gluconeogenesis (and glycolysis) at the level of the triose phosphates. The glycerol for gluconeogenesis in the liver is derived from triglyceride hydrolysis in adipose tissue. *RBC,* Red blood cell.

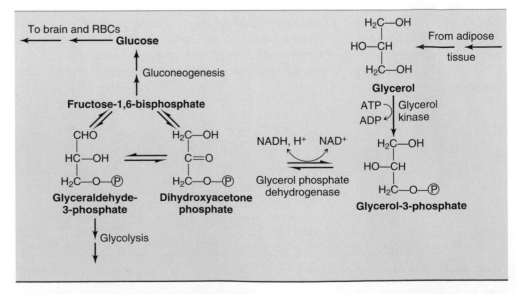

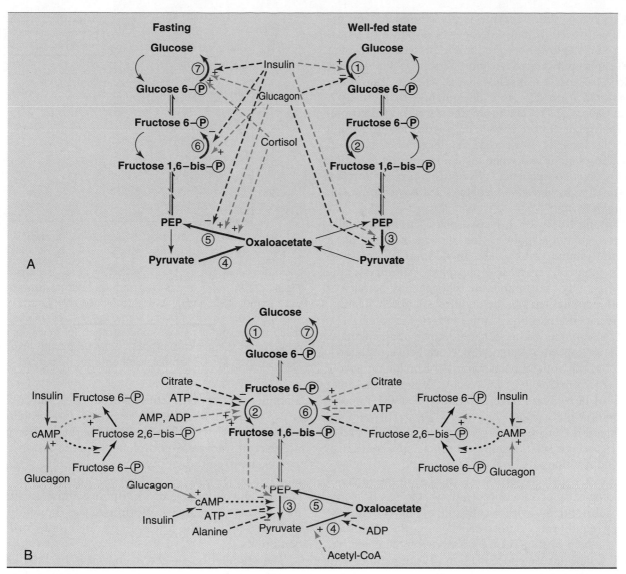

Figure 22.6 Reciprocal regulation of glycolysis and gluconeogenesis in the liver. ①, Glucokinase; ②, phosphofructokinase; ③, pyruvate kinase; ④, pyruvate carboxylase; ⑤, phosphoenolpyruvate (*PEP*)-carboxykinase; ⑥, fructose-1,6-bisphosphatase; ⑦, glucose-6-phosphatase. ⇢, Stimulation; →, inhibition. **A,** Substrate flow during fasting and in the well-fed state, and the effects of hormones on the amounts of glycolytic and gluconeogenic enzymes. Regulation of enzyme synthesis and degradation is the most important long-term (hours to days) control mechanism. In most cases, the hormone acts by changing the rate of transcription or by affecting the stability of the messenger RNA. Some of the insulin effects shown here require the presence of glucose. **B,** Short-term regulation of glycolysis and gluconeogenesis by reversibly binding effectors and by phosphorylation/dephosphorylation. – – –►, Allosteric and competitive effects; ·····►, phosphorylation. Only pyruvate kinase and phosphofructo-2-kinase/fructose-2,6-bisphosphatase are regulated by cyclic AMP (*cAMP*)-dependent phosphorylation. *CoA,* Coenzyme A.

stimulation. Pyruvate kinase is also inhibited by cAMP-induced phosphorylation.

PEP-carboxykinase is not known to be subject to short-term regulation, but **pyruvate carboxylase** is allosterically activated by acetyl-CoA and competitively inhibited by ADP. This ensures that gluconeogenesis is launched only when sufficient metabolic energy is available.

ATP and citrate stimulate **fructose-1-6-bisphosphatase** but inhibit **PFK.** Therefore high energy charge and the availability of metabolites favor gluconeogenesis over

glycolysis. The most potent modulator of these two enzymes, however, is **fructose-2,6-bisphosphate.** This regulatory metabolite, not to be confused with the glycolytic intermediate fructose-1,6-bisphosphate, is an activator of PFK and an inhibitor of fructose-1,6-bisphosphatase.

Fructose-2,6-bisphosphate is both synthesized from and degraded to fructose-6-phosphate by a unique bifunctional enzyme that combines the activities of a 6-phosphofructo-2-kinase (PFK-2) and a fructose-2, 6-bisphosphatase on the same polypeptide.

This bifunctional enzyme is phosphorylated by the cAMP-activated protein kinase A in response to glucagon and is dephosphorylated in the presence of insulin. The dephosphorylated enzyme acts as a kinase that makes fructose-2,6-bisphosphate, whereas the phosphorylated form acts as a phosphatase that breaks it down (*Fig. 22.7*). Therefore the level of fructose-2,6-bisphosphate in the liver is high when insulin is high and glucagon is low, and the level of fructose-2,6-bisphosphate is low when insulin is low and glucagon is high. As a consequence, *glycolysis is turned on when insulin is high, and gluconeogenesis is turned on when glucagon is high.*

Through fructose-2,6-bisphosphate, insulin and glucagon regulate glycolysis and gluconeogenesis on a minute-to-minute time scale. In addition to this hormonal control, fructose-6-phosphate stimulates the kinase activity and inhibits the phosphatase activity of the bifunctional enzyme by an allosteric mechanism.

The glucose-phosphorylating enzyme in the liver is isoenzyme 4 of hexokinase, better known as **glucokinase.** The most important kinetic difference between glucokinase and the other isoenzymes of hexokinase is the Michaelis constant (K_m) for glucose. Whereas the other forms of hexokinase have K_m values near 0.1 mmol/L (2 mg/dl), glucokinase has a K_m near 10 mmol/L (200 mg/dl). Glucokinase also shows a sigmoidal rather than hyperbolic relationship between glucose concentration and reaction rate (*Fig. 22.8*).

Because the steep part of the curve is in the range of physiological glucose concentrations, the reaction rate rises substantially with rising glucose level. Glucose rapidly equilibrates across the hepatocyte membrane with the help of the GLUT2 transporter; therefore, the intracellular glucose concentration rises in parallel with the blood glucose concentration after a carbohydrate-rich meal.

Glucokinase is inhibited by the CoA thioesters of long-chain fatty acids. These products are most abundant during fasting, when the liver metabolizes large

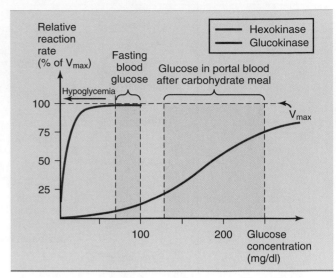

Figure 22.8 Approximate reaction rates of hexokinase (isoenzymes 1, 2, and 3) and glucokinase at different substrate concentrations. The sigmoidal relationship between reaction rate and substrate concentration for glucokinase accentuates the increase of the reaction rate with increased glucose level. V_{max}, Maximal reaction rate.

amounts of fatty acids from adipose tissue. Glucokinase is also regulated by a **glucokinase regulatory protein** that inhibits its activity and sequesters it in the nucleus in the presence of fructose-6-phosphate. Glucose and fructose-1-phosphate (a product of fructose metabolism) activate glucokinase by binding to this regulatory protein.

Like glucokinase, glucose-6-phosphatase is affected by substrate availability. With a K_m of 3 mmol/L for glucose-6-phosphate, it is not saturated under ordinary conditions.

The stimulation of gluconeogenesis by high energy charge and high concentrations of citrate and acetyl-CoA is counterintuitive. Gluconeogenesis is active in the fasting state. Why would the levels of ATP and metabolites be increased rather than decreased in a starving organism?

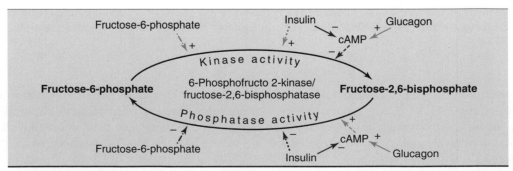

Figure 22.7 Synthesis and degradation of fructose-2,6-bisphosphate, the most important regulator of phosphofructokinase and fructose-1,6-bisphosphatase. This regulatory metabolite is synthesized and degraded by a bifunctional enzyme that combines the kinase and phosphatase activities on the same polypeptide. Cyclic AMP (*cAMP*)-induced phosphorylation inhibits the kinase activity and stimulates the phosphatase activity of the bifunctional enzyme. --▸, Phosphorylation; ⋯▸, dephosphorylation; ---▸, allosteric effect; ⊥▸, stimulation; ⟶▸, inhibition.

The reason is that gluconeogenesis takes place mainly in the liver, and the liver receives large quantities of fatty acids from adipose tissue during fasting. Fatty acid oxidation is less tightly controlled by feedback inhibition than is glucose oxidation, and the levels of ATP and acetyl-CoA in the liver actually are elevated during fasting. Thus *the energy for gluconeogenesis is supplied by fatty acid oxidation.*

CARBOHYDRATE IS STORED AS GLYCOGEN

Glycogen granules are seen in many cell types, but the most important stores are in liver and skeletal muscle. In the well-fed state, the glycogen content of the liver is up to 8% of the fresh weight: 100 to 120 g in the adult. The glycogen concentration in skeletal muscle is 1% or a bit less, but because most people have more muscle than liver, the total amount of muscle glycogen exceeds that in the liver.

Glycogen is a branched polymer of between 10,000 and 40,000 glucose residues held together by α-1,4 glycosidic bonds. Approximately one in 12 glucose residues serves as a branch point by forming an α-1,6 glycosidic bond with another glucose residue (**Fig. 22.9**). With a molecular weight between 10^6 and 10^7 D, it is as big as a complete human ribosome (4.2×10^6 D).

Theoretically, the molecule has only one reducing end with a free hydroxyl group at carbon 1 but a large number of nonreducing ends with a free hydroxyl group at carbon 4. The enzymes of glycogen synthesis and glycogen degradation are nested between the outer branches of the molecule and act only on the nonreducing ends. Therefore *the many nonreducing end branches of glycogen facilitate its rapid synthesis and degradation.*

GLYCOGEN IS READILY SYNTHESIZED FROM GLUCOSE

The steps in the synthesis of glycogen from glucose are outlined in **Figures 22.10** and **22.11**. Glucose-6-phosphate is isomerized to glucose-1-phosphate by **phosphoglucomutase**. There are about 20 molecules of glucose-6-phosphate for every molecule of glucose-1-phosphate at equilibrium. Glucose-1-phosphate then reacts with uridine triphosphate (UTP) to form **UDP-glucose**. This otherwise reversible reaction is driven to completion by the subsequent hydrolysis of pyrophosphate. *UDP-glucose is the activated form of glucose for biosynthetic reactions.*

UDP is attached to C-1 of glucose; therefore, it is this carbon that forms the glycosidic bond. The bond between glucose and UDP is energy rich. With a free energy content of 7.3 kcal/mol, it rivals the phosphoanhydride bonds

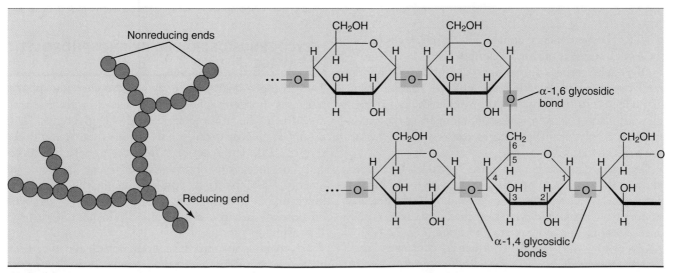

Figure 22.9 Structure of glycogen. *Left,* Overall structure. Note the large number of nonreducing ends, which are required as substrates for the enzymes of glycogen metabolism. *Right,* Structure around a branch point.

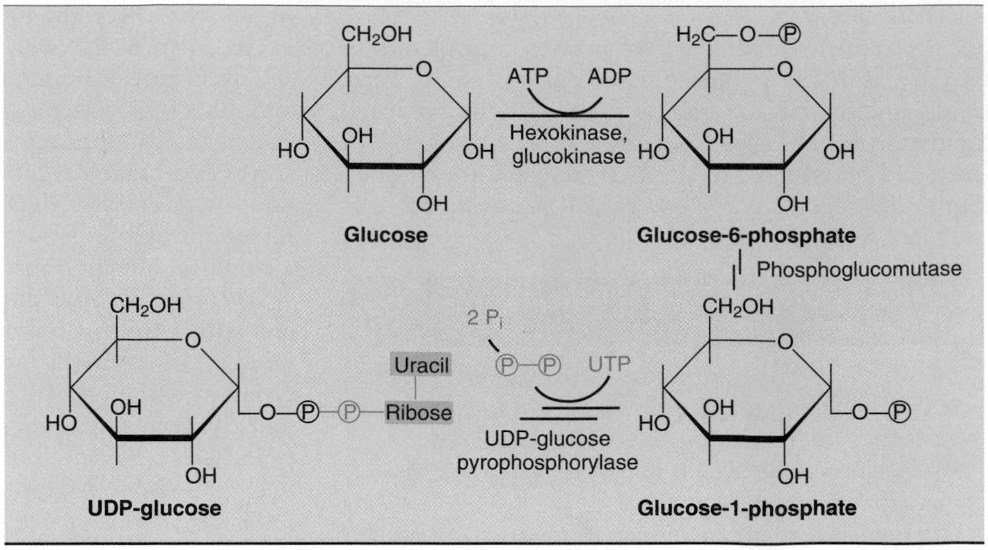

Figure 22.10 Synthesis of uridine diphosphate (*UDP*)-glucose. UDP-glucose is the activated form of glucose for glycogen synthesis but also for the synthesis of other complex carbohydrates (see *Table 8.3*).

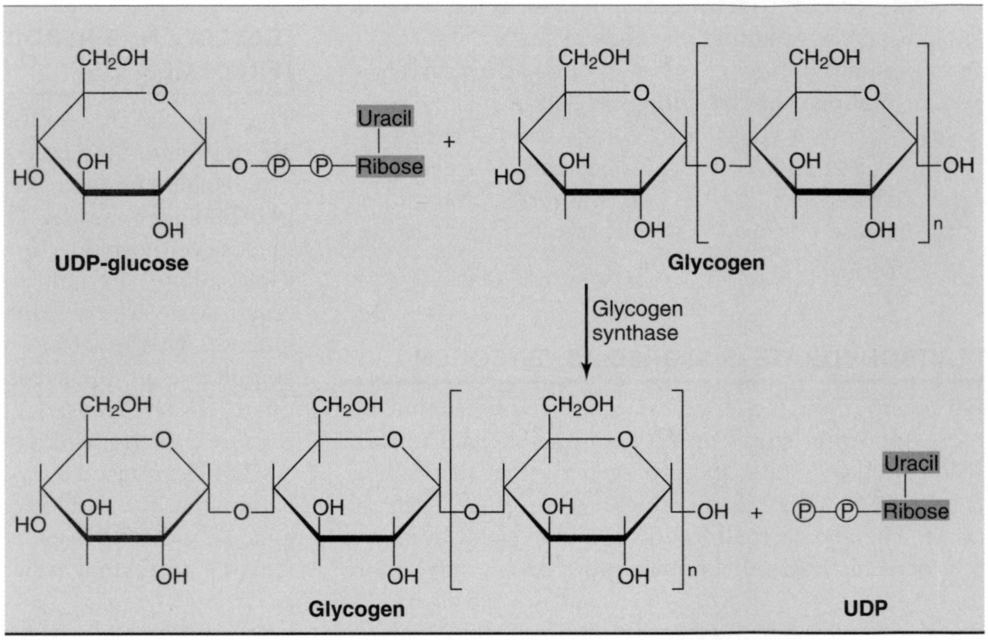

Figure 22.11 Glycogen synthase reaction. *UDP,* Uridine diphosphate.

in ATP. The free energy content of an α-1,4 glycosidic bond in glycogen is only 4.5 kcal/mol.

Glycogen synthase forms the α-1,4 glycosidic bonds in glycogen by transferring the glucose residue from UDP-glucose to the 4-hydroxyl group at the nonreducing end of the glycogen molecule, elongating the outer branches of glycogen by one glucose residue at a time (see *Fig. 22.11*).

Glycogen synthase cannot form the α-1,6 glycosidic bonds at the branch points. Branching requires a **branching enzyme,** which transfers a string of about seven glucose residues from the end of an unbranched chain to C-6 of a glucose residue in a more interior location (*Fig. 22.12*).

Glycogen synthesis from glucose consumes *two phosphoanhydride bonds for each glucose residue:* one in ATP for the hexokinase reaction and one in UTP for the formation of UDP-glucose.

GLYCOGEN IS DEGRADED BY PHOSPHOROLYTIC CLEAVAGE

The glycogen-degrading enzyme **glycogen phosphorylase** uses inorganic phosphate to cleave a glucose residue from the nonreducing end of glycogen. This produces glucose-1-phosphate rather than free glucose (*Fig. 22.13*). The reaction is reversible, with 3.6 molecules of inorganic phosphate for every molecule of glucose-1-phosphate at equilibrium. In the living cell, however, it proceeds in the direction of glycogen breakdown because the cellular [phosphate]/[glucose-1-phosphate] ratio is at least 100.

Glycogen phosphorylase does not cleave the α-1,6 glycosidic bonds at the branch points. It does not even go near the branch points; it stops four residues before. At this point, the **debranching enzyme** takes over.

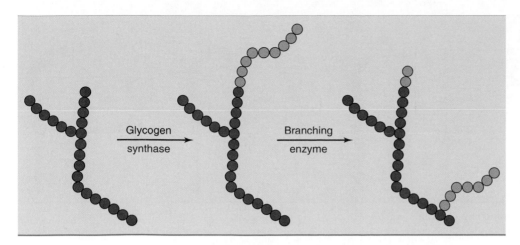

Figure 22.12 Action of the branching enzyme.

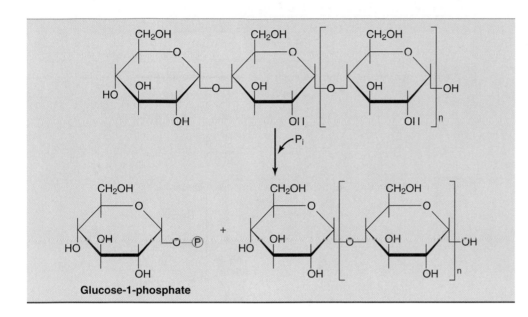

Glucose-1-phosphate

Figure 22.13 Glycogen phosphorylase reaction.

It first transfers a block of three glucose residues from the end of the chain to the C-4 end of another chain, leaving a single glucose at the branch point. It then removes this last glucose residue by hydrolysis, producing a molecule of free glucose. Thus, the debranching enzyme has two enzymatic activities: a transferase activity and a hydrolase activity (***Fig. 22.14***). Overall, *about 92% of the glucose residues in glycogen form glucose-1-phosphate and 8% form free glucose.* Glucose-1-phosphate is metabolized through glucose-6-phosphate.

Glycogen breakdown serves different purposes in liver and muscle. *The liver synthesizes glycogen after a carbohydrate meal and degrades it to free glucose during fasting.* The glucose-6-phosphate from glycogen breakdown is cleaved to free glucose by glucose-6-phosphatase, and the glucose is released into the blood for use by needy tissues, including brain and blood cells (***Fig. 22.15***).

Skeletal muscle synthesizes glycogen at rest and degrades it during exercise. Muscles cannot produce free glucose because they have no glucose-6-phosphatase. They metabolize glucose-6-phosphate by glycolysis, forming lactate. Because glycogen degradation produces glucose-6-phosphate without consuming ATP, *anaerobic glycolysis from glycogen produces three rather than two molecules of ATP for each glucose residue.*

Liver glycogen is synthesized and degraded in response to feeding and fasting, so its level fluctuates widely in the course of a typical day (***Fig. 22.16***). Muscle glycogen, in contrast, is fairly constant and becomes depleted only during vigorous and prolonged physical exercise.

GLYCOGEN METABOLISM IS REGULATED BY HORMONES AND METABOLITES

Glycogen synthesis and glycogen degradation should not be active at the same time to avoid an ATP-consuming futile cycle. This is achieved by phosphorylation of the key enzymes glycogen synthase and glycogen

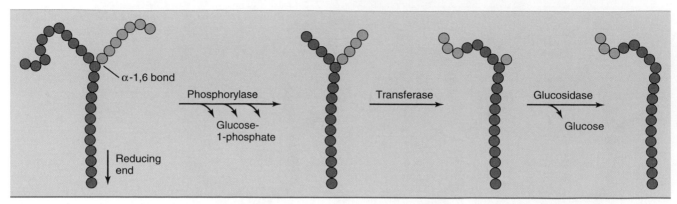

Figure 22.14 Action of the debranching enzyme.

Figure 22.15 Metabolic fates of glycogen in liver (**A**) and muscle (**B**). Note that the liver possesses glucose-6-phosphatase, which forms free glucose both in gluconeogenesis (see *Fig. 22.1*) and from glycogen. This enzyme is not present in muscle tissue.

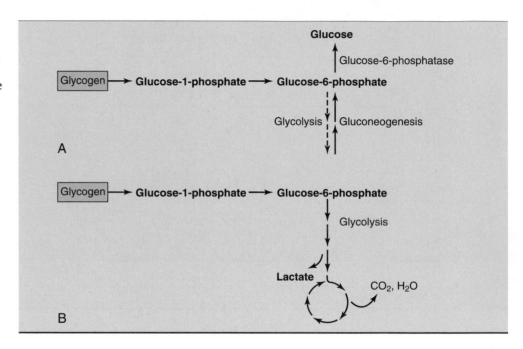

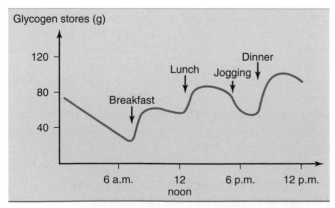

Figure 22.16 Changes in the glycogen stores of the liver during the course of a day. Glycogen metabolism in the liver regulates the blood glucose level in the short term, and gluconeogenesis is important for long-term regulation after more than 12 to 24 hours of fasting.

phosphorylase (*Fig. 22.17*). Both enzymes are phosphorylated in response to the same stimuli, but glycogen synthase is active in the dephosphorylated state, whereas glycogen phosphorylase is active in the phosphorylated state. Therefore *simultaneous phosphorylation of both enzymes switches the cell from glycogen synthesis to glycogen degradation.* In both cases, the active form of the enzyme is designated by the letter *a* and the less active form by *b*.

The phosphorylation state of the enzymes is controlled by hormones and their second messengers. Broadly, glucagon and the catecholamines induce phosphorylation of the regulated enzymes, and insulin induces their dephosphorylation (*Fig. 22.18*).

1. **Glucagon** stimulates glycogen degradation in the liver during fasting, when glycogen-derived glucose is needed to maintain the blood glucose level. Its

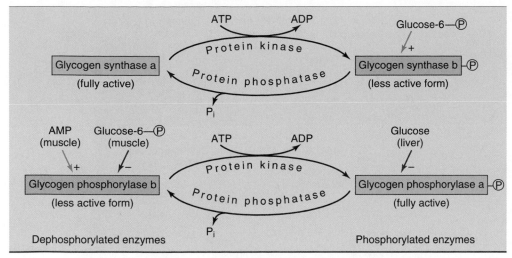

Figure 22.17   Regulation of glycogen synthase and glycogen phosphorylase by covalent modification and allosteric effectors. Note that simultaneous phosphorylation of the two enzymes leads to glycogen degradation, and their dephosphorylation leads to glycogen synthesis. ⎯+⟶, Allosteric activation; ⎯−⟶, allosteric inhibition.

effects are mediated by cAMP. The cAMP-activated protein kinase A phosphorylates and thereby inactivates glycogen synthase. It also phosphorylates and activates **phosphorylase kinase,** which in turn phosphorylates both glycogen phosphorylase and glycogen synthase. *All regulated enzymes of glycogen metabolism become phosphorylated by the cAMP-induced phosphorylation cascade.*

2. **Catecholamines** (norepinephrine and epinephrine) stimulate glycogen breakdown in liver and muscle during physical exertion, when fuels need to be mobilized for the energy needs of the muscles. They stimulate cAMP synthesis through β-adrenergic receptors and raise the cytoplasmic calcium concentration through α_1-adrenergic receptors. α_1-Adrenergic receptors prevail in the liver, whereas β-adrenergic receptors are more important in muscle tissue. Calcium stimulates phosphorylase kinase synergistically with cAMP.

3. **Insulin** stimulates glycogen synthesis in liver and skeletal muscle. It ensures that excess carbohydrate is stored away as glycogen after a meal. Through the protein kinase B cascade (see Chapter 17), it regulates glycogen metabolism by at least three mechanisms:

- *It reduces the level of cAMP* by activating the cAMP-degrading phosphodiesterase **PDE3B.**
- *It inhibits* **glycogen synthase kinase-3** (**GSK3**), one of the protein kinases that phosphorylate and inactivate glycogen synthase.
- *It stimulates* **protein phosphatase-1,** which reverses the cAMP-induced phosphorylations.

Protein phosphatase-1 dephosphorylates glycogen synthase, glycogen phosphorylase, and phosphorylase

kinase. As a result, *protein phosphatase-1 switches the cell from glycogen breakdown to glycogen synthesis.*

Phosphatase-1 is activated by an insulin-triggered phosphorylation and inactivated by the phosphorylation of a different site by protein kinase A. In addition it is allosterically inhibited by the cAMP-activated phosphoprotein **inhibitor-1** (see *Fig. 22.18, B*).

Glucose-6-phosphate is an allosteric activator of glycogen synthase *b* and phosphatase-1, and an inhibitor of glycogen phosphorylase in muscle. Thus glycogen synthesis is favored when substrate is available. **AMP** is an allosteric activator of glycogen phosphorylase in muscle and other extrahepatic tissues. This ensures that *glycogen is rapidly degraded in metabolic emergencies.* In hypoxia, it is the major substrate of anaerobic glycolysis.

Glucose is an inhibitor of glycogen phosphorylase in the liver. In addition to inhibiting the enzyme, the binding of glucose exposes the covalently bound phosphate to the action of the protein phosphatase. Because the intracellular glucose concentration in the liver approximates the blood glucose level, *a high blood glucose level inhibits glycogen breakdown in the liver.*

The effects of the second messengers on glycogen metabolism are similar in muscle and liver, but the stimuli that regulate them are different. Epinephrine rather than glucagon is the major cAMP-elevating hormone in skeletal muscle; and whereas calcium levels in the liver are raised by epinephrine through α_1-adrenergic receptors, cytoplasmic calcium in the muscle fiber rises when calcium is released from the sarcoplasmic reticulum during muscle contraction.

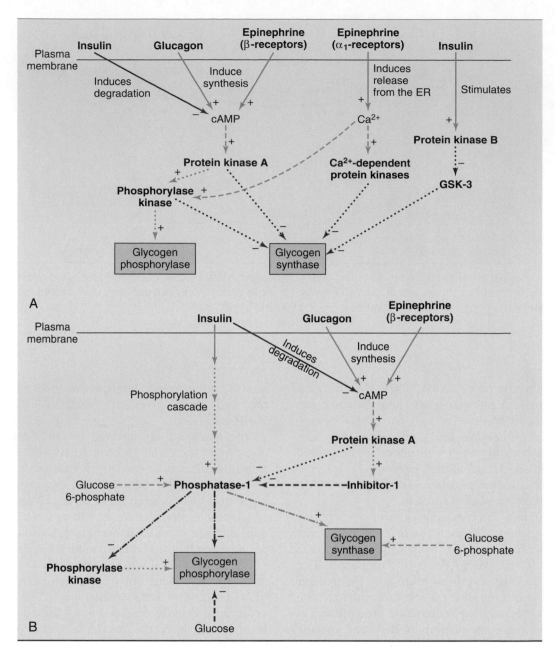

Figure 22.18 Regulation of glycogen metabolism in the liver. Note that the hormones affect glycogen synthase and glycogen phosphorylase through the protein kinases and the protein phosphatase (phosphatase-1) that regulate their phosphorylation state. ---►, Allosteric effects; ·····►, phosphorylation; —·—►, dephosphorylation; _+_►, activation; _–_►, inhibition. **A,** Hormonal effects on the phosphorylation of the glycogen-metabolizing enzymes by protein kinases in the liver. *ER,* Endoplasmic reticulum; *GSK-3,* glycogen synthase kinase-3. **B,** Hormonal effects on the dephosphorylation of the glycogen-metabolizing enzymes by protein phosphatase-1 and the effects of allosteric effectors.

CLINICAL EXAMPLE 22.2: von Gierke Disease

Of all glycogen storage diseases, deficiency of glucose-6-phosphatase (von Gierke disease) leads to the most severe fasting hypoglycemia, starting 2 to 4 hours after the last meal. This has to be expected because glucose-6-phosphatase is required for the formation of glucose by glycogen breakdown as well as gluconeogenesis.

Patients present with life-threatening hypoglycemia and acidosis within months after birth. The acidosis is caused by the overproduction of both lactic acid and the "ketone bodies" (acetoacetic acid and β-hydroxybutyric acid). Lactic acidosis develops because the liver is unable to convert lactic acid into glucose, and ketoacidosis develops because the severe hypoglycemia reduces

CLINICAL EXAMPLE 22.2: von Gierke Disease—cont'd

insulin secretion while stimulating sympathetic nervous activity. This combination causes excessive fat breakdown in adipose tissue and conversion of the fatty acids to ketone bodies in the liver (see Chapter 23). The liver is massively enlarged with accumulating glycogen and fat.

Patients can be kept alive only by regular carbohydrate feeding day and night. von Gierke disease shows that *without the synthesis of glucose by the liver, we would die of hypoglycemia within hours after the last meal.*

GLYCOGEN ACCUMULATES IN SEVERAL ENZYME DEFICIENCIES

Glycogen storage diseases are rare (overall incidence 1:40,000), recessively inherited diseases in which the deficiency of a glycogen-degrading enzyme causes the abnormal accumulation of glycogen. Because different isoenzymes are present in different tissues, most deficiencies are limited to one or a few organ systems. The most useful distinction is among *hepatic, myopathic,* and *generalized* types (*Table 22.1* and *Clinical Examples 22.2 through 22.4*).

Hepatic glycogen storage diseases present with fasting hypoglycemia. This is expected because the primary function of liver glycogen is maintenance of an adequate blood glucose level during fasting. The myopathic forms present with muscle weakness and muscle cramps during exertion, but no symptoms during rest. This is expected because during vigorous exercise, glycogen is a major fuel for both oxidative metabolism and lactate formation.

CLINICAL EXAMPLE 22.3: McArdle Disease

Deficiency of glycogen phosphorylase in skeletal muscle, known as McArdle disease, leads to muscle weakness and painful cramps on exertion. Patients are otherwise in good health, although some experience acute episodes of myoglobinuria, and some develop persistent muscle weakness and muscle wasting as they grow older. This disease shows that *muscle glycogen is not essential for life but is necessary for normal performance during physical exercise.*

Patients with McArdle disease do not show the expected rise in blood level of lactic acid after muscular activity. This demonstrates that *the most important source of lactic acid during muscular activity is not glucose from the blood but stored muscle glycogen.*

CLINICAL EXAMPLE 22.4: Pompe Disease

Although most glycogen is degraded by glycogen phosphorylase, a small amount is ingested by lysosomes and degraded by a lysosomal α-glucosidase ("**acid maltase**"). Like most lysosomal enzymes, acid maltase does not have tissue-specific isoenzymes. Therefore its deficiency leads to glycogen accumulation in virtually all tissues.

In classic cases, diagnosed as **Pompe disease,** the enzyme is virtually absent, and affected infants die of cardiac failure before age 3 years. Milder forms with significant residual activity of acid maltase present with proximal muscle weakness that can start at any age and, if fatal, progresses to death by respiratory failure.

Table 22.1 Glycogen Storage Diseases

Type	Enzyme Deficiency	Organ(s) Affected	Clinical Course
I (von Gierke disease)	Glucose-6-phosphatase	Liver, kidney	Severe hepatomegaly, severe hypoglycemia, lactic acidosis, ketosis, hyperuricemia
II (Pompe disease)	α-1,4-Glucosidase ("acid maltase")	All organs	Death from cardiac failure in infants
III (Cori disease)	Debranching enzyme	Muscle, liver	Like type I but much milder
IV (Andersen disease)	Branching enzyme	Liver, myocardium	Death from liver cirrhosis usually before age 2 years
V (McArdle disease)	Phosphorylase	Muscle	Muscle cramps and pain on exertion, easy fatigability, normal life expectancy
VI (Hers disease)	Phosphorylase	Liver	Like type I but milder, with less severe hypoglycemia
VII (Tarui disease)	Phosphofructokinase	Muscle, red blood cells	Like type V
VIII	Phosphorylase kinase*	Liver	Mild hepatomegaly and hypoglycemia

*There is also an X-linked form of phosphorylase kinase deficiency that affects muscle and several autosomal recessive forms that affect liver, muscle plus liver, or muscle plus heart. The enzyme contains four different subunits, one of which is encoded by a gene on the X chromosome.

FRUCTOSE IS CHANNELED INTO GLYCOLYSIS/GLUCONEOGENESIS

Free fructose is present in honey and in many fruits, but most of the dietary fructose comes in the form of the disaccharide sucrose (table sugar) and the high-fructose corn syrup in soft drinks. This dietary fructose has to be channeled into the major pathways of glucose metabolism.

Fructose is less rapidly absorbed from the intestine than is glucose, but once in the blood, it is more rapidly metabolized. Its plasma half-life after intravenous injection is only half that of glucose (18 minutes vs 43 minutes). Some of the fructose is phosphorylated to the glycolytic intermediate fructose-6-phosphate by hexokinase. But because the K_m of hexokinase for fructose is more than 3 mmol/L, this pathway is important only when the fructose concentration is very high.

Most of the dietary fructose is phosphorylated by **fructokinase** in liver, kidneys, and intestines. The liver alone accounts for almost half of the total fructose metabolism. Fructokinase produces fructose-1-phosphate, which is not a glycolytic intermediate (*Fig. 22.19*). Fructose-1-phosphate is cleaved to dihydroxyacetone phosphate and glyceraldehyde by **aldolase B**, an isoenzyme of aldolase that can cleave both fructose-1,6-bisphosphate and fructose-1-phosphate. The products of aldolase B are further metabolized by glycolysis or gluconeogenesis.

EXCESS FRUCTOSE IS TOXIC

The rate-limiting glucokinase and PFK reactions are bypassed by fructose, and pyruvate kinase is stimulated by fructose-1-phosphate as it is by fructose-1,6-bisphosphate

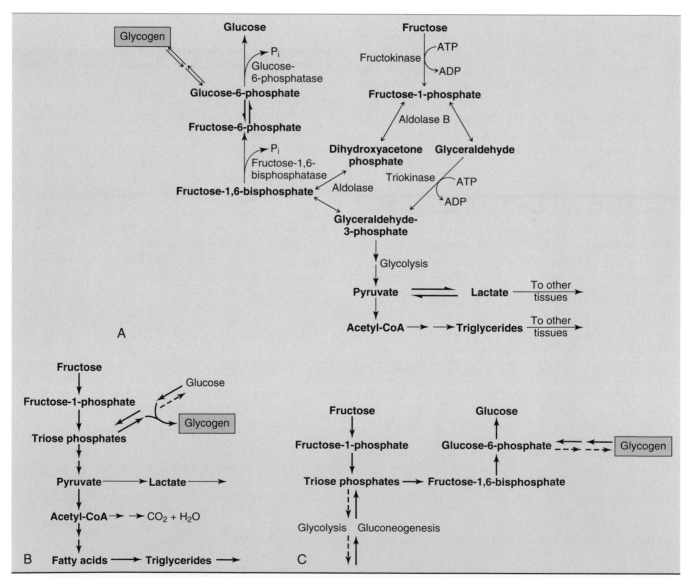

Figure 22.19 Metabolism of fructose in the liver. **A,** Pathways. **B,** Substrate flow after a good meal. **C,** Substrate flow when the blood glucose level is low. *CoA,* Coenzyme A; *Pᵢ,* inorganic phosphate.

Table 22.2   Kinetic Properties of Fructose-Metabolizing Enzymes in the Liver and the Glucose-Metabolizing Enzyme Glucokinase for Comparison

Enzyme	V$_{max}$ (μmol/min per gram of tissue)	K$_m$ for Carbohydrate Substrate (mmol/L)
Glucokinase	1*	10
Fructose carrier (in plasma membrane)	30	67–200[†]
Fructokinase	10	0.5
Aldolase B		
Cleavage of fructose-1-phosphate	2–3	1
Cleavage of fructose-1,6-bisphosphate	2–3	0.004–0.012
Triokinase	2	0.01
Fructose-1,6-bisphosphatase	4*	1[‡]
Glucose-6-phosphatase	10*	2.5–3[†]

*Depends on nutritional state.
[†]After a sweet meal, the fructose concentration in the portal vein reaches approximately 2 to 3 mmol/L. The usual glucose-6-phosphate concentration in the liver is approximately 0.2 mmol/L (higher during fasting, lower after a meal).
[‡]Depends on allosteric effectors.

(see ***Fig. 22.6, B***). Therefore *the liver metabolizes fructose faster than glucose,* and because the activity of fructokinase exceeds that of aldolase B in the liver (***Table 22.2***), *fructose-1-phosphate tends to accumulate.*

Natural foods contain fructose together with glucose. Therefore it is not surprising that *fructose promotes glucose metabolism in the liver.* Fructose-1-phosphate stimulates glucokinase by binding to the glucokinase-regulating protein. It also stimulates the otherwise inactive phosphorylated form of glycogen synthase but has no effect on PFK. Therefore *fructose-1-phosphate directs dietary glucose into glycogen synthesis.*

Although fructose helps the liver to dispose of excess glucose, the large amounts of fructose present in soft drinks and other sweetened foods are considered problematic. The tissue concentration of fructose-1-phosphate in the liver can reach 10 μmol/g after a sugary meal. This ties up a substantial portion of the inorganic phosphate in the cell, leading to impairment of oxidative phosphorylation.

Fructose has been used as a substitute for glucose in parenteral nutrition, and diabetic diets were formulated in which a large portion of the dietary carbohydrate is supplied as fructose, based on the reasoning that the insulin-dependent PFK reaction is bypassed. However, it was soon found that excess fructose is apt to damage the liver and to raise the plasma levels of lactic acid, triglycerides, and uric acid.

These effects can be attributed to the depletion of inorganic phosphate and to the rapid conversion of excess fructose to lactic acid and triglyceride in the liver. Uric acid is increased because fructose is metabolized to glucose-6-phosphate in the liver. Some of the glucose-6-phosphate is converted to ribose-5-phosphate, a substrate of purine biosynthesis. Excess purines are degraded to uric acid (see Chapter 28).

CLINICAL EXAMPLE 22.5: Hereditary Fructose Intolerance

Fructokinase deficiency leads to **essential fructosuria,** a benign condition in which fructose appears in the urine after a fructose-containing meal. Urinalysis shows a positive test for "reducing sugar" (fructose), although enzymatic glucose tests are negative. Most of the fructose is metabolized slowly by hexokinase in muscle and adipose tissue.

More serious is **hereditary fructose intolerance** caused by aldolase B deficiency. Affected children present with nausea and vomiting after a fructose-containing meal, along with signs of hypoglycemia (weakness, trembling, and sweating). Repeated episodes can cause liver damage.

When fructose-1-phosphate accumulates in the liver, it ties up phosphate. The shortage of inorganic phosphate impairs ATP synthesis, thereby damaging the cells and preventing gluconeogenesis. Activation of glucokinase and glycogen synthase by fructose-1-phosphate contributes to the hypoglycemia.

Deficiency of the gluconeogenic enzyme fructose-1,6-bisphosphatase results in fructose intolerance similar to aldolase B deficiency, but patients also develop hypoglycemia during long-term fasting because gluconeogenesis is interrupted.

Fructose intolerance is treated by excluding fructose from the diet. Indeed, affected children spontaneously avoid sweets. This is an example of a *conditioned taste aversion,* which develops whenever illness and malaise are experienced after eating. It is an evolved learning predisposition that protects humans from poisonous food. On the bright side: Adults with fructose intolerance have excellent teeth.

CLINICAL EXAMPLE 22.6: Galactosemia

Galactosemia, with an incidence at birth of 1:40,000, is a recessively inherited deficiency of galactose-1-phosphate-uridyl transferase. Symptoms appear only after the ingestion of milk or other galactose-containing foods and are accompanied by the accumulation of galactose in the blood and of galactose-1-phosphate in the cells.

The first sign of the disease is vomiting after feeding, evident within weeks after birth. Untreated patients can develop liver cirrhosis, cataracts (clouding of the lens), and mental deficiency. Accumulating galactose-1-phosphate, like fructose-1-phosphate in hereditary fructose intolerance (see *Clinical Example 22.5*), damages the liver by tying up inorganic phosphate and thereby reducing ATP synthesis.

In the case of one galactosemic child, most signs of the disease were eliminated after liver transplantation,

but nausea and vomiting after milk consumption persisted. Presumably, nausea and vomiting are caused by the accumulation of galactose-1-phosphate, depletion of inorganic phosphate, and impairment of ATP synthesis in the intestinal mucosa. When you have eaten something that prevents ATP synthesis, you better vomit it out fast!

A diagnosis of galactosemia is suggested by the presence of reducing material (galactose) in the urine and negative results of enzymatic tests for glucose. It is confirmed by the absence of galactose-1-phosphate-uridyl transferase in red blood cells. Unaffected heterozygotes have approximately 50% of the normal enzyme activity. Galactosemia is included in many newborn screening programs because after early diagnosis, all clinical manifestations can be prevented by placing the infant on a milk-free diet.

EXCESS GALACTOSE IS CHANNELED INTO THE PATHWAYS OF GLUCOSE METABOLISM

Most dietary galactose is metabolized in liver and intestinal mucosa by the pathway shown in *Figure 22.20*. **Galactokinase** phosphorylates galactose to galactose-1-phosphate, which then reacts with UDP-glucose to form UDP-galactose. UDP-galactose is epimerized to UDP-glucose. This pathway amounts to the *ATP-dependent conversion of galactose to glucose-1-phosphate*. Because of its reversibility, the epimerase reaction is also a source of UDP-galactose for the synthesis of glycolipids, glycoproteins, and proteoglycans.

Inherited deficiencies of galactose-metabolizing enzymes are seen occasionally. **Galactokinase deficiency** is a relatively benign condition leading to elevated blood galactose levels after consumption of milk and milk products. Cataracts (clouding of the lens) develop in those

who consume milk despite their enzyme deficiency. Aldose reductase, the same enzyme that reduces glucose to sorbitol (see *Fig. 22.23*), reduces galactose to galactitol in the lens. The accumulating galactitol damages the lens, probably through its osmotic activity. The deficiency of galactose-1-phosphate-uridyl transferase is far more serious (see *Clinical Example 22.6*).

THE PENTOSE PHOSPHATE PATHWAY SUPPLIES NADPH AND RIBOSE-5-PHOSPHATE

The "minor" pathways of carbohydrate metabolism provide specialized products for biosynthesis. The cytoplasmic **pentose phosphate pathway,** also known as the **hexose monophosphate shunt,** makes two important products: ribose-5-phosphate and NADPH (reduced form of nicotinamide adenine dinucleotide phosphate).

Ribose-5-phosphate is a precursor for the synthesis of purine and pyrimidine nucleotides, and NADPH is a redox coenzyme. NADPH has the same standard redox potential as NADH, but its functions are different. Whereas NADH feeds its hydrogen/electrons into the respiratory chain, NADPH is used for *reductive biosynthesis of fatty acids and cholesterol* and for *defense against oxidative damage.*

The **oxidative branch** of the pentose phosphate pathway synthesizes NADPH (*Fig. 22.21*). **Glucose-6-phosphate dehydrogenase** catalyzes the committed and rate-limiting step. The reaction sequence is irreversible, and this enables the cell to maintain a high [NADPH]/[NADP$^+$] ratio. Cells generally contain far more NADPH than NADP$^+$; this is in contrast to NADH whose concentration is generally far lower than the NAD$^+$ concentration. For this reason, *the cells use NADPH rather than NADH whenever a strong reducing agent is required.*

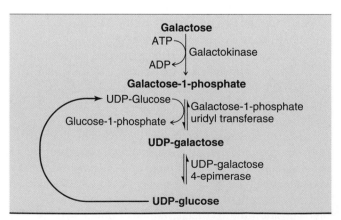

Figure 22.20 Galactose metabolism. *ADP,* Adenosine diphosphate; *ATP,* adenosine triphosphate; *UDP,* uridine diphosphate.

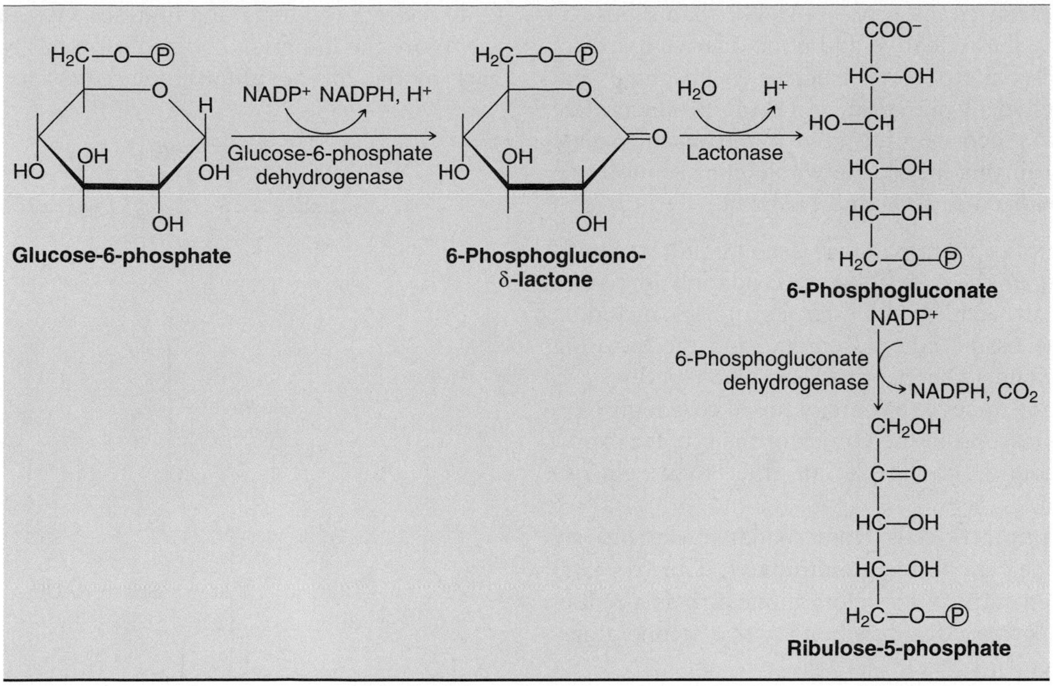

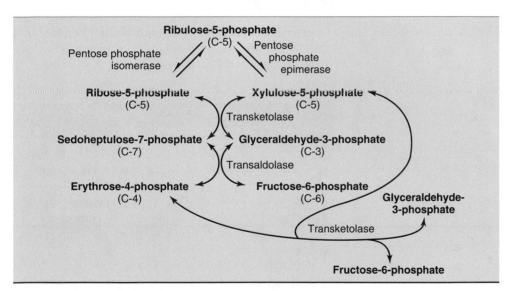

Figure 22.21 Oxidative branch of the pentose phosphate pathway. $NADP^+$, Nicotinamide adenine dinucleotide phosphate; *NADPH,* reduced form of nicotinamide adenine dinucleotide phosphate.

Figure 22.22 Nonoxidative branch of the pentose phosphate pathway in adipose tissue.

The **nonoxidative branch** of the pentose phosphate pathway links ribulose-5-phosphate, the product of the oxidative branch, to glycolysis and gluconeogenesis (*Fig. 22.22*). The most important enzymes in this reversible reaction sequence are **transketolase** and **transaldolase**. Transketolase transfers a two-carbon unit, and transaldolase transfers a three-carbon unit. Transketolase (but not transaldolase) contains enzyme-bound thiamin pyrophosphate, which functions as a transient carrier of the two-carbon unit.

The overall balance of the pentose phosphate pathway (see *Figs. 22.21* and *22.22*) can be written as

$$3 \text{ Glucose-6-phosphate} + 6 \text{ NADP}^+$$
$$\downarrow$$
$$2 \text{ Fructose-6-phosphate} + \text{Glyceraldehyde-3-phosphate} + 6 \text{ NADPH} + 6 \text{ H}^+ + 3 \text{ CO}_2$$

In addition to the glycolytic intermediates, *two molecules of NADPH are formed for each carbon released as CO_2.* However, the pentose phosphate pathway can run in different modes.

1. When the cell needs more ribose-5-phosphate than NADPH, ribose-5-phosphate is formed not only through the oxidative branch but also by reversal of the reactions in the nonoxidative branch.

2. When the cell needs more NADPH than ribose-5-phosphate, the oxidative and nonoxidative branches work in series to form fructose-6-phosphate and glyceraldehyde-3-phosphate. These products are recycled to glucose-6-phosphate in the gluconeogenic reactions. In this mode, the whole glucose molecule can be oxidized to CO_2 and NADPH.

The pentose phosphate pathway accounts for a significant portion of the total glucose oxidation in tissues with active fatty acid or cholesterol synthesis, including liver, adipose tissue, adrenal cortex, and the lactating mammary gland. The pentose phosphate pathway is also important in cells that are exposed to a high oxygen partial pressure. In the cornea of the eye, for example, it accounts for 60% of the total glucose consumption.

NADPH protects cells from oxidative damage by maintaining the tripeptide **glutathione** (γ-Glu-Cys-Gly) in the reduced state. When glutathione acts as a reducing agent, it forms a disulfide bond with a second glutathione molecule:

$$
\begin{array}{ccc}
\gamma - \text{Glu} & & \gamma - \text{Glu} \\
| & & | \\
\text{Cys} - \text{SH} + \text{HS} - \text{Cys} \\
| & & | \\
\text{Gly} & & \text{Gly}
\end{array}
$$

$$
2\,[H] \quad \big\Updownarrow \quad 2\,[H]
$$

$$
\begin{array}{ccc}
\gamma - \text{Glu} & & \gamma - \text{Glu} \\
| & & | \\
\text{Cys} - \text{S} - \text{S} - \text{Cys} \\
| & & | \\
\text{Gly} & & \text{Gly}
\end{array}
$$

It can, for example, destroy hydrogen peroxide in a reaction that is catalyzed by **glutathione peroxidase**:

$$
2\quad
\begin{array}{c}
\gamma - \text{Glu} \\
| \\
\text{Cys} - \text{SH} + H_2O_2 \\
| \\
\text{Gly}
\end{array}
$$

Glutathione peroxidase

$$
\downarrow
$$

$$
\begin{array}{ccc}
\gamma - \text{Glu} & & \gamma - \text{Glu} \\
| & & | \\
\text{Cys} - \text{S} - \text{S} - \text{Cys} + 2H_2O \\
| & & | \\
\text{Gly} & & \text{Gly}
\end{array}
$$

Only the reduced form of glutathione is an antioxidant. Therefore the dimeric, oxidized form has to be reduced back by the enzyme **glutathione reductase**:

$$
\begin{array}{ccc}
\gamma - \text{Glu} & & \gamma - \text{Glu} \\
| & & | \\
\text{Cys} - \text{S} - \text{S} - \text{Cys} + \text{NADPH} + H^+ \\
| & & | \\
\text{Gly} & & \text{Gly}
\end{array}
$$

Glutathione reductase

$$
\downarrow
$$

$$
2\quad
\begin{array}{c}
\gamma - \text{Glu} \\
| \\
\text{Cys} - \text{SH} + \text{NADP}^+ \\
| \\
\text{Gly}
\end{array}
$$

The amounts of glucose-6-phosphate dehydrogenase and phosphogluconate dehydrogenase are increased in the well-fed state, and this effect probably is mediated by insulin. In the short term, glucose-6-phosphate dehydrogenase is inhibited by a high [NADPH]/[NADP$^+$] ratio. Therefore *increased NADPH consumption increases the activity of the oxidative branch.*

CLINICAL EXAMPLE 22.7: Glucose-6-Phosphate Dehydrogenase Deficiency

Erythrocytes cannot replace defective proteins by new synthesis. Therefore they must protect their proteins from oxidative damage by maintaining a reducing environment in the cell. This requires reduced glutathione. NADPH, obtained from the pentose phosphate pathway, is needed to keep glutathione in the reduced state.

Partial deficiencies of glucose-6-phosphate dehydrogenase, inherited as an X-linked trait, lead to hemolytic episodes after exposure to drugs that either are oxidants or give rise to oxidizing products during their metabolism. The offending drugs include the antimalarial primaquine, the sulfonamides sulfanilamide and sulfamethoxazole, the antimicrobial drug nalidixic acid, and the urinary antiseptic nitrofurantoin. Hemolytic attacks can also occur during infections. Even broad beans (*Vicia faba*) are dangerous, causing severe attacks of hemolysis within 1 to 2 days of eating the beans ("favism"). In the sixth century BC, Pythagoras strongly advised against the eating of beans, possibly because of the high prevalence of favism in Greece.*

Although the enzyme deficiency is present in all tissues, only the erythrocytes are seriously affected

CLINICAL EXAMPLE 22.7: Glucose-6-Phosphate Dehydrogenase Deficiency—cont'd

because they have no alternative routes for NADPH synthesis, and they cannot compensate for low enzyme activity by synthesizing more enzyme.

The abnormal forms of glucose-6-phosphate dehydrogenase have either reduced catalytic activity (decreased V_{max} or increased K_m) or, more commonly, a shortened lifespan. More than 400 genetic variants have been described, more than for any other human enzyme. Mutant enzymes with zero activity are not seen in patients, presumably because they would be lethal.

After exposure to oxidants, a large amount of glutathione becomes oxidized, and a large amount of NADPH is required to reduce it. In this situation, the mutant glucose-6-phosphate dehydrogenase cannot keep up with the increased demand. Without sufficient NADPH and reduced glutathione, membrane proteins become covalently cross-linked, aggregates of oxidized proteins become visible in the cells as **Heinz bodies,** and a hemolytic crisis develops within 2 to 3 days after the initial exposure to the drug. Glucose-6-phosphate dehydrogenase deficiency is common in people of South Asian, Mediterranean, or African descent, presumably because this trait provided improved malaria resistance.

*According to some scholars, however, Pythagoras' injunction against beans stems from the belief that beans contain the souls of dead people. Pythagoras was one of the first European philosophers to believe in the transmigration of the soul.

FRUCTOSE IS THE PRINCIPAL SUGAR IN SEMINAL FLUID

Seminal fluid contains up to 11 mmol/L (200 mg/dl) of free fructose. It is the major energy source for the sperm cells in their all-important race for the ovum. The advantage of fructose over glucose may be that many bacteria, which compete with the sperm cells for the available nutrient, prefer glucose to other energy sources.

However, trying to boost male fertility by eating fructose would be futile. The fructose in seminal fluid comes not from the diet but from synthesis in the seminal vesicles by the **polyol pathway** (*Fig. 22.23*).

Glucose is reduced by NADPH, and sorbitol is oxidized by NAD^+. Therefore the high ratios of [NADPH]/[NADP$^+$] and [NAD$^+$]/[NADH] in the cell ensure that the pathway proceeds from glucose to fructose rather than from fructose to glucose. This pathway is active not only in seminal vesicles but in many other tissues as well, including the lens, retina, blood vessels, and peripheral nerves.

AMINO SUGARS AND SUGAR ACIDS ARE MADE FROM GLUCOSE

The carbohydrate in glycolipids, glycoproteins, and proteoglycans is derived from nucleotide-activated precursors (*Table 22.3*). These "activated" sugar derivatives are made from glucose. The synthesis of the activated **amino sugars** is shown in *Figure 22.24*.

UDP-glucuronic acid, which is required for the synthesis of proteoglycans and for conjugation reactions in the liver, is made by NAD^+-dependent oxidation of carbon 6 in UDP-glucose (*Fig. 22.25*). The free glucuronic acid produced during degradation of proteoglycans (reaction 3 in *Fig. 22.25*) is metabolized to an intermediate of the pentose phosphate pathway.

Most mammals can convert the intermediate gulonic acid to **ascorbic acid** (**vitamin C**). Only primates, guinea pigs, and fruit bats cannot make their own vitamin C and therefore are prone to scurvy. Ancestors of modern humans could afford this genetic defect because they had a dependable supply of ascorbic acid from the fruits they ate.

Essential pentosuria is caused by an enzymatic block in the conversion of L-xylulose to xylitol (reaction 6 in *Fig. 22.25*). This harmless inherited condition is sometimes misdiagnosed as diabetes mellitus because the L-xylulose that patients excrete in the urine yields a positive test result for "reducing sugar." Enzymatic tests, such as the glucose oxidase method, are necessary to distinguish between the sugars.

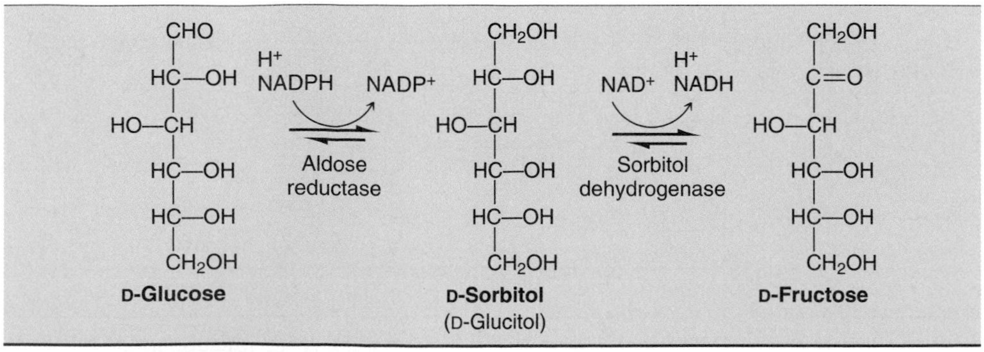

Figure 22.23 Polyol pathway. *NAD,* Nicotinamide adenine dinucleotide.

Table 22.3 Sugars in Glycolipids, Glycoproteins, and Proteoglycans

Sugar	Type	Activated Form	Occurrence
Mannose	Hexose	GDP-Man	Glycoproteins (especially *N*-linked)
Galactose	Hexose	UDP-Gal	Glycoproteins, glycolipids, proteoglycans
Glucose	Hexose	UDP-Glc	Glycoproteins (rare), glycolipids
Fucose	Deoxyhexose	GDP-Fuc	Glycoproteins, glycolipids
N-acetylglucosamine	Aminohexose	UDP-GlcNAc	Glycoproteins, proteoglycans
N-acetylgalactosamine	Aminohexose	UDP-GalNAc	Glycoproteins, glycolipids, proteoglycans
Glucuronic acid	Uronic acid	UDP-GlcUA	Proteoglycans
Iduronic acid	Uronic acid	None*	Proteoglycans
N-acetylneuraminic acid	Sialic acid	CMP-NANA	Glycoproteins, glycolipids

*Formed by epimerization of glucuronic acid in the proteoglycan. CMP, Cytidine monophosphate; GDP, guanosine diphosphate; UDP, uridine diphophate.

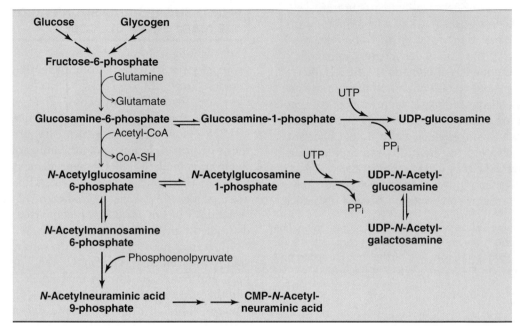

Figure 22.24 Synthesis of amino sugars. *CMP*, Cytidine monophosphate; *CoA*, coenzyme A; PP$_i$, inorganic pyrophosphate; *UDP*, uridine diphosphate; *UTP*, uridine triphosphate.

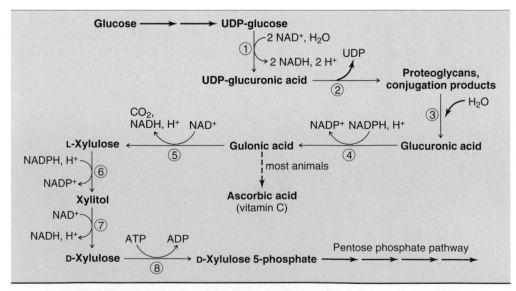

Figure 22.25 Uronic acid pathway. *NAD*, Nicotinamide adenine dinucleotide; *NADP*, nicotinamide adenine dinucleotide phosphate; *UDP*, uridine diphosphate.

SUMMARY

Because glucose is a required fuel for brain and erythrocytes, a blood glucose level of 70 to 100 mg/dl has to be maintained at all times. In the fasting state, the liver has to produce glucose by two pathways: gluconeogenesis and glycogen degradation.

Gluconeogenesis produces glucose from amino acids, lactate, and glycerol. This pathway uses the reversible reactions of glycolysis while bypassing the irreversible ones. It is the only source of glucose during long-term fasting.

Glycogen degradation in the liver is the major source of blood glucose during short-term fasting. Extrahepatic tissues use their glycogen not for blood glucose regulation but as an energy reserve during oxygen deficiency, and in skeletal muscle it is used during strenuous exercise.

Glucose metabolism is regulated by hormones. Insulin stimulates the glucose-consuming pathways of glycolysis and glycogen synthesis, whereas glucagon and epinephrine stimulate the glucose-producing pathways of gluconeogenesis and glycogen degradation.

The dietary monosaccharides fructose and galactose are channeled into glycolysis. These reactions take place mainly in the liver. The "minor pathways" of carbohydrate metabolism supply specialized products: The *pentose phosphate pathway* provides ribose-5-phosphate and NADPH, and other specialized reaction sequences produce fructose, galactose, amino sugars, and sugar acids.

Further Reading

Agius L: Glucokinase and molecular aspects of liver glycogen metabolism, *Biochem J* 414:1–18, 2008.

Anderka O, Boyken J, Aschenbach U, et al: Biophysical characterization of the interaction between hepatic glucokinase and its regulatory protein, *J Biol Chem* 283:31333–31340, 2008.

Armoni M, Harel C, Karnieli E: Transcriptional regulation of the GLUT4 gene: from PPAR-γ and FOXO1 to FFA and inflammation, *Trends Endocrinol Metab* 18:100–107, 2007.

Beer NL, Tribble ND, McCulloch LJ, et al: The P446L variant in *GCKR* associated with fasting plasma glucose and triglyceride levels exerts its effects through increased glucokinase activity in liver, *Hum Mol Genet* 18:4081–4088, 2009.

Cheng A, Saltiel AR: More TORC for the gluconeogenic engine, *BioEssays* 28:231–234, 2006.

Cohen P: The twentieth century struggle to decipher insulin signaling, *Nat Rev Mol Cell Biol* 7:867–873, 2006.

Dolan LC, Potter SM, Burdock GA: Evidence-based review on the effect of normal dietary consumption of fructose on development of hyperlipidemia and obesity in healthy, normal weight individuals, *Crit Rev Food Sci Nutr* 50:53–84, 2010.

Foufelle F, Ferré P: New perspectives in the regulation of hepatic glycolytic and lipogenic genes by insulin and glucose: a role for the transcription factor sterol regulatory element binding protein–1c, *Biochem J* 366:377–391, 2002.

Havel PJ: Dietary fructose: implications for dysregulation of energy homeostasis and lipid/carbohydrate metabolism, *Nutr Rev* 63:133–157, 2005.

Jitrapakdee S, Maurice M, Rayment I, et al: Structure, mechanism and regulation of pyruvate carboxylase, *Biochem J* 413:369–387, 2008.

Kellett GL, Brot-Laroche E, Mace OJ, et al: Sugar absorption in the intestine: the role of GLUT2, *Annu Rev Nutr* 28:35–54, 2008.

Koeberl DD, Kishnani PS, Bali D, et al: Emerging therapies for glycogen storage disease type I, *Trends Endocrinol Metab* 20:252–258, 2009.

Liu Y, Dentin R, Chen D, Hedrick S, et al: A fasting inducible switch modulates gluconeogenesis via activator/coactivator exchange, *Nature* 456:269–273, 2008.

Nordlie RC, Foster JD, Lange AJ: Regulation of glucose production by the liver, *Annu Rev Nutr* 19:379–406, 1999.

Orho-Melander M, Melander O, Guiducci C, Perez-Martinez P, et al: Common missense variant in the glucokinase regulatory protein gene is associated with increased plasma triglyceride and C-reactive protein but lower fasting glucose concentrations, *Diabetes* 57:3112–3121, 2008.

Rider MH, Bertrand L, Vertommen D, et al: 6-phosphofructo-2-kinase/fructose-2,6-bisphosphatase: head-to-head with a bifunctional enzyme that controls glycolysis, *Biochem J* 381:561–579, 2004.

Ruxton CHS, Gardner EJ, McNulty HM: Is sugar consumption detrimental to health? A review of the evidence 1995-2006, *Crit Rev Food Sci Nutr* 50:1–19, 2010.

Towle HC: Glucose as a regulator of eukaryotic gene transcription, *Trends Endocrinol Metab* 16:489–494, 2005.

Watford M: Small amounts of dietary fructose dramatically increase hepatic glucose uptake through a novel mechanism of glucokinase activation, *Nutr Rev* 60:253–264, 2002.

Weedon MN, Clark VJ, Qian Y, Ben-Shlomo Y, et al: A common haplotype of the glucokinase gene alters fasting glucose and birth weight: association in six studies and population-genetics analyses, *Am J Hum Genet* 79:991–1001, 2006.

Yang J, Reshef L, Cassuto H, et al: Aspects of the control of phosphoenolpyruvate carboxykinase gene transcription, *J Biol Chem* 284:27031–27035, 2009.

QUESTIONS

1. Ischemic tissues have an increased rate of glycolysis. Most of this is not fueled by glucose but by locally stored glycogen that is degraded in response to ischemia. This response depends on the activation of glycogen phosphorylase by

   A. ATP
   B. AMP
   C. Low pH
   D. Carbon dioxide
   E. Glucose-6-phosphate

2. Several inborn errors of carbohydrate metabolism cause fasting hypoglycemia. The *most severe* fasting hypoglycemia has to be expected in deficiencies of

   A. Phosphofructokinase
   B. Aldolase
   C. Glycogen phosphorylase
   D. Fructose-1,6-bisphosphatase
   E. Glucose-6-phosphatase

3. A medical student of Middle Eastern ethnic background develops an episode of hemoglobinuria 24 hours after injecting himself with a street drug of unknown composition. He probably has a low activity of the red blood cell enzyme

   A. Glucose-6-phosphate dehydrogenase
   B. Hexokinase
   C. Phosphofructokinase
   D. Fructokinase
   E. Glucose-6-phosphatase

4. Liver glycogen is normally synthesized after a meal and degraded during fasting. What pharmacological manipulation would enhance glycogen degradation in the liver?

   A. An inhibitor of α-adrenergic receptors
   B. An inhibitor of β-adrenergic receptors
   C. The injection of insulin
   D. A drug that activates protein phosphatase-1
   E. A drug that inhibits the degradation of cAMP

5. Glycogen degradation is an important energy source for exercising muscle. How many high-energy phosphate bonds are synthesized by converting one glucose residue in glycogen to lactic acid?

   A. 1
   B. 2
   C. 3
   D. 4
   E. 5

Chapter 23
THE METABOLISM OF FATTY ACIDS AND TRIGLYCERIDES

Triglycerides (fat) supply 35% to 40% of the total calories in typical Western diets. Ninety-five percent of this energy is contributed by the fatty acids and only 5% by the glycerol. The human body uses triglycerides as the principal storage form of energy, and most people carry between 5 and 20 kg of fat in their adipose tissue. With a basal metabolic rate of 1800 kcal/day, a 10-kg store of fat (93,000 kcal) can keep a human alive for 52 days without food. Fat metabolism includes the following processes:

1. Digestion, absorption, and transport of dietary fat
2. Generation of metabolic energy from this fat
3. Storage of excess fat in adipose tissue
4. Metabolic links between triglycerides and other biomolecules, including carbohydrates and ketone bodies

FATTY ACIDS DIFFER IN THEIR CHAIN LENGTH AND NUMBER OF DOUBLE BONDS

A "standard" fatty acid is an unbranched hydrocarbon chain with a carboxyl group at one end. Most naturally occurring fatty acids have an even number of carbons. Chain lengths of 16 and 18 are the most common.

In **saturated fatty acids**, the carbons are linked exclusively by single bonds. Of the fatty acids listed in *Table 23.1*, **acetic acid** does not occur in natural fats and oils, but vinegar contains about 5% of free (unesterified) acetic acid. **Butyric acid** is also rare in natural

fats except milk fat. It is notorious for its smell, which resembles that of malodorous feet. In the production of some types of cheese, butyric acid is released from milk fat by the action of microbial lipases and contributes to the flavor of the product. **Myristic acid** is abundant in nutmeg, coconut, and palm kernel oil. **Palmitic acid** and **stearic acid** are the most common saturated fatty acids in animal fat, accounting for 30% to 40% of the fatty acids in human adipose tissue.

The carbons of the fatty acids are numbered, starting with the carboxyl carbon. Alternatively, they are designated by Greek letters. As in the amino acids, the α-carbon is the one next to the carboxyl carbon, the β-carbon is carbon 3, and so forth. The last carbon in the chain is the ω-carbon, as in the example of stearic acid:

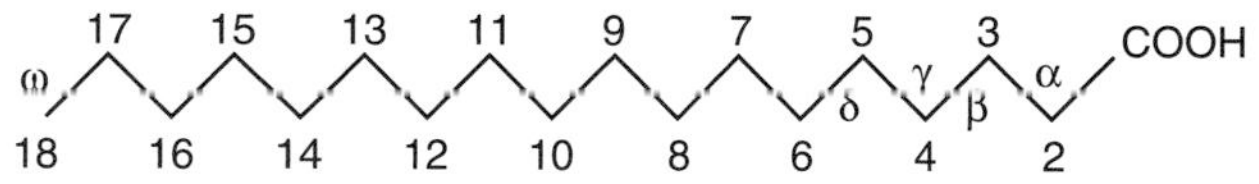

Monounsaturated fatty acids have one carbon-carbon double bond, and **polyunsaturated fatty acids** have more than one. The double bonds of the polyunsaturated fatty acids are always three carbons apart, with a single methylene (—CH_2—) group in between. The positions of the double bonds are specified by their distance from the carboxyl end. A Δ^9 double bond, for example, is between carbons 9 and 10. Alternatively, the distance from the ω carbon can be specified.

The latter designation is useful because fatty acids can be elongated and shortened only at the carboxyl

Table 23.1 Structures of Some Naturally Occurring Saturated Fatty Acids

No. of Carbons	Fatty Acid	Structure	
2	Acetic acid	H_3C—COOH	
4	Butyric acid	H_3C—$(CH_2)_2$—COOH	
14	Myristic acid	H_3C—$(CH_2)_{12}$—COOH	
16	Palmitic acid	H_3C—$(CH_2)_{14}$—COOH	
18	Stearic acid	H_3C—$(CH_2)_{16}$—COOH	
20	Arachidic acid	H_3C—$(CH_2)_{18}$—COOH	
22	Behenic acid	H_3C—$(CH_2)_{20}$—COOH	
24	Lignoceric acid	H_3C—$(CH_2)_{22}$—COOH	

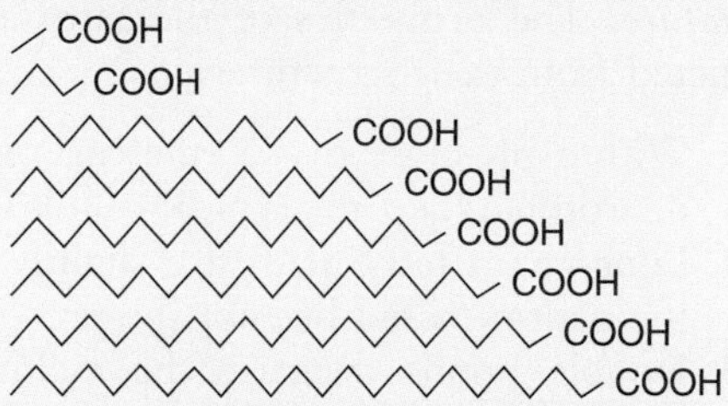

Table 23.2 Structures of Some Unsaturated Fatty Acids

Fatty Acid	Biosynthetic Class	Formula*	Structure	Nutritionally Essential
Palmitoleic acid	ω^7	16:1;9	$H_3C-(CH_2)_5-CH=CH-(CH_2)_7-COOH$	No
Oleic acid	ω^9	18:1;9	$H_3C-(CH_2)_7-CH=CH-(CH_2)_7-COOH$	No
Linoleic acid	ω^6	18:2;9,12	$H_3C-(CH_2)_3-(CH_2-CH=CH)_2-(CH_2)_7-COOH$	Yes
α-Linolenic acid	ω^3	18:3;9,12,15	$H_3C-(CH_2-CH=CH)_3-(CH_2)_7-COOH$	Yes
Arachidonic acid	ω^6	20:4;5,8,11,14	$H_3C-(CH_2)_3-(CH_2-CH=CH)_4-(CH_2)_3-COOH$	No[†]

*Number of carbons: number of double bonds; positions of double bonds
[†]Can be synthesized from dietary linoleic acid.

end. For example, if oleic acid (*Table 23.2*) is elongated by two carbons at the carboxyl end, the product is no longer a Δ^9 fatty acid but Δ^{11}, but it is still an ω^9 fatty acid. *Humans cannot introduce new double bonds beyond Δ^9.* Therefore some of the polyunsaturated fatty acids, notably linoleic acid and possibly α-linolenic acid, are *nutritionally essential.* The structures of unsaturated fatty acids can be described by a formula indicating chain length, number of double bonds, and locations of the double bonds (see *Table 23.2*).

There is no free rotation around the carbon-carbon double bond, and the substituents are fixed in *cis* or *trans* configuration:

cis   or   *trans*

Whereas the *trans* configuration favors an extended shape of the hydrocarbon chain, a *cis* double bond forms an angle of 120 degrees:

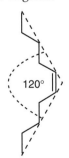

120°

Only fatty acids with cis *double bonds are common in nature.* The properties of the fatty acids can be predicted from their structures:

1. With a pK close to 4.8, the carboxyl group is 99% deprotonated at the typical cellular pH of 6.8.
2. Long-chain fatty acids are slightly water soluble in the deprotonated but not the protonated state.
3. Double bonds decrease the melting points of the fatty acids. For example, stearic acid has a melting point of 70°C, oleic acid 16°C, linoleic acid −5°C, and α-linolenic acid −11°C, even though these 18-carbon fatty acids all have nearly the same molecular weight. Fats and oils that are solid at room temperature contain mainly saturated (or transunsaturated) fatty acids, and those that remain liquid even in the refrigerator contain mainly unsaturated fatty acids.

CHYLOMICRONS TRANSPORT TRIGLYCERIDES FROM THE INTESTINE TO OTHER TISSUES

The main products of fat digestion are *2-monoacylglycerol* and *free fatty acids* (see Chapter 19). After their absorption, the fatty acids are activated to **acyl-coenzyme A** (acyl-CoA) in the endoplasmic reticulum (ER) of the intestinal mucosal cell:

$$R-COO^- + HS-CoA$$

ATP

Acyl-CoA synthetase

AMP, PP$_i$

$$R-\overset{\overset{\displaystyle O}{\|}}{C}-S-CoA$$

This is always the first reaction of intracellular fatty acid metabolism, much as phosphorylation by hexokinase is always the first reaction of intracellular glucose metabolism. Like the phosphorylated sugars, *the CoA-activated fatty acids are strictly intracellular metabolites.* They do not cross the plasma membrane and are not transported in the blood.

The synthesis of acyl-CoA is made irreversible by hydrolysis of the inorganic pyrophosphate that is formed in the reaction. The acyl-CoA then reacts with 2-monoacylglycerol to form triglyceride (*Fig. 23.1*).

Why are triglycerides hydrolyzed in the intestinal lumen only to be resynthesized in the mucosal cell? The reason is that triglycerides are too insoluble. Only

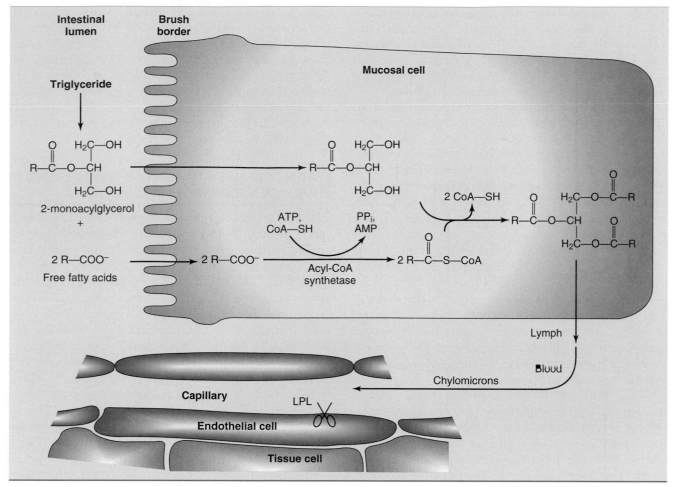

Figure 23.1 Absorption and transport of dietary fat. *LPL,* Lipoprotein lipase.

free fatty acids and monoglycerides are sufficiently water soluble to diffuse to the cell surface for absorption.

In the ER of the intestinal mucosal cell, the triglycerides are assembled into small fat droplets (diameter 1 μm). These droplets, known as **chylomicrons,** also contain other dietary lipids and a small amount of ER-synthesized proteins. After processing through the secretory pathway, the chylomicrons are released into the extracellular space. Because the endothelium of intestinal capillaries has no fenestrations, *chylomicrons are collected by the lymph rather than by the blood.* They are carried to the left brachiocephalic vein by the thoracic duct.

The triglycerides in chylomicrons are utilized by adipose tissue, heart, skeletal muscle, lactating mammary glands, and, to a lesser extent, by spleen, lungs, kidneys, endocrine glands, and aorta. These tissues (but not the liver and brain) possess **lipoprotein lipase** (LPL), an enzyme that is attached to heparan sulfate proteoglycans on the surface of the capillary endothelium. As the chylomicrons pass through the capillaries, they bind to LPL. Their triglycerides are hydrolyzed to free fatty acids and 2-monoacylglycerol, and these products are taken up by the cells.

LPL expression is regulated. Feeding raises LPL activity in adipose tissue but reduces it in skeletal muscle and myocardium. This ensures that dietary fat is directed mainly to adipose tissue in the well-fed state but to the muscles during fasting. During lactation, LPL activity declines in adipose tissue but rises massively in the mammary gland. These effects are orchestrated by hormones, including insulin, epinephrine, glucocorticoids, and prolactin.

Injected heparin detaches LPL from the capillary wall and increases its enzymatic activity. Therefore LPL activity can be determined in the laboratory by measuring serum lipase activities before and after heparin injection.

ADIPOSE TISSUE IS SPECIALIZED FOR THE STORAGE OF TRIGLYCERIDES

Triglyceride is the best storage form of energy because of its high energy density. It has a caloric value of 9.3, as opposed to 4.0 for glycogen, and whereas fat can be stored without accompanying water, each gram of glycogen binds 2 g of water. Therefore the energy value of 15 kg of fat is equivalent to 100 kg of hydrated glycogen.

After a mixed meal containing fat, carbohydrate, and protein, adipose tissue obtains most of its fatty acids from the action of LPL on chylomicron triglycerides. These fatty acids are transported into the cell and are activated to their CoA-thioesters before they can be used for triglyceride synthesis.

The glycerol of the triglycerides is derived from **glycerol-3-phosphate.** Adipose tissue has low levels of glycerol kinase. Therefore most glycerol phosphate is made not from free glycerol but from the glycolytic intermediate dihydroxyacetone phosphate. The NADH-dependent **glycerol phosphate dehydrogenase** that catalyzes this reaction is the same enzyme that participates in the glycerol phosphate shuttle (see Chapter 21) and in gluconeogenesis from glycerol (see Chapter 22). Dihydroxyacetone phosphate is derived from glucose after a carbohydrate meal or from lactate during fasting and after a high-fat, low-carbohydrate meal (*Fig. 23.2*).

Fat breakdown (lipolysis) in adipose tissue requires three lipases: adipose tissue triglyceride lipase, diglyceride lipase, and monoglyceride lipase. The diglyceride lipase traditionally has been described as the **hormone-sensitive adipose tissue lipase,** although the triglyceride lipase is responsive to hormones as well.

Unlike liver and intestine, *adipose tissue releases lipid not in the form of lipoproteins but as "free" (unesterified) fatty acids.* These fatty acids are transported to distant sites in reversible binding to serum albumin. The albumin-bound fatty acids have a plasma half-life of only 3 minutes. The other product of fat breakdown, glycerol, is used for gluconeogenesis by the liver.

A good deal of futile cycling occurs during fat metabolism. Approximately 40% of the fatty acids released by lipolysis during fasting does not leave the tissue but is resynthesized into storage triglyceride. This futile cycling consumes about 3% of the energy in the triglyceride, but it permits better regulation of lipolysis by controlling both the lipases that release the fatty acids and the enzymes needed for resynthesis of triglyceride from the released fatty acids.

FAT METABOLISM IN ADIPOSE TISSUE IS UNDER HORMONAL CONTROL

Hormones control both the adipose tissue triglyceride lipase and the "hormone-sensitive" diglyceride lipase:

Norepinephrine (noradrenaline) from sympathetic nerve terminals and **epinephrine** (adrenaline) from the adrenal medulla are released during physical exercise and stress. They stimulate lipolysis through β-adrenergic receptors and cyclic AMP (cAMP). *Figure 23.3* shows the mechanism for stimulation of the hormone-sensitive diglyceride lipase by the catecholamines and other cAMP-elevating hormones. The catecholamines also stimulate the adipose tissue triglyceride lipase by unknown mechanisms.

Synaptically released norepinephrine is more important than circulating epinephrine. In animal experiments, sympathetic denervation causes excessive fat accumulation in the denervated portions of adipose tissue. This is most obvious under conditions of food deprivation or cold exposure, when fat is degraded in the surrounding innervated tissue.

Figure 23.2 Sources of glycerol 3-phosphate for fat synthesis in adipose tissue. After a carbohydrate meal (high insulin), most glycerol phosphate is derived from glucose. Glyceroneogenesis from pyruvate is the major source during fasting, leading to substantial futile cycling.

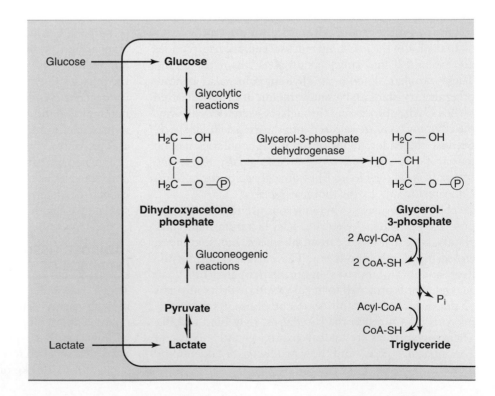

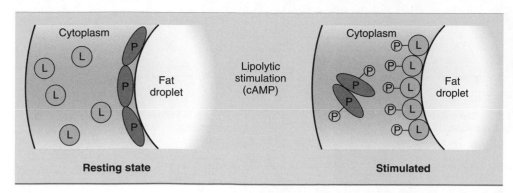

Figure 23.3 Hormonal control of the hormone-sensitive adipose tissue lipase. Both the lipase (*L*) and the fat-associated protein perilipin (*P*) become phosphorylated by the cyclic AMP-dependent protein kinase A. This enables the lipase to bind to the fat droplet and hydrolyze the triglycerides.

Insulin is released by glucose and amino acids after an opulent meal. A high insulin level signals the abundance of dietary nutrients that are eligible for storage. Conversely, a low insulin level signals a shortage of nutrients during fasting and a need for fat breakdown.

Insulin reduces lipolysis in adipose tissue. Part of this effect is mediated by activation of the cAMP-degrading phosphodiesterase PDE3B. Another effect is a reduction in the synthesis of the adipose tissue triglyceride lipase.

Insulin increases the uptake of glucose into the cell by the GLUT4 transporter. The metabolism of glucose stimulates fat synthesis by providing the precursor glycerol phosphate. In addition, insulin stimulates LPL in the capillaries of adipose tissue and induces glycerol phosphate-acyltransferase, the enzyme that adds the first fatty acid to glycerol phosphate in the biosynthetic pathway (see *Fig. 23.2*).

Tumor necrosis factor-α (**TNF-α**) stimulates lipolysis through multiple signaling cascades, leading to long-term stimulation of lipolysis that is mediated mainly by increased synthesis of the lipolytic enzymes. As a cytokine that is released during chronic infections and other severe diseases, *TNF-α is in large part responsible for the mobilization of fat stores during severe chronic diseases.*

Glucocorticoids, growth hormone, and **thyroid hormones** facilitate lipolysis by inducing the synthesis of lipolytic proteins. Glucocorticoids also reduce the reesterification of free fatty acids by *repressing* phosphoenolpyruvate (PEP) carboxykinase in adipose tissue, although they *induce* this gluconeogenic enzyme in the liver. This reduces futile cycling in times of stress and fasting, when the body needs all the energy it can get.

Not all kinds of adipose tissue respond equally to glucocorticoids. Patients with Cushing syndrome (excess glucocorticoids) lose fat in the extremities but develop truncal obesity and a "buffalo hump."

FATTY ACIDS ARE TRANSPORTED INTO THE MITOCHONDRION

Neurons and erythrocytes depend on glucose because they cannot oxidize fatty acids. For most other cells, however, fatty acid oxidation by the mitochondrial pathway of **β-oxidation** is a major energy source.

Fatty acids are activated to their CoA-thioesters by enzymes on the ER membrane and the outer mitochondrial membrane. They then pass through the pores in the outer mitochondrial membrane and are shuttled across the inner mitochondrial membrane with the help of **carnitine**:

$$H_3C - \overset{\overset{\displaystyle CH_3}{|}}{\underset{|}{N^+}} - CH_3$$
$$|$$
$$CH_2$$
$$|$$
$$HO - CH$$
$$|$$
$$CH_2$$
$$|$$
$$COO^-$$

Carnitine

On the outer surface of the inner mitochondrial membrane, the fatty acid is transferred from CoA to carnitine, forming acyl-carnitine:

$$H_3C - (CH_2)_{14} - \overset{\overset{\displaystyle O}{\|}}{C} - O - \overset{}{CH}$$

Palmitoyl-carnitine

Acyl-carnitine crosses the membrane in exchange for free carnitine. In the mitochondrial matrix, the fatty acid is transferred back to CoA. The reversible enzymatic reactions are catalyzed by two carnitine-acyltransferases (*Fig. 23.4*).

Fatty acids with a chain length of 12 carbons or fewer do not depend on carnitine. They diffuse

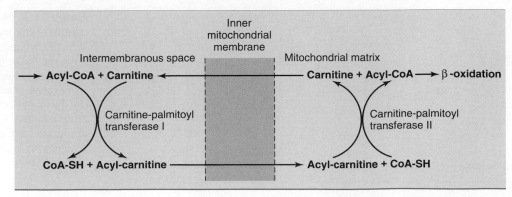

Figure 23.4   Transport of long-chain fatty acids into the mitochondrion. The carnitine-palmitoyltransferase reaction is freely reversible. *Acyl-CoA*, Acyl-coenzyme A.

passively across the membrane and subsequently are activated in the mitochondrion.

β-OXIDATION PRODUCES ACETYL-CoA, NADH, AND FADH$_2$

The major pathway of fatty acid oxidation is called β-oxidation because it oxidizes the β-carbon (carbon 3). Eventually, it slices the whole fatty acid into two-carbon fragments in the form of acetyl-CoA. Each cycle of β-oxidation produces NADH and the reduced form of flavin adenine dinucleotide (FADH$_2$) in addition to acetyl-CoA (*Fig. 23.5*). These reduced coenzymes feed into the respiratory chain.

The stoichiometry for β-oxidation of palmitate is as follows:

$$\text{Palmitoyl-CoA} + 7\ \text{FAD} + 7\ \text{NAD}^+ + 7\ \text{CoA} + 7\ \text{H}_2\text{O}$$

$$\downarrow$$

$$8\ \text{Acetyl-CoA} + 7\ \text{FADH}_2 + 7\ \text{NADH} + 7\ \text{H}^+$$

The energy yield can be calculated as

8 acetyl-CoA	→	96 ATP
7 FADH$_2$	→	14 ATP
7 NADH	→	21 ATP
		131 ATP
		−2 ATP
		129 ATP

Two ATP molecules are subtracted because the initial activation of palmitate to palmitoyl-CoA requires two high-energy phosphate bonds in ATP. *The energy yield is close to 40%*, which is about the same as for glucose oxidation.

Within rather wide limits, the use of fatty acids by the tissues is proportional to the plasma free fatty acid level. Therefore *fatty acid oxidation is regulated mainly at the level of lipolysis in adipose tissue.*

In addition, *carnitine-palmitoyltransferase I is allosterically inhibited by malonyl-CoA.* Malonyl-CoA is

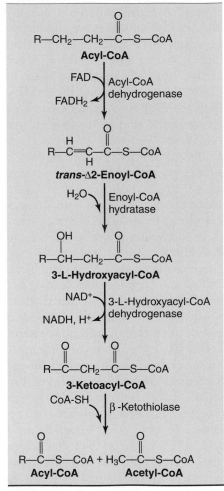

Figure 23.5   Reaction sequence of β-oxidation. These reactions take place in the mitochondrial matrix of most cells. *Acetyl-CoA*, Acetyl-coenzyme A; *Acyl-CoA*, acyl-coenzyme A; *CoA-SH*, free coenzyme A; *FAD*, flavin adenine dinucleotide; *NAD*, nicotinamide adenine dinucleotide.

formed in the regulated step of fatty acid biosynthesis (see section on Fatty acids Are Synthesized from Acetyl-CoA). Therefore *fatty acid oxidation is inhibited when fatty acid synthesis is active.* This prevents excessive futile cycling.

CLINICAL EXAMPLE 23.1: Carnitine Deficiency

Carnitine deficiency can be caused by impaired carnitine biosynthesis in the kidneys and liver or by impaired uptake into the cells. Carnitine is also depleted in many organic acidurias, including methylmalonic aciduria (see Chapter 26) and medium-chain acyl-CoA dehydrogenase deficiency (see *Clinical Example 23.3*) because the accumulating acids form carnitine esters that are excreted in the urine. Ordinarily, the body uses this mechanism for the disposal of unwanted organic acids from dietary sources.

Carnitine deficiency in the liver leads to *hypoketotic hypoglycemia during periods of extended fasting*. During fasting, β-oxidation is needed to produce acetyl-CoA for ketogenesis and ATP for gluconeogenesis. Therefore both pathways are compromised in carnitine deficiency. The combined deficiency of ketone bodies and glucose is especially bad for the brain because the brain depends on a mix of glucose and ketone bodies during prolonged fasting.

Carnitine deficiency in skeletal muscle causes *muscle weakness and muscle cramps on exertion*. Many patients with generalized carnitine deficiency show an unusual abundance of fat droplets in muscle and liver, and some develop fatty degeneration of the liver. This is because excess acyl-CoA that cannot be transported into the mitochondrion is diverted into triglyceride synthesis.

Carnitine deficiency can be treated with oral carnitine, and some athletes use carnitine in an attempt to boost their β-oxidation. However, carnitine is poorly absorbed, and intestinal bacteria metabolize it under formation of trimethylamine. Although otherwise harmless, this product causes an embarrassing effect: a body odor like rotten fish.

CLINICAL EXAMPLE 23.2: Medium-Chain Acyl-CoA Dehydrogenase Deficiency

The most common inherited defect in the β-oxidation sequence is **medium-chain acyl-CoA dehydrogenase deficiency**. The affected enzyme catalyzes the first reaction in the β-oxidation of medium-chain fatty acids (C-5 to C-12). Two other acyl-CoA dehydrogenases catalyze this reaction with short-chain and long-chain fatty acids, respectively.

Most patients with this deficiency present with *fasting hypoglycemia* during infancy or childhood, often during an infectious illness, when the child eats little. Many cases go undiagnosed, but some infants die of their first hypoglycemic attack under circumstances suggestive of sudden infant death syndrome. The condition is most common in northwestern Europe, where a single mutation accounts for nearly 90% of cases. Therefore early diagnosis by neonatal screening is an attractive option. Once the condition is diagnosed, patients can be kept healthy simply by avoiding prolonged fasting.

SPECIAL FATTY ACIDS REQUIRE SPECIAL REACTIONS

Mitochondrial β-oxidation oxidizes unbranched saturated fatty acids with an even number of carbons and a chain length up to 18 or 20 carbons. Fatty acids that do not fit this description require additional enzymatic reactions.

1. **Unsaturated fatty acids** require modifications of their double bonds before β-oxidation, as shown for linoleic acid in *Figure 23.6*.
2. **α-Oxidation** is a peroxisomal pathway that is required for fatty acids with a methylated β-carbon (see *Clinical Example 23.4*). It oxidizes carbon 2 (the α-carbon) and releases carbon 1 as CO_2, thereby shortening the fatty acid by one carbon at a time.
3. **ω-Oxidation** is a microsomal system that oxidizes the last carbon of medium-chain fatty acids (the ω-carbon) to a carboxyl group, producing a dicarboxylic acid. The dicarboxylic acids can be activated at either end, followed by β-oxidation.
4. **Peroxisomal β-oxidation** is similar to mitochondrial β-oxidation, but an H_2O_2-producing flavoprotein is used for the first reaction. The peroxisomal system is designed for fatty acids with chain lengths of 20 carbons or more, which are poor substrates for mitochondrial β-oxidation. Peroxisomal β-oxidation can proceed only to the stage of octanoyl-CoA.
5. **Odd-chain fatty acids** produce propionyl-CoA rather than acetyl-CoA in the last cycle of β-oxidation. Propionyl-CoA is converted to succinyl-CoA via methylmalonyl-CoA (*Fig. 23.7*). The reaction sequence requires both biotin and deoxyadenosyl-cobalamin, a coenzyme form of vitamin B_{12}. Unlike acetyl-CoA, propionyl-CoA is a substrate of gluconeogenesis.

CLINICAL EXAMPLE 23.3: Ackee

The ackee fruit is part of the local cuisine in Jamaica, but vendors on the local markets warn the naïve tourist that this fruit needs to be cooked well because it is poisonous when eaten raw. The heat-labile alkaloid hypoglycin in this fruit causes fasting hypoglycemia by blocking the acyl-CoA dehydrogenases of β-oxidation. Therefore it is most dangerous when it is eaten without carbohydrate when glycogen stores in the liver are depleted.

CLINICAL EXAMPLE 23.4: Refsum Disease

Phytanic acid is a branched-chain fatty acid that is derived from the alcohol phytol, a constituent of chlorophyll in green vegetables that accumulates in the fat of ruminants:

Continued

CLINICAL EXAMPLE 23.4: Refsum Disease—cont'd

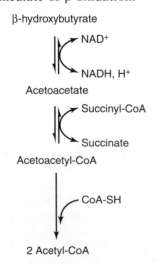

Phytanic acid

The methylated β-carbon of phytanic acid cannot be β-oxidized. α-Oxidation is needed to shorten phytanic acid by one carbon, followed by a round of β-oxidation that yields propionyl-CoA rather than acetyl-CoA.

Refsum disease is a recessively inherited defect in α-oxidation that leads to the progressive accumulation of phytanic acid in triglycerides and membrane lipids. The presenting sign is a slowly progressive peripheral neuropathy with weakness and muscle wasting, combined with blindness. Patients respond to dietary restriction of green vegetables and of ruminant milk and meat, but treatment must be started early, before the neurological damage has become irreversible.

THE LIVER CONVERTS EXCESS FATTY ACIDS TO KETONE BODIES

The ketone bodies include the three biosynthetically related products **acetoacetate**, **β-hydroxybutyrate**, and **acetone**. *Ketone bodies are formed only in the liver.* The pathway of ketogenesis in liver mitochondria is shown in *Figure 23.8*.

A very small amount of acetone is formed by the nonenzymatic decarboxylation of acetoacetate. It serves no recognized biological function and is exhaled through the lungs. In diabetic ketoacidosis, *acetone imparts a characteristic smell to the patient's breath.*

Acetoacetate and β-hydroxybutyrate, however, are useful products. They are sent from the liver to other tissues for oxidation. Even the brain can cover part of its energy requirement from ketone bodies during fasting. The tissues that oxidize the ketone bodies use succinyl-CoA to activate acetoacetate to acetoacetyl-CoA, an intermediate of β-oxidation:

β-hydroxybutyrate

NAD⁺

NADH, H⁺

Acetoacetate

Succinyl-CoA

Succinate

Acetoacetyl-CoA

CoA-SH

2 Acetyl-CoA

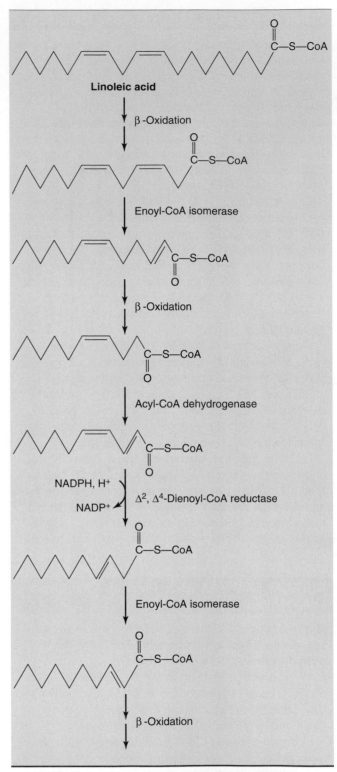

Figure 23.6 β-Oxidation of linoleic acid. Note that the Δ^2 double bond that is formed in each round of β-oxidation is in *trans* configuration, whereas those in the original fatty acid are in *cis* transformation. *CoA*, Coenzyme A; *NADP*, nicotinamide adenine dinucleotide phosphate.

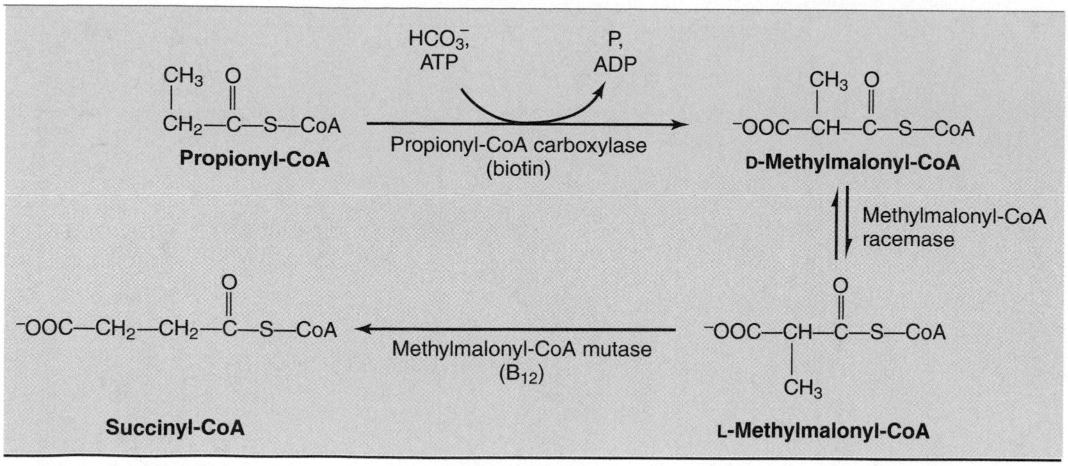

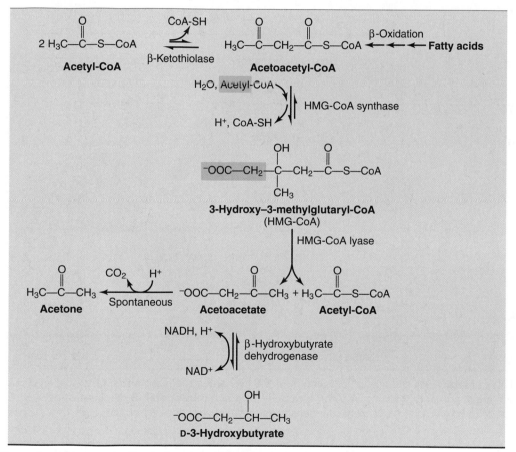

Figure 23.7 Reactions that channel propionyl-coenzyme A (CoA) into the tricarboxylic acid cycle. *Pi,* Inorganic phosphate.

Figure 23.8 Formation of ketone bodies in liver mitochondria. *CoA-SH,* Free coenzyme A; *HMG-CoA,* 3-hydroxy-3-methylglutaryl coenzyme A.

In theory, any substrate that is degraded to acetyl-CoA in the liver can be turned into ketone bodies. Actually, however, *ketogenesis is associated with fatty acid oxidation.* When dietary carbohydrate is plentiful, the liver channels only a moderate amount of glucose through glycolysis. Most of this is released as lactate, converted to fat, or oxidized in the tricarboxylic acid (TCA) cycle.

During fasting, however, the hormonal stimulation of adipose tissue lipolysis provides a large amount of free fatty acids. The liver has a very high capacity for fatty acid oxidation, and *mitochondrial fatty acid uptake and β-oxidation are less tightly regulated than are glycolysis and the pyruvate dehydrogenase reaction.* The acetyl-CoA formed by β-oxidation is not readily used for biosynthesis during fasting. Its oxidation by

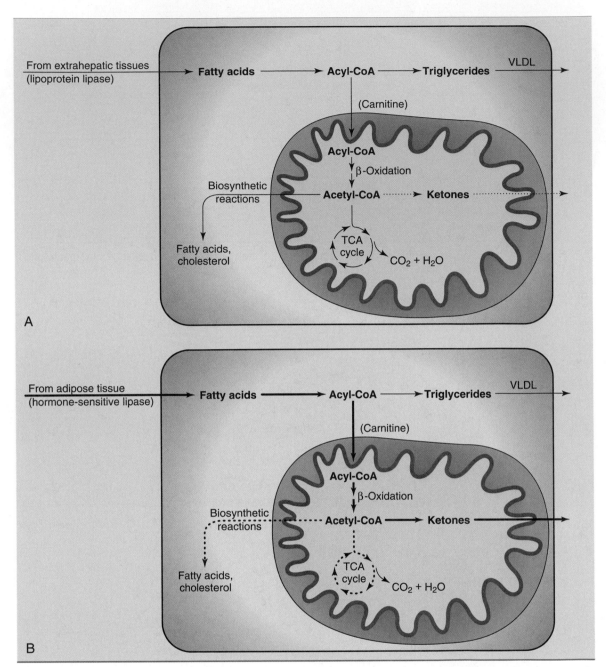

Figure 23.9 Fates of fatty acids and acetyl-coenzyme A in the liver when the plasma free fatty acid level is low (after a carbohydrate-rich meal) and during fasting. **A,** After a carbohydrate-rich mixed meal. **B,** During fasting. *Acyl-CoA,* Acyl-coenzyme A; *TCA,* tricarboxylic acid; *VLDL,* very-low-density lipoprotein.

the TCA cycle is limited as well because the NADH and FADH$_2$ formed during β-oxidation provide enough fuel for the respiratory chain (*Fig. 23.9*).

Enzyme induction also is important. The synthesis of 3-hydroxy-3-methylglutaryl (HMG)-CoA synthase, the rate-limiting enzyme of ketogenesis, is powerfully stimulated by fasting, dietary fat, and insulin deficiency. Fatty acids, in particular, are excellent inducers of this enzyme.

FATTY ACIDS ARE SYNTHESIZED FROM ACETYL-CoA

Fatty acids cannot be converted into carbohydrates, but excess carbohydrate is converted into fat after a carbohydrate-rich meal. Therefore people can get fat on a carbohydrate-rich diet. This is achieved by turning glucose into acetyl-CoA, and acetyl-CoA into fatty acids.

Triglycerides are synthesized mainly in liver, adipose tissue, and lactating mammary glands. These tissues are also able to synthesize the fatty acids that become incorporated into the triglyceride. Adipose tissue synthesizes triglycerides for storage, the mammary gland secretes them into milk, and the liver exports them in **very-low-density lipoprotein (VLDL)**. VLDL triglycerides are utilized in the same way as the dietary triglycerides in chylomicrons, by the action of LPL.

In the first step of fatty acid biosynthesis, acetyl-CoA is carboxylated to malonyl-CoA by **acetyl-CoA carboxylase (ACC)**:

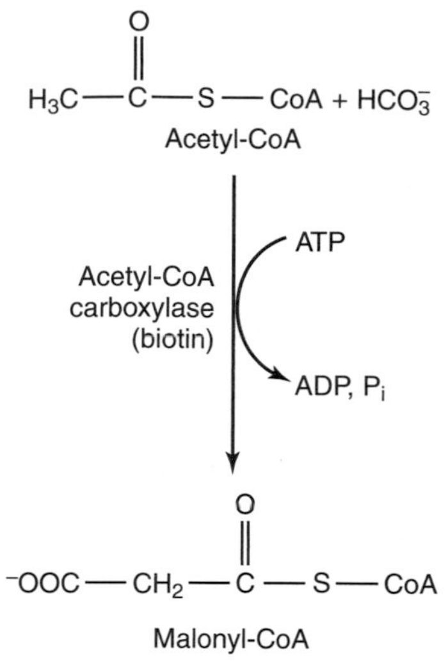

$$H_3C-\overset{\overset{O}{\|}}{C}-S-CoA + HCO_3^-$$

Acetyl-CoA

Acetyl-CoA carboxylase (biotin)

ATP

ADP, P_i

$$^-OOC-CH_2-\overset{\overset{O}{\|}}{C}-S-CoA$$

Malonyl-CoA

This ATP-dependent carboxylation requires enzyme-bound biotin. Because its product malonyl-CoA is not used in other metabolic pathways, *this reaction is the committed step of fatty acid biosynthesis.*

The other reactions of fatty acid synthesis are catalyzed by the cytoplasmic **fatty acid synthase complex**. This complex is a dimer of two identical polypeptide chains, with diverse enzymatic activities located on the same polypeptide (*Fig. 23.10*). It contains two important sulfhydryl groups that carry the growing fatty acid during its synthesis. One belongs to a cysteine side chain and the other to the covalently bound coenzyme **phosphopantetheine** (*Fig. 23.11*).

The first elongation cycle of fatty acid synthesis is shown in *Figure 23.12*. It includes two reductive reactions that require NADPH as the reductant. The second cycle continues with the transfer of another malonyl group to phosphopantetheine. The reactions are repeated until a chain length of 16 carbons is reached. At this point, the thioesterase domain of the fatty acid synthase (see *Fig. 23.10*) catalyzes the release of the end product palmitic acid.

The stoichiometry for the synthesis of palmitic acid is

Acetyl-CoA + 7 Malonyl-CoA + 14 NADPH + 14 H$^+$

↓

Palmitate + 7CO$_2$ + 14 NADP$^+$ + 8 CoA-SH + 6 H$_2$O

Malonyl-CoA is formed from acetyl-CoA in the reaction

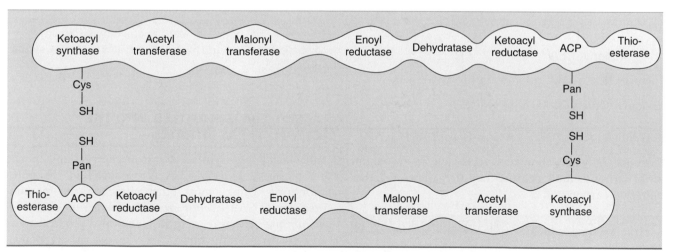

Figure 23.10 Structure of the mammalian fatty acid synthase complex. During fatty acid synthesis, acyl groups are transferred between the cysteine side chain of one subunit and the phosphopantetheine group of the other subunit. *ACP*, Acyl carrier protein.

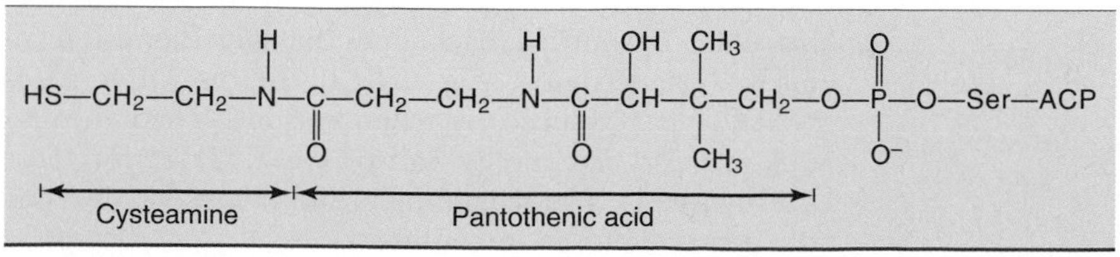

Figure 23.11 Phosphopantetheine group in the fatty acid synthase complex. It resembles coenzyme A in its structure and in its ability to form a thioester bond with organic acids. *ACP*, Acyl carrier protein.

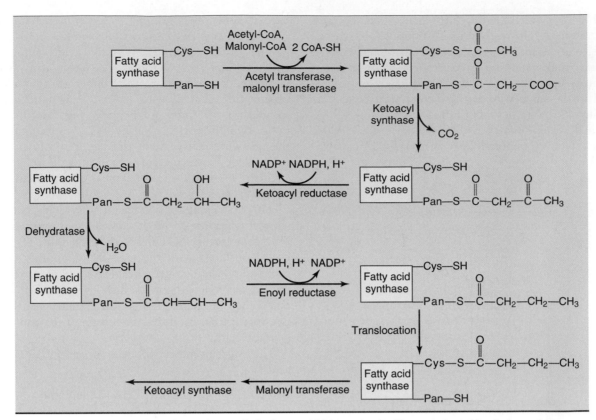

Figure 23.12 Reactions of the first elongation cycle in fatty acid biosynthesis. The cysteine side chain and the phosphopantetheine group actually belong to two separate polypeptides in the fatty acid synthase complex. *CoA*, Coenzyme A; *NADP*, nicotinamide adenine dinucleotide phosphate.

$$\text{Acetyl-CoA} + CO_2 + ATP + H_2O$$
$$\downarrow$$
$$\text{Malonyl-CoA} + ADP + P_i + H^+$$

Therefore the overall reaction can be written as

$$8\ \text{Acetyl-CoA} + 7\ ATP + 14\ NADPH + 6\ H^+ + H_2O$$
$$\downarrow$$
$$\text{Palmitate} + 14\ NADP^+ + 8\ \text{CoA-SH} + 7\ ADP + 7\ P_i$$

Most naturally occurring fatty acids have an even number of carbons simply because they are patched together from two-carbon units.

CLINICAL EXAMPLE 23.5: Peroxisomal Diseases

The most severe type of inherited peroxisomal disease is **Zellweger syndrome.** It is caused by defects in the protein import system of peroxisomes, which leave the peroxisomes "empty." Affected infants die shortly after birth with severe abnormalities of brain, liver, and kidneys.

Other peroxisomal diseases are more specific. In **adrenoleukodystrophy,** a defect in peroxisomal β-oxidation leads to the accumulation of very-long-chain fatty acids with up to 26 carbons. This X-linked recessive disease causes blindness, behavioral changes, mental deficiency, and death in childhood. Refsum disease (see *Clinical Example 23.4*) also is a peroxisomal disease.

ACETYL-CoA IS SHUTTLED INTO THE CYTOPLASM AS CITRATE

Fatty acids are synthesized from acetyl-CoA in the cytoplasm, but acetyl-CoA is produced in the mitochondrion. Unlike most other mitochondrial metabolites, *acetyl-CoA cannot cross the inner mitochondrial membrane.* However, citrate can cross. To transport acetyl-CoA from the mitochondrion into the cytoplasm, acetyl-CoA is converted to citrate first. Citrate is transported into the cytoplasm, where it is cleaved back to acetyl-CoA and oxaloacetate by the cytoplasmic **ATP-citrate lyase.**

Acetyl-CoA is used for fatty acid synthesis, and oxaloacetate is shuttled back into the mitochondrion as malate or pyruvate (*Fig. 23.13*). In the latter case, NADPH is produced by **malic enzyme.** Theoretically, this reaction can supply half of the NADPH for fatty acid synthesis. The remaining NADPH must come from the pentose phosphate pathway.

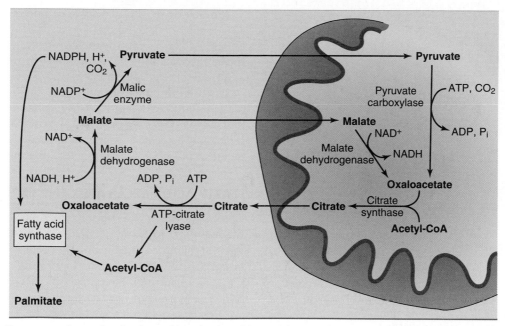

Figure 23.13 Transport of acetyl units from the mitochondrion to the cytoplasm. The inner mitochondrial membrane has carriers for citrate, pyruvate, and malate but not for acetyl-CoA and oxaloacetate. *CoA*, Coenzyme A; *NADP*, nicotinamide adenine dinucleotide phosphate.

FATTY ACID SYNTHESIS IS REGULATED BY HORMONES AND METABOLITES

On a day-to-day basis, fatty acid synthesis is regulated by adjustments in the synthesis of acetyl-CoA carboxylase (ACC), fatty acid synthase, ATP-citrate lyase, and glucose-6-phosphate dehydrogenase. These enzymes are induced by carbohydrate feeding and repressed by a fat-based diet and starvation.

On a time scale of minutes, fatty acid synthesis is controlled by ACC. This enzyme occurs in two forms. ACC1 is a cytoplasmic enzyme in liver, adipose tissue, and lactating mammary glands, where it supplies malonyl-CoA for fatty acid synthesis. ACC2 is an enzyme of the outer mitochondrial membrane, where it produces malonyl-CoA for the regulation of carnitine-palmitoyltransferase 1. ACC2 is most important in the nonlipogenic tissues, including heart and skeletal muscle. Both forms are allosterically activated by citrate and inhibited by the CoA-thioesters of long-chain fatty acids. The well-fed liver has a higher citrate level and a lower acyl-CoA level than does the fasting liver.

In addition, *ACC is stimulated by insulin and inhibited by glucagon and epinephrine.* Glucagon and epinephrine induce the phosphorylation and partial inactivation of ACC by the cAMP-dependent protein kinase A. Insulin opposes this effect by activating the cAMP-degrading phosphodiesterase 2B.

ACC is also subject to inhibitory phosphorylation by the **AMP-activated protein kinase.** As its name implies, this kinase is activated in metabolic emergencies when the cellular energy charge is dangerously low. It helps the cell to survive the energy shortage by switching off nonessential biosynthetic pathways, including fatty acid synthesis. In the liver, the AMP-activated protein kinase is inhibited by insulin (*Fig. 23.14*).

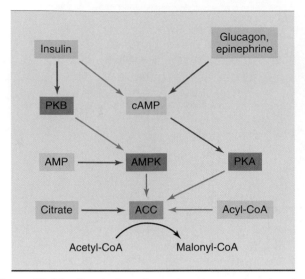

Figure 23.14 Regulation of acetyl-coenzyme A carboxylase (*ACC*) by hormones, protein kinases, and allosteric effectors. *Green arrow*, Stimulation; *red arrow*, inhibition. *AMP*, Adenosine monophosphate; *AMPK*, AMP-activated protein kinase; *cAMP*, cyclic AMP; *CoA*, coenzyme A; *PKA*, protein kinase A; *PKB*, protein kinase B (Akt).

MOST FATTY ACIDS CAN BE SYNTHESIZED FROM PALMITATE

The fatty acid synthase complex produces palmitate, a saturated 16-carbon fatty acid. However, the fatty acids in human triglycerides and membrane lipids have chain lengths up to 24 or 26 carbons, with C-18 fatty acids being the most common. Also, only about 50% of human fatty acids is saturated; another 40% is monounsaturated, and 10% is polyunsaturated. Most of these fatty acids can be synthesized from palmitate in the human body.

Chain elongation takes place in the ER and the mitochondrion. Like the fatty acid synthase complex, *the elongation systems add two carbons at a time*. The mitochondrial system prefers fatty acids with fewer than 16 carbons, but microsomal chain elongation works best with palmitate. Both unsaturated and saturated fatty acids can be elongated.

Desaturation requires membrane-bound desaturase enzymes in the ER. The desaturases are monooxygenases that use molecular oxygen as the oxidant and either NADH or NADPH as a cofactor.

The first double bond is introduced in position Δ^9 of palmitic or stearic acid, producing palmitoleic acid or oleic acid, respectively. Oleic acid is the most abundant unsaturated fatty acid in human lipids. Additional double bonds can be introduced between the carboxyl group and the first double bond, but not beyond Δ^9. Most polyunsaturated fatty acids can be synthesized from dietary palmitic or stearic acid by a combination of desaturation and chain elongation. These belong to the ω^7 and ω^9 classes.

Linoleic acid (18:2;9,12) and α-**linolenic acid** (18:3;9, 12,15; see *Table 23.2*) are the parent compounds of the ω^6 and ω^3 classes of polyunsaturated fatty acids, respectively. They cannot be synthesized in the human body and therefore are *nutritionally essential*.

Essential fatty acid deficiency is characterized by dermatitis and poor wound healing. It has been observed in patients who were kept on total parenteral nutrition for long time periods, in patients suffering from severe fat malabsorption, and in infants fed low-fat milk formulas.

FATTY ACIDS REGULATE GENE EXPRESSION

The synthesis of metabolic enzymes has to be adjusted to the supply of dietary nutrients. Carbohydrates induce most of their gene regulatory effects indirectly, by stimulating the release of insulin. The insulin signaling pathways, in turn, impinge on nuclear transcription factors to induce the enzymes of carbohydrate metabolism.

Dietary fatty acids use a more direct route, by *binding to nuclear transcription factors*. This mechanism resembles the effects of steroid hormones. However, the receptors for dietary lipids are less selective for their ligands than are the hormone receptors. These receptors are sometimes described as **orphan receptors** because knowledge of their physiological ligands is uncertain.

The **peroxisome proliferator-activated receptors** (**PPARs**), as their name implies, cause the proliferation of peroxisomes and of the lipid-metabolizing peroxisomal pathways. However, they have many other metabolic effects as well.

PPAR-α is expressed mainly in the liver. It is activated by many monounsaturated and polyunsaturated fatty acids as well as some oxidized arachidonic acid derivatives from both the cyclooxygenase and lipoxygenase pathways (see Chapter 16). Binding of these ligands to PPAR-α stimulates the peroxisomal pathways profoundly and mitochondrial β-oxidation to a lesser extent.

Knockout mice without PPAR-α have grossly abnormal lipid metabolism. Plasma triglycerides are elevated, and fat accumulates in the liver. Rather than oxidizing the fatty acids in mitochondria and peroxisomes, the liver esterifies them into triglycerides. The triglyceride either is exported as a constituent of lipoproteins or accumulates in the liver. Lipid-lowering drugs of the **fibrate** class (bezafibrate, gemfibrozil) are potent activators of PPAR-α.

PPAR-γ is most important in adipose tissue. It is required for the differentiation of adipose cells during embryogenesis, and it stimulates the synthesis of many proteins involved in lipid metabolism. Its activation by polyunsaturated fatty acids induces the synthesis of many proteins that are involved in fat synthesis in adipose tissue. Pharmacological activation of PPAR-γ has beneficial effects in type 2 diabetes (*Clinical Example 23.7*).

CLINICAL EXAMPLE 23.7: Treatment of Diabetes Mellitus with Rosiglitazone

The "insulin sensitizer" rosiglitazone (Avandia) has been used extensively for the treatment of type 2 diabetes. Rosiglitazone regulates gene expression in adipose tissue by activating the transcription factor **PPAR-γ**. This results in increased levels of hormone-sensitive lipase, the fatty acid transport protein CD36, and many other enzymes of lipid metabolism.

By inducing PEP carboxykinase, PPAR-γ increases the conversion of pyruvate/lactate to glycerol-3-phosphate in adipose tissue. It also stimulates the transcription of the genes for glycerol phosphate dehydrogenase and glycerol kinase. These enzymes provide glycerol-3-phosphate as a substrate for triglyceride synthesis even when insulin is low and little glycerol-3-phosphate is formed from glucose.

The improved supply of glycerol phosphate increases the esterification of fatty acids that are released from stored triglycerides during fasting or from chylomicrons after a fatty meal, reducing the levels of free fatty acids in blood and tissues. *Many tissues, including muscle and liver, metabolize fatty acids in preference to glucose when fatty acids are abundant.* Therefore excessive amounts of free (unesterified) fatty acids reduce glucose metabolism and contribute to hyperglycemia in diabetes mellitus.

PPAR-γ is activated not only by drugs. Under physiological conditions it responds to many monounsaturated and polyunsaturated fatty acids. In theory, a diet high in unsaturated fatty acids could be used to treat insulin resistance in type 2 diabetes.

POLYUNSATURATED FATTY ACIDS CAN BE OXIDIZED NONENZYMATICALLY

In the presence of oxygen, polyunsaturated fatty acids are subject to nonenzymatic **auto-oxidation** or **peroxidation**. When this occurs outside the body, it causes fat to become rancid. In the body, it can damage the cells.

Polyunsaturated fatty acids auto-oxidize when a hydrogen atom is abstracted from the methylene group between two double bonds (reaction ① in *Fig. 23.15*). The initiator is a free radical that is derived either from another polyunsaturated fatty acid (reaction ④ in *Fig. 23.15*) or from partially reduced oxygen, such as the superoxide radical:

$$O_2^- \xrightarrow[\text{Reaction ①(Fig. 23.15)}]{\substack{\text{[H] from}\\ \text{fatty acid}}} O_2H^- \xrightarrow{H^+} H_2O_2$$

The initiator can also be a peroxide radical generated from hydrogen peroxide with the aid of a metal ion:

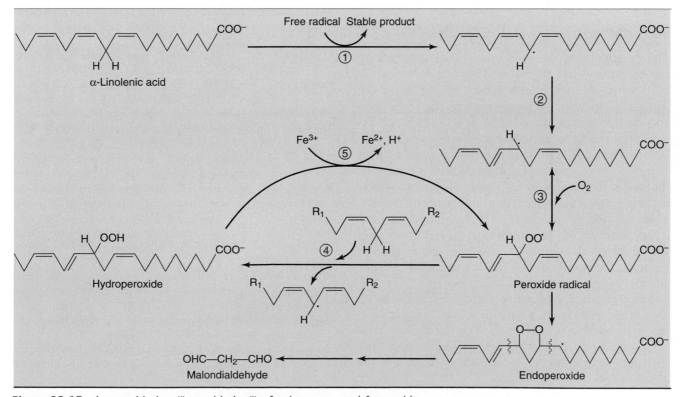

Figure 23.15 Auto-oxidation ("peroxidation") of polyunsaturated fatty acids.

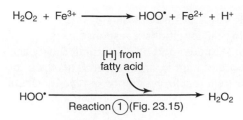

$$H_2O_2 + Fe^{3+} \longrightarrow HOO^{\bullet} + Fe^{2+} + H^+$$

By the same mechanism, hydroperoxide derivatives of polyunsaturated fatty acids can be converted back into reactive peroxide radicals (reaction ⑤ in *Fig. 23.15*). This implies the possibility of *a branching chain reaction leading to an avalanche of free radicals.*

The fatty acid itself can finally be fragmented into smaller products. If at least three double bonds (which are always three carbons apart) are present, **malondialdehyde** is a prominent product. Malondialdehyde is chemically reactive. It cross-links proteins and other molecules, resulting in membrane damage and the accumulation of yellow **lipofuscin,** a poorly degradable polymeric product formed from partially decomposed fatty acids and cross-linked, denatured proteins. It accumulates as "age pigment" in the lysosomes of elderly persons.

The enzymes **catalase, superoxide dismutase,** and **glutathione peroxidase** are the body's major defenses against lipid peroxidation. They destroy dangerous products of oxidative metabolism. Some vitamins, metabolites, and phytochemicals act as free radical scavengers by reacting with free radicals, forming harmless products. They include, among many others, **vitamin E,** the **retinoids, uric acid,** and **vitamin C.**

SUMMARY

The intestinal mucosa resynthesizes triglycerides from the products of fat digestion. These triglycerides are transported in lymph and blood by chylomicrons. Their utilization by the tissues requires the endothelial enzyme lipoprotein lipase (LPL).

Adipose tissue is an important destination for dietary triglycerides. With the help of insulin, the adipose cells synthesize storage fat after a meal. Conversely, the hydrolysis of stored fat is stimulated by norepinephrine and epinephrine but inhibited by insulin. Thus the storage fat that is synthesized after a meal is degraded during fasting, when insulin is low, and during physical exertion, when the catecholamines are high. Fatty acids from adipose tissue are the major energy source for the body during fasting.

Fatty acids are oxidized to acetyl-CoA by the mitochondrial pathway of β-oxidation, which is active in the mitochondria of most cells. The fasting liver converts a major portion of the fatty acid–derived acetyl-CoA into ketone bodies, which are released into the blood as fuel for other tissues.

On a high-carbohydrate, low-fat diet, carbohydrates are converted into fat by the sequential action of glycolysis, pyruvate dehydrogenase, fatty acid biosynthesis, and esterification of the fatty acids with glycerol. This sequence is most active in liver and adipose tissue.

Further Reading

Costanzi S, Neumann S, Gershengorn MC: Seven transmembrane-spanning receptors for free fatty acids as targets for diabetes mellitus: pharmacological, phylogenetic, and drug discovery aspects, *J Biol Chem* 283: 16269–16273, 2008.

Duncan RE, Ahmadian M, Jaworski K, et al: Regulation of lipolysis in adipocytes, *Annu Rev Nutr* 27:79–101, 2007.

Goldberg IJ, Eckel RH, Abumrad NA: Regulation of fatty acid uptake into tissues: lipoprotein lipase- and CD36-mediated pathways, *J Lipid Res* 2009:S86–S90, 2009.

Granneman JG, Moore H-PH: Location, location: protein trafficking and lipolysis in adipocytes, *Trends Endocrinol Metab* 19:3–9, 2007.

Gregersen N, Bross P, Andresen BS: Genetic defects in fatty acid β-oxidation and acyl-CoA dehydrogenases, *Eur J Biochem* 271:470–482, 2004.

Hue L, Rider MH: The AMP-activated protein kinase: more than an energy sensor, *Essays Biochem* 43:121–137, 2007.

Jaworski K, Sarkadi-Nagy E, Duncan RE, et al: Regulation of triglyceride metabolism. IV. Hormonal regulation of lipolysis in adipose tissue, *Am J Physiol Gastrointest Liver Physiol* 293:G1–G4, 2007.

Neels JG, Olefsky JM: A new way to burn fat, *Science* 312:1756–1758, 2006.

Nye C, Kim J, Kalhan SC, et al: Reassessing triglyceride synthesis in adipose tissue, *Trends Endocrinol Metab* 19:356–361, 2008.

Saggerson D: Malonyl-CoA, a key signaling molecule in mammalian cells, *Annu Rev Nutr* 28:253–272, 2008.

Sampath H, Ntambi JM: Polyunsaturated fatty acid regulation of genes of lipid metabolism, *Annu Rev Nutr* 25:317–340, 2005.

Tontonoz P, Spiegelman BM: Fat and beyond: the diverse biology of PPARγ, *Annu Rev Biochem* 77:289–312, 2008.

Wakil SJ, Abu-Elheiga LA: Fatty acid metabolism: target for metabolic syndrome, *J Lipid Res* 2009:S138–S143, 2009.

Wanders RJA, Waterham HR: Biochemistry of mammalian peroxisomes revisited, *Annu Rev Biochem* 75:295–332, 2006.

Watt MJ, Steinberg GR: Regulation and function of triacylglycerol lipases in cellular metabolism, *Biochem J* 414: 313–325, 2008.

Wintour EM, Henry BA: Glycerol transport: an additional target for obesity therapy? *Trends Endocrinol Metab* 17:77–78, 2006.

Wolf G: Brown adipose tissue: the molecular mechanism of its formation, *Nutr Rev* 67:167–171, 2009.

Zechner R, Kienesberger PC, Haemmerle G, et al: Adipose triglyceride lipase and the lipolytic catabolism of cellular fat stores, *J Lipid Res* 50:3–21, 2009.

QUESTIONS

1. **Like many other tissues, the myocardium can use the triglycerides in chylomicrons for its own energy needs. The utilization of these triglycerides requires the enzyme**

   A. Acetyl-CoA carboxylase
   B. Glucose-6-phosphate dehydrogenase
   C. Phospholipase A_2
   D. LPL
   E. Hormone-sensitive lipase

2. **The excessive formation of ketone bodies occurs in many diseases. The *most important* regulated step determining the rate of ketogenesis is catalyzed by**

   A. Acyl-CoA dehydrogenase
   B. Pyruvate kinase
   C. Adipose tissue triglyceride lipase
   D. Acetyl-CoA carboxylase
   E. Glucose-6-phosphate dehydrogenase

3. **Medium-chain acyl-CoA dehydrogenase deficiency is the most common inherited defect of β-oxidation. Most patients with this condition present initially with**

   A. Liver cirrhosis
   B. Fasting hypoglycemia
   C. Ketoacidosis
   D. Hypertriglyceridemia
   E. Slowly developing ataxia (poor motor coordination)

4. **A pharmaceutical company wants to develop an antiobesity drug that acts directly on adipose tissue metabolism. The most promising drug type would be agents that**

   A. Stimulate β-adrenergic receptors
   B. Inhibit adenylate cyclase
   C. Stimulate glucose uptake into adipose cells
   D. Inhibit the hormone-sensitive adipose tissue lipase
   E. Stimulate insulin receptors in adipose tissue

Chapter 24

THE METABOLISM OF MEMBRANE LIPIDS

Biological membranes contain phosphoglycerides, sphingolipids, and cholesterol (see Chapter 12). All of these membrane lipids can be synthesized in the body, and most are made in the cells in which they are used. However, considerable quantities are transported in the blood as constituents of plasma lipoproteins. This chapter discusses the biosynthesis and degradation of the membrane lipids.

PHOSPHATIDIC ACID IS AN INTERMEDIATE IN PHOSPHOGLYCERIDE SYNTHESIS

Phosphoglycerides are synthesized in the cytoplasm and endoplasmic reticulum (ER) of all cells. **Phosphatidic acid,** which is synthesized from glycerol phosphate, is the key intermediate. Its biosynthesis is shown in **Figure 24.1**.

De novo synthesis of phosphoglycerides occurs via two pathways. In the **phosphatidic acid pathway,** phosphatidate is activated as cytidine diphosphate (CDP)-diacylglycerol. This strategy is used for the synthesis of phosphatidylinositol (**Fig. 24.2**) and cardiolipin.

In the **salvage pathway,** phosphate is removed from phosphatidate to form 1,2-diacylglycerol. As shown in **Figure 24.3** for the synthesis of phosphatidylcholine, choline is activated as the CDP derivative, and phosphocholine is then attached to the 3-hydroxyl group of 1,2-diacylglycerol. Phosphatidylethanolamine is synthesized in a similar way. Use of CDP-activated precursors for the synthesis of membrane lipids is analogous to use of uridine diphosphate–activated precursors for the synthesis of glycogen and other complex carbohydrates.

However, in the case of the phosphoglycerides, one of the two phosphates in the CDP derivative remains in the product.

PHOSPHOGLYCERIDES ARE REMODELED CONTINUOUSLY

Phospholipases are used to remodel the phosphoglycerides by changing the fatty acids in positions 1 and 2 (**Fig. 24.4**). They are named according to their cleavage specificity:

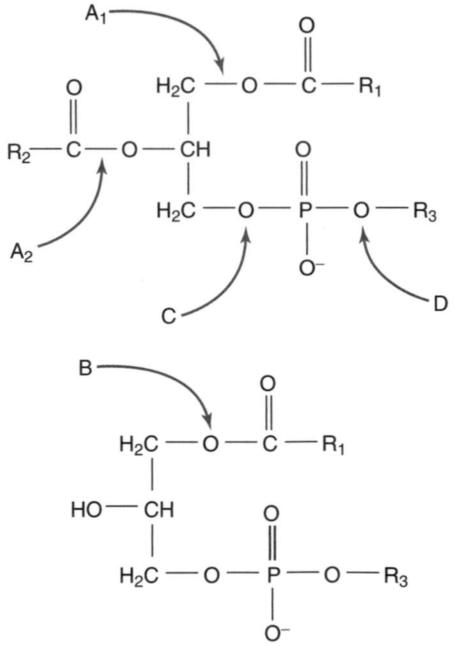

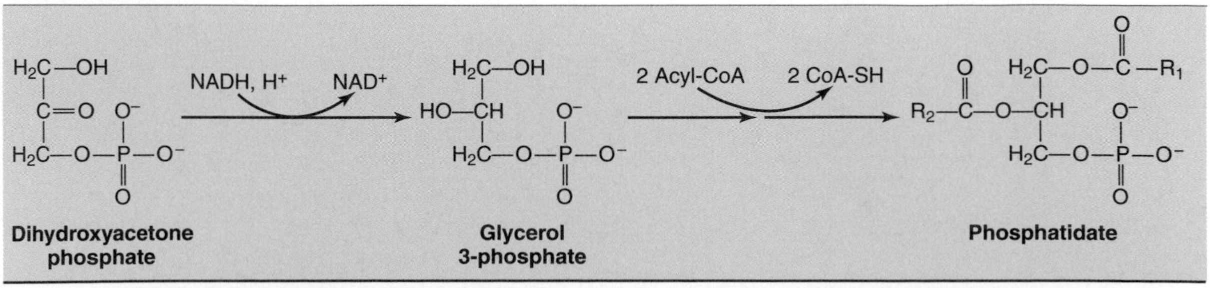

Figure 24.1 Synthesis of phosphatidic acid.

The acyltransferases that replace the cutout fatty acid usually place a saturated fatty acid in position 1 and an unsaturated fatty acid in position 2. The unsaturated fatty acid is most often arachidonic acid for phosphatidylinositol and oleic acid or linoleic acid for the other phosphoglycerides.

The alcoholic substituent of phosphatidic acid is exchangeable as well. Most phosphatidylserine is synthesized by base exchange with ethanolamine in human tissues:

Phosphatidylethanolamine + Serine

↓

Phosphatidylserine + Ethanolamine

Phosphatidylethanolamine can be made by decarboxylation of phosphatidylserine, whereas phosphatidylcholine can be formed by methylation of phosphatidylethanolamine (*Fig. 24.5*).

Plasmalogens, which constitute up to 10% of the phosphoglycerides in muscle and brain, have an unsaturated fatty alcohol instead of a fatty acid in position 1 of the glycerol. Their synthesis is shown in *Figure 24.6*.

Platelet-activating factor (PAF) (see *Fig. 24.6*) is formed by white blood cells as a mediator of hypersensitivity reactions and acute inflammation. In concentrations as low as 10^{-11} to 10^{-10} mol/L, it induces platelet adhesion, vasodilation, and chemotaxis of polymorphonuclear leukocytes. The presence of an acetyl group in position 2, instead of a long-chain acyl group, makes PAF sufficiently water soluble to diffuse through an aqueous medium.

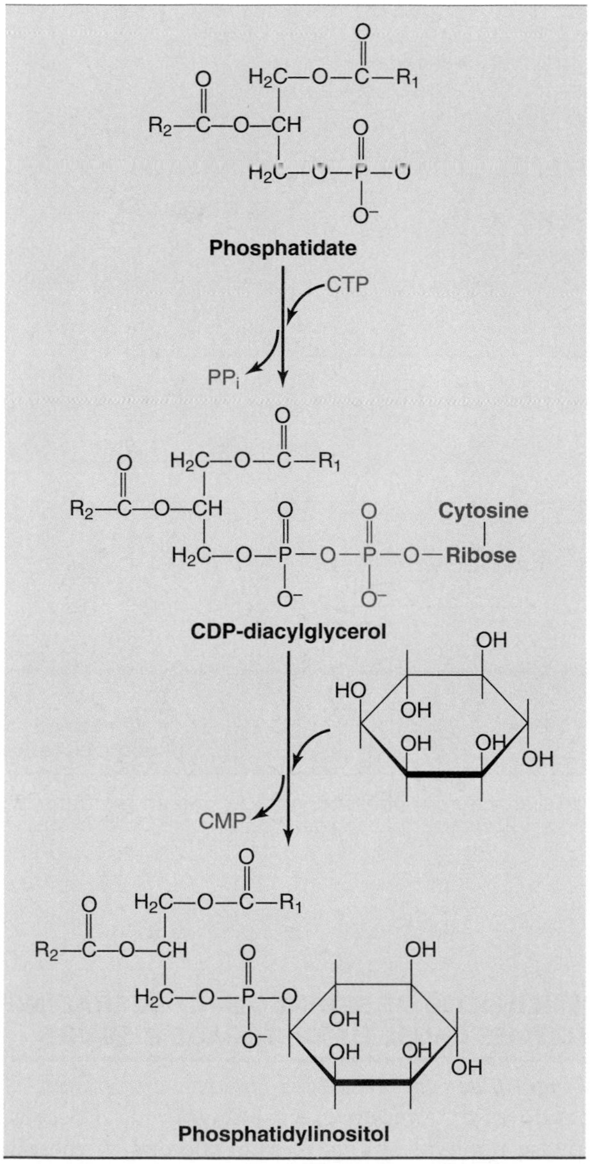

SPHINGOLIPIDS ARE SYNTHESIZED FROM CERAMIDE

Ceramide, consisting of sphingosine and a long-chain fatty acid, is the core structure of the sphingolipids:

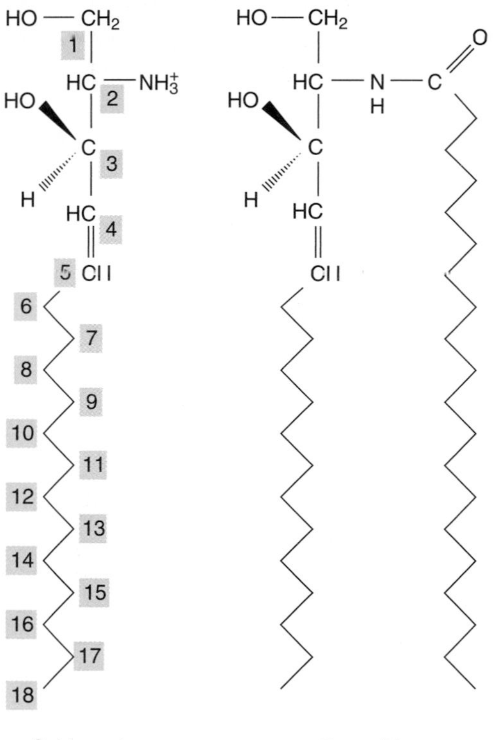

Sphingosine   Ceramide

The primary hydroxyl group at C-1 of the sphingosine moiety carries either phosphocholine (in sphingomyelin) or carbohydrate (in the glycosphingolipids) (see *Fig. 12.5*). Sphingosine is synthesized in the ER of most cells from palmitoyl-CoA and serine, and the fatty acid is introduced from its CoA-thioester. The fatty acid usually is saturated and can be very long, with 22 or 24 carbons.

During the synthesis of sphingolipids in the ER and Golgi apparatus, *the hydroxyl group at C-1 of sphingosine*

Figure 24.2 Synthesis of phosphatidylinositol by the phosphatidic acid pathway.

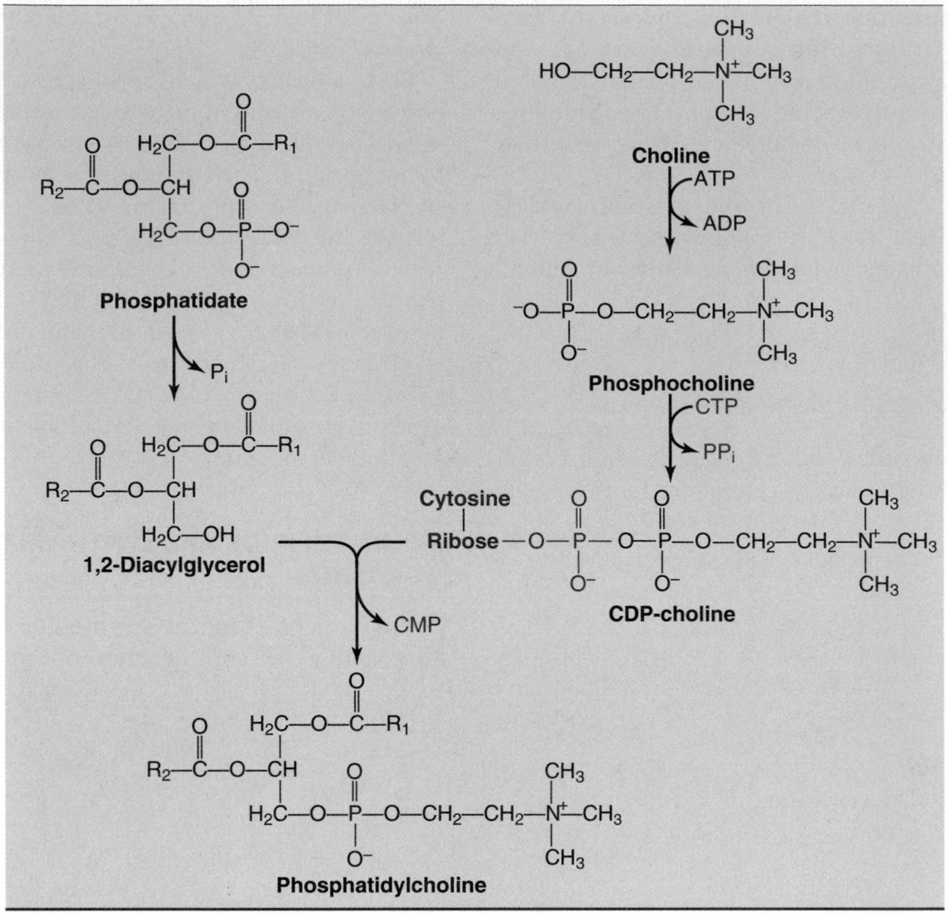

Figure 24.3 Synthesis of phosphatidylcholine by the salvage pathway.

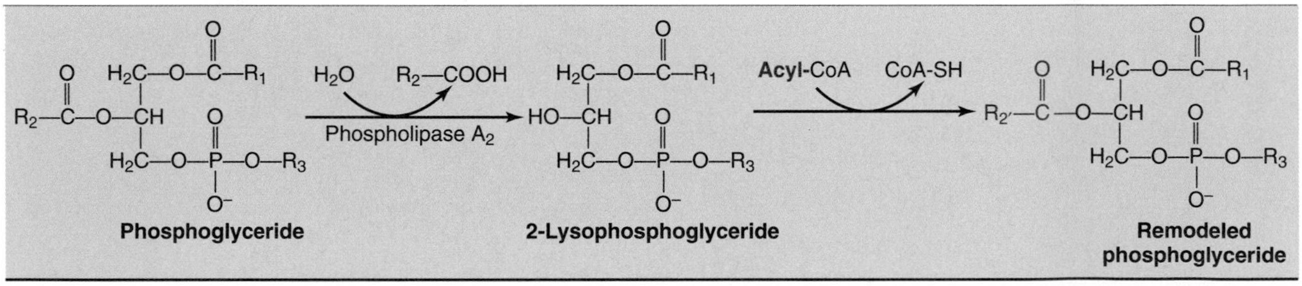

Figure 24.4 Exchange of a fatty acid in a phosphoglyceride by successive action of phospholipase A_2 and an acyltransferase. *CoA*, Coenzyme A; *CoA-SH*, uncombined CoA.

is not activated. Instead, its substituent is introduced from an activated precursor. For example, sphingomyelin is synthesized with the help of phosphatidylcholine:

Ceramide + Phosphatidylcholine
↓
Sphingomyelin + 1, 2-Diacylglycerol

The oligosaccharide chains of the glycosphingolipids are synthesized by stepwise addition of monosaccharides from their activated precursors.

DEFICIENCIES OF SPHINGOLIPID-DEGRADING ENZYMES CAUSE LIPID STORAGE DISEASES

Sphingolipids are degraded in the lysosomes. The breakdown of complex glycosphingolipids proceeds by stepwise removal of sugars from the end of the oligosaccharide (***Fig. 24.8***). Each of these enzymes is specific for the monosaccharide that it removes and the type of glycosidic bond that it cleaves.

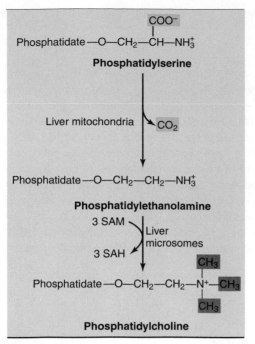

Figure 24.5 Synthesis of phosphatidylethanolamine and phosphatidylcholine from phosphatidylserine. *SAH,* S-adenosyl homocysteine; *SAM,* S-adenosyl methionine.

A deficiency of any of these enzymes leads to the accumulation of its substrate in the lysosomes. The resulting disease is called a **lipid storage disease** or **sphingolipidosis** (***Table 24.1***). *The enzyme deficiency is expressed in all tissues.* The nervous system is seriously affected in essentially all cases because of its high sphingolipid content and turnover. Hepatosplenomegaly is another common finding in these diseases because phagocytic cells in spleen and liver remove erythrocytes from the circulation, and nondegradable lipid from the red blood cell membrane accumulates in these tissues.

The inheritance is autosomal recessive except for Fabry disease, which is X-linked recessive. For diagnosis and genetic counseling, enzyme activities are determined in cultured leukocytes, skin fibroblasts, or, for prenatal diagnosis, amniotic cells. In the more severe diseases, affected homozygotes have near-zero enzyme activity. These diseases are progressive and lead to early death. In milder variants of lipid storage diseases, affected homozygotes have greatly reduced but not completely absent enzyme activity. Heterozygotes can be identified because their enzyme activity is reduced to about half of normal.

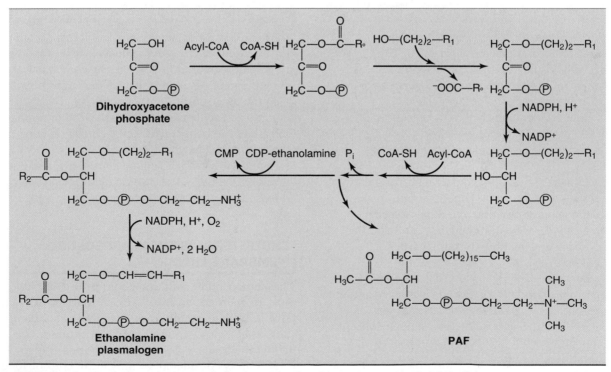

Figure 24.6 Synthesis of plasmalogens and platelet-activating factor (*PAF*). *CDP,* Cytidine diphosphate; *CMP,* cytidine monophosphate; *CoA-SH,* uncombined coenzyme A; P_i, inorganic phosphate.

CLINICAL EXAMPLE 24.1: ABO Incompatibility

Blood group substances are genetically polymorphic antigens on the surface of the erythrocyte membrane. People cannot form antibodies to their own blood group substances, but they can form antibodies against those of other people. This can result in dangerous transfusion reactions.

The antigens of the ABO blood group system are glycosphingolipids whose antigenic specificities are caused by variations in the terminal sugar of the oligosaccharide (*Fig. 24.7*). The glycosyl transferase that adds the last monosaccharide comes in three alleles. The A allele codes for an enzyme that adds *N*-acetylgalactosamine, the B allele codes for an enzyme that adds galactose, and the O allele has a nonsense mutation and produces no enzyme.

Only the A and B substances are effective antigens. Therefore the A and B alleles are genetically codominant, and the O allele is recessive. People have preformed antibodies against blood group substances that they do not have themselves, and a serious transfusion reaction results when the A or B substance is present in the donor but not the recipient of a blood transfusion. In this case the recipient's antibodies will agglutinate the donated blood cells.

The ABO oligosaccharide is found on some glycoproteins as well as on ceramide, and it is present on most cells in the human body. Therefore ABO matching is required for organ transplantation as well as for blood transfusions.

Figure 24.7 Synthesis of the ABO blood group substances. *N*-acetylgalactosamine (*GalNAc*) transferase (present in people with blood group A) and galactose (*Gal*) transferase (present in people with blood group B) are encoded by allelic variants of the same gene. A third variant of this gene does not produce an active enzyme. Homozygosity for this nonfunctional allele produces blood group O (only the H substance is present). *Cer*, Ceramide; *Fuc*, fucose.

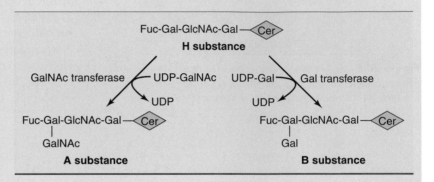

CLINICAL EXAMPLE 24.2: Tay-Sachs Disease

Tay-Sachs disease is caused by a complete deficiency of hexosaminidase A (reaction ② in *Fig. 24.8*), leading to an accumulation of ganglioside G_{M2}. Although affected children appear normal at birth, they develop mental and neurological deterioration along with hepatomegaly within the first year of life. The disease progresses relentlessly until death at or before age 3 years.

The old name "amaurotic idiocy" refers to the apparent blindness of these patients (from Greek αμαυροσ meaning "obscure"). Ophthalmoscopy reveals a cherry-red spot in the fovea centralis. This actually represents its normal color, which is accentuated by the gray appearance of the surrounding lipid-laden ganglion cells. However, this finding is not diagnostic for Tay-Sachs disease because it is seen in other lipid storage diseases as well. Tay-Sachs disease is very rare except among Ashkenazi Jews, among whom it occurs with a frequency of 1:3600 births.

CLINICAL EXAMPLE 24.3: Gaucher Disease

Gaucher disease occurs in different forms according to the extent of the enzyme deficiency. In the infantile form, glucocerebrosidase is missing completely and the clinical course resembles that of Tay-Sachs disease.

In the adult-onset form, patients have residual enzyme activity between 10% and 20% of normal. Therefore the patients are not mentally retarded but present in midlife with splenomegaly, thrombocytopenia, abdominal discomfort, and bone erosion. Like Tay-Sachs disease, adult-onset Gaucher disease is most prevalent among Ashkenazi Jews.

CHOLESTEROL IS THE LEAST SOLUBLE MEMBRANE LIPID

The human body contains about 140 g of cholesterol, most of it in the form of "free" (unesterified) cholesterol in cellular membranes. It is most abundant in tissues that also contain large amounts of other membrane lipids, especially the nervous system. Therefore brain is considered an unhealthy kind of food.

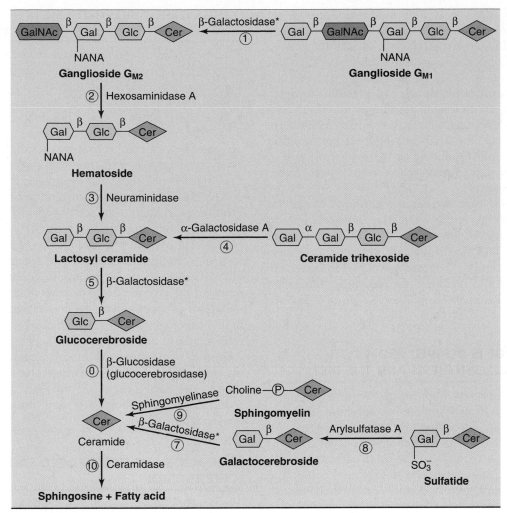

Figure 24.8 Lysosomal degradation of sphingolipids. The numbered reactions refer to the storage diseases listed in *Table 24.1*. There are two different β-galactosidases, one for ganglioside G$_{M1}$ (reaction 1) and the other for galactocerebroside (reaction ⑦). Lactosyl ceramide (*Cer*) is degraded by both (reaction ⑤). *Gal*, Galactose; *GalNAc*, N-acetylgalactosamine; *Glc*, glucose; *NANA*, N-acetylneuraminic acid.

Table 24.1 Examples of Lipid Storage Diseases

Disease	Enzyme Deficiency*	Incidence	Clinical Course
Generalized gangliosidosis	1	Unknown	Mental retardation, hepatomegaly, skeletal abnormalities
Tay-Sachs	2	1:3600 (Ashkenazi Jews)	Mental retardation, blindness, hepatosplenomegaly, death in infancy
Gaucher	6	Infantile: rare; adult: 1:600 (Ashkenazi Jews)	Infantile form: similar to Tay-Sachs; adult-onset form: without mental retardation
Fabry	4	1:40,000	Skin rash, renal failure, heart failure
Krabbe (globoid leukodystrophy)	7	1:50,000 (Sweden); lower elsewhere	Mental retardation, myelin nearly absent
Metachromatic leukodystrophy	8	1:100,000	Demyelination, mental deterioration; different degrees of severity
Niemann-Pick	9	Rare	Hepatosplenomegaly, mental retardation, early death
Farber	10	Rare	Hoarse voice, mental retardation, dermatitis, skeletal abnormalities, early death

*Numbers refer to numbered reactions in Figure 24.8.

Cholesterol is poorly soluble in water. Only 0.2 mg dissolves in 100 ml of water at 25°C. The concentration of unesterified cholesterol that circulates in the plasma in the form of lipoproteins is 300 times higher than this value.

Seventy percent of the cholesterol in plasma lipoproteins is esterified with long-chain fatty acids. These cholesterol esters are even less soluble than cholesterol itself. In addition, the lipid droplets that are found in the cells of steroid-producing endocrine glands and in some macrophages contain cholesterol esters rather than free cholesterol.

Only animals form significant amounts of cholesterol. Therefore *a vegan diet is essentially cholesterol free.* Plants contain **phytosterols** instead. Ergosterol (in fungi) and β-sitosterol (in higher plants) are examples of phytosterols. They are poorly absorbed from dietary sources and therefore are present in only small amounts in the human body. Bacteria do not produce steroids.

CHOLESTEROL IS DERIVED FROM BOTH ENDOGENOUS SYNTHESIS AND THE DIET

Cholesterol is derived both from the diet and from endogenous synthesis. Cholesterol synthesis amounts to 0.5 to 1 g/day, depending on the dietary supply. All nucleated cells can synthesize cholesterol, but the liver accounts for at least 50% of the total. Steroid-producing endocrine glands, including the adrenal cortex and the corpus luteum, have very high rates of cholesterol synthesis.

The dietary supply is variable, but most people in modern societies eat close to 1 g of cholesterol per day. In the presence of bile salts, approximately half of this is absorbed in the intestine.

In the intestinal mucosa, most of the absorbed cholesterol is converted to cholesterol esters by the microsomal enzyme **acyl-CoA–cholesterol acyltransferase** (**ACAT**). Together with triglycerides, some free cholesterol, and other dietary lipids, *the cholesterol esters are packaged into chylomicrons.*

Most of the triglyceride is removed by lipoprotein lipase in peripheral tissues, and the cholesterol-rich remnant particles thus formed are taken up by the liver. Therefore *most of the dietary triglyceride goes to extrahepatic tissues, but most of the cholesterol goes to the liver.*

The liver releases cholesterol as a constituent of very-low-density lipoprotein (VLDL), which becomes remodeled into low-density lipoprotein (LDL) in the blood. *LDL is the principal external source of cholesterol for most cells.* The transport of cholesterol from the extrahepatic tissues to the liver requires high-density lipoprotein (HDL) along with other lipoproteins. Details of lipoprotein function and metabolism are described in Chapter 25.

CHOLESTEROL BIOSYNTHESIS IS REGULATED AT THE LEVEL OF HMG-CoA REDUCTASE

All 27 carbons of cholesterol are derived from the acetyl group in acetyl-CoA. The enzymes of the biosynthetic pathway, which number close to 30, are in the cytosol and the ER. *Figure 24.9* shows the pathway in a very abbreviated form. The first reactions, up to 3-hydroxy-3-methylglutaryl-coenzyme A (HMG-CoA), are shared with the synthesis of ketone bodies. However, ketogenesis is mitochondrial, whereas the HMG-CoA synthase of cholesterol synthesis is cytoplasmic.

The NADPH-dependent formation of mevalonate by HMG-CoA reductase (reaction ② in *Fig. 24.9*) is the committed and regulated step of cholesterol synthesis. *HMG-CoA reductase is feedback inhibited by free cholesterol.* Cholesterol reduces the transcription of the HMG-CoA reductase gene, and it accelerates the breakdown of the enzyme protein. HMG-CoA reductase has a lifespan of approximately 4 hours; therefore, a change in its rate of synthesis or degradation can affect cholesterol synthesis rather rapidly.

Insulin stimulates HMG-CoA reductase, most likely by inhibiting the AMP-activated protein kinase. Like acetyl-CoA carboxylase (see Chapter 23), HMG-CoA reductase is phosphorylated and inactivated by this insulin-inhibited enzyme.

BILE ACIDS ARE SYNTHESIZED FROM CHOLESTEROL

The steroid ring system of cholesterol cannot be degraded in the human body. Cholesterol has to be disposed of by the biliary system, either as such or after conversion to bile acids.

Bladder bile contains approximately 400 mg/dl of nonesterified cholesterol. Because only approximately half of this is absorbed by the intestine, *nearly 500 mg of unmetabolized cholesterol can be eliminated from the body per day.* Intestinal bacteria metabolize cholesterol to various "neutral sterols."

Approximately half of the cholesterol eventually is metabolized to the **primary bile acids** in the liver. They include **cholic acid** and **chenodeoxycholic acid,** with cholic acid being the more abundant. The liver secretes the bile acids not in the free form but as conjugation products with glycine or taurine (*Fig. 24.10*). The ratio of glycine conjugates to taurine conjugates is about 3:1. Bile acids are not useless excretory products; they serve a vital function in lipid absorption (see Chapter 19).

BILE ACID SYNTHESIS IS FEEDBACK-INHIBITED

The committed step in bile acid synthesis is catalyzed by the microsomal enzyme **7α-hydroxylase** (*Fig. 24.11*). This monooxygenase reaction requires molecular oxygen, NADPH, and cytochrome P-450. Ascorbate

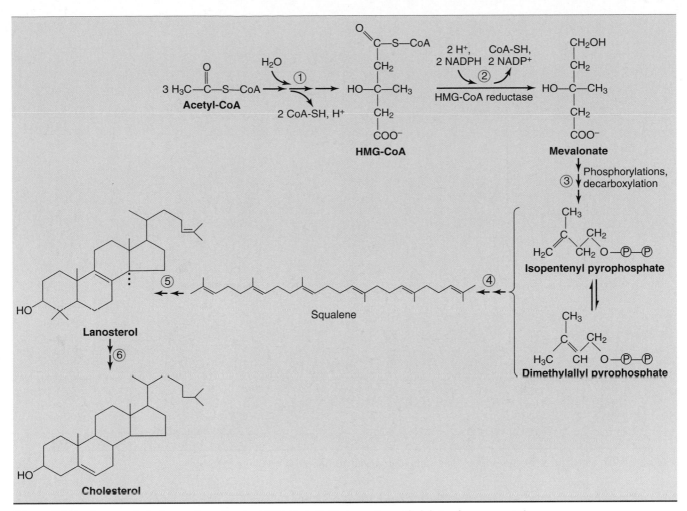

Figure 24.9 Stages of cholesterol synthesis. *HMG-CoA*, 3-Hydroxy-3-methylglutaryl coenzyme A.

also seems to be involved. Ascorbate deficiency (scurvy) impairs the formation of bile acids and causes cholesterol accumulation and atherosclerosis, at least in guinea pigs.

Bile acids reduce the level of 7α-hydroxylase by inhibiting transcription of its gene. Interestingly, bile acids also reduce the activity of HMG-CoA reductase. Cholesterol, in contrast, induces 7α-hydroxylase synthesis in addition to inhibiting HMG-CoA reductase. These regulatory effects ensure the maintenance of an adequate pool of free cholesterol in the liver.

Thyroid hormones induce the synthesis of 7α-hydroxylase. This effect contributes to the increased plasma cholesterol level in patients with hypothyroidism.

BILE ACIDS ARE SUBJECT TO EXTENSIVE ENTEROHEPATIC CIRCULATION

As the primary bile acids reach the lower parts of the small intestine, they are modified by bacterial enzymes. First, the glycine or taurine is cleaved off. This is followed by the reductive removal of the 7α-hydroxyl group. The **secondary bile acids** formed in these reactions are **deoxycholic acid** and **lithocholic acid** (*Fig. 24.12*).

Ninety-five percent of the bile acids is absorbed by a sodium cotransport mechanism in the ileum and returned to the liver. The liver conjugates these bile acids and secretes them again in the bile. Because of this *enterohepatic circulation* (*Fig. 24.13*), both primary and secondary bile acids are present in the bile.

The enterohepatic circulation ensures that enough bile acids are available for fat absorption. Only 0.5 g is synthesized per day, and between 3 and 5 g is present in liver, bile, and intestines at any time. Overall, however, 20 to 30 g of bile acids is secreted per day. Each bile acid molecule is recycled five to eight times every day, and it remains in the system for an average of 1 week before it finally is excreted.

Bile acids are synthesized and secreted round the clock by the liver, but their release into the intestine from the gallbladder is intermittent, being stimulated by the intestinal hormone cholecystokinin after a fatty meal. The gallbladder concentrates the bile in addition to storing it. Inorganic ions are actively removed across the gallbladder epithelium, followed by passive water

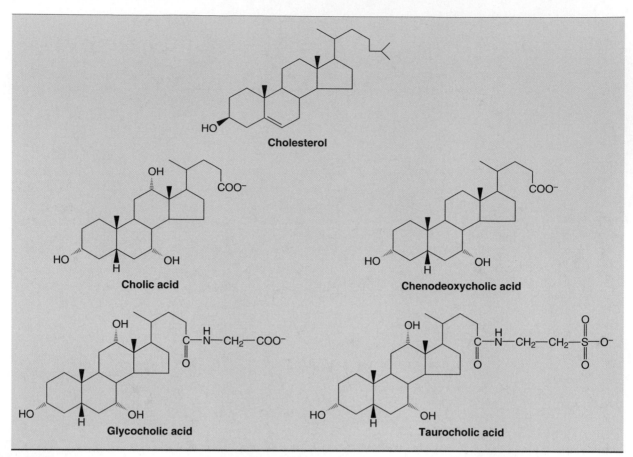

Figure 24.10 Structures of the primary bile salts (bile acids) compared with cholesterol.

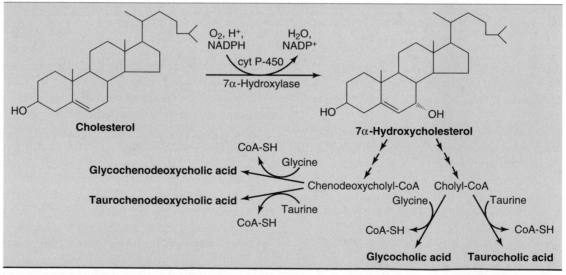

Figure 24.11 Synthesis of the primary bile acids by endoplasmic reticulum-associated enzymes in hepatocytes. *cyt*, Cytochrome.

flux. Therefore *all solids except inorganic ions are more concentrated in bladder bile than in hepatic bile.*

A very small portion of the bile acids that is absorbed from the ileum fails to return to the liver but escapes into the peripheral circulation. Plasma bile acid levels are elevated in patients with biliary obstruction because bile backs up, and the bile acids enter the blood from the liver. Plasma bile acid levels are also elevated in liver cirrhosis and portal hypertension when portal blood is shunted around the cirrhotic liver. Although otherwise not very toxic, the bile acids can cause a most distressing itching (pruritus) in these patients.

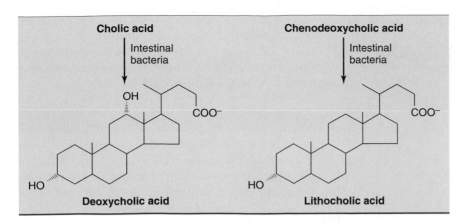

Figure 24.12 Synthesis of the secondary bile acids by intestinal bacteria.

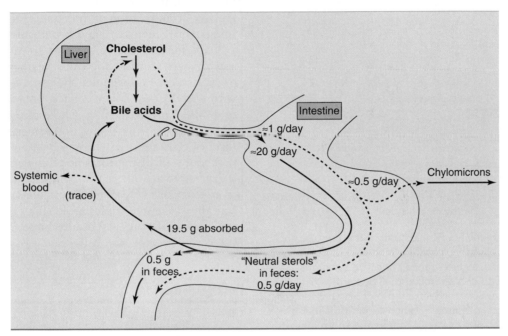

Figure 24.13 Disposition of bile acids and cholesterol in the enterohepatic system.

CLINICAL EXAMPLE 24.4: Treatment of Gallstone Disease

In theory, cholesterol-containing gallstones can be treated by reducing the cholesterol concentration of the bile or by raising the concentration of bile acids. Dietary changes that reduce the plasma cholesterol level tend to reduce biliary cholesterol as well, but the effect is small and few patients adhere to the recommended diets.

A more promising approach is the oral administration of large amounts of chenodeoxycholic acid or ursodeoxycholic acid. Through the enterohepatic circulation, these bile acids are incorporated into the bile and gradually dissolve the cholesterol stones. Although effective, this treatment is unpopular because it can cause diarrhea and because it raises the plasma cholesterol level by reducing the conversion of cholesterol to bile acids.

This leaves cholecystectomy as the preferred treatment. Postoperatively, lipid absorption is only mildly abnormal because bile acids still can reach the small intestine. Only the accurate timing of their release is no longer possible, and this limits the tolerance for fatty foods.

MOST GALLSTONES CONSIST OF CHOLESTEROL

The bile contains cholesterol, bile acids, phosphatidylcholine (lecithin), and the heme-derived bile pigments. *Cholesterol is the least soluble constituent of bile.* Although less abundant than some of the other components (*Table 24.2*), *cholesterol can be kept in solution only by being incorporated into mixed bile salt/phospholipid micelles.*

When the cholesterol level in the bile is too high or when the levels of the emulsifying lipids are too low,

Table 24.2 Approximate Composition of Hepatic Bile and Bladder Bile

Component	Hepatic Bile	Bladder Bile
Total solids	2.5%	10%
Inorganic salt	0.85%	0.85%
Bile acids	1.2%	6%
Cholesterol	0.06%	0.4%
Lecithin	0.04%	0.3%
Bile pigments	0.2%	1.5%
pH	7.4	5.0–6.0

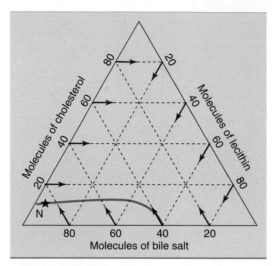

Figure 24.14 Solubility of cholesterol in the presence of bile acids and phosphatidylcholine ("lecithin"). If the relative composition of bile is above the *red line,* the system is supersaturated with cholesterol, and cholesterol is likely to precipitate. A total lipid concentration of 10% is assumed. Point *N* represents a "normal" composition of bladder bile, with 10 molecules of cholesterol for every 5 molecules of lecithin and 85 molecules of bile acid.

cholesterol precipitates and forms **gallstones.** The "solubility triangle" (**Fig. 24.14**) shows the solubility of cholesterol at different concentrations of bile salts and lecithin. *Most patients with gallstone disease have an elevated cholesterol level in their bile.*

Gallstones afflict about 20% of all people in Western countries at some point in their lives, occurring most commonly in fat, fertile females. The risk rises with increasing age. Some gallstones contain both cholesterol and bile pigments, but others are pure cholesterol. Only 10% of all gallstones consist mainly of substances other than cholesterol, usually bilirubin and other bile pigments.

Most gallstones form in the gallbladder and then are flushed into the common bile duct with the bile flow. Two thirds of patients with gallstones are asymptomatic. However, the stones can cause colic pain by inducing spasm of the smooth muscle in the wall of the common bile duct, and they can even obstruct the bile flow.

Unlike kidney stones, most gallstones are not calcified and therefore are not visible on plain x-ray films. The most important procedure for their diagnosis is ultrasonography. The treatment of gallstone disease is discussed in *Clinical Example 24.4.*

SUMMARY

The membrane phosphoglycerides are synthesized from CDP-activated precursors. They are remodeled and finally degraded with the help of several phospholipases.

Sphingolipids are synthesized in the ER and Golgi apparatus. Their degradation requires lysosomal endoglycosidases. Deficiencies of sphingolipid-degrading enzymes result in lysosomal storage diseases, with progressive accumulation of the nondegradable lipid, neurological degeneration, and hepatosplenomegaly.

Cholesterol is derived in part from dietary sources and in part from endogenous synthesis in liver and other tissues. Endogenous cholesterol synthesis starts with acetyl-CoA. It is feedback inhibited at the level of HMG-CoA reductase. Cholesterol is transported as a constituent of plasma lipoproteins, mainly in the form of cholesterol esters.

About half of the total body cholesterol eventually is converted to bile acids. The bile acids are subject to an extensive enterohepatic circulation. The bile also contains some free cholesterol. This biliary cholesterol can form gallstones, especially in people with an elevated cholesterol level in the bile.

Further Reading

Clarke JTR: Narrative review: Fabry disease, *Ann Intern Med* 146:425–433, 2007.

Desnick RJ: Prenatal diagnosis of Fabry disease, *Prenat Diagn* 27:693–694, 2007.

Dietschy JM: Central nervous system: cholesterol turnover, brain development and neurodegeneration, *Biol Chem* 390:287–293, 2009.

Gupta G, Surolia A: Glycosphingolipids in microdomain formation and their spatial organization, *FEBS Lett* 584:1634–1641, 2010.

Hosoi E: Biological and clinical aspects of ABO blood group system, *J Med Invest* 55:174–182, 2008.

Kosters A, Jirsa M, Groen AK: Genetic background of cholesterol gallstone disease, *Biochim Biophys Acta* 1637:1–19, 2003.

Linthorst GE, Bouwman MG, Wijburg FA, et al: Screening for Fabry disease in high-risk populations: a systematic review, *J Med Genet* 47:217–222, 2010.

Merrill AH: De novo sphingolipid biosynthesis: a necessary, but dangerous, pathway, *J Biol Chem* 277:25843–25846, 2002.

Murphy RC, Johnson KM: Cholesterol, reactive oxygen species, and the formation of biologically active mediators, *J Biol Chem* 283:15521–15525, 2008.

Raghow R, Yellaturu C, Deng X, et al: SREBPs: the crossroads of physiological and pathological lipid homeostasis, *Trends Endocrinol Metab* 19:65–73, 2008.

Russell DW: The enzymes, regulation, and genetics of bile acid synthesis, *Annu Rev Biochem* 72:137–174, 2003.

Sandhoff K, Kolter T: Biosynthesis and degradation of mammalian glycosphingolipids, *Phil Trans R Soc Lond B* 358:847–861, 2003.

Settembre C, Fraldi A, Jahreiss L, Spampanato C, et al: A block of autophagy in lysosomal storage disorders, *Hum Mol Genet* 17:119–129, 2008.

Spada M, Pagliardini S, Yasuda M, Tukel T, et al: High incidence of later-onset Fabry disease revealed by newborn screening, *Am J Hum Genet* 79:31–40, 2006.

Vance DE, Li Z, Jacobs RL: Hepatic phosphatidylethanolamine N-methyltransferase, unexpected roles in animal biochemistry and physiology, *J Biol Chem* 282: 33237–33241, 2007.

Vance JE, Vance DE: Phospholipid biosynthesis in mammalian cells, *Biochem Cell Biol* 82:113–128, 2004.

Wang D Q-H, Cohen DE, Carey MC: Biliary lipids and cholesterol gallstone disease, *J Lipid Res* 2009:S406–S411, 2009.

QUESTIONS

1. **The ABO blood group substances are oligosaccharides in plasma membrane glycolipids of erythrocytes and other cells. The biosynthetic enzymes that are encoded by the ABO gene can be characterized as**

   A. Glycosidases
   B. Glycosyltransferases
   C. Lipases
   D. Glycolipases
   E. Phospholipases

2. **Gallstones can easily form when the bile contains an increased amount of**

   A. Free (unesterified) fatty acids
   B. Bile salts
   C. Phospholipids
   D. Cholesterol
   E. Calcium

3. **An 8-month-old child of Jewish parents is examined for failure to thrive and abnormal neurological development. The child is found to have hepatosplenomegaly and a cherry-red spot on the macula of the eye. Chromatography of lipids from cultured leukocytes shows abnormally high levels of ganglioside G_{M2}. This child has**

   A. Refsum disease
   B. Tay-Sachs disease
   C. Gaucher disease
   D. Metachromatic leukodystrophy
   E. Hurler disease

Chapter 25
LIPID TRANSPORT

The plasma levels of the major lipids are not only higher than the normal blood glucose level of 100 mg/dl (*Table 25.1*), but they fluctuate over a wider range, depending on nutrition, lifestyle, and individual constitution. This is possible because none of the major tissues depends on lipids as its only energy source, although some tissues depend on glucose.

Unesterified ("free") fatty acids are transported in noncovalent binding to serum albumin, but triglycerides, phospholipids, and cholesterol esters form noncovalent aggregates with proteins called **lipoproteins**. The four pathways of lipid transport in the human body are as follows:

1. *Transport of fatty acids from adipose tissue to other tissues*

2. *Transport of dietary lipids from the intestine to other tissues*
3. *Transport of endogenously synthesized lipids from the liver to other tissues*
4. *Reverse transport of cholesterol from extrahepatic tissues to the liver.* This pathway is required because cholesterol cannot be degraded locally and must be transported to the liver for biliary excretion.

MOST PLASMA LIPIDS ARE COMPONENTS OF LIPOPROTEINS

The general structure of a lipoprotein (*Fig. 25.1*) can be predicted from the solubility properties of the lipids. *The hydrophobic triglycerides and cholesterol esters always avoid contact with water.* They form the core of the lipoprotein. *The amphipathic phospholipids prefer the water-lipid interface.* They form a monolayer that covers the surface of the particle. The protein components, or **apolipoproteins**, are also amphipathic and reside on the surface of the particle. Large lipoprotein particles with a high volume/surface ratio have a high content of nonpolar lipids, and small particles contain mainly polar lipids and protein.

The composition of lipoproteins keeps changing. Most lipids and apolipoproteins can be transferred from one lipoprotein particle to another, and lipids can be acquired from cells, processed by enzymes while in the lipoprotein,

Table 25.1 "Normal" Concentrations of Plasma Lipids in the Adult, Determined in the Postabsorptive State 8 to 12 Hours after the Last Meal

Lipid	Normal Range (mg/dl)
Total lipid	400–800
Triglycerides	40–280
Total cholesterol	120–280
LDL cholesterol	65–200
HDL cholesterol	30–90
Phospholipids	125–275
Free fatty acids	8–25

HDL, High-density lipoprotein; *LDL,* low-density lipoprotein.

Figure 25.1 General structure of a lipoprotein.

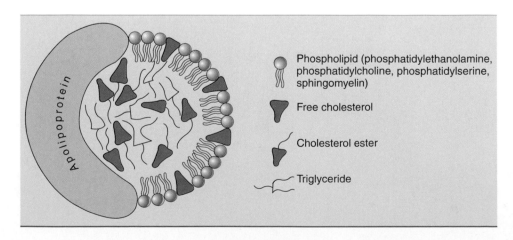

Phospholipid (phosphatidylethanolamine, phosphatidylcholine, phosphatidylserine, sphingomyelin)

Free cholesterol

Cholesterol ester

Triglyceride

and given off to cells. For their final destruction, many lipoproteins are taken up into cells by receptor-mediated endocytosis, followed by lysosomal hydrolysis of their constituents.

The plasma lipoproteins can be separated by **electrophoresis**, along with the other plasma proteins (see Chapter 15). In fasting serum or plasma, the two most prominent lipoprotein bands are in the α_1 and β fractions. They are designated as **α-** and **β-lipoproteins**. A weaker band, the **pre–β-lipoproteins**, moves slightly ahead of the β-lipoproteins. The **chylomicrons**, found only after a fatty meal, do not move upon electrophoresis.

Density gradient centrifugation separates the lipoproteins according to their protein/lipid ratio. Nonpolar lipids have densities near 0.9 g/cm^3. For lipoprotein particles, the densities increase from 0.95 g/cm^3 in the most lipid-rich particles to well above 1.0 g/cm^3 in the protein-rich types (*Table 25.2*). Based on their order of density and protein content, we can distinguish **chylomicrons**, very-low-density lipoprotein (**VLDL**), low-density lipoprotein (**LDL**), and high-density lipoprotein (**HDL**). The correspondence of these density classes to the electrophoretic separation pattern is shown in *Figure 25.2*.

LIPOPROTEINS HAVE CHARACTERISTIC LIPID AND PROTEIN COMPOSITIONS

Table 25.2 lists the approximate compositions of the lipoprotein classes. In the fasting state, *most of the plasma triglyceride is in VLDL, whereas 70% of the total cholesterol is in LDL*. Therefore, elevations of plasma triglycerides usually are caused by increased VLDL, and elevations of cholesterol usually are caused by increased LDL.

Each lipoprotein class has its own characteristic apolipoproteins (*Table 25.3*). Chylomicrons contain apoB-48; LDL and VLDL contain apoB-100; and HDL contains the A-apolipoproteins. However, with the exception of the B-apolipoproteins, most apolipoproteins can be exchanged among the lipoprotein classes. The apolipoproteins

- regulate lipid-metabolizing enzymes in the blood
- facilitate the transfer of lipids between lipoprotein classes and between lipoproteins and cells
- mediate the endocytosis of lipoproteins by binding to cell surface receptors

DIETARY LIPIDS ARE TRANSPORTED BY CHYLOMICRONS

Approximately 100 g of dietary triglycerides is transported daily from the small intestine to other tissues. As discussed in Chapter 23, they are transported as constituents of **chylomicrons**. *Chylomicrons are present only after a fatty meal*. The fate of chylomicrons is shown in *Figure 25.3*. They are formed with **apoB-48** and the A-apolipoproteins as their only apolipoproteins. ApoE and the C-apolipoproteins are acquired in the blood by transfer from HDL.

Lipoprotein lipase (**LPL**) removes 80% to 90% of the chylomicron triglycerides, most of this in muscle and adipose tissue. LPL is activated by **apoC-II** on the surface of the chylomicron and is inhibited by **apoC-III**. During triglyceride hydrolysis, some surface phospholipids and apolipoproteins peel off from the surface of the shrinking particle and are transferred to HDL. Phospholipid transfer requires a specialized **phospholipid transfer**

Table 25.2 Typical Compositions of Plasma Lipoproteins

Lipoprotein Class	Source	Diameter (nm)	Density (g/cm^3)	Protein (%)	Lipid (%)			
					Triglycerides	Phospholipid	Cholesterol Esters	Cholesterol
Chylomicrons	Intestine	100–1000	0.95	1–2	86	8	3	2
Very-low-density lipoprotein (VLDL)	Liver	30–80	0.95–1.006	6–10	55	18	13	7
Intermediate-density lipoprotein (IDL)	VLDL	25–30	1.006–1.019	15–20	25	21	28	9
Low-density lipoprotein (LDL)	VLDL, IDL	20–25	1.019–1.063	22	9	20	40	8
High-density lipoprotein	Liver, intestine							
HDL$_2$		9–12	1.063–1.125	35–45	5	33	17	5
HDL$_3$		5–9	1.125–1.21	50–55	3	28	12	3

Figure 25.2 Electrophoretic mobilities and density classes of plasma lipoproteins. Intermediate-density lipoprotein is included here in low-density lipoprotein (*LDL*). *HDL*, High-density lipoprotein; *VLDL*, very-low-density lipoprotein

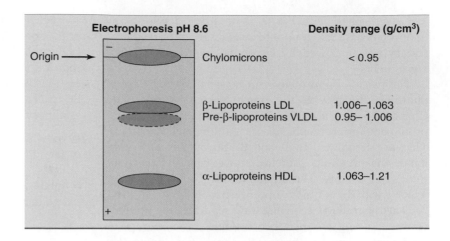

Electrophoresis pH 8.6		Density range (g/cm³)
Origin →	Chylomicrons	< 0.95
	β-Lipoproteins LDL	1.006–1.063
	Pre-β-lipoproteins VLDL	0.95– 1.006
	α-Lipoproteins HDL	1.063–1.21

Table 25.3   Characteristics of the Apolipoproteins

Apolipoprotein	Molecular Weight (D)	Plasma Concentration (mg/dl)	Lipoproteins	Source	Function
A-I	29,000	130	}HDL,	Liver,	Major structural proteins of HDL, also in
A-II	17,000	40	} chylomicrons	intestine	chylomicrons; apo A-I activates LCAT
B-48	241,000	Variable	Chylomicrons	Intestine	Structural protein of chylomicrons
B-100	513,000	80	VLDL, LDL	Liver	Structural protein of VLDL, IDL, LDL; only apoprotein of LDL; mediates tissue uptake of LDL
C-I	6,600	6	}Most		Readily transferred between lipoprotein
C-II	8,900	3	}lipoproteins	Liver	classes
C-III	8,800	12			C-II activates and C-III inhibits LPL
D	19,000	10	HDL		Unknown
E	34,000	5	VLDL, IDL, chylomicrons	Liver	Mediates uptake of chylomicron remnants and IDL by liver

HDL, High-density lipoprotein; *IDL*, intermediate-density lipoprotein; *LCAT*, lecithin-cholesterol acyl transferase; *LDL*, low-density lipoprotein; *LPL*, lipoprotein lipase; *VLDL*, very-low-density lipoprotein.

protein. Thus the large chylomicron, with a diameter of about 1 μm, is reduced to a far smaller **chylomicron remnant.**

The remnant particles bind to lipoprotein receptors in the liver with the help of **apoE,** followed by *receptor-mediated endocytosis into the hepatocytes.* In the cell, lipids and apolipoproteins are hydrolyzed by lysosomal enzymes.

The lifespan of a chylomicron, from its secretion by the intestinal cell to the uptake of the remnant by the liver, is less than 1 hour. Once in the bloodstream, the life expectancy of the chylomicron triglycerides is only 5 to 10 minutes.

VLDL IS A PRECURSOR OF LDL

The liver synthesizes 25 to 50 g of triglycerides and smaller amounts of other lipids per day. These lipids are released as **VLDL.** Like the chylomicrons, VLDL is synthesized in the endoplasmic reticulum (ER) and Golgi apparatus and is released by exocytosis

(*Fig. 25.4*). The liver sinusoids have a fenestrated endothelium that allows the passage of lipoproteins into the sinusoidal blood.

VLDL is released with **apoB-100,** small amounts of apoE and the C-apolipoproteins, and a modest amount of cholesterol esters. Like the chylomicrons, it acquires more C-apolipoproteins and apoE from HDL. Additional cholesterol esters are acquired from circulating HDL. This requires a **cholesterol ester transfer protein** (**CETP**).

The major apolipoprotein of VLDL, apoB-100, is a single polypeptide of 4536 amino acids. It is encoded by the same gene as apoB-48, the major apolipoprotein of chylomicrons. Indeed, apoB-48 consists of the first 2152 amino acids of apoB-100, counting from the N-terminus. In the intestine, a CAA codon that codes for glutamine in position 2153 is posttranscriptionally changed into the stop codon UAA. This is an example of *tissue-specific editing of an RNA transcript.*

Like the chylomicrons, *VLDL is metabolized by LPL,* although VLDL triglycerides are hydrolyzed a

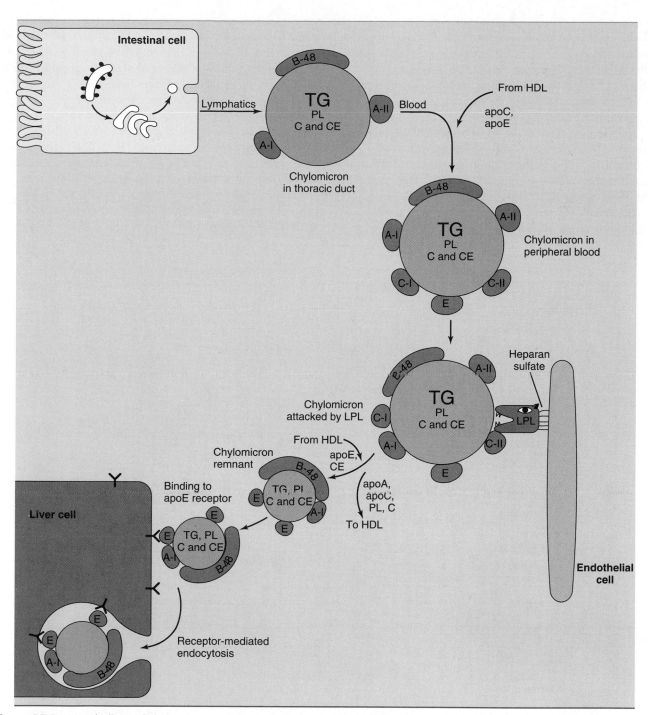

Figure 25.3 Metabolism of chylomicrons. *C,* Free cholesterol; *CE,* cholesterol ester; *HDL,* high-density lipoprotein; *LPL,* lipoprotein lipase; *PL,* phospholipid; *TG,* triglyceride.

bit more slowly than those in chylomicrons (see *Fig. 25.4*). Like chylomicrons, VLDL transfers C-apolipoproteins to HDL during triglyceride hydrolysis but retains most of its apoE.

About half of the VLDL remnants, especially larger specimens with multiple copies of apoE, are taken up by the liver. Smaller remnant particles appear initially as **intermediate-density lipoprotein (IDL)** and eventually are remodeled to **LDL**. This requires the hydrolysis of excess triglyceride and phospholipid by the **hepatic lipase (HL)** and the transfer of excess apolipoproteins to HDL (see *Fig. 25.4*).

HL is anchored to the surface of hepatocytes by heparan sulfate proteoglycans. Like LPL, it is released by heparin; however, unlike LPL, it is not activated by apoC-II and does not attack triglycerides in chylomicrons and VLDL. *HL hydrolyzes triglycerides and, to some extent, phosphoglycerides in IDL and HDL.* It also facilitates the uptake of remnant particles into hepatocytes.

CLINICAL EXAMPLE 25.1: ApoC-III Mutations and Plasma Lipids

Elevated levels of VLDL as well as LDL increase the risk of atherosclerosis. Therefore genetic traits and pharmacological manipulations that enhance the activity of LPL are expected to reduce the incidence and progression of atherosclerosis.

Ordinarily, apoC-II activates and apoC-III inhibits LPL. Among the Old Order Amish of Pennsylvania, approximately 5% of the population is heterozygous for a null mutation in the gene for apoC-III, which reduces the level of this apolipoprotein by 50%.

As a result, the fasting and postprandial plasma triglyceride levels are 45% lower in carriers than in noncarriers. In addition, the mutation raises HDL cholesterol and lowers LDL cholesterol by approximately 20% each. As expected, carriers have a reduced risk of atherosclerotic lesions in their coronary arteries.

Whereas the Amish mutation is rare, a common polymorphism has been observed in Ashkenazi Jews. In this population, homozygosity for an SNP variant 641 base pairs upstream of the transcriptional start site leads to reduced transcription of the *APOC3* gene and reduced levels of circulating apoC-III. Homozygosity for this promoter variant was found in 25% of centenarians but in only 10% of controls.

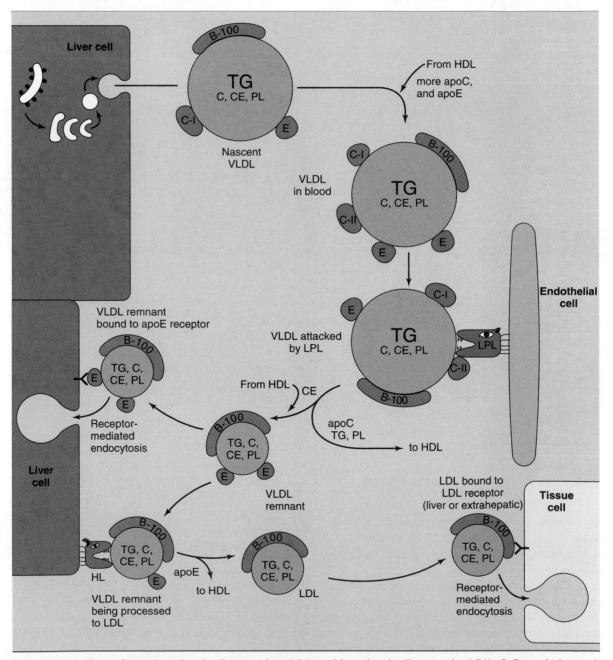

Figure 25.4 Metabolism of very-low-density lipoprotein (*VLDL*) and low-density lipoprotein (*LDL*). *C*, Free cholesterol; *CE*, cholesterol esters; *HDL*, high-density lipoprotein; *HL*, hepatic lipase; *LPL*, Lipoprotein lipase; *PL*, phospholipid; *TG*, triglyceride.

LDL IS REMOVED BY RECEPTOR-MEDIATED ENDOCYTOSIS

LDL has a well-defined structure. Its only apolipoprotein is a solitary apo B-100 molecule, and its lipid component includes a high proportion of cholesterol and cholesterol esters (see *Table 25.2*).

Unlike VLDL and chylomicrons, which are metabolized within minutes to hours, LDL circulates in the plasma for an average of 3 days. Eventually, *LDL is removed by receptor-mediated endocytosis*. This requires the binding of apoB-100 to the **LDL receptor** (apoB-100/apoE receptor). The endocytosed LDL is directed to the lysosomes, and its apolipoproteins, cholesterol esters, and other lipids are hydrolyzed by lysosomal enzymes.

Approximately two thirds of the LDL ends up in the liver. However, for the extrahepatic tissues, *LDL acquired through the LDL receptor is the major external source of cholesterol.*

Not all LDL is cleared by the LDL receptor. Macrophages and some endothelial cells possess alternative lipoprotein receptors, collectively known as **scavenger receptors**. They have a four to seven times higher Michaelis constant (K_m), or lower affinity, for LDL than does the regular LDL receptor. Therefore their contribution to LDL metabolism is greatest when the plasma LDL concentration is high.

LDL that has been chemically modified by acetylating or oxidizing agents or by exposure to the cross-linking agent malondialdehyde (formed during lipid peroxidation; see Chapter 23) has a higher affinity for scavenger receptors than does virgin LDL. Therefore one likely function of these receptors is the *removal of aberrant or aged lipoproteins* that are no longer good ligands for the other lipoprotein receptors. The scavenger receptors bind not only lipoproteins but also other particles with negative surface charges, including some bacteria. Therefore they can participate in the defense against infections.

More than 90% of LDL uptake is through the LDL receptor in liver, ovaries, adrenal glands, lungs, and kidneys. However, 44% of LDL uptake is independent of the LDL receptor in the intestine and 72% in the spleen. These organs contain many macrophages, which remove LDL with their scavenger receptors.

CHOLESTEROL REGULATES ITS OWN METABOLISM

The concentration of free cholesterol in the cellular membranes is tightly regulated. To this effect, free (unesterified) cholesterol regulates the synthesis of three important proteins (*Fig. 25.5*):

1. *It induces acyl-coenzyme A (CoA)–cholesterol acyl transferase (ACAT).* This enzyme converts excess cholesterol into highly insoluble cholesterol esters that are stored in the cell:

$$\text{Cholesterol} + \text{Acyl-CoA}$$
$$\downarrow$$
$$\text{Cholesterol ester} + \text{CoA-SH}$$

2. *It represses transcription of the gene for 3-hydroxy-3-methylglutaryl-coenzyme A (HMG-CoA) reductase.* HMG-CoA reductase is the rate-limiting enzyme of cholesterol biosynthesis.

3. *It represses transcription of the gene for the LDL receptor.* This reduces the uptake of LDL cholesterol from the blood.

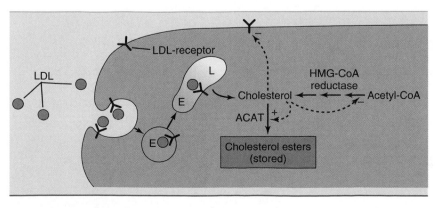

Figure 25.5 Regulation of cholesterol metabolism by low-density lipoprotein (*LDL*)-derived cholesterol in extrahepatic cells. *ACAT,* Acyl-coenzyme A–cholesterol acyl transferase; *E,* endosome; *HMG-CoA,* 3-hydroxy-3-methylglutaryl-coenzyme A; *L,* lysosome.

Cholesterol regulates gene expression through the **sterol response element binding protein (SREBP)**. In the presence of cholesterol, SREBP is located in the ER membrane. However, when cholesterol is depleted, SREBP is transferred to the Golgi apparatus, where it is cleaved by proteases. The proteases generate an active fragment that translocates into the nucleus, where it binds to the **sterol response element** in the promoters of genes. It induces the transcription of the genes for HMG-CoA reductase, the LDL receptor, and other proteins of cholesterol metabolism.

Unlike the LDL receptor, the scavenger receptors of macrophages are not down-regulated when cellular cholesterol is abundant. As a consequence, *macrophages accumulate cholesterol when the LDL level is high.*

CLINICAL EXAMPLE 25.3: Tangier Disease

Tangier disease is a near-complete absence of HDL, caused by *absence of the membrane protein ABCA1,* which transfers free cholesterol from cells to lipid-poor HDL. The A-apolipoproteins never acquire their lipid component, and no full-fledged HDL particles can be formed.

The LDL level is also reduced to about one third of normal, probably because cholesterol esters cannot be transferred from HDL to VLDL remnants, but VLDL is normal or mildly elevated.

Affected patients have deposits of cholesterol esters in macrophages, bone marrow, and Schwann cells. They develop peripheral neuropathy, hepatosplenomegaly, and lymphadenopathy. A telltale orange discoloration of the tonsils is caused by cholesterol esters that are colored by dietary carotene. Despite the HDL deficiency, patients have only a mild tendency for early atherosclerosis.

HDL IS NEEDED FOR REVERSE CHOLESTEROL TRANSPORT

ApoA-I, the major apolipoprotein of HDL, is released from the liver either without lipid or with a small amount of phospholipid (*Fig. 25.6*). Initially, it forms small particles that look like little shreds of phospholipid bilayer with apoA-I at the edge. These particles can acquire apoA-II, apoE, and the C-apolipoproteins from other lipoproteins.

Once in the circulation, *lipid-poor HDL attracts free, unesterified cholesterol both from other lipoproteins and from cells.* Through apoA-I or apoE, HDL particles can dock to cell surfaces. The cellular membrane protein ATP-binding cassette protein-A1 (**ABCA1**) then drains free cholesterol from the plasma membrane into HDL. This cell-derived cholesterol is processed in two steps:

1. **Lecithin-cholesterol acyltransferase (LCAT)** turns cholesterol into cholesterol esters:

Cholesterol + Phosphatidylcholine
↓
Cholesterol ester + 2-Lysophosphatidylcholine

This reaction takes place on the surface of the HDL particle. Lysophosphatidylcholine (lysolecithin) is transferred to albumin, and the hydrophobic cholesterol esters sink into the center of the HDL particle. The originally flat HDL bulges into a spherical particle with a hydrophobic core of cholesterol esters.

2. **Cholesterol ester transfer protein (CETP)** transfers cholesterol esters from HDL to other lipoproteins, either alone or in exchange for triglycerides. This happens especially during the processing of chylomicrons and VLDL by LPL. The remnant particles carry the cholesterol esters to the liver.

In the liver sinusoids, part of the triglycerides and phospholipids in HDL are hydrolyzed by **HL**. This converts larger HDL particles, known as HDL_2, to the smaller HDL_3. Whereas triglycerides and phospholipids are removed by HL, cholesterol esters are transferred selectively to the cells with the help of scavenger receptor class B type I (**SR-BI**).

There is a fundamental difference between cholesterol delivery to cells by LDL and HDL. *LDL is endocytosed in one piece, whereas HDL remains intact while giving off cholesterol esters to the cells.* Only a few of the larger HDL particles acquire multiple copies of apoE, leading to their endocytosis by hepatocytes. It now is apparent that cholesterol from the extrahepatic tissues can reach the liver by three routes:

- *Apo-E–mediated endocytosis of remnant particles,* which have obtained part of their cholesterol esters from HDL
- *Direct transfer of cholesterol esters from HDL during lipolysis by HL, mediated by SR-BI*
- *Endocytosis of large apoE-coated HDL particles in the liver.*

The roles of various apolipoproteins, lipoprotein receptors, and enzymes of lipoprotein metabolism are summarized in *Table 25.4.*

CLINICAL EXAMPLE 25.4: LCAT Deficiencies

In recessively inherited **familial LCAT deficiency**, lipoprotein cholesterol cannot be processed to cholesterol esters. HDL particles have abnormal shapes, and most of the lipoprotein cholesterol is in the form of free cholesterol rather than cholesterol esters. The accumulation of free cholesterol in the tissues results in corneal clouding, mild anemia, and proteinuria that tends to progress to renal failure. There is only a mild tendency for early atherosclerosis.

Partial LCAT deficiencies lead to **fish eye disease**, with corneal clouding but without progressive kidney disease.

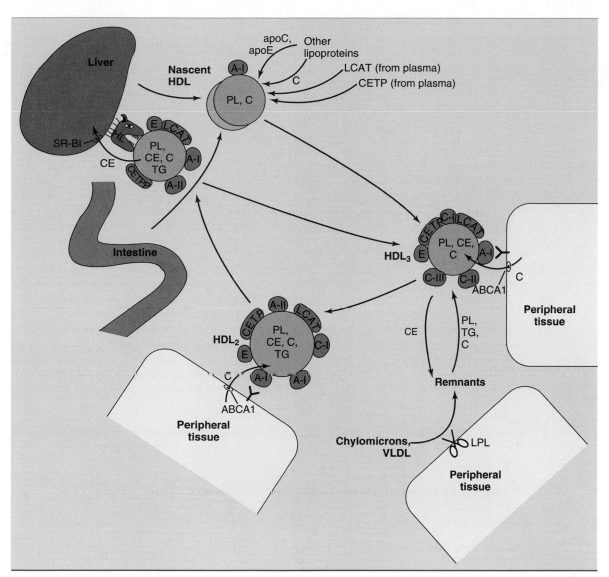

Figure 25.6   Metabolism of high-density lipoprotein (*HDL*). All HDL apolipoproteins can be exchanged with other lipoprotein classes. *ABCA1*, ATP-binding cassette protein-A1; *A-I*, apolipoprotein A-I; *A-II*, apolipoprotein A-II; *C*, cholesterol; *CE*, cholesterol esters; *CETP*, cholesterol ester transfer protein; *C-I*, apolipoprotein C-I; *C-II*, apolipoprotein C-II; *C-III*, apolipoprotein C-III; *E*, apolipoprotein E; *HL*, hepatic lipase; *LCAT*, lecithin-cholesterol acyltransferase; *LPL*, lipoprotein lipase; *PL*, phospholipid; *SR-BI*, scavenger receptor B-I; *TG*, triglyceride; *VLDL*, very-low-density lipoprotein.

CLINICAL EXAMPLE 25.5: CETP Deficiency

CETP deficiency is a benign condition in which the cholesterol esters formed by LCAT cannot be transferred from HDL to other lipoproteins. Affected homozygotes have a fourfold elevation of HDL cholesterol (100–250 mg/dl), but LDL cholesterol is normal or low (35–150 mg/dl). The HDL particles are oversized, with abundant cholesterol ester and very little triglyceride. Even heterozygotes have mildly elevated HDL cholesterol. Reverse cholesterol transport is possible even in homozygotes because cholesterol esters still can reach the liver by direct transfer from HDL through SR-BI and by endocytosis of apo-E–coated HDL particles.

One percent of Japanese persons are heterozygous for a CETP allele that causes a complete lack of cholesterol ester transfer in homozygotes, and 5% are heterozygous for an allele that causes moderately increased HDL cholesterol. These genetic traits have no major effect on the risk of coronary heart disease (CHD). Likewise, pharmacological inhibitors of CETP do not protect against coronary heart disease, although they raise the "good" HDL cholesterol.

LIPOPROTEINS CAN INITIATE ATHEROSCLEROSIS

Atherosclerosis is a disease of large arteries that can present as coronary heart disease (CHD) and acute myocardial infarction, gangrene, stroke, and even as senile dementia ("multi-infarct dementia"). The complications

Table 25.4 Important Determinants for Hyperlipidemia and Atherosclerosis

Risk Factor	Normal Function	Relation to Plasma Lipids and Atherosclerosis
Lipoprotein lipase (LPL)	Hydrolysis of triglycerides in chylomicrons and VLDL	Deficiency leads to hyperchylomicronemia but not atherosclerosis
ApoC-II	Stimulates LPL	Deficiency leads to hyperchylomicronemia
ApoC-III	Inhibits LPL	Partial deficiency lowers plasma triglyceride, raises HDL, lowers LDL
Hepatic lipase (HL)	Hydrolysis of triglycerides and phosphoglycerides in HDL and remnant particles; possibly facilitates hepatic uptake of chylomicron remnants and transfer of cholesterol esters from HDL to liver	Activity inversely related to plasma HDL concentration; lower in females than males; complete deficiency causes severe hypercholesterolemia, hypertriglyceridemia, possibly increased atherosclerosis
ApoB-100	Major structural apolipoprotein of VLDL, LDL; ligand of "LDL receptor"	High in patients with type II or IV hyperlipoproteinemia; high levels associated with high atherosclerosis risk
ApoA-I	Major apolipoprotein of HDL; mediates binding of HDL to cells, facilitates transfer of unesterified cholesterol from cells to HDL	High level of apoA-I (but not apoA-I *and* apoA-II) containing HDL is associated with decreased atherosclerosis risk; higher in females than males; low in patients with CHD and their relatives; high in octogenarians
ApoE	Cellular uptake of remnant particles; stimulation of cholesterol transfer from cells to HDL	Homozygosity for apoE-2 causes dysbetalipoproteinemia; knockout mice lacking apoE have impaired flux of cholesterol from cells to HDL and develop rampant atherosclerosis
LDL receptor (apoB-100/ apoE receptor)	Cellular uptake of LDL in liver, extrahepatic tissues	Deficiency leads to high LDL, atherosclerosis
Lecithin-cholesterol acyltransferase (LCAT)	Formation of cholesterol esters in HDL	Homozygous deficiency leads to moderately increased atherosclerosis risk
Cholesterol ester transfer protein (CETP)	Transfer of cholesterol esters from HDL to triglyceride-rich lipoproteins; activated in presence of LPL	Inversely related to plasma HDL level; induced by hypercholesterolemia
ABCA1	Transfer of free cholesterol from cells to HDL	Homozygous deficiency causes Tangier disease
SR-BI	Transport of cholesterol esters from HDL into cells	Unknown

CHD, Coronary heart disease; *HDL,* high-density lipoprotein; *LDL,* low-density lipoprotein; *VLDL,* very-low-density lipoprotein.

of atherosclerosis account for at least one third of all deaths in affluent societies.

The characteristic lesion of atherosclerosis is the **atheromatous plaque** in the intima of the artery. Typical plaques contain a core of cholesterol esters surrounded by an area of fibrosis, often with calcification. The plaque impairs blood flow by narrowing the lumen of the artery, and it can lead to hemorrhage into the plaque and thrombosis.

The accumulation of cholesterol esters in subendothelial macrophages, which take up lipoproteins through their scavenger receptors, is considered an early event in the development of atherosclerotic lesions. When lipid-laden macrophages, known as **foam cells,** die, the lipid becomes extracellular (*Fig. 25.7*). The resulting **fatty streaks** initially are reversible. They are seen even in children, and most regress spontaneously.

However, the insoluble extracellular lipid is hard to metabolize. It acts as a proinflammatory stimulus on surrounding cells, causing the release of cytokines and growth factors. Cytokines attract additional monocytes that become tissue macrophages, and growth factors cause the abnormal proliferation of fibroblasts and smooth muscle cells that deposit extracellular matrix. The inflammatory nature of the process is revealed by mild, chronic elevations of C-reactive protein (see Chapter 15) in patients with extensive atherosclerosis.

Lipids and cytokines induce the expression of cell adhesion molecules on the surface of endothelial cells that attract additional monocytes into the vessel wall. This is most likely to occur at places where the endothelium is otherwise stressed or damaged, for example, by hypertension or by rheological stress at arterial bifurcations. Platelets that become activated at sites of endothelial damage release platelet-derived growth factor, which attracts even more fibroblasts and smooth muscle cells.

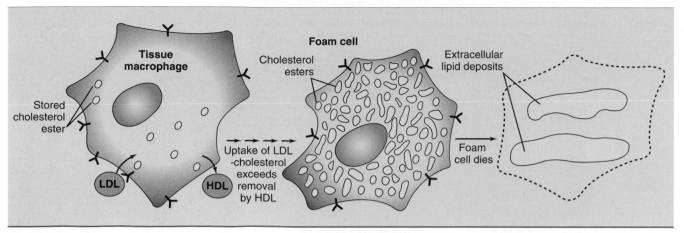

Figure 25.7 Hypothetical model for the formation of a fatty streak. The extracellular lipid deposits of the fatty streak are thought to induce a fibroproliferative response, leading eventually to the formation of an atheromatous plaque. Y indicates a scavenger receptor. *HDL*, High-density lipoprotein; *LDL*, low-density lipoprotein.

LIPOPROTEINS RESPOND TO DIET AND LIFESTYLE

The most important risk factors of atherosclerosis and coronary heart disease (CHD) are *advanced age, male gender, smoking, diabetes mellitus, hypertension,* and *hypercholesterolemia. Figure 25.9* shows the relationship between total plasma cholesterol level and incidence of death from CHD. Because two thirds of the plasma cholesterol is in LDL, the total cholesterol level reflects mainly the level of LDL cholesterol.

LDL cholesterol is the "bad cholesterol" that promotes atherosclerosis, in contrast to the "good cholesterol" in HDL. Presumably, LDL is bad because it brings cholesterol into the arterial wall, and HDL is good because it removes excess cholesterol. *A fatty streak develops when the amount of cholesterol supplied by LDL exceeds the amount of cholesterol removed by HDL* (see *Fig. 25.7*).

In the clinical laboratory, the total cholesterol and triglyceride levels are determined directly from fresh plasma or serum. HDL cholesterol is determined after selective precipitation of LDL and VLDL by phosphotungstate or some other polyanion. LDL cholesterol (in mg/dl) is estimated with the formula

$$\text{LDL cholesterol} = \text{Total cholesterol} - (\text{HDL cholesterol} + 0.16 \times \text{Triglycerides})$$

The reagents used for routine cholesterol determination contain a cholesterol esterase. Therefore the measured "cholesterol" includes both free and esterified cholesterol.

CLINICAL EXAMPLE 25.6: Familial Hypercholesterolemia

Familial hypercholesterolemia (FH) is caused by *deficiency of LDL receptors in liver and extrahepatic tissues*. The number of functional LDL receptors is reduced to 50% of normal in heterozygotes, which is sufficient to double the level of circulating LDL cholesterol to between 200 and 350 mg/dl. The cells, unable to obtain sufficient cholesterol from LDL, respond by increasing the rate of endogenous synthesis (see *Fig. 25.5*).

Tendon xanthomas develop after age 20 years. Xanthomas are visible subcutaneous lipid deposits that occur not only in FH but in many other hyperlipidemic states as well. They are important for the differential diagnosis of lipoprotein disorders.

CHD develops early in life. In a study in England, 5% of male FH heterozygotes suffered their first myocardial infarction by age 30 years, 51% by age 50 years, and 85% by age 60 years. *Five percent of all myocardial infarctions before age 60 years occur in patients with FH.* The diagnosis is based on the presence of plasma total cholesterol levels greater than 260 mg/dl, tendon xanthomas, and a positive family history for CHD.

Heterozygous FH has an incidence at birth of 1:500. The rare homozygous state leads to plasma cholesterol levels of 600 to 1200 mg/dl and rampant atherosclerosis before age 20 years (*Fig. 25.8*).

The LDL receptor mutations in FH include complete and partial gene deletions, receptors that are not translocated from the ER to the plasma membrane, receptors that cannot bind LDL, and receptors that fail to trigger endocytosis after binding LDL. These mutations are common because in the heterozygous state, there is not much selection against them. They kill their victims only after the reproductive age, when the mutation has already been transmitted to the offspring.

Continued

CLINICAL EXAMPLE 25.6: Familial Hypercholesterolemia—cont'd

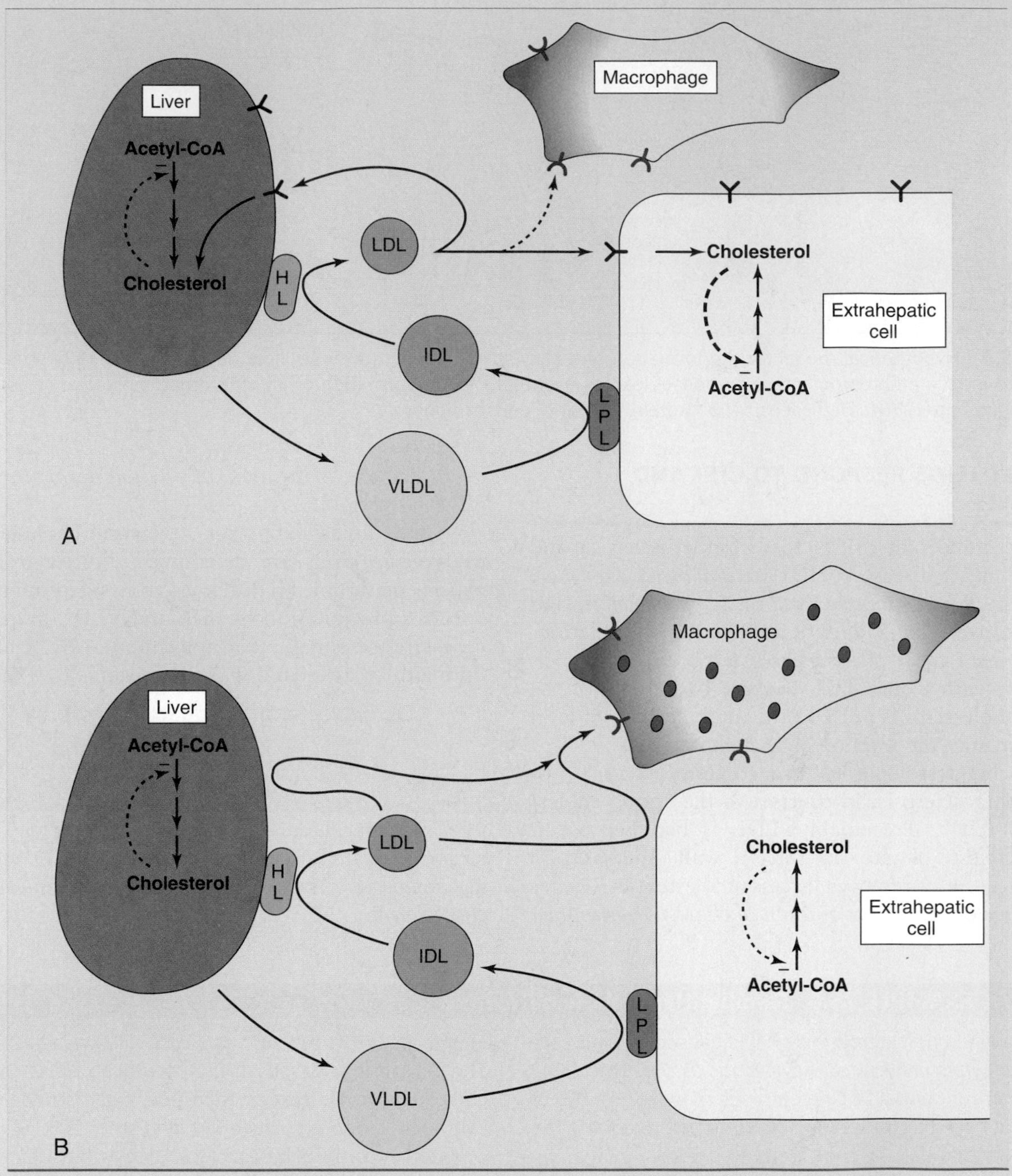

Figure 25.8 Metabolism of low-density lipoprotein (*LDL*) in normal individuals and in patients with homozygous familial hypercholesterolemia. **A,** Normal. Both liver and extrahepatic tissues obtain most of their cholesterol from receptor-mediated LDL uptake. LDL-derived cholesterol inhibits endogenous synthesis at the level of 3-hydroxy-3-methylglutaryl-coenzyme A (*HMG-CoA*) reductase. Y, LDL receptor; Y, scavenger receptor. *HL,* Hepatic lipase; *IDL,* intermediate-density lipoprotein; *LPL,* lipoprotein lipase; *VLDL,* very-low-density lipoprotein. **B,** Familial hypercholesterolemia, homozygous. LDL is redirected from parenchymal cells in liver and extrahepatic tissues to tissue macrophages, which become foam cells. These foam cells contribute to the formation of xanthomas, fatty streaks, and atherosclerotic lesions.

In addition to LDL cholesterol, elevated VLDL triglycerides are an independent risk factor for atherosclerosis.

Some environmental effects on LDL and HDL cholesterol are summarized in *Table 25.5*. Dietary cholesterol raises the lipoprotein cholesterol only mildly because it suppresses endogenous cholesterol synthesis. The type of fat consumed is more important. Monounsaturated and polyunsaturated fatty acids, and especially the long-chain ω3 fatty acids in fish oil, are recommended. Most saturated fatty acids raise LDL cholesterol except stearic acid, which is converted to

CLINICAL EXAMPLE 25.7: Lipoprotein(a)

Lipoprotein(a) [Lp(a)] is a variant of LDL that contains a molecule of the glycoprotein **apolipoprotein(a) [apo(a)]** disulfide-bonded to apoB-100. Apo(a) occurs in different sizes in different individuals who are determined by copy number variations of two adjacent exons in the apo(a)-encoding *LPA* gene. This structural variation affects the plasma level of apo(a). Generally, shorter forms of apo(a) are present in higher concentrations. The plasma level of Lp(a) can range from less than 5 to more than 100 mg/dl.

Elevated Lp(a) concentrations are an independent risk factor for atherosclerosis. The mechanism of the atherogenic effect is uncertain. It has been attributed either to effects on lipoprotein metabolism or to a prothrombotic effect of apo(a). Unlike ordinary LDL, Lp(a) does not seem to respond to dietary manipulations.

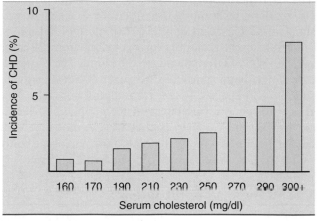

Figure 25.9 Relationship between the plasma cholesterol level and death from coronary heart disease (CHD).

monounsaturated oleic acid in the body. Fatty acids appear to influence lipoproteins by regulating gene expression.

Thyroid hormones lower LDL cholesterol by inducing the synthesis of LDL receptors and 7α-hydroxylase in the liver. Otherwise, little is known about the mechanisms by which hormones, lifestyle factors, and dietary manipulations affect lipoprotein levels. Evidence indicates that many interventions that reduce LDL or raise HDL actually reduce the risk of CHD.

Other risk factors are less easily manipulated. Premenopausal women have less CHD than do men, possibly because their HDL level is 20% higher. Mother Nature is not politically correct. She discriminates against males, and even more against senior citizens.

Table 25.5 Effects of Various Manipulations on Plasma Lipid Levels and the Risk of CHD

Manipulation	LDL Cholesterol	HDL Cholesterol	VLDL Triglycerides	Risk of CHD	Other Effects
Weight gain	(↑)	↓	↑	↑	High CETP
Weight reduction	(↓)	↑	↓	↓	
Stearic acid (C18)	↔	↑	↔	↔	
C12-C16 saturated fat	↑↑	↑↑	(↑)	↑	
Monounsaturated fat	↔	↑	(↓)	↓	↓ Lipid peroxidation (?), improved insulin sensitivity
Polyunsaturated fat	↓	↔	(↓)	↓	↑ Lipid peroxidation (?)
Carbohydrate	↔	↓	↑	↔	
Fish oil	(↑)	↔	↓↓	↓↓	↑ Lipid peroxidation (?), antithrombotic effect
Dietary cholesterol	↑	(↑)	↔	↑	
Regular alcohol consumption	(↑)	↑	↑	(↓)	Can cause alcoholic cardiomyopathy
Cigarette smoking	↔	↓	↔	↑	Causes oxidative damage of lipoproteins
Regular exercise	↔	↑	↔	↓	High lipoprotein lipase, low hepatic lipase
Diabetes mellitus	(↑)	(↓)	↑↑	↑	
Hypothyroidism	↑	↔	↔	↑	
Estrogen-rich birth control pills	(↑)	↑	↑	(↓)	
Progesterone-rich birth control pills	(↑)	↓	↑	(↑)	
Antioxidant vitamins (C and E)	↔	↔	↔	(↓)	Prevent oxidative damage of lipoproteins

↑, Increase; ↓, decrease; ↔, no change. Weak and/or inconsistent effects are in parentheses.
CETP, Cholesterol ester transfer protein; *CHD*, coronary heart disease; *HDL*, high-density lipoprotein; *LDL*, low-density lipoprotein; *VLDL*, very-low-density lipoprotein.

HYPERLIPOPROTEINEMIAS ARE GROUPED INTO FIVE PHENOTYPES

The hyperlipidemias are said to have a combined prevalence of 5% to 20% in affluent societies, but the cutoff between normal and abnormal is more than a bit arbitrary. Five types are distinguished, depending on the lipoprotein class that is affected (*Table 25.6*). They are not diseases but phenotypes that occur in a variety of contexts. In rare instances, as in familial hypercholesterolemia (FH), the condition can be blamed on a single faulty gene. More commonly, it is related to a chronic disease, diet and lifestyle, and/or multifactorial genetic predisposition.

Type I Hyperlipoproteinemia

Type I hyperlipoproteinemia, or **hyperchylomicronemia,** is a rare condition (prevalence, 1:10,000) caused by impaired hydrolysis of chylomicron triglycerides. It is caused by inherited deficiencies of lipoprotein lipase (LPL) or its activator, apoC-II. The plasma triglyceride level can reach 1000 mg/dl, but LDL is reduced to 20% of normal or less, and most cholesterol is present in VLDL rather than LDL. This shows the importance of VLDL lipolysis for the formation of LDL. Patients have eruptive cutaneous xanthomas, abdominal pain after fatty meals, and recurrent attacks of pancreatitis, but no excessive atherosclerosis. Treatment consists of a low-fat diet.

Type II Hyperlipoproteinemia

Type II hyperlipoproteinemia, or **hypercholesterolemia,** is an elevation of LDL. FH is included as **type IIa,** but multifactorial and secondary forms (**type IIb**) are at least 10 times more common. In some type IIb patients, VLDL and LDL are elevated. Weight gain and obesity, diabetes mellitus, and a diet high in cholesterol and saturated fat are the main culprits, but genetic factors other than a deficiency of LDL receptors are also involved. *This pattern is a major risk factor for atherosclerosis and coronary heart disease (CHD).*

Type III Hyperlipoproteinemia

Type III hyperlipoproteinemia, or **dysbetalipoproteinemia,** is caused by homozygosity for apoE-2, a genetic variant of apoE that does not bind to hepatic apoE receptors. This results in the accumulation of chylomicron remnants and IDL-like VLDL remnants in the blood. The phagocytosis of remnant particles by macrophages leads to xanthomas on palms, knees, elbows, and buttocks. Atherosclerosis shows a predilection for peripheral arteries, but the CHD risk is increased as well. Although 1% of the population has the offending apoE genotype, only 2% to 10% of these persons become hyperlipidemic.

Type IV Hyperlipoproteinemia

Type IV hyperlipoproteinemia, or **hypertriglyceridemia,** is defined by elevated VLDL. Triglyceride is elevated to a greater extent than is cholesterol, and *the atherosclerosis risk is increased.* This is a common type that is related to obesity, type II diabetes mellitus, alcoholism, progesterone-rich contraceptives, and excess dietary carbohydrate (especially sugar).

Table 25.6 Five Hyperlipoproteinemia Phenotypes

Type	Name	Plasma Lipids		Fraction Elevated	Incidence	Causes
		Triglyceride	**Cholesterol**			
I	Hyperchylomicronemia	↑↑↑	(↑)	Chylomicrons	Rare	Inherited deficiency of LPL or apoC-II, systemic lupus erythematosus, unknown
II	Hypercholesterolemia	(↑)	↑↑	LDL	Common	Primary: familial hypercholesterolemia Secondary: obesity, poor dietary habits, hypothyroidism, diabetes mellitus, nephrotic syndrome
III	Dysbetalipoproteinemia	↑	↑	Chylomicron remnants, VLDL remnants	Rare	Homozygosity for apoE-2 (does not bind to hepatic apoE receptors), combined with poor dietary habits
IV	Hypertriglyceridemia	↑↑	↑	VLDL	Common	Diabetes mellitus, obesity, alcoholism, poor dietary habits
V	—	↑↑	↑	Chylomicrons, VLDL	Rare	Obesity, diabetes mellitus, alcoholism, oral contraceptives

Elevations of lipid levels range from minimal (↑) to massive ↑↑↑.
LDL, Low-density lipoprotein; *LPL,* lipoprotein lipase; *VLDL,* very-low-density lipoprotein.

Table 25.7 Most Commonly Used Antihyperlipidemic Drugs

Drug Type	Mechanism of Action	Uses	Lipoprotein Effects
Statins (e.g., lovastatin)	Inhibition of HMG-CoA reductase	First-line treatment of hypercholesterolemia	↓↓ LDL
Bile acid binding resins (e.g., cholestyramine)	Interruption of enterohepatic circulation of bile acids	Hypercholesterolemia	↓ LDL
Niacin	Reduces lipolysis in adipose tissue and VLDL formation in the liver	Type II and IV hyperlipoproteinemia, but many side effects	↓ VLDL ↓ LDL ↑ HDL
Fibrates (e.g., clofibrate, gemfibrozil)	PPAR-α agonists increase LPL, apoA-I, and apoA-II, and decrease apoC-III	Hypertriglyceridemia	↓↓ VLDL ↑ HDL

HDL, High-density lipoprotein; *HMG-CoA*, 3-hydroxy-3-methylglutaryl-coenzyme A; *LDL*, low-density lipoprotein; *LPL*, lipoprotein lipase; *PPAR*, peroxisome proliferator-activated receptor; *VLDL*, very-low-density lipoprotein.

Type V Hyperlipoproteinemia

Type V **hyperlipoproteinemia** consists of combined elevations of chylomicrons and VLDL. In addition to genetic factors that impair lipolysis by LPL, it is associated with uncontrolled diabetes mellitus, alcoholism, obesity, and kidney disease.

HYPERLIPIDEMIAS ARE TREATED WITH DIET AND DRUGS

Most hyperlipoproteinemias respond to dietary management. Hypertriglyceridemias tend to be more responsive than hypercholesterolemias. The recommendation for hypertriglyceridemic patients is *reduction of caloric intake, alcohol, and simple carbohydrates, and consumption of fish oil.* For hypercholesterolemia, the recommendation is *less cholesterol and saturated fat, and more unsaturated fat and dietary fiber.* In many obese patients, a balanced weight-reduction diet normalizes the lipoproteins without the need for further treatment.

Dietary treatment is of little practical use because of poor patient compliance; pill popping is far easier. Therefore hyperlipidemias usually are treated with drugs. Two important drug classes reduce the plasma cholesterol level by interfering with critical steps in cholesterol metabolism:

1. **Statins** are inhibitors of HMG-CoA reductase. Endogenous cholesterol synthesis is blocked, and the reduced level of free cholesterol in the cells induces the synthesis of LDL receptors (***Fig. 25.10, C***; see also ***Fig. 25.5***). By this mechanism, *statins reduce LDL cholesterol but not HDL cholesterol.*
2. **Cholestyramine** is an insoluble, nonabsorbable anion exchanger that binds bile acids in the lumen of the small intestine, preventing their absorption from the ileum. The bile acids are excreted in the stools, rather than returning to the liver. Therefore there is less feedback inhibition of 7α-hydroxylase in the

liver, and *more cholesterol is converted to bile acids.* This depletes the cellular cholesterol pool, which in turn leads to *up-regulation of hepatic LDL receptors* and reduction of LDL (but not HDL) in the plasma (see *Fig. 25.10, B*). A high-fiber diet lowers LDL cholesterol by the same mechanism as cholestyramine: by impairing the absorption of bile acids from the ileum.

Some other lipid-lowering drugs are listed in ***Table 25.7***. **Antioxidant vitamins** slow down the oxidation of LDL. Because oxidized LDL is a preferred substrate for macrophage scavenger receptors, they reduce cholesterol accumulation in macrophages without lowering the plasma LDL level.

SUMMARY

The three highways of lipoprotein-based lipid transport are as follows:

1. Lipids of dietary origin are transported from the intestine to other tissues as constituents of chylomicrons. Lipolysis by extrahepatic lipoprotein lipase (LPL) produces remnant particles that undergo endocytosis by hepatocytes through apoE receptors.
2. Lipids from endogenous synthesis in the liver are carried by VLDL. After hydrolysis of the VLDL triglycerides by LPL, some of the remnant particles are processed to cholesterol-rich LDL. LDL undergoes endocytosis in liver and extrahepatic tissues.
3. HDL plays a key role in the reverse transport of cholesterol from peripheral tissues to the liver.

The deposition of cholesterol esters in the arterial wall can initiate atherosclerosis. A high level of LDL favors lipid deposition and atherosclerosis, and a high level of HDL is protective. Genes, diet, and lifestyle all are important in determining plasma lipoprotein levels and the development of vascular disease.

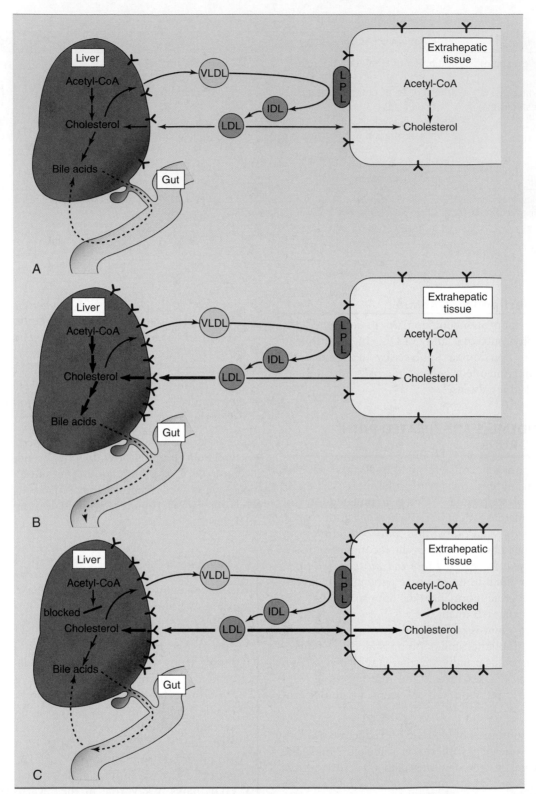

Figure 25.10 Effects of a bile acid binding resin (cholestyramine) and a 3-hydroxy-3-methylglutaryl-coenzyme A (HMG-CoA) reductase inhibitor (lovastatin) on cholesterol metabolism. **A,** Normal or hyperlipidemic. **Y,** Low-density lipoprotein (LDL) receptor. *IDL,* intermediate-density lipoprotein; *LPL,* extrahepatic lipoprotein lipase; *VLDL,* very-low-density lipoprotein. **B,** Effect of cholestyramine. Hepatic LDL receptors are up-regulated. The liver removes an increased amount of LDL to obtain cholesterol for bile acid synthesis. **C,** Effect of lovastatin. LDL receptors are up-regulated in all tissues. The cells require an increased amount of LDL cholesterol because they are unable to obtain cholesterol from endogenous synthesis.

Further Reading

Atzmon G, Rincon M, Schechter CB, et al: Lipoprotein genotype and conserved pathway for exceptional longevity in humans, *PLoS Biol* 4(4):e113, 2006.

Aulchenko YS, Ripatti S, Lindqvist I, Boomsma D, et al: Loci influencing lipid levels and coronary heart disease risk in 16 European population cohorts, *Nat Genet* 41:47–55, 2009.

Baldán A, Bojanic DD, Edwards PA: The ABCs of sterol transport, *J Lipid Res* 2009:S80–S85, 2009.

Brouwer IA, Wanders AJ, Katan MB: Effect of animal and industrial trans fatty acids on HDL and LDL cholesterol levels in humans—a quantitative review, *PLoS ONE* 5 (3):e9434, 2010.

Brown MS, Goldstein JL: Cholesterol feedback: from Schoenheimer's bottle to Scap's MELADL, *J Lipid Res* 50(Suppl): S15–S27, 2009.

Chasman DI, Paré G, Mora S, Hopewell JC, et al: Forty-three loci associated with plasma lipoprotein size, concentration, and cholesterol content in genome-wide analysis, *PLoS Genet* 5(11):e1000730, 2009.

Feng H, Li X-A: Dysfunctional high-density lipoprotein, *Curr Opin Endocrinol Diabetes Obes* 16:156–162, 2009.

Fernandez ML, Webb D: The LDL to HDL cholesterol ratio as a valuable tool to evaluate coronary heart disease risk, *J Am Coll Nutr* 27:1–5, 2008.

Galli C, Risé P: Fish consumption, omega 3 fatty acids and cardiovascular disease: the science and the clinical trials, *Nutr Health* 20:11–20, 2009.

Goldberg RB, Sabharwal AK: Fish oil in the treatment of dyslipidemia, *Curr Opin Endocrinol Diabetes Obes* 15:167–174, 2008.

Greaves DR, Gordon S: The macrophage scavenger receptor at 30 years of age: current knowledge and future challenges, *J Lipid Res* 50(Suppl):S282–S286, 2009.

Griel AE, Kris-Etherton PM: Beyond saturated fat: the importance of the dietary fatty acid profile on cardiovascular disease, *Nutr Rev* 64:257–262, 2006.

Hegele RA: Plasma lipoproteins: genetic influences and clinical implications, *Nat Rev Genet* 10:109–121, 2009.

Jenkins DJA, Josse AR, Dorian P, et al: Heterogeneity in randomized controlled trials of long chain (fish) omega-3 fatty acids in restenosis, secondary prevention and ventricular arrhythmias, *J Am Coll Nutr* 27:367–378, 2008.

Kamstrup PR, Benn M, Tybjærg-Hansen A, et al: Extreme lipoprotein(a) levels and risk of myocardial infarction in the general population, *Circulation* 117:176–184, 2008.

Karmally W: Balancing unsaturated fatty acids: what's the evidence for cholesterol lowering? *J Am Dietetic Assoc* 105:1068–1070, 2005.

Kathiresan S, Willer CJ, Peloso GM, Demissie S, et al: Common variants in 30 loci contribute to polygenic dyslipidemia, *Nat Genet* 41:56–65, 2009.

Lecerf J-M: Fatty acids and cardiovascular disease, *Nutr Rev* 67:273–283, 2009.

Linsel-Nitschke p, Götz A, Erdmann J, Braenne I, et al: Life-long reduction of LDL-cholesterol related to a common variant in the LDL-receptor gene decreases the risk of coronary artery disease—a Mendelian randomization study, *PLoS ONE* 3(8)e2986.

Majeed F, Miller M: Low high-density lipoprotein cholesterol: an important consideration in coronary heart disease risk assessment, *Curr Opin Endocrinol Diabetes Obes* 15:175–181, 2008.

Masson D, Jiang X-C, Lagrost L, et al: The role of plasma lipid transfer proteins in lipoprotein metabolism and atherogenesis, *J Lipid Res* 50(Suppl):S201–S206, 2009.

Mohlke KL, Boehnke M, Abecasis GR: Metabolic and cardiovascular traits: an abundance of recently identified common genetic variants, *Hum Mol Genet* 17:R102–R108, 2008.

Mozaffarian D, Micha R, Wallace S: Effects on coronary heart disease of increasing polyunsaturated fat in place of saturated fat: a systematic review and meta-analysis of randomized controlled trials, *PLoS Med* 7(3):e1000252, 2010.

Nicholls SJ, Wilson Tang WH, Scoffone H, et al: Lipoprotein (a) levels and long-term cardiovascular risk in the contemporary era of statin therapy, *J Lipid Res* 51(10): 3055–3061, 2010.

Ooi EMM, Barrett PHR, Chan DC, et al: Apolipoprotein C-III: understanding an emerging cardiovascular risk factor, *Clin Sci* 114:611–624, 2008.

Pollin TI, Damcott CM, Shen H, Ott SH, et al: A null mutation in human *APOC3* confers a favorable plasma lipid profile and apparent cardioprotection, *Science* 322: 1702–1705, 2008.

Rader DJ, Alexander ET, Weibel GL, et al: The role of reverse cholesterol transport in animals and humans and relationship to atherosclerosis, *J Lipid Res* 50(Suppl):S189–S194, 2009.

Remig V, Franklin B, Margolis S, et al: *Trans* fats in America: a review of their use, consumption, health implications, and regulation, *J Am Diet Assoc* 110:585–592, 2010.

Riediger ND, Othman RA, Suh M, et al: A systemic review of the roles of n-3 fatty acids in health and disease, *J Am Diet Assoc* 109:668–679, 2009.

Rousset X, Vaisman B, Amar M, et al: Lecithin: cholesterol acyltransferase – from biochemistry to role in cardiovascular disease, *Curr Opin Endocrinol Diabetes Obes* 16:163–171, 2009.

Rye K-A, Bursill CA, Lambert G, et al: The metabolism and anti-atherogenic properties of HDL, *J Lipid Res* 50(Suppl): S195–S200, 2009.

Wall R, Ross RP, Fitzgerald GF, et al: Fatty acids from fish: the anti-inflammatory potential of long-chain omega-3 fatty acids, *Nutr Rev* 68:280–289, 2010.

QUESTIONS

1. **A pharmaceutical company wants to develop a drug for the treatment of type IV hyperlipoproteinemia. The most promising approach would be an agent that**

   A. Increases the synthesis of apoB-100 in the liver
   B. Prevents the synthesis of apoE
   C. Stimulates the hormone-sensitive adipose tissue lipase
   D. Inhibits LPL
   E. Inhibits triglyceride synthesis in the liver

2. **Cholestyramine can reduce the level of LDL cholesterol by increasing the activity of the liver enzyme**

   A. HMG-CoA reductase
   B. LPL
   C. HL
   D. 7α-hydroxylase
   E. LCAT

3. **The statins inhibit the endogenous synthesis of cholesterol, thereby reducing the level of free cholesterol in the cell. The reduced level of cellular cholesterol, in turn, leads to**

   A. Increased activity of ACAT
   B. Increased synthesis of LDL receptors in most tissues
   C. Reduced synthesis of LDL receptors in most tissues
   D. Increased transfer of cholesterol esters from the cell to HDL
   E. Increased synthesis of bile acids by the liver

4. **If you are looking for ways to increase the reverse transport of cholesterol from peripheral tissues to the liver, the best bet would be a drug that**

   A. Inhibits the synthesis of LDL receptors
   B. Inhibits hepatic lipase
   C. Inhibits lipoprotein lipase
   D. Stimulates the transcription of the apoB gene
   E. Stimulates the transcription of the gene for the ABCA1 protein

Chapter 26
AMINO ACID METABOLISM

Amino acids are used for three major purposes:

1. *They are substrates for the generation of metabolic energy.* Most people in affluent countries obtain 15% to 20% of their metabolic energy from protein.
2. *They are substrates for protein synthesis.* Human body proteins are degraded and resynthesized continuously. Therefore pools of free amino acids must be maintained in all nucleated cells.
3. *They are substrates for the synthesis of many products,* including heme, purines, pyrimidines, several coenzymes, melanin, and the biogenic amines.

Only 11 of the 20 amino acids can be synthesized in the human body, either from common metabolic intermediates or from other amino acids. Those that cannot be synthesized are called **essential amino acids.** The essential amino acids are valine, leucine, isoleucine, phenylalanine, tryptophan, methionine, lysine, histidine, and threonine.

This chapter describes the fate of the amino nitrogen during amino acid catabolism, the pathways by which amino acids are degraded to simple nitrogen-free metabolic intermediates, and the biosynthesis of the nonessential amino acids.

AMINO ACIDS CAN BE USED FOR GLUCONEOGENESIS AND KETOGENESIS

The adult human body contains approximately 10 kg of protein in addition to small quantities of free amino acids in tissues and body fluids. The plasma concentrations of the 20 amino acids combined are only 20 to 30 mg/dl, one fourth of the blood glucose level.

Figure 26.1 shows an overview of amino acid and protein metabolism. A typical dietary protein intake is 100 g/day. Another 250 to 300 g of amino acids comes from protein breakdown, but the same amount is consumed for protein synthesis. Different proteins turn over at different rates. Most metabolic enzymes have a life expectancy of one or a few days, but most plasma proteins circulate for 1 to 3 weeks. Hemoglobin survives for 120 days, collagen lasts up to several years in some tissues, and the lens proteins last for a lifetime.

Glucogenic amino acids are degraded to intermediates of tricarboxylic acid cycle or glycolysis. They are used for gluconeogenesis during fasting. **Ketogenic amino acids** are degraded to acetyl-coenzyme A (acetyl-CoA). They are used for ketogenesis during fasting. Only leucine and lysine are purely ketogenic. Some of the larger amino acids, including isoleucine and the three aromatic amino acids phenylalanine, tyrosine, and tryptophan, are both. All other amino acids are glucogenic.

THE NITROGEN BALANCE INDICATES THE NET RATE OF PROTEIN SYNTHESIS

One hundred grams of dietary protein contains approximately 16 g of nitrogen. Eighty-three percent of this ingested nitrogen eventually leaves the body as urea, 7% as ammonium ion and 10% as organic waste products, including uric acid and creatinine. Ninety-five percent of the urea and a large majority of the other nitrogenous wastes are excreted in the urine, but 1 to 2 g of nitrogen from undigested protein is excreted in the stools.

The **nitrogen balance** is the difference between the nitrogen entering the body and that leaving it. A normal adult with adequate protein intake should be in **nitrogen equilibrium** (*Fig. 26.2*). This means that the amount of outgoing nitrogen matches exactly the amount of

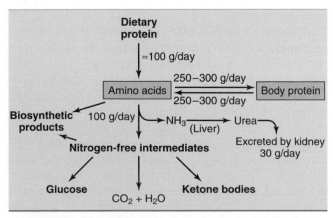

Figure 26.1 Metabolic interrelationships of amino acids.

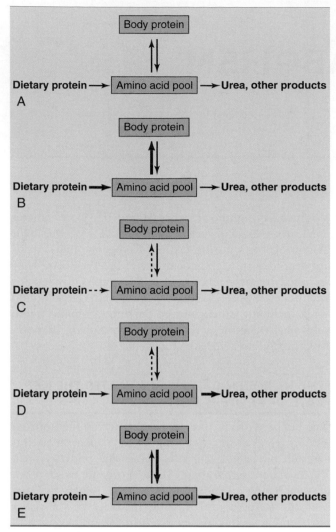

Figure 26.2 Nitrogen balance in different normal and abnormal states. **A,** Normal adult: nitrogen equilibrium. **B,** Growth, pregnancy: positive nitrogen balance. **C,** Protein deficiency: negative nitrogen balance. **D,** Essential amino acid deficiency: negative nitrogen balance. **E,** Wasting diseases, burns, trauma: negative nitrogen balance.

incoming nitrogen, and the amount of body protein remains constant.

A **positive nitrogen balance** is observed when nitrogen intake exceeds nitrogen excretion. It implies that the amount of body protein increases. Growing children, pregnant women, bodybuilders, and patients recovering from severe illnesses have a positive nitrogen balance. Therefore they have an increased requirement for dietary protein.

A **negative nitrogen balance** is observed in dietary protein deficiency. Even the protein-starved body degrades 30 to 40 g of amino acids every day. This amount defines the dietary requirement. Essential amino acid deficiency has the same effect because protein synthesis is impaired even if only one of the essential amino acids is missing.

Patients with chronic infections, cancer, or other severe diseases have a negative nitrogen balance because *glucocorticoids and other stress hormones favor protein degradation over protein synthesis*, thereby supplying amino acids for gluconeogenesis. Some **cytokines**—biologically active proteins released by white blood cells in many diseases—have catabolic effects similar to those of the stress hormones.

THE AMINO GROUP OF AMINO ACIDS IS RELEASED AS AMMONIA

During amino acid catabolism, some of the amino acid nitrogen is released as ammonia. The most important ammonia-forming reaction is the oxidative deamination of glutamate by **glutamate dehydrogenase** in liver and other tissues (*Fig. 26.3, A*). This reversible reaction can function in both the synthesis and the degradation of glutamate. The enzyme uses mainly nicotinamide adenine dinucleotide (NAD^+) for glutamate degradation and reduced nicotinamide adenine dinucleotide phosphate (NADPH) for glutamate synthesis. The glutamate dehydrogenase reaction implies that *glutamate is both nonessential and glucogenic*.

Most other amino acids do not form ammonia directly. *They transfer their α-amino group to α-ketoglutarate to form glutamate.* The enzymes that catalyze these reversible amino group transfers are called **transaminases** or **aminotransferases**. Examples are shown in *Figure 26.3, B*.

At least a dozen transaminases have been described in human tissues. Most of them use glutamate/α-ketoglutarate as one of their substrates/products. *All amino acids except threonine, lysine, and proline can be transaminated.* The α-amino groups of these amino acids are turned into ammonia by the transamination reactions to form glutamate followed by oxidative deamination of the glutamate:

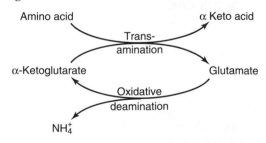

Alternatively, the glutamate that accumulates from these transaminase reactions can be used to make aspartate via aspartate transaminase operating in the reverse direction (*Fig. 26.3, B*). Both ammonia and aspartate are sources of nitrogen for the synthesis of urea (see section about urea cycle).

All transaminases contain **pyridoxal phosphate (PLP)**, the coenzyme form of vitamin B_6, as a prosthetic group. PLP is bound to the active site of the enzyme by

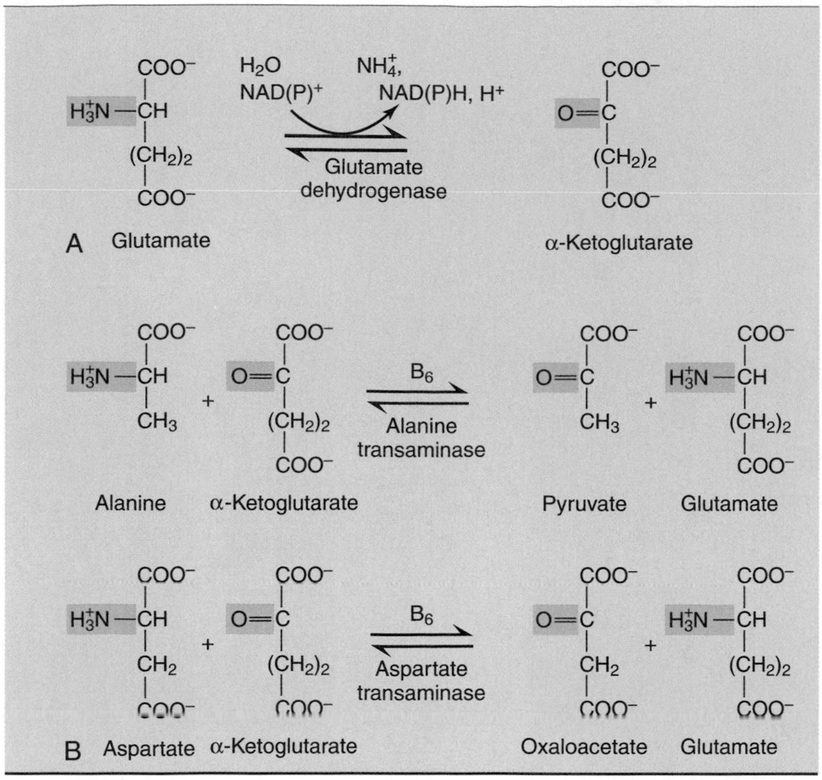

Figure 26.3 Fate of the amino group during amino acid catabolism. **A,** Release of ammonia from glutamate in the glutamate dehydrogenase reaction. Although reversible, this reaction functions in glutamate degradation under most conditions. *NAD(P),* Nicotinamide adenine dinucleotide (phosphate); *NAD(P)H,* reduced form of NAD(P). **B,** Transamination of alanine and aspartate. These reversible reactions transfer the amino group to α-ketoglutarate, forming glutamate. From glutamate, the nitrogen can be released as ammonia in the glutamate dehydrogenase reaction.

electrostatic interactions and by a Schiff base (aldimine) bond with a lysine side chain of the apoprotein. PLP participates directly in the reaction as shown in *Figure 26.4*.

AMMONIA IS DETOXIFIED TO UREA

Ammonia is a hazardous waste. It is neurotoxic even in low concentrations, so it must be disposed of quickly. Being unable to excrete ammonia fast enough, humans turn it into nontoxic, water-soluble, and therefore easily excretable urea.

Urea is the diamide of carbonic acid. This dry statement implies that *urea can be cleaved into carbonic acid and ammonia*. The reaction is catalyzed by the bacterial enzyme **urease:**

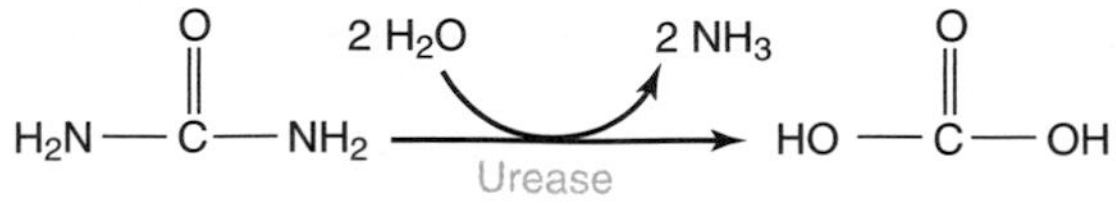

Humans do not possess urease, but some bacteria do. The bacterium *Proteus mirabilis* causes urinary tract infections in which the bacterial urease produces large amounts of ammonia. The ammonia alkalinizes the urine, causing the formation of large kidney stones ("staghorn calculi") consisting of magnesium ammonium phosphate. Also, the sharp smell of latrines is ammonia formed by urease-producing bacteria.

Because urea contains 48% nitrogen by weight and proteins contain 16%, *3 g of dietary protein forms 1 g of urea*—a total of 33 g urea on a diet of 100 g protein per day.

The blood urea level is measured as **blood urea nitrogen (BUN).** In health, the level is 8 to 20 mg/dl. *The BUN rises sharply in renal failure.* This condition is called **uremia.** Urea is not responsible for most of the clinical manifestations of uremia, but BUN is a convenient measure for the retention of nitrogenous wastes.

UREA IS SYNTHESIZED IN THE UREA CYCLE

Most amino acid catabolism takes place in the liver, and the liver is also the only important site for the synthesis of urea in the urea cycle. Nitrogen enters the cycle in the form of **carbamoyl phosphate,** which is synthesized in liver mitochondria from ammonia, carbon dioxide, and ATP:

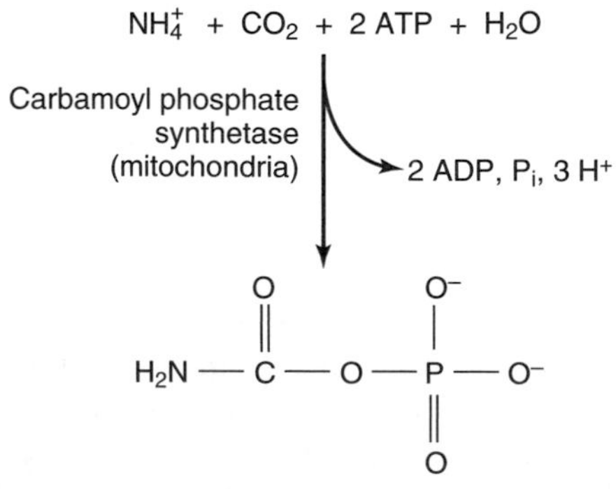

The use of two ATP molecules makes this reaction irreversible. The carbamoyl phosphate synthetase requires

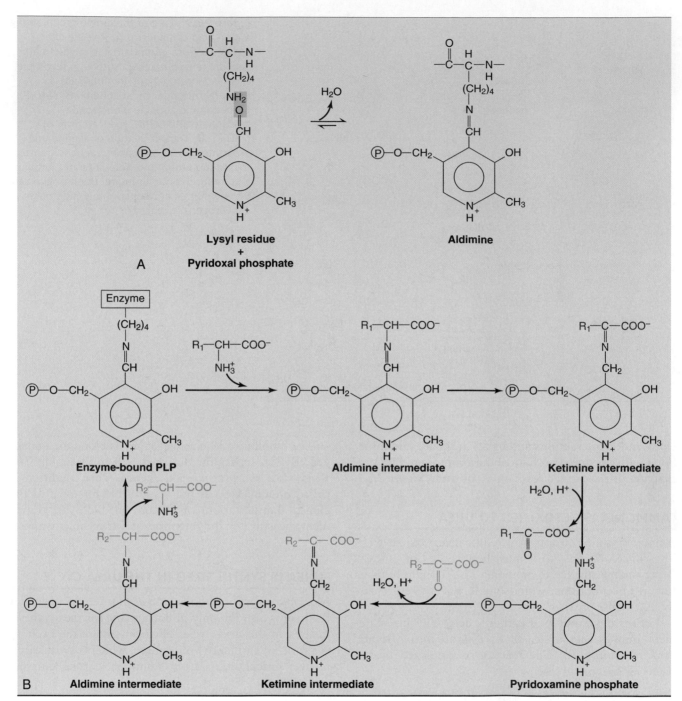

Figure 26.4 Mechanism of transamination reactions. **A,** Pyridoxal phosphate (*PLP*) is bound to a lysine side chain in the apoprotein by an aldimine ("Schiff base") bond. **B,** Catalytic cycle. Transamination is a sequence of two reactions in which the prosthetic group of the enzyme participates as a reactant.

N-acetylglutamate as an activator. This regulatory metabolite is formed by a separate enzyme from glutamate and acetyl-CoA. *N*-acetylglutamate is formed when glutamate is increased and indicates that the urea cycle should be turned on to get rid of nitrogen. Carbamoyl phosphate synthetase has a very high affinity for its substrate ammonia ($K_m = 250\ \mu mol/L$) and therefore can maintain the

ammonia concentration at a low level of 30 to 60 μmol/L at all times.

The reactions of the urea cycle proper are shown in *Figure 26.5*. *One of the two nitrogen atoms in urea comes from ammonia via carbamoyl phosphate and the other from aspartate.* Most of the aspartate nitrogen is derived from transamination reactions in the liver (*Fig. 26.6*).

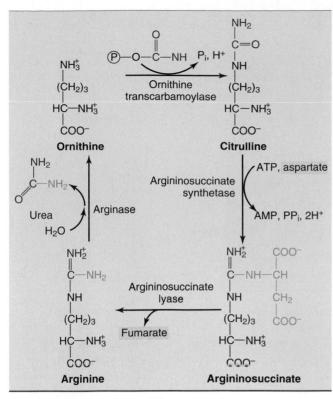

Figure 26.5 Reactions of the urea cycle.

Synthesis of one urea molecule requires four high-energy phosphate bonds. Two ATP molecules are converted to ADP in the carbamoyl phosphate synthetase reaction, and two additional phosphate bonds are consumed for the formation of argininosuccinate, when one ATP molecule is hydrolyzed to AMP and inorganic pyrophosphate. *The nitrogen is committed to urea synthesis because the two reactions that introduce it into the cycle are made irreversible by ATP hydrolysis.*

Failure of the urea cycle leads to ammonia toxicity and encephalopathy. Inherited urea cycle enzyme deficiencies (see ***Clinical Example 26.1***) are rare conditions with a combined incidence of 1:8000. In addition to ammonia, glutamine is elevated because excess ammonia is diverted into glutamine synthesis. The substrate of the defective enzyme also accumulates. Death in infancy or severe disability is inevitable when a urea cycle enzyme deficiency is complete, but partial enzyme deficiencies lead to milder impairments.

A far more common cause of hyperammonemia is liver failure. Patients develop a form of encephalopathy that is caused in large part by ammonia toxicity but also is related to other aspects of impaired liver function (*Clinical Example 26.2*).

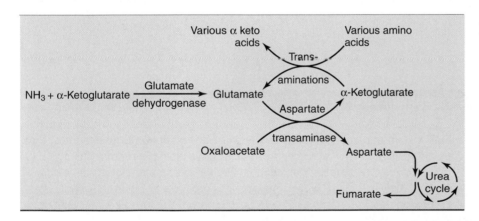

Figure 26.6 Sources of nitrogen for the argininosuccinate synthetase reaction of the urea cycle.

CLINICAL EXAMPLE 26.1: Ornithine Transcarbamoylase Deficiency

With an estimated incidence of 1:14,000, X-linked ornithine transcarbamoylase deficiency is the most common inherited urea cycle enzyme deficiency. In classic cases, affected males become lethargic and anorexic between 1 and 3 days after birth. Vomiting, hypothermia, and hyperventilation may be present, and laboratory investigations show respiratory alkalosis. Cerebral edema develops because of the osmotic activity of glutamine accumulating in astrocytes, and many patients die within weeks after birth.

The diagnosis is established by findings of elevated blood ammonia, glutamine, and ornithine and reduced blood urea nitrogen. Orotic acid appears in blood and urine because accumulating carbamoyl phosphate leaks from the mitochondria into the cytoplasm, where it is a precursor of orotic acid in the pathway of pyrimidine synthesis (see Chapter 28).

Treatment includes dietary protein restriction, combined with sufficient carbohydrate to prevent the breakdown of body protein for gluconeogenesis. Patients are fed high doses of **benzoic acid** and **phenylacetic**

Continued

CLINICAL EXAMPLE 26.1: Ornithine Transcarbamoylase Deficiency—cont'd

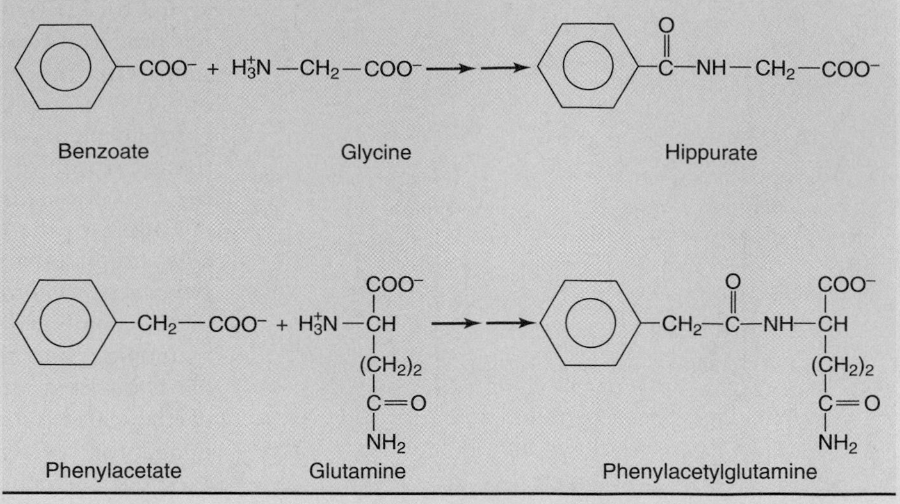

Figure 26.7 Use of benzoate and phenylacetate for treatment of hyperammonemia in liver cirrhosis and inherited urea cycle enzyme deficiencies. The amino acid conjugates of these organic acids provide alternative routes of nitrogen excretion.

Benzoate + Glycine → Hippurate

Phenylacetate + Glutamine → Phenylacetylglutamine

acid, which are excreted in the urine as conjugation products with glycine and glutamine, respectively (*Fig. 26.7*). Ordinarily, these reactions are detoxification reactions that convert the unwanted acids into water-soluble excretable products. In this context, however, they are exploited as alternative routes of nitrogen excretion. Arginine or, preferably, citrulline is administered because the urea cycle functions as a biosynthetic pathway for arginine. *For patients with urea cycle enzyme deficiencies, arginine is an essential amino acid.*

Incomplete deficiencies lead to mild forms of the disease that become symptomatic in older children or adults, usually during episodes of dieting or starvation, when a large amount of body protein is degraded to provide substrate for gluconeogenesis. In addition, some carrier females develop signs of encephalopathy in these situations.

CLINICAL EXAMPLE 26.2: Hepatic Encephalopathy

Liver cirrhosis is defined by *progressive loss of hepatocytes, which are replaced by fibrous connective tissue.* It is an end point of many pathological processes, with alcoholism being the most common cause.

The proliferating connective tissue impairs blood flow through the liver. This leads to **portal hypertension** and the development of a collateral circulation. Venous channels in the lower esophagus and in the periumbilical, rectal, and retroperitoneal areas dilate, shunting blood from the portal vein to the systemic circulation. Portal hypertension is dangerous because it can result in the rupture of veins and fatal hemorrhage, especially in the lower esophagus.

The biochemical derangements in liver cirrhosis cause **hepatic encephalopathy,** also called **portal systemic encephalopathy** because the shunting of blood around the cirrhotic liver contributes to the problem. It manifests with slurring of speech, blurring of vision, motor incoordination (ataxia), a characteristic coarse flapping tremor (asterixis), and mental derangements. The condition can progress to **hepatic coma** and death. Although other biochemical abnormalities have been implicated as well, *hyperammonemia is a major cause of the central nervous system disorder.*

Foul-smelling breath is an important diagnostic sign. It is caused by volatile sulfhydryl compounds (mercaptans) that are formed from dietary cysteine and methionine by intestinal bacteria. Ordinarily, the mercaptans are oxidized to nonvolatile, odorless products in the liver. In liver cirrhosis, however, they reach the lungs and are exhaled.

A low-protein, alcohol-free diet is the best long-term treatment of liver cirrhosis. The replacement of essential amino acids by their corresponding α-keto acids is an effective (but expensive) way of reducing the total nitrogen intake without precipitating essential amino acid deficiencies. Because of the transamination reactions, most of the essential amino acids are no longer essential when their corresponding α-keto acids are present in the diet.

Intestinal bacteria are an important source of ammonia. They ferment undigested proteins under formation of ammonia, and they cleave the urea that is present in digestive secretions into carbonic acid and ammonia. Therefore hepatic encephalopathy can be treated with sterilization of the gastrointestinal tract by broad-spectrum antibiotics, although there is a danger of overgrowth by drug-resistant bacteria with resulting enterocolitis.

SOME AMINO ACIDS ARE CLOSELY RELATED TO COMMON METABOLIC INTERMEDIATES

Some amino acids are close relatives of intermediates in the major metabolic pathways. **Alanine** is related to pyruvate through the reversible **alanine transaminase** reaction:

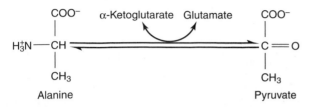

Glutamate is similarly interconvertible with α-ketoglutarate, both by transamination and the glutamate dehydrogenase reaction. **Glutamine** is both synthesized from and degraded to glutamate:

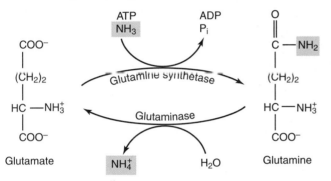

Aspartate is interconvertible with oxaloacetate by transamination. **Asparagine** is related to aspartate:

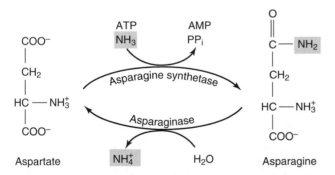

CLINICAL EXAMPLE 26.3: Asparaginase for Treatment of Leukemia

Parenterally administered asparaginase is used to treat cases of acute lymphocytic leukemia in which the malignant cells have lost the ability to synthesize asparagine. These cancer cells depend on asparagine from the blood. By destroying asparagine in the blood, the asparaginase deprives the malignant cells of an essential nutrient. This treatment achieves remission in many patients and cure in some, especially when asparaginase is combined with traditional chemotherapy.

GLYCINE, SERINE, AND THREONINE ARE GLUCOGENIC

Serine is both synthesized from and degraded to the glycolytic-gluconeogenic intermediate 3-phosphoglycerate (**Fig. 26.8**).

Serine is also converted to pyruvate by **serine dehydratase** and to glycine by **serine hydroxymethyl transferase** (**Fig. 26.9**). The latter reaction is an important source of one-carbon units for tetrahydrofolate.

The major reaction of glycine degradation (and another source of one-carbon units for tetrahydrofolate) is the **glycine cleavage reaction**:

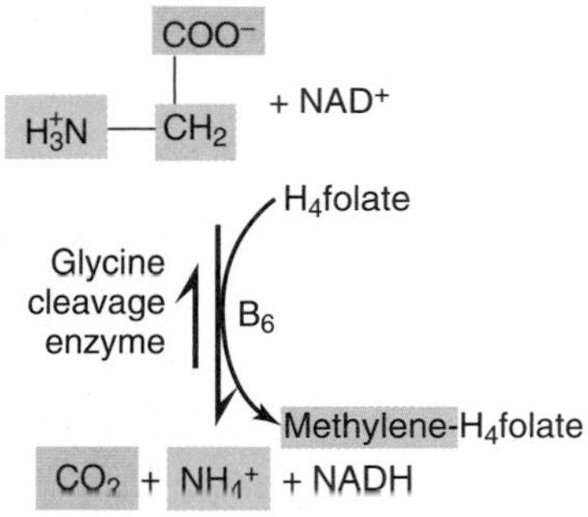

A specialized metabolic product formed from glycine in bacteria (but not humans) is **trimethylamine**:

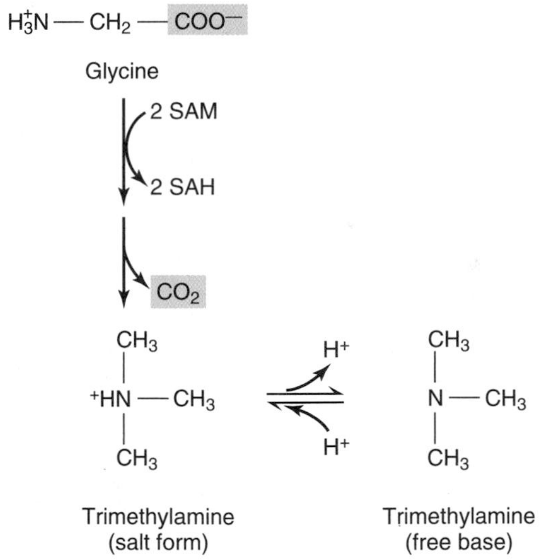

where SAH = *S*-adenosyl homocysteine and SAM = *S*-adenosyl methionine. Trimethylamine is distinguished by its scent, which resembles that of stale fish. It is formed during the bacterial decomposition of many protein-rich substrates. The typical smell is most noticeable under alkaline conditions (e.g., in the presence of soap) when the volatile free base is released from the protonated form.

Threonine cannot be synthesized in the human body, but there are several pathways for its degradation (**Fig. 26.10**). **Figure 26.11** summarizes the metabolic relationships of serine, glycine, and threonine.

Figure 26.8 Metabolic interconversion of serine and the glycolytic intermediate 3-phosphoglycerate.

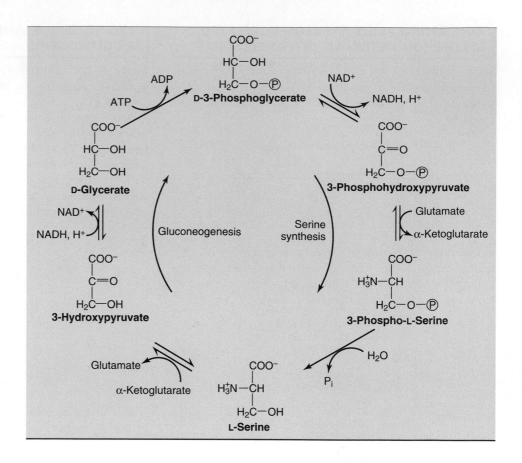

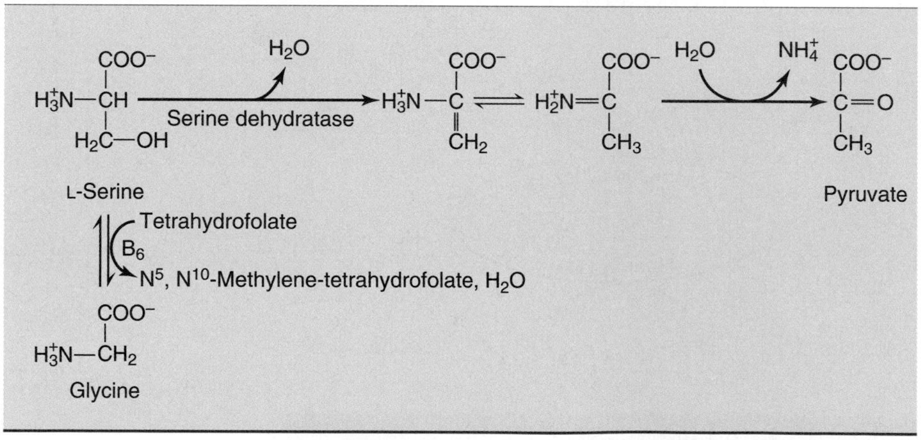

Figure 26.9 Catabolism of serine.

CLINICAL EXAMPLE 26.4: Nonketotic Hyperglycinemia

Nonketotic hyperglycinemia is a rare, recessively inherited disease (1:250,000 liveborn infants) caused by functional absence of the glycine-cleaving enzyme. It presents with coma or seizures during the first weeks of life, and many affected infants die before the diagnosis can be established. Survival is possible if the infant is treated with high doses of anticonvulsants and benzoic acid. The latter is used in an attempt to eliminate excess glycine from the body (see *Fig. 26.7*). Despite treatment, the not-so-lucky survivors are left with profound mental and neurological deficits. The mechanism of these effects most likely involves glycine's role as an inhibitory neurotransmitter and as a modulator of glutamate effects on the NMDA glutamate receptor.

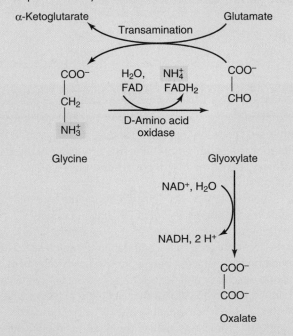

Figure 26.10 Catabolism of threonine. *TPP,* Thiamin pyrophosphate.

CLINICAL EXAMPLE 26.5: Oxalate Stones

Between 5% and 15% of people in modern societies develop kidney stones at one or another point in their lives. *Eighty percent of all kidney stones consist of calcium oxalate.* Some of the oxalate is derived from spinach, rhubarb, and other dietary sources, but only 10% of the 50 to 200 mg of oxalic acid in the daily diet is absorbed in the intestine. Another portion is formed in the body from glycine with the help of the enzyme **D-amino acid oxidase:**

Normally, the total urinary oxalate excretion is less than 45 mg/day. Oxalate stones can be prevented by reducing the dietary intake of oxalic acid and possibly protein, but the preferred method is increased fluid intake, to provide sufficient solvent for the calcium oxalate.

PROLINE, ARGININE, ORNITHINE, AND HISTIDINE ARE DEGRADED TO GLUTAMATE

Proline, arginine, and **ornithine** are degraded to glutamate (*Fig. 26.12*). Proline can be synthesized freely from glutamate or arginine and therefore is not nutritionally essential. Arginine is nonessential because it can be synthesized from glutamate via ornithine, using the reactions of the urea cycle.

Histidine is degraded to glutamate by an unrelated pathway (*Fig. 26.13*). The last reaction in the pathway contributes a formimino group to tetrahydrofolate. The folate requirement of this reaction is exploited in a laboratory test for folate deficiency. After an oral histidine load, the excess is normally degraded without the accumulation of metabolic intermediates. In folate deficiency, however, formiminoglutamate is no longer converted to glutamate and can be demonstrated in the urine.

This test is of limited usefulness because some people lack the formiminotransferase and habitually excrete formiminoglutamate as an end product of histidine degradation. This enzyme deficiency is benign.

Although histidine cannot be synthesized in the human body, people can subsist on a histidine-free diet for many weeks without ill effects. The reason is that histidine can be formed from the dipeptide **carnosine** (β-alanyl-histidine), which is present in large quantity in muscle tissue:

Carnosine is a pH buffer that limits the effect of lactic acid on tissue pH during anaerobic contraction.

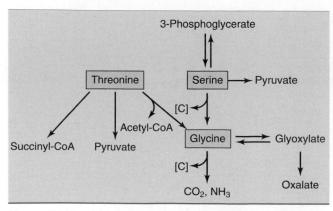

Figure 26.11 Metabolism of serine, glycine, and threonine.

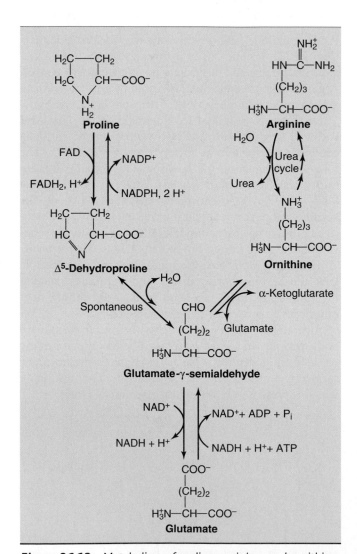

Figure 26.12 Metabolism of proline, arginine, and ornithine.

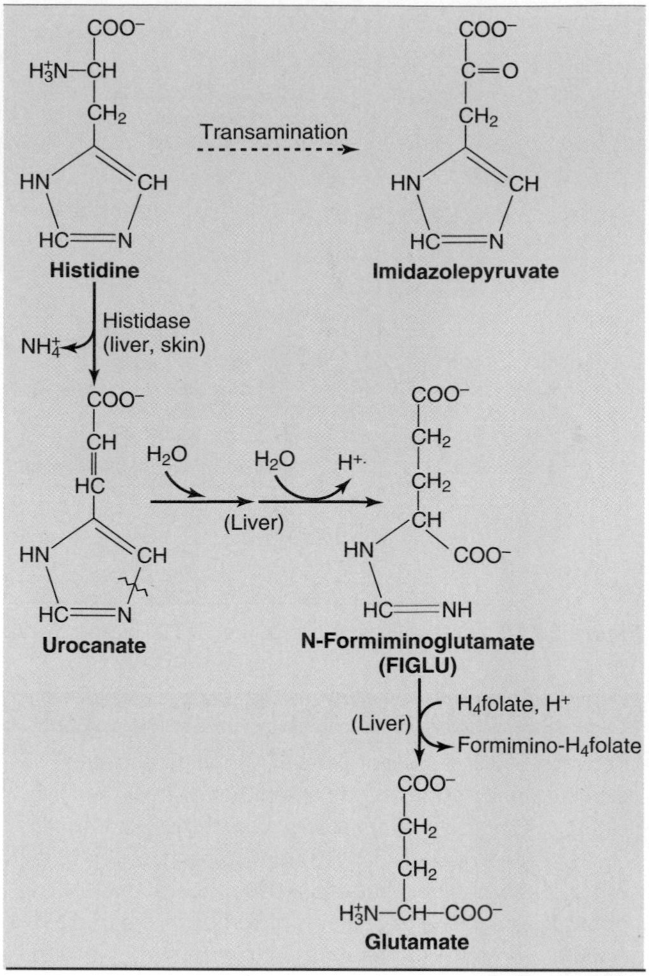

Figure 26.13 Catabolism of histidine.

CLINICAL EXAMPLE 26.6: Histidinemia

Histidinemia is a rare (incidence 1:12,000), recessively inherited condition in which histidase is deficient. In this situation transamination, which is otherwise a minor pathway, becomes the major reaction of histidine catabolism.

Histidinemia first was detected during the screening of newborns for phenylketonuria (PKU) when urinary imidazolepyruvate produced a false-positive color reaction in the ferric chloride test for urinary phenylpyruvate. The condition is considered benign, despite early reports of mental deficiency and speech disorders in some affected children. Dietary treatment by histidine restriction, which corrects the biochemical abnormality, is not required. Diagnostic procedures include the determination of serum histidine, enzyme determination in skin biopsy, and measurement of the urocanate concentration in sweat. Histidase is present only in skin and liver, and urocanate is a normal constituent of sweat.

METHIONINE AND CYSTEINE ARE METABOLICALLY RELATED

The essential amino acid **methionine** is a precursor of the methyl group donor **S-adenosylmethionine (SAM)** (see Chapter 5). SAM is synthesized from methionine and ATP in an unusual reaction in which all three phosphates of ATP are released (*Fig. 26.14*). By donating its methyl group during methylation reactions,

SAM becomes **S-adenosylhomocysteine (SAH)**. SAH forms **homocysteine** and finally methionine. The methylation of homocysteine to methionine requires both folate (as methyl-tetrahydrofolate) and vitamin B_{12} (as methylcobalamin).

Figure 26.14 also shows how **cysteine** is made from the carbon skeleton of serine and the sulfur of methionine. Cysteine catabolism releases the sulfur as inorganic sulfite, which is rapidly oxidized and excreted in the urine as sulfate.

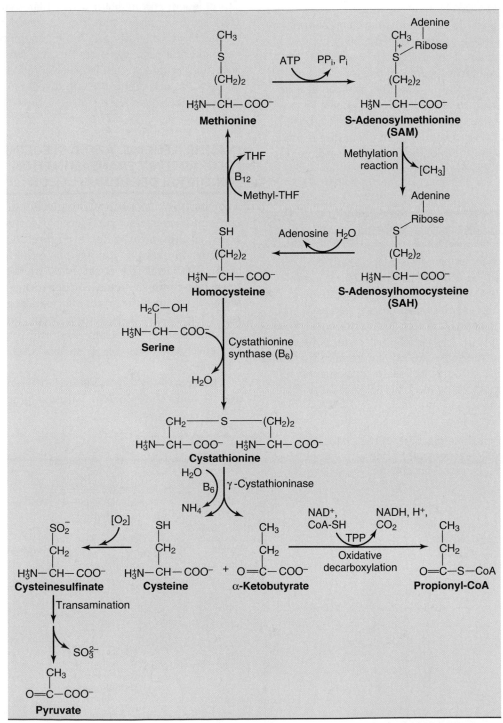

Figure 26.14 Metabolism of methionine and cysteine. B_6, Pyridoxal phosphate; *THF*, tetrahydrofolate; *TPP*, thiamin pyrophosphate.

CLINICAL EXAMPLE 26.7: Homocystinuria

Homocystinuria is a rare (incidence of 1:200,000), recessively inherited deficiency of cystathionine synthase. Homocysteine, homocystine, and methionine accumulate. Patients show thinning and lengthening of the long bones, osteoporosis, lens dislocation, thrombosis, and mental deficiency. These abnormalities are caused by accumulation of homocysteine, not methionine.

Homocystinuria can be treated by restriction of dietary methionine. Some patients have an abnormal cystathionine synthase with reduced affinity for pyridoxal phosphate. They respond to megadoses of vitamin B_6, the dietary precursor of pyridoxal phosphate. Supplements of vitamin B_{12} and folic acid can also be tried in an attempt to boost the homocysteine → methionine reaction. Betaine (*N,N,N*-trimethylglycine), which is a methyl group donor in an alternative reaction for the synthesis of methionine from homocysteine, can be used with the same reasoning.

CLINICAL EXAMPLE 26.8: Homocysteine as Risk Factor for Cardiovascular Disease

Based on the observation of vascular disease in homocystinuria (see *Clinical Example 26.7*), several studies explored the role of plasma homocysteine in cardiovascular disease. Most studies showed a significant association. A rise of homocysteine from 10 to 15 µmol/L appears to raise the risk of cardiovascular disease to about the same extent as a rise of cholesterol level from 180 to 200 mg/dl. Folate supplements reduce the homocysteine level, probably because folate

is required for the homocysteine → methionine reaction, and such supplements may reduce the risk of cardiovascular disease.

However, plasma homocysteine levels are affected by renal function. People with low glomerular filtration rate tend to have elevated plasma homocysteine. When measures of vascular disease were studied in relation to glomerular filtration rate and plasma homocysteine, renal function but not homocysteine was found to be an independent predictor of vascular changes. This raises the possibility that homocysteine is not a risk factor for vascular disease in the general population but a marker for renal function. Possibly some aspect of impaired renal function is causally related to vascular disease. At this point, the controversy remains unresolved.

VALINE, LEUCINE, AND ISOLEUCINE ARE DEGRADED BY TRANSAMINATION AND OXIDATIVE DECARBOXYLATION

The first three steps in the degradation of valine, leucine, and isoleucine are identical for all three amino acids, as shown for valine in *Figure 26.15*.

Transamination is followed by oxidative decarboxylation. The latter step is catalyzed by the mitochondrial **branched-chain α-ketoacid dehydrogenase** complex, which resembles the pyruvate dehydrogenase complex (see Chapter 21) in structure, coenzyme requirements, and reaction mechanism. The third reaction in the sequence resembles the first step of β-oxidation (see Chapter 23).

The remaining reactions are different for the three amino acids (*Fig. 26.16*). Valine is glucogenic, leucine

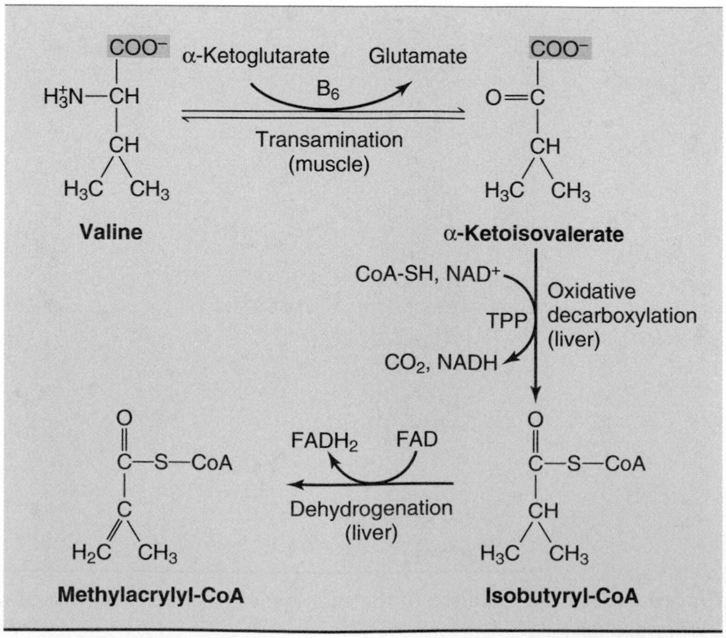

Figure 26.15 First three reactions in the catabolism of valine. Analogous reactions take place with leucine and isoleucine. B_6, Pyridoxal phosphate; *TPP*, thiamin pyrophosphate.

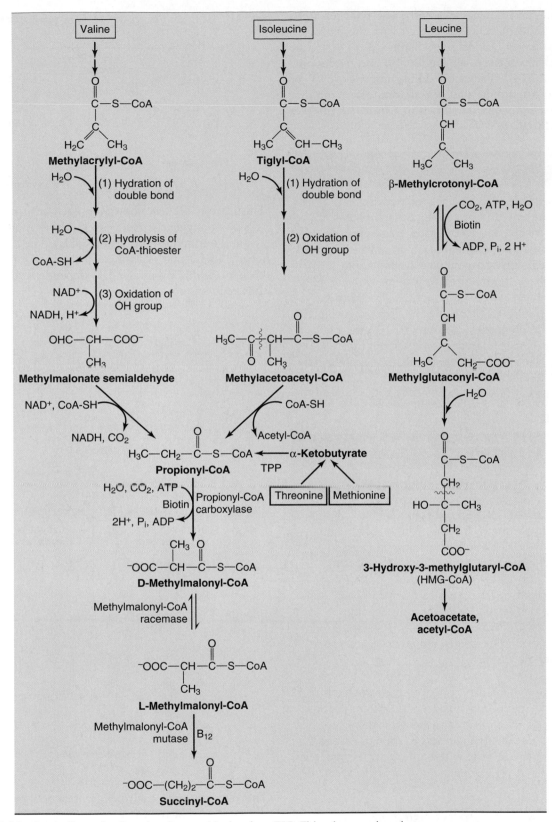

Figure 26.16 Catabolism of valine, leucine, and isoleucine. *TPP*, Thiamin pyrophosphate.

is ketogenic, and isoleucine is both. The final reactions for valine and isoleucine are shared with the pathways of odd-chain fatty acids (see Chapter 23), threonine (threonine dehydratase; see *Fig. 26.10*) and methionine (see *Fig. 26.14*). The most important disorders of branched-chain amino acid degradation affect the first and the last reactions, as shown in *Clinical Examples 26.9* and *26.10*.

CLINICAL EXAMPLE 26.9: Maple Syrup Urine Disease

Deficiency of the branched-chain α-keto acid dehydrogenase, which oxidatively decarboxylates all three branched-chain α-keto acids, causes **maple syrup urine disease**. The disease presents in infants with severe neurological damage, acidosis, and sweet-smelling urine. Untreated patients with complete enzyme deficiency die within months after birth. Dietary restriction of valine, leucine, and isoleucine improves the prognosis but is not always effective in preventing mental retardation and episodes of metabolic acidosis. Megadoses of thiamin are effective in a few patients. The incidence at birth is approximately 1:200,000.

CLINICAL EXAMPLE 26.10: Methylmalonic Aciduria

A recessively inherited defect in the vitamin B_{12}-dependent methylmalonyl-CoA mutase reaction (incidence at birth of 1:50,000) leads to the accumulation of methylmalonic acid in blood and urine. Being an acid, methylmalonic acid causes serious and often fatal acidosis in affected infants. It also leads to hypoglycemia, ketosis, and hyperammonemia. Treatment can be attempted by the cautious restriction of valine, isoleucine, threonine, and methionine. However, substantial restrictions of these essential amino acids will cause signs of protein deficiency.

Some cases are caused not by a defective enzyme protein but by an inability to convert dietary vitamin B_{12} to the coenzyme form deoxyadenosylcobalamin. These patients respond to injected adenosylcobalamin. Predictably, a deficiency of dietary vitamin B_{12} raises the methylmalonic acid level in the absence of any genetic defect.

PHENYLALANINE AND TYROSINE ARE BOTH GLUCOGENIC AND KETOGENIC

The ring systems of the aromatic amino acids cannot be synthesized in the body. Nevertheless tyrosine is considered nonessential because it is synthesized from phenylalanine in the **phenylalanine hydroxylase** reaction:

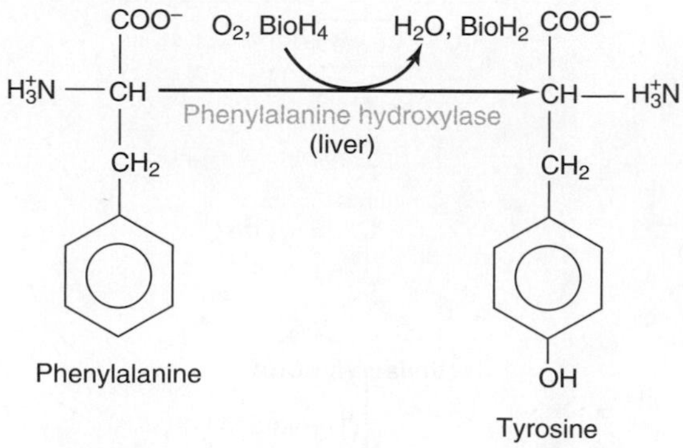

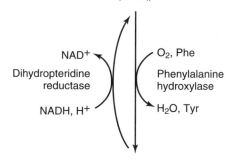

This irreversible reaction takes place only in the liver. It is a monooxygenase reaction requiring molecular oxygen and **tetrahydrobiopterin (BioH$_4$)**. The dihydrobiopterin (BioH$_2$) that is formed in the reaction is reduced back to BioH$_4$ by an NADH-dependent **dihydropteridine reductase**:

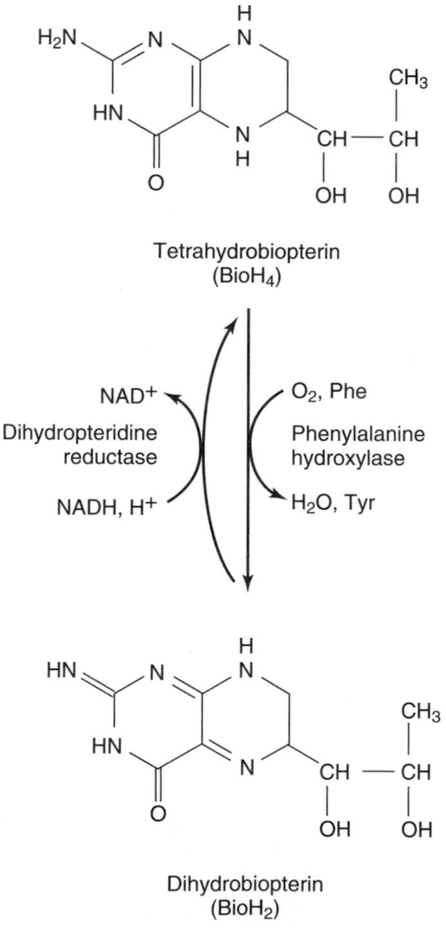

The phenylalanine hydroxylase reaction mechanism is the same as that for the tyrosine hydroxylase and tryptophan hydroxylase reactions discussed in Chapter 16.

The importance of the phenylalanine hydroxylase is shown in *Clinical Example 26.11*. *Figure 26.17* shows the catabolism of tyrosine in the liver. Inherited enzyme deficiencies in this pathway give rise to several rare diseases, as shown in *Clinical Example 26.12*.

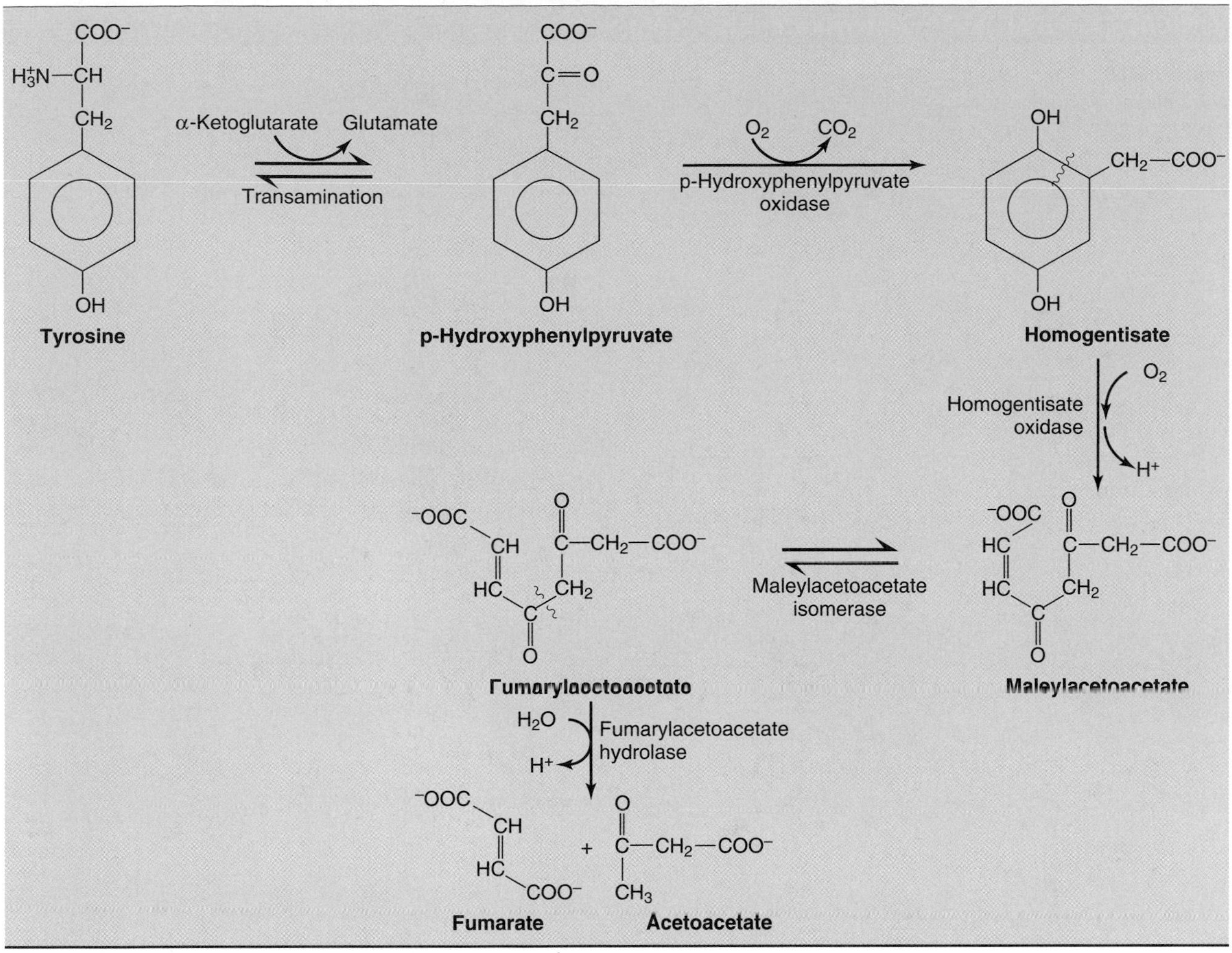

Figure 26.17   Degradation of tyrosine.

CLINICAL EXAMPLE 26.11: Phenylketonuria

Classic phenylketonuria (PKU) is caused by a complete deficiency of phenylalanine hydroxylase. *Phenylalanine accumulates, and most of the accumulating phenylalanine is eventually transaminated to phenylpyruvate.* Transamination is otherwise a very minor pathway of phenylalanine metabolism. Phenylpyruvate is converted to other products that are excreted in the urine along with phenylalanine and phenylpyruvate (*Fig. 26.18*).

Although normal at birth, serum phenylalanine and urinary phenylpyruvate rise within a few days after birth. *Untreated patients develop mental retardation.* Some patients develop spasticity, seizures, or other neurological signs. Hypopigmentation is present because normal melanocytes use phenylalanine hydroxylase to turn phenylalanine into the melanin precursor tyrosine, and high levels of phenylalanine inhibit the use of tyrosine for melanin synthesis.

Mental retardation in PKU can be prevented by the restriction of dietary phenylalanine. Patients have to cover most of their protein needs from a phenylalanine-free mix of synthetic amino acids. The artificial sweetener **aspartame** (*N*-aspartyl-phenylalanine methylester) must be avoided. Tyrosine is an essential amino acid for phenylketonuric patients, but dietary supplements are not needed. The diet must be started shortly after birth to prevent irreversible brain damage. Although there is no risk of severe brain damage in adults, lifelong continuation of dietary management is recommended.

Newborn screening for PKU is performed in nearly all affluent societies. Early screening programs used the **ferric chloride test** for urinary phenylpyruvate or the determination of blood phenylalanine, but today most newborn screening programs use **tandem mass spectrometry.** This method permits simultaneous

Continued

CLINICAL EXAMPLE 26.11: Phenylketonuria—cont'd

Figure 26.18 Phenylalanine metabolism in phenylketonuria (PKU).

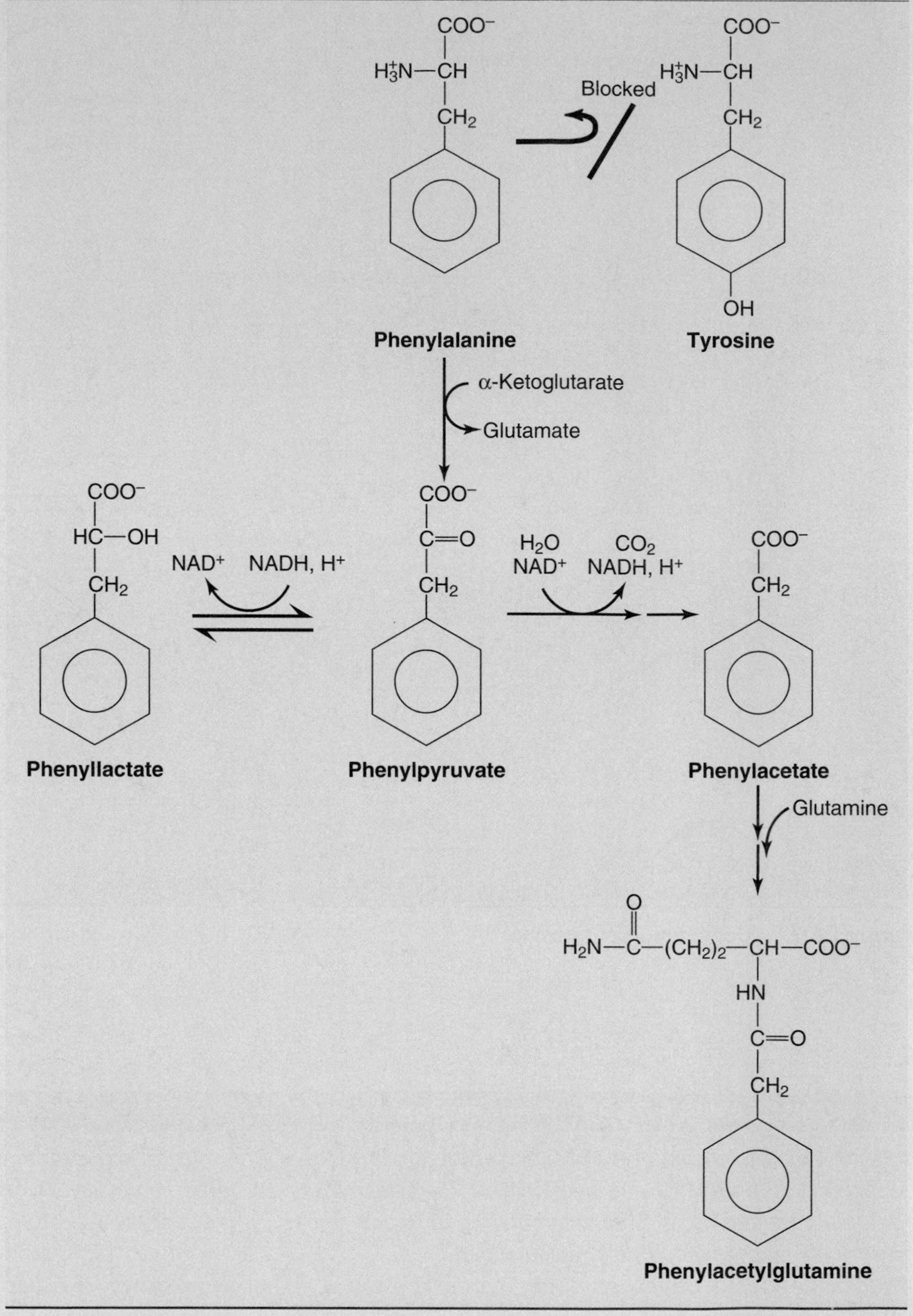
Blocked
Phenylalanine
Tyrosine
α-Ketoglutarate
Glutamate
NAD+ NADH, H+
H2O CO2
NAD+ NADH, H+
Phenyllactate
Phenylpyruvate
Phenylacetate
Glutamine
Phenylacetylglutamine

testing for dozens of inborn errors of metabolism. PKU testing should be done no less than 2 days after birth because false-negative results are common during the first 24 or even 48 hours. PKU is most common in people of European ancestry, with highest frequency (1:6000) in Britain and Ireland. It is far less common in other racial groups (e.g., 1:200,000 in Japan).

Heterozygotes have about half of the normal enzyme activity. Diagnosis by determination of enzyme activity is difficult because phenylalanine hydroxylase is expressed mainly in liver and melanocytes. For example, amniotic cells do not express this enzyme. DNA-based methods are of limited value because many different mutations have been identified in different families.

The children of phenylketonuric mothers are mentally retarded, although most of them do not have the homozygous PKU genotype. This is because phenylalanine and its metabolites are transferred from the mother to the fetus and impair fetal brain development. Therefore strict dietary control during pregnancy is required.

CLINICAL EXAMPLE 26.12: Disorders of Tyrosine Degradation

Alkaptonuria is a rare inborn error of tyrosine degradation in which homogentisate accumulates. Homogentisate in the urine is oxidized and polymerized to black products on exposure to light and air. Although the ink-colored diapers of affected babies look alarming, the condition is relatively benign. Black pigment gradually accumulates in cartilage and other connective tissues, a condition known as **ochronosis**. Older patients develop painful arthritis.

Type I tyrosinemia is caused by a deficiency of fumarylacetoacetate hydrolase (see *Fig. 26.17*). Fumarylacetoacetate and related organic acids inhibit the early steps in tyrosine degradation and cause a cabbage-like smell, impairment of renal tubular absorption, and liver failure. The incidence at birth is 1:100,000 in most parts of the world but up to 1:2000 in some French Canadian groups.

MELANIN IS SYNTHESIZED FROM TYROSINE

Melanin is the dark pigment of skin, hair, iris, and retinal pigment epithelium. *Melanin protects the skin* by absorbing not only visible light but also the ultraviolet component of sunlight. Ultraviolet radiation, especially at wavelengths of 280 to 320 nm, is dangerous because it damages DNA, causing sunburn and skin cancer. In the eye, the melanin of the pigment epithelium underlying the sensory cells of the retina absorbs stray light, thereby enhancing visual acuity and preventing overstimulation of the photoreceptors.

Melanin is synthesized from tyrosine. In the melanocytes, tyrosine is oxidized first to L-dopa and then to dopaquinone by the copper-containing enzyme **tyrosinase** (*Fig. 26.19*). These oxidation products polymerize nonenzymatically to form melanin.

Recessively inherited defects of melanin synthesis are the cause of **oculocutaneous albinism**. Some albinos lack tyrosinase, whereas others have a defect in the carrier that transports tyrosine across the melanosome membrane.

LYSINE AND TRYPTOPHAN HAVE LENGTHY CATABOLIC PATHWAYS

Lysine is degraded to acetoacetyl-CoA in a pathway with nine enzymatic reactions. Therefore it is a ketogenic amino acid. **Carnitine**, which transports long-chain fatty acids into the mitochondrion (see Chapter 23), is synthesized from protein-bound trimethyllysine. After degradation of the protein, trimethyllysine is converted to carnitine (*Fig. 26.20*).

Tryptophan is both glucogenic and ketogenic. The indole ring is ketogenic, and the side chain forms the

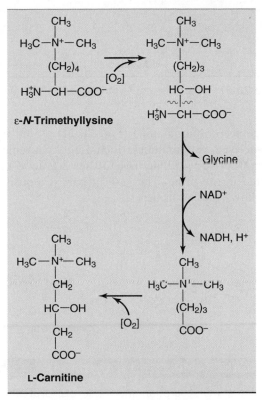

Figure 26.20 Biosynthesis of carnitine from ε-*N*-trimethyllysine. Trimethyllysine is formed in some proteins as a posttranslational modification of lysine.

Figure 26.19 Synthesis of melanin from tyrosine.

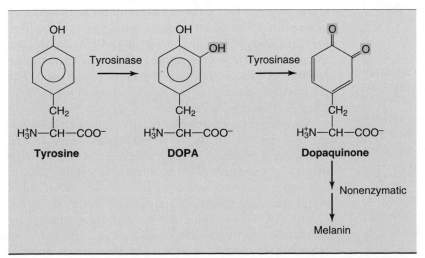

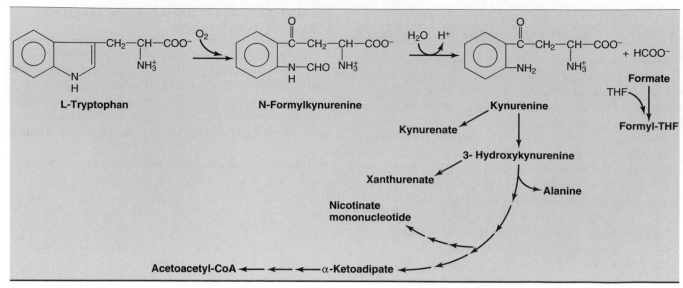

Figure 26.21 Catabolism of tryptophan. *THF*, Tetrahydrofolate.

glucogenic product alanine (*Fig. 26.21*). Some tryptophan-derived isoquinolines, including kynurenic acid and xanthurenic acid, are not further degraded but are excreted in the urine. They are in part responsible for the yellow color of urine:

Kynurenate

Xanthurenate

CLINICAL EXAMPLE 26.13: Cystinuria

Both intestinal absorption and renal reabsorption of amino acids require sodium cotransporters in the apical plasma membrane of the epithelial cells. Cystinuria (not to be confused with homocystinuria) is caused by a recessively inherited defect in the intestinal absorption and renal reabsorption of the dibasic amino acids lysine, arginine, ornithine, and cystine. Although lysine is nutritionally essential, signs of amino acid deficiency are not common in this condition, probably because amino acids can still be absorbed from the small intestine as dipeptides and tripeptides.

Cystine, however, is problematic. It is poorly soluble under acidic conditions. Therefore *cysteine forms kidney stones*. The diagnosis of cystinuria is established by the demonstration of abnormal quantities of dibasic amino acids in the urine. Cystinuria has an incidence of 1:7000, and it accounts for a fairly small proportion of kidney stones in the population. Treatment consists of measures to maintain a large urine volume and a neutral or alkaline urinary pH.

THE LIVER IS THE MOST IMPORTANT ORGAN OF AMINO ACID METABOLISM

Nearly half of the protein in the human body is in muscle tissue, but *enzymes of amino acid catabolism are most abundant in the liver*. This makes sense because, during fasting, amino acids have to be channeled into the hepatic pathways of gluconeogenesis (glucogenic amino acids) and ketogenesis (ketogenic amino acids).

After a meal (*Fig. 26.22, A*), most of the dietary glutamine and glutamate is metabolized in the intestinal mucosa. Most of the other amino acids go to the liver. Some are used for synthesis of plasma proteins, but most are catabolized. Only valine, leucine, and isoleucine pass through the liver and are transaminated in muscle and other peripheral tissues. The resulting branched-chain α-keto acids return to the liver for further catabolism except during physical exercise, when they are catabolized in the muscles.

Muscle tissue is the major source of plasma amino acids in the fasting state (see *Fig. 26.22, B*). Alanine accounts for 50% of the released amino acids and glutamine for 25%. Most of the alanine goes to the liver for gluconeogenesis, and most of the glutamine goes to kidneys and intestine. In the kidneys, the glutaminase reaction produces ammonia for urinary excretion. For the intestine, glutamine is a major substrate for the generation of metabolic energy.

Nitrogen is transported to the liver both as a constituent of amino acids and as free ammonia (*Fig. 26.23*). Ammonia is produced by glutamate dehydrogenase (most tissues), glutaminase (kidney, intestine), histidase (skin), and other enzymes. Intestinal bacteria contribute additional ammonia from urea and leftover dietary protein.

Most of the ammonia for the carbamoyl phosphate synthetase reaction of the urea cycle is imported from other organs, but most of the nitrogen that is brought

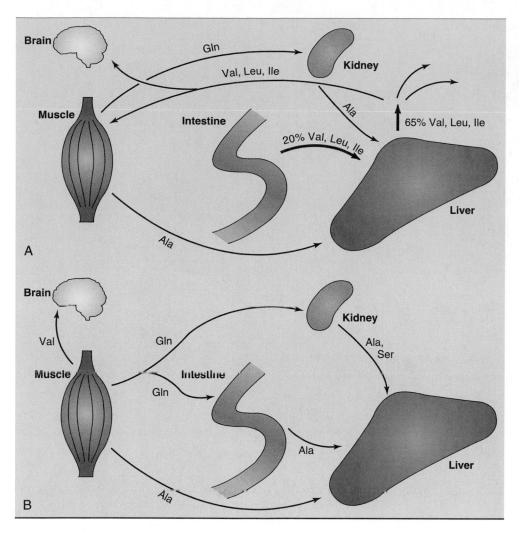

Figure 26.22 Interorgan exchange of amino acids. **A,** After protein-containing meal. All amino acids except valine (Val), leucine (Leu), and isoleucine (Ile) are metabolized extensively during their first passage through the liver. *Ala,* Alanine; *Gln,* glutamine. **B,** Postabsorptive state. Muscle tissue is the main source of plasma amino acids. Alanine and glutamine are quantitatively most important. *Ser,* Serine.

into the urea cycle by aspartate comes from transamination reactions in the liver. The perivenous cells of the hepatic lobules possess **glutamine synthetase,** which mops up most of the ammonia that escaped from the carbamoyl phosphate synthetase in the periportal hepatocytes (see *Fig. 26.23, B*).

CLINICAL EXAMPLE 26.14: Hartnup Disease

Hartnup disease is a recessively inherited defect in the intestinal absorption and renal reabsorption of large neutral amino acids. The clinical signs are similar to those of pellagra (niacin deficiency; see Chapter 29), with dermatitis and neurological abnormalities in the form of intermittent ataxia. These signs are caused by *decreased availability of tryptophan.* Normally, part of the human niacin requirement is covered by endogenous synthesis from tryptophan. Therefore tryptophan deficiency can cause signs of niacin deficiency.

Hartnup disease is a relatively benign disorder. The biochemical abnormality has a prevalence of 1:25,000, but only a minority of these individuals develops clinical signs. Treatment consists of a diet containing adequate protein, and oral niacin supplements.

GLUTAMINE PARTICIPATES IN RENAL ACID-BASE REGULATION

The blood has a pH between 7.35 and 7.40, and *the long-term maintenance of this pH is the task of the kidneys.* In acidosis, the kidneys excrete excess protons; in alkalosis, they retain protons. Therefore the urinary pH can range anywhere between 4 and 8. *Figure 26.24* shows how the kidneys use glutamine-derived ammonia as a vehicle for the excretion of excess protons during chronic acidosis.

In the tubular epithelium, blood-derived glutamine is deaminated first to glutamate and then to α-ketoglutarate. Being small and uncharged, the ammonia (NH_3) formed in these reactions diffuses passively into the urine of the tubular lumen. The urine is more acidic than the cytoplasm because the epithelial cells secrete protons through a sodium-proton antiporter. Therefore the ammonia in the urine combines with a proton to form the ammonium ion (NH_4^+). Being charged, the ammonium ion cannot diffuse back into the cell and is flushed down the sewage system of the urinary tract. Although NH_3 equilibrates across the membrane, *ammonium ions accumulate in the urine as long as the urine is more acidic than the cytoplasm of the epithelial cells.*

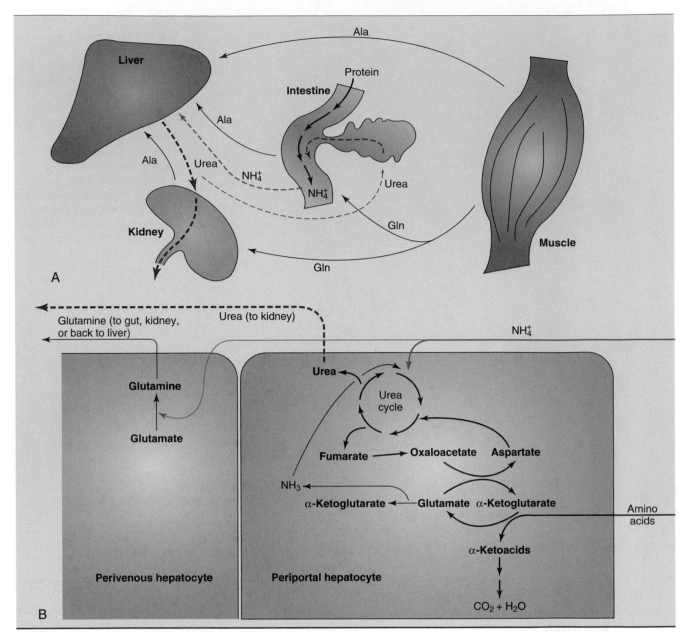

Figure 26.23 Transport of nitrogen to the liver. **A,** Extrahepatic pathways. Only the intestine supplies nitrogen for urea synthesis mainly in the form of ammonia, which is derived from the glutaminase reaction and from bacterial enzymes acting on urea in digestive secretions and on amino acids from undigested dietary proteins. Other tissues supply most of their nitrogen in the form of nontoxic amino acids, mainly alanine (Ala) and glutamine (Gln). **B,** Intrahepatic pathways. Ammonia detoxification is compartmentalized between the periportal and perivenous hepatocytes in the hepatic lobule. The urea cycle is most active in the periportal cells. Residual ammonia is scavenged by glutamine synthetase in the perivenous cells.

The glutamine-derived α-ketoglutarate is converted to glucose by gluconeogenesis in the kidneys. This process absorbs four protons for each molecule of glucose formed according to the following equation:

$$2\,C_5H_4O_5{}^{2-} + 4\,H_2O + 4\,H^+$$
α-Ketoglutarate
$$\downarrow$$
$$C_6H_{12}O_6 + 4\,CO_2 + 8\,[H]$$
Glucose

The eight hydrogen atoms ([H]) in this equation are exchanged with NAD and FAD in the α-ketoglutarate dehydrogenase, succinate dehydrogenase, malate dehydrogenase, and glyceraldehyde-3-phosphate dehydrogenase reactions.

The excretion of ammonium ions—but not urea—as an end product of amino acid metabolism is accompanied by the removal of protons. Even without the details shown in *Figure 26.24*, this is apparent from the stoichiometry for the oxidation of a typical amino acid such as alanine:

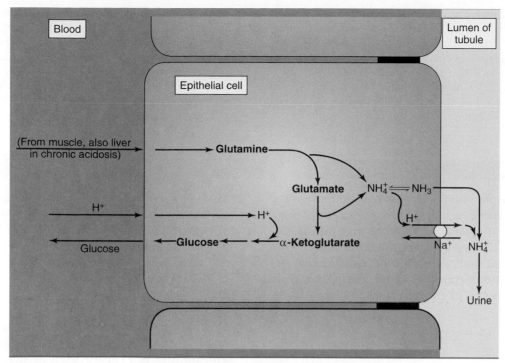

Figure 26.24 Glutamine metabolism and acid-base regulation in the renal tubules. The reactions shown here are most active during chronic acidosis, when a large proportion of the total nitrogen is excreted as the ammonium ion rather than as urea.

$$C_3H_7O_2N + 3\,O_2 + H^+$$
Alanine

$$\downarrow$$

$$NH_4^+ + 3\,CO_2 + 2\,H_2O$$
Ammonium ion

and

$$2\,C_3H_7O_2N + 6\,O_2$$
Alanine

$$\downarrow$$

$$CH_4N_2O + 5\,CO_2 + 5\,H_2O$$
Urea

During acidosis, the liver diverts an increasing fraction of the incoming ammonia from urea synthesis in the periportal cells to glutamine synthesis in the perivenous cells (see **Fig. 26.23, B**). The liver becomes a net producer of glutamine, which is forwarded to the kidneys. In the kidneys, acidosis induces glutaminase, glutamate dehydrogenase, and the gluconeogenic enzyme PEP carboxykinase. As a result, *up to 50% of the nitrogen is excreted as ammonium ion rather than urea during chronic acidosis.*

SUMMARY

Amino acids are degraded to carbon dioxide, water, and urea. These reactions take place mainly in the liver. Urea formation requires transamination reactions, oxidative deamination of glutamate, and the

reactions of the urea cycle. Patients with advanced liver cirrhosis cannot turn ammonia into urea. They develop encephalopathy and coma resulting from the accumulation of toxic ammonia.

Excretion of the ammonium ion rather than urea is accompanied by elimination of excess protons from the body. The kidneys increase ammonium excretion during acidosis in an attempt to eliminate excess protons.

The carbon skeletons of the amino acids are channeled either into gluconeogenesis (glucogenic amino acids) or into ketogenesis (ketogenic amino acids). Many deficiencies of amino acid–degrading enzymes are known. The clinical manifestations of these inborn errors of amino acid metabolism are caused by the abnormal accumulation of the affected amino acid or its metabolites.

Further Reading

Cagnon L, Braissant O: Hyperammonemia-induced toxicity for the developing central nervous system, *Brain Res Rev* 56:183–197, 2007.

Maillot F, Lilburn M, Baudin J, et al: Factors influencing outcomes in the offspring of mothers with phenylketonuria during pregnancy: the importance of variation in maternal blood phenylalanine, *Clin Nutr* 88:700–705, 2008.

Maron BA, Loscalzo J: The treatment of hyperhomocysteinemia, *Annu Rev Med* 60:39–54, 2009.

McCabe LL, McCabe ERB: Expanded newborn screening: implications for genomic medicine, *Annu Rev Med* 59:163–175, 2008.

Meleady R, Graham I: Plasma homocysteine as a cardiovascular risk factor: causal, consequential, or of no consequence? *Nutr Rev* 57:299–305, 2009.

Morris SM: Regulation of enzymes of the urea cycle and arginine metabolism, *Annu Rev Nutr* 22:87–105, 2002.

Potter K, Hankey GJ, Green DJ, et al: Homocysteine or renal impairment: which is the real cardiovascular risk factor? *Arterioscler Thromb Vasc Biol* 28:1158–1164, 2008.

Richards NGJ, Kilberg MS: Asparagine synthetase chemotherapy, *Annu Rev Biochem* 75:629–654, 2006.

Watford M: Glutamine metabolism and function in relation to proline synthesis and the safety of glutamine and proline supplementation, *J Nutr* 138:2003S–2007S, 2008.

Yamaguchi Y, Brenner M, Hearing VJ: The regulation of skin pigmentation, *J Biol Chem* 282:27557–27561, 2007.

QUESTIONS

1. **A 4-month-old child is evaluated for irritability, vomiting after feeding, and delayed motor development. Blood tests show an ammonia level 10 to 20 times higher than the upper limit of normal, as well as marked elevations of ornithine and glutamine. Most likely, this child has a deficiency of the enzyme**

   A. Arginase
   B. Ornithine decarboxylase
   C. Glutaminase
   D. Ornithine transcarbamoylase
   E. Ornithine transglutaminase

2. **A 55-year-old alcoholic is brought to the hospital in a confused state. The emergency room physician notes that the patient's breath has a foul smell, but the patient has no sign of acute alcohol intoxication. A blood test shows an abnormally high ammonia level. The *worst* treatment for this patient would be to give him**

   A. A lot of good, protein-rich food
   B. Benzoic acid or phenylacetic acid
   C. A diet low in proteins but with plenty of vitamins
   D. A broad-spectrum antibiotic to eliminate intestinal bacteria

3. **The urine of untreated phenylketonuric patients contains all of the following substances, *except***

   A. Phenylalanine
   B. Tyrosine
   C. Phenylpyruvate
   D. Phenyllactate

4. **Under normal conditions, the kidneys excrete a small amount of nitrogen in the form of the ammonium ion rather than as urea. The amount of urinary ammonium ion is greatly increased in patients who suffer from**

   A. Phenylketonuria
   B. Fat malabsorption
   C. Hartnup disease
   D. Glutaminase deficiency
   E. Chronic acidosis

5. **All transamination reactions require the coenzyme**

   A. Tetrahydrofolate
   B. Thiamin pyrophosphate
   C. Pyridoxal phosphate
   D. Biotin
   E. SAM

Chapter 27
HEME METABOLISM

Heme is a tightly bound prosthetic group of hemoglobin, myoglobin, the cytochromes, and other proteins. It is bound to its apoproteins either noncovalently, as in hemoglobin and myoglobin, or by a covalent bond, as in cytochrome *c*. Heme consists of a porphyrin, known as **protoporphyrin IX,** with an iron chelate in its center. The porphyrin system consists of four pyrrole rings linked by methine (—CH=) bridges:

Heme
(Fe-protoporphyrin IX)

The conjugated (alternating) double bonds absorb visible light. Therefore *the heme proteins are colored.* **Porphyrinogens** are important intermediates in heme biosynthesis. Their pyrrole rings are connected by methylene (—CH$_2$—) bridges, and they do not absorb light because the double bonds do not alternate with single bonds over the whole system:

Protoporphyrinogen IX
(a porphyrinogon)

Porphyrinogens are prone to nonenzymatic oxidation to the corresponding porphyrins.

Although a small amount of dietary heme is absorbed in the small intestine, *essentially all the heme in the human body is derived from endogenous synthesis.* This chapter describes the pathways for the biosynthesis and degradation of heme and the diseases in which these pathways are disrupted.

BONE MARROW AND LIVER ARE THE MOST IMPORTANT SITES OF HEME SYNTHESIS

The 800 to 900 g of hemoglobin in the adult body contains 30 to 35 g of heme. From 250 to 300 mg of heme is synthesized in the red bone marrow every day, most of this in the erythroblasts and proerythroblasts. *The bone marrow accounts for 70% to 80% of the total heme synthesis in the body.*

The second most important site is the liver because of its high content of cytochrome P-450, which accounts for 65% of the total heme in the liver (see Chapter 30). P-450 enzymes are concerned with the inactivation of drugs and other foreign molecules, and the transcription of their genes is stimulated by many drugs. These enzymes have far shorter half-lives than does hemoglobin. Therefore hepatic heme synthesis is quite productive, accounting for approximately 15% of the total.

HEME IS SYNTHESIZED FROM SUCCINYL-COENZYME A AND GLYCINE

Heme biosynthesis starts with the formation of Δ-aminolevulinate from succinyl-coenzyme A (succinyl-CoA) and glycine, catalyzed by the heme-containing, vitamin B_6–dependent enzyme **δ-aminolevulinate (ALA) synthase.** This is the committed step of the pathway shown in *Figure 27.1.*

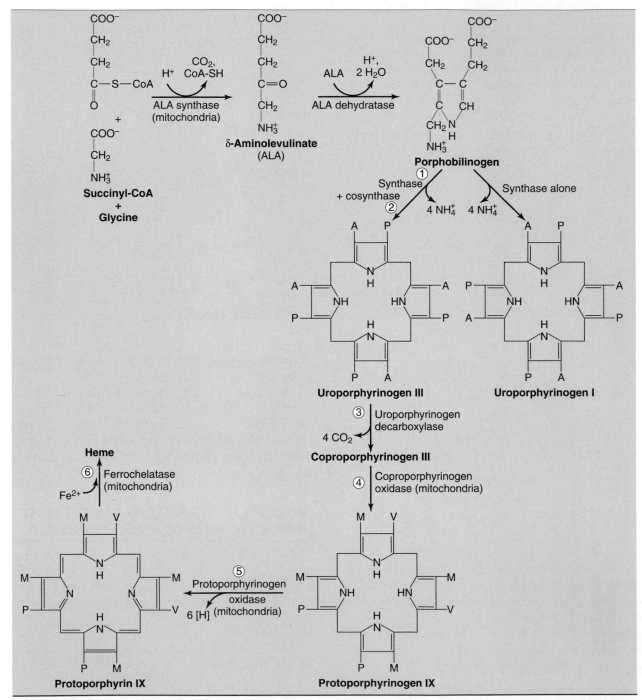

Figure 27.1 Pathway of heme biosynthesis. The numbered reactions refer to numbers listed in *Table 27.1. A,* Acetate (carboxymethyl) group; *M,* methyl group; *P,* propionate (carboxyethyl) group; *V,* vinyl group.

The second reaction, catalyzed by **ALA dehydratase,** forms the pyrrole ring of **porphobilinogen.** The third enzyme, **uroporphyrinogen I synthase** (also called **porphobilinogen deaminase),** links together four molecules of porphobilinogen. Left on its own, the synthase produces **uroporphyrinogen I.** In the cell, however, a second protein, **uroporphyrinogen III cosynthase,** channels the reaction into the formation of the isomer **uroporphyrinogen III.** All naturally occurring porphyrins, including heme, belong to the III series. Uroporphyrinogen III is processed to heme by the reactions shown in *Figure 27.1.*

The first reaction and the last three reactions of the pathway are mitochondrial. The others are cytoplasmic. *ALA synthase is the regulated enzyme.* ALA synthase has an unusually short biological half-life of 1 to 3 hours in the liver, and *its synthesis is very effectively suppressed by heme.* Only free, nonprotein-bound heme acts as a feedback inhibitor.

PORPHYRIAS ARE CAUSED BY DEFICIENCIES OF HEME-SYNTHESIZING ENZYMES

The porphyrias (*Table 27.1*) are caused by a *partial deficiency of one of the heme-synthesizing enzymes other than ALA synthase.* Any one of the numbered enzymes shown in *Figure 27.1* can be affected. A complete deficiency would be fatal, and the offending mutations are generally expressed as autosomal dominant traits; affected heterozygotes have 50% of the normal enzyme activity. Clinically, we can distinguish between *hepatic porphyrias* and *erythropoietic porphyrias.*

Clinical abnormalities in the porphyrias are caused not by heme deficiency but by the accumulation of metabolic intermediates. The substrate of the partly deficient enzyme accumulates in situations in which ALA synthase activity is high. Two types of toxic effect are especially common:

1. *Neurological abnormalities* are seen in many porphyrias because some intermediates of heme biosynthesis are neurotoxic. Abdominal pain is a frequent symptom, most likely because visceral pain fibers are stimulated by the accumulating metabolic intermediates.

2. *Cutaneous photosensitivity* is typical for porphyrias in which porphyrins or porphyrinogens accumulate. The porphyrinogens are oxidized nonenzymatically to the corresponding porphyrins. In the skin, the porphyrins become photoexcited by the action of sunlight, which leads to the formation of highly reactive and therefore toxic singlet oxygen. These porphyrias frequently result in unusually dark or colorful urine. The color deepens when the urine is exposed to light and air because of the nonenzymatic oxidation of the porphyrinogens to porphyrins.

Two enzymes of heme synthesis, ALA dehydratase and ferrochelatase, are sensitive to inhibition by lead. This results in increased levels of urinary ALA and an increased concentration of protoporphyrin IX in erythrocytes. Some of the neurological impairments in lead poisoning are attributed to the accumulation of these metabolites in nervous tissue.

Table 27.1   The Porphyrias

Enzyme Deficiency[†]	Disease (Class)	Inheritance	Signs and Symptoms*			
			Visceral	**Neurological**	**Cutaneous**	**Laboratory Tests**
1	Acute intermittent (hepatic)	AD	++	++	−	Urinary ALA, urinary PBG
2	Congenital erythropoietic (erythropoietic)	AR			+++	Urinary uroporphyrin,[‡] urinary coproporphyrin,[‡] fecal coproporphyrin[‡]
3	Porphyria cutanea tarda (hepatic)	AD[§]			++	Urinary uroporphyrin, urinary uroporphyrin, coproporphyrin
4	Hereditary coproporphyria (hepatic)	AD	+	+	(+)	Urinary ALA, urinary PBG, urinary coproporphyrin, urinary uroporphyrin
5	Variegate porphyria (hepatic)	AD	++	++	+	Urinary ALA, urinary PBG, urinary coproporphyrin, fecal protoporphyrin, fecal coproporphyrin
6	Protoporphyria (erythropoietic)	AD			+	Fecal protoporphyrin, RBC protoporphyrin

*Severity ranging from minimal (+) to profound (+++).
[†]Numbers refer to numbered reactions in Figure 27.1.
[‡]Type I uroporphyrin and coproporphyrin are elevated.
[§]In many cases, no specific inheritance can be demonstrated.
AD, Autosomal dominant; *ALA,* δ-aminolevulinate; *AR,* autosomal recessive; *PBG,* porphobilinogen; *RBC,* red blood cell.

CLINICAL EXAMPLE 27.1: Acute Intermittent Porphyria

Acute intermittent porphyria (AIP) is caused by a dominantly inherited deficiency of uroporphyrinogen I synthase (porphobilinogen deaminase). The enzyme activity is reduced to 50% of normal in all tissues, but clinical manifestations are related to impaired heme synthesis in the liver because the activity of this enzyme, in relation to the other heme biosynthetic enzymes, is rather low in this organ.

Only 10% of individuals with the genetic trait ever show clinical manifestations. They experience episodes of abdominal pain, constipation, muscle weakness, and cardiovascular abnormalities. Agitation, seizures, or mental derangement may be present. These episodes last from a few days to several months and are attributed to the accumulation of aminolevulinic acid (ALA) and porphobilinogen in blood and cerebrospinal fluid. Although these metabolites originate in the liver, they cause most of the symptoms by acting on the central and peripheral nervous systems.

Acute attacks of AIP can be precipitated by barbiturates, phenytoin, griseofulvin, and other drugs that induce the synthesis of **cytochrome P-450.** When the P-450 proteins are induced by drugs, the small amount of free, unbound heme in the liver rapidly binds to the newly synthesized apoenzymes. This depletes the pool of free, unbound heme, and heme depletion derepresses ALA synthase. ALA and porphobilinogen accumulate when the activity of ALA synthase exceeds the activity of uroporphyrinogen I synthase.

The symptoms of AIP are not accompanied by specific physical findings and are often misdiagnosed as "psychosomatic." The patient is treated symptomatically with sedative-hypnotics, tranquilizers, or anticonvulsants. These drugs aggravate the condition by inducing cytochrome P-450 synthesis in the liver. Patients have died of this treatment.

Adequate treatment consists of the withdrawal of any offending drugs and the infusion of **hematin,** a stable derivative of heme in which the heme iron is in the ferric form. Like heme, hematin represses the synthesis of ALA synthase. A carbohydrate-rich diet is prescribed for long-term management because it represses the synthesis of ALA synthase. Conversely, attacks of porphyria can be precipitated by dieting.

CLINICAL EXAMPLE 27.2: Porphyria Cutanea Tarda

The most common porphyria is porphyria cutanea tarda. Although some cases are caused by a dominantly inherited defect of uroporphyrinogen decarboxylase, this disease is expressed mainly in people with alcoholism or liver damage. Iron overload is an important factor because the affected enzyme is sensitive to inhibition by iron salts.

This porphyria produces no neurological or abdominal symptoms, but *the patient presents with cutaneous photosensitivity.* The condition is most common in older men during the summer months. It is treated by the avoidance of sunlight, abstinence from alcohol, and phlebotomy for the reduction of iron overload.

HEME IS DEGRADED TO BILIRUBIN

From 300 to 400 mg of heme is degraded in the human body every day, and close to 80% of this is derived from hemoglobin. The splenic macrophages that dispose of senile erythrocytes convert heme first to the green pigment **biliverdin** and then to yellow **bilirubin.** The heme oxygenase that catalyzes the first of these reactions is the only known CO-forming enzyme in the human body (*Fig. 27.2*).

The stages of heme degradation can be observed in the color changes of a hematoma (e.g., when a punch to the face leaves a "black eye"). After rupture of the capillaries, red blood cells are stranded in the interstitial spaces, in which their hemoglobin becomes deoxygenated. Deoxyhemoglobin is blue. Within a few days, the erythrocytes are scavenged by tissue macrophages, and the heme is degraded first to biliverdin and then to bilirubin. The blue coloration disappears and is replaced by first a greenish and then a yellow color.

BILIRUBIN IS CONJUGATED AND EXCRETED BY THE LIVER

From the macrophages, bilirubin is transported to the liver in tight, noncovalent binding to serum albumin. It enters the hepatocytes on a facilitated-diffusion type carrier of high capacity and is then conjugated to bilirubin diglucuronide by two successive reactions with uridine diphosphate (UDP)-glucuronic acid. The water-soluble bilirubin diglucuronide is actively secreted into the bile canaliculi against a steep concentration gradient. From 60% to 80% of the bilirubin in the bile is bilirubin diglucuronide, and 20% to 40% is bilirubin monoglucuronide.

In the intestine, bacteria deconjugate the biliary bilirubin and reduce it to uncolored **urobilinogens.** Some of the urobilinogens are oxidized to urobilins and other colored products, which are responsible for the brown color of the stools. A small amount of urobilinogen is absorbed in the terminal ileum, returned to the liver, and secreted in the bile. Less than 4 mg/day finds its way to the kidneys, to be excreted in the urine.

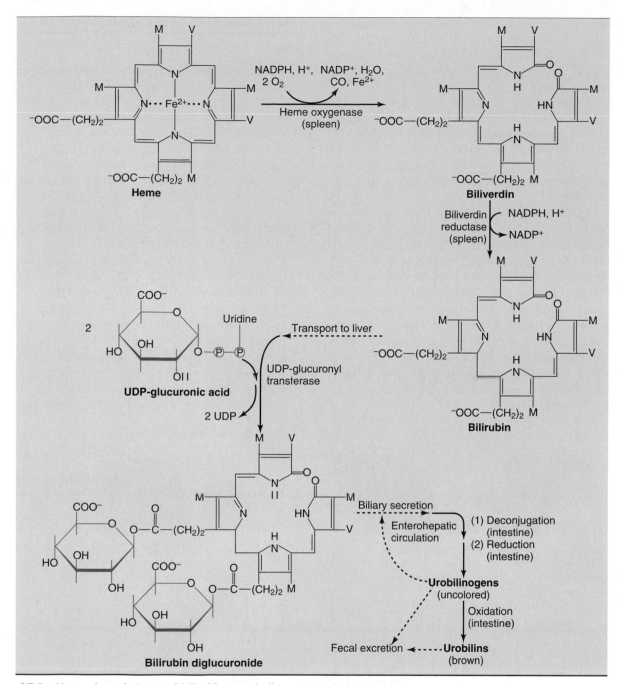

Figure 27.2 Heme degradation and bilirubin metabolism. *M*, Methyl; *V*, vinyl.

ELEVATIONS OF SERUM BILIRUBIN CAUSE JAUNDICE

Normal blood contains less than 17 μmol/L (1 mg/dl) of bilirubin. Most of this is unconjugated bilirubin in transit from the spleen to the liver. Elevations of either conjugated or unconjugated bilirubin are called **hyperbilirubinemia**. Both types of hyperbilirubinemia lead to the deposition of bilirubin in the skin and the sclera of the eye. The resulting yellow discoloration is called **jaundice** or **icterus**. It appears when the serum bilirubin level rises above 70 μmol/L (4 mg/dl). The sclera of the eye is affected early because of its high content of elastin, for which bilirubin has a high affinity. However, there are two important differences between conjugated and unconjugated bilirubin:

1. *Only unconjugated bilirubin, which is lipid soluble, can enter the brain*, especially in infants. Bilirubin deposition in the basal ganglia can cause irreversible brain damage, a condition known as **kernicterus** (from German *kern* meaning "nucleus"). Kernicterus in infants can be rapidly fatal. Many survivors suffer permanent neurological impairments, including an athetoid motor disorder, oculomotor palsy, ataxia, spasticity, and mental deficiency. At a normal

albumin concentration of 4 g/dl, up to 25 mg/dl of bilirubin is transported in tight, noncovalent association with a high-affinity binding site on this plasma protein. Kernicterus develops only at bilirubin levels above this limit.

2. *Only conjugated bilirubin is excreted by the kidneys.* Unconjugated bilirubin cannot be excreted because it is tightly bound to albumin, but conjugated bilirubin is water soluble and not protein bound. Therefore it is excreted in the urine, to which it imparts a yellow-brown coloration. This is called **choluric jaundice.**

Rarely, hyperbilirubinemia is caused by an inherited defect of bilirubin metabolism. Complete deficiency of the bilirubin-UDP glucuronyl transferase leads a rare condition called **Crigler-Najjar syndrome type I.** It is characterized by unconjugated bilirubin in excess of 20 mg/dl and kernicterus. Partial deficiencies of the enzyme, diagnosed as **Crigler-Najjar syndrome type II,** have a better prognosis. Inherited defects affecting the secretion of conjugated bilirubin, including **Dubin-Johnson syndrome,** and **Rotor syndrome,** are benign conditions with conjugated hyperbilirubinemia. *Clinical Examples 27.3* through *27.5* describe more common forms of hyperbilirubinemia.

MANY DISEASES CAN CAUSE JAUNDICE

Jaundice can originate at three levels (*Fig. 27.3*):

1. **Prehepatic jaundice,** also called **hemolytic jaundice,** is the consequence of severe hemolytic conditions in which a large amount of bilirubin is formed from heme. The excess bilirubin is unconjugated bilirubin in transit from the spleen to the liver. Because an increased amount of bilirubin diglucuronide reaches the intestine, more urobilinogen is formed by intestinal bacteria, and the levels of urobilinogen in blood and urine are increased. Most livers have a substantial spare capacity for the conjugation and excretion of bilirubin. Therefore the bilirubin level rarely exceeds 3 to 4 mg/dl.

2. **Hepatic jaundice** is caused by parenchymal liver diseases. Viral hepatitis is the most common cause of acute hepatic jaundice, and liver cirrhosis can lead to chronic jaundice. Because both bilirubin conjugation and the energy-dependent secretion of conjugated bilirubin into the bile are impaired, both forms of bilirubin are elevated to variable extents. As long as bile flow is uninterrupted, urobilinogen is elevated in blood and urine because the diseased liver loses its ability to scavenge urobilinogen from the portal

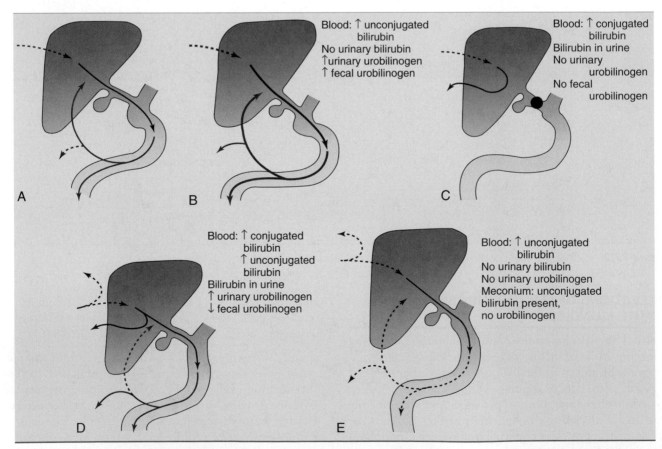

Figure 27.3 Bilirubin and urobilinogen in different types of jaundice. *Dashed black line* represents unconjugated bilirubin; *solid line* represents conjugated bilirubin; *red line* represents urobilinogen. **A,** Normal pattern. **B,** Hemolysis. **C,** Biliary obstruction. **D,** Hepatitis (no cholestasis). **E,** Physiological jaundice of the newborn.

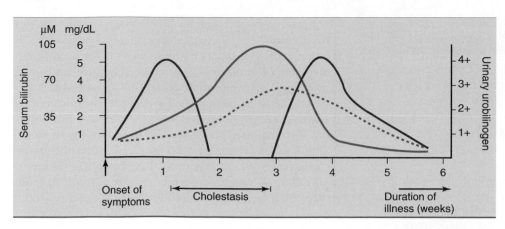

Figure 27.4 Levels of serum bilirubin and urinary urobilinogen in a patient with acute viral hepatitis. *Dashed blue line* represents unconjugated bilirubin; *solid blue line* represents conjugated bilirubin; *red line* represents urobilinogen. Urobilinogen is increased as long as the disease does not lead to cholestasis but disappears as soon as cholestasis develops.

circulation. However, if cholestasis occurs in the course of the illness, urobilinogen disappears (*Fig. 27.4*).

3. **Posthepatic jaundice,** also called **cholestatic jaundice,** is caused by biliary obstruction, either at the level of the common bile duct or at the level of the bile canaliculi in the liver. It can result from an impacted gallstone, cancer in the head of the pancreas compressing the common bile duct, liver diseases that are severe enough to prevent the formation of bile, or autoimmune destruction of the bile canaliculi (*Clinical Example 27.5*). Bilirubin still is conjugated, but the conjugated bilirubin cannot reach the intestine. It overflows into the blood. Urobilinogen, normally formed from bilirubin by intestinal bacteria, disappears from blood, stool, and urine. In complete biliary obstruction, the stools lose their normal brown color, which is caused by urobilins and their polymerization products, and appear clay colored. However, the urine is colored yellow-brown by bilirubin diglucuronide. *Liver function is unimpaired in acute biliary obstruction, but long-standing cholestasis causes irreversible liver damage.*

CLINICAL EXAMPLE 27.3: Physiological Jaundice of the Newborn

In most infants, the serum bilirubin concentration rises from 1 to 2 mg/dl at birth to about 5 to 6 mg/dl at day 3. The level then gradually declines to 1 mg/dl over the following week. Up to 50% of all newborns become visibly jaundiced during the first 5 days after birth; in 16%, the serum bilirubin concentration reaches 10 mg/dl or higher; and in 5%, the serum bilirubin rises above 15 mg/dl.

Physiological jaundice of the newborn is caused by *immaturity of the bilirubin-metabolizing system of the liver.* The uptake of unconjugated bilirubin, the activity of the conjugating enzymes, the intracellular level of UDP-glucuronic acid, and the biliary secretion of conjugated bilirubin all are low in the neonate. To make matters worse, bilirubin diglucuronide is deconjugated by β-glucuronidase in the intestine and in breast milk,

but no bacterial flora is present in the intestine to convert bilirubin to urobilinogen. Some of this unconjugated bilirubin is absorbed and contributes to the hyperbilirubinemia.

The milder forms of physiological jaundice require no treatment. However, *there is a risk of kernicterus.* Therefore increases of serum bilirubin above 15 mg/dl must be prevented. In **phototherapy,** the baby is put under bright light. This safe, noninvasive treatment causes a photochemical isomerization of bilirubin in the skin. The geometrical isomers thus formed are more water soluble than native bilirubin and can be excreted in the bile without conjugation.

Administration of **phenobarbital** is indicated when the bilirubin level remains dangerously high despite phototherapy. This drug induces the synthesis of the bilirubin-conjugating enzymes.

Factors that increase the likelihood and severity of neonatal jaundice include breastfeeding, glucose-6-phosphate dehydrogenase deficiency, and Gilbert syndrome (see *Clinical Example 27.4*). Hemolytic conditions are especially dangerous. In **rhesus incompatibility,** a maternal immunoglobulin G antibody to a fetal blood group antigen causes severe hemolysis in the newborn. In some cases, exchange transfusion is required immediately after birth or even before birth.

CLINICAL EXAMPLE 27.4: Gilbert Syndrome

Gilbert syndrome is a benign condition in which mildly elevated unconjugated bilirubin is the only abnormality. It is caused by homozygosity for a mutation in the TATA box of the gene for bilirubin-UDP glucuronyl transferase. Affected individuals have only 30% of the enzyme. Nine percent of Europeans are homozygous for the promoter variant, and 50% are heterozygous. However, only some homozygotes have hyperbilirubinemia.

CLINICAL EXAMPLE 27.5: Primary Biliary Cirrhosis

In some cases, intrahepatic biliary obstruction results from an autoimmune disease called primary biliary cirrhosis. It is characterized by antimitochondrial antibodies and inflammation in the epithelium of small intrahepatic bile ducts. Markers of biliary obstruction, including plasma levels of bile acids, conjugated bilirubin, alkaline phosphatase, and γ-glutamyltransferase, are elevated. If untreated, most cases progress to liver cirrhosis.

Primary biliary cirrhosis affects mainly middle-aged women. Treatment is based on the administration of **ursodeoxycholic acid**, either alone or with an antiinflammatory and immunosuppressant steroid. Ursodeoxycholic acid is a minor bile acid in humans. It is less cytotoxic than the major bile acids, and it stimulates bile flow.

SUMMARY

Heme is synthesized in bone marrow, liver, and other tissues that produce heme proteins. The pathway starts with the formation of δ-aminolevulinic acid (ALA) from succinyl-CoA and glycine. This reaction, catalyzed by ALA synthase, is feedback inhibited by free, nonprotein-bound heme. In the porphyrias, one of the biosynthetic enzymes other than ALA synthase is impaired by genetic or environmental insults. Toxic intermediates of heme biosynthesis accumulate, leading to neurological symptoms or cutaneous photosensitivity.

The heme of hemoglobin is degraded to bilirubin by macrophages in the spleen and other organs. The bilirubin is transported to the liver in tight binding to serum albumin. The liver conjugates bilirubin to bilirubin diglucuronide for secretion into the bile. Elevations of serum bilirubin, known as hyperbilirubinemia, result in jaundice. Unconjugated hyperbilirubinemia occurs under hemolytic conditions and in otherwise normal newborns; conjugated hyperbilirubinemia results from conditions in which bile flow is blocked (cholestasis). Mixed hyperbilirubinemia is typical for nonspecific liver diseases, including viral hepatitis and toxic liver damage.

Further Reading

Kumagi T, Heathcote EJ: Primary biliary cirrhosis, *Orphanet J Rare Dis* 3(1) 2008 (online).

Lindor K: Ursodeoxycholic acid for the treatment of primary biliary cirrhosis, *N Engl J Med* 357:1524–1529, 2007.

Phillips JD, Kushner JP: Fast track to the porphyrias, *Nat Med* 11:1049–1050, 2005.

Puy H, Gouya L, Deybach JC: Porphyrias, *Lancet* 375:924–937, 2010.

QUESTIONS

1. **Porphyrias can be caused by a reduced activity of any of the following enzymes** *except*

   A. Ferrochelatase
   B. Uroporphyrinogen decarboxylase
   C. Uroporphyrinogen synthase
   D. ALA synthase
   E. Protoporphyrinogen oxidase

2. **A combination of elevated conjugated bilirubin, near-normal unconjugated bilirubin, and absence of fecal urobilinogen in a jaundiced patient suggests**

   A. Mild hepatitis
   B. Cholestasis
   C. Hemolysis
   D. Absence of bilirubin-UDP glucuronyl transferase
   E. Gilbert syndrome

Chapter 28
THE METABOLISM OF PURINES AND PYRIMIDINES

The purine and pyrimidine bases (*Fig. 28.1*) are constituents of nucleotides and nucleic acids. The **ribonucleotides** adenosine triphosphate (ATP), guanosine triphosphate (GTP), uridine triphosphate (UTP), and cytidine triphosphate (CTP) are present in millimolar concentrations in the cell. They serve important coenzyme functions in addition to being precursors of RNA synthesis. The **deoxyribonucleotides** deoxyadenosine triphosphate (dATP), deoxyguanosine triphosphate (dGTP), deoxycytidine triphosphate (dCTP), and deoxythymidine triphosphate (dTTP) are present in micromolar concentrations and are required only for DNA replication and DNA repair. Their cellular concentrations are highest during S phase of the cell cycle.

Dietary nucleic acids and nucleotides are digested to nucleosides and free bases in the intestine, but the products are poorly absorbed. Especially the absorbed purine bases are extensively degraded in the intestinal mucosa. Therefore *humans depend on the endogenous synthesis of purines and pyrimidines*. This chapter discusses the pathways for the synthesis and degradation of the nucleotides.

PURINE SYNTHESIS STARTS WITH RIBOSE-5-PHOSPHATE

De novo synthesis of purines is most active in the liver, which exports the bases and nucleosides to other tissues. Most tissues have a limited capacity for de novo purine synthesis, although they can synthesize the nucleotides from externally supplied bases.

The pathway of purine biosynthesis is shown in *Figure 28.2*. It starts with ribose-5-phosphate, a product of the pentose phosphate pathway (see Chapter 22). In the reactions of the pathway, all of them cytoplasmic, *the purine ring system is built up step by step, with C-1 of ribose-5-phosphate used as a primer.*

The first enzyme, **5-phosphoribosyl-1-pyrophosphate (PRPP) synthetase,** transfers a pyrophosphate group from ATP to C-1 of ribose-5-phosphate, forming **PRPP.** *PRPP is the activated form of ribose for nucleotide synthesis.* The next enzyme, **PRPP amidotransferase,** replaces the pyrophosphate group of PRPP with a nitrogen from the side chain of glutamine. *This reaction is the committed step of purine biosynthesis.* In the following reactions, the purine ring is constructed from simple building blocks:

where THF = tetrahydrofolate. The first nucleotide formed in the pathway is **inosine monophosphate (IMP),** which contains the base **hypoxanthine.** IMP is a branch point in the synthesis of AMP and GMP (*Fig. 28.3*). These nucleoside monophosphates are in equilibrium with their corresponding diphosphates and triphosphates through kinase reactions.

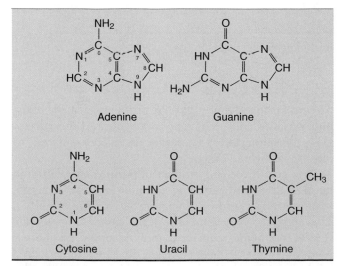

Figure 28.1 Structures of the purine and pyrimidine bases.

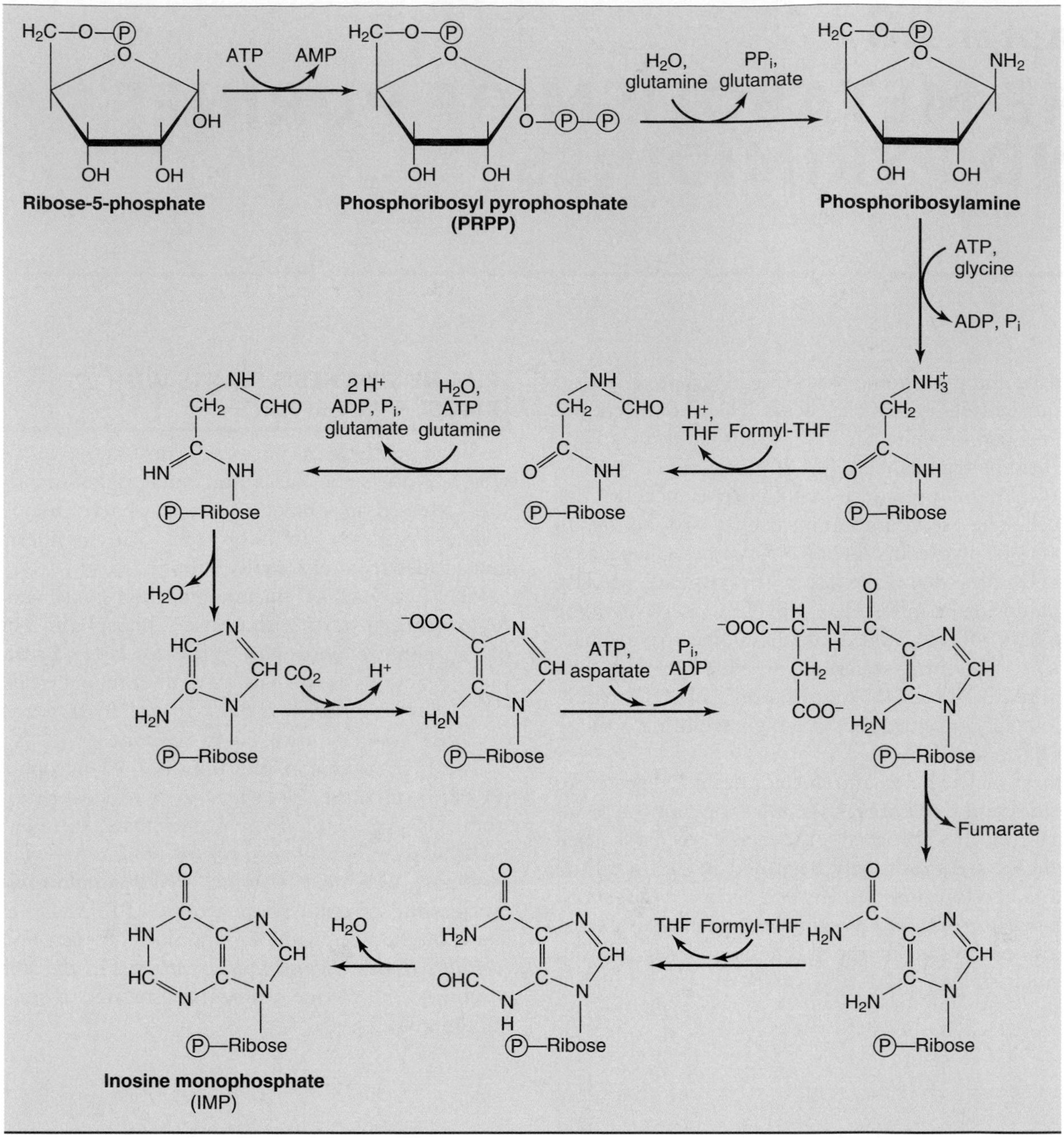

Figure 28.2 De novo pathway of purine biosynthesis. *THF*, Tetrahydrofolate.

As expected, purine synthesis is regulated by feedback inhibition (*Fig. 28.4*). *The first two enzymes of the pathway, PRPP synthetase and PRPP amidotransferase, are inhibited by the purine nucleotides.* In addition, the reactions leading from IMP to AMP and GMP are feedback inhibited by the end products.

PURINES ARE DEGRADED TO URIC ACID

The degradation of purine nucleotides starts with the hydrolytic removal of phosphate from the nucleotides. The nucleosides thus formed are then cleaved into free base and ribose-1-phosphate by **purine nucleoside phosphorylase**. Adenosine is a poor substrate of the nucleoside phosphorylase. Therefore it is deaminated to inosine first (*Fig. 28.5*).

Uric acid is the end product of purine degradation in humans. It is synthesized by **xanthine oxidase** via hypoxanthine and xanthine (reaction ⑥ in *Figure 28.5*). This enzyme contains flavin adenine dinucleotide (FAD), nonheme iron, and molybdenum. Like other nonmitochondrial flavoproteins, it regenerates its FAD by transferring hydrogen from $FADH_2$ to molecular oxygen, forming hydrogen peroxide.

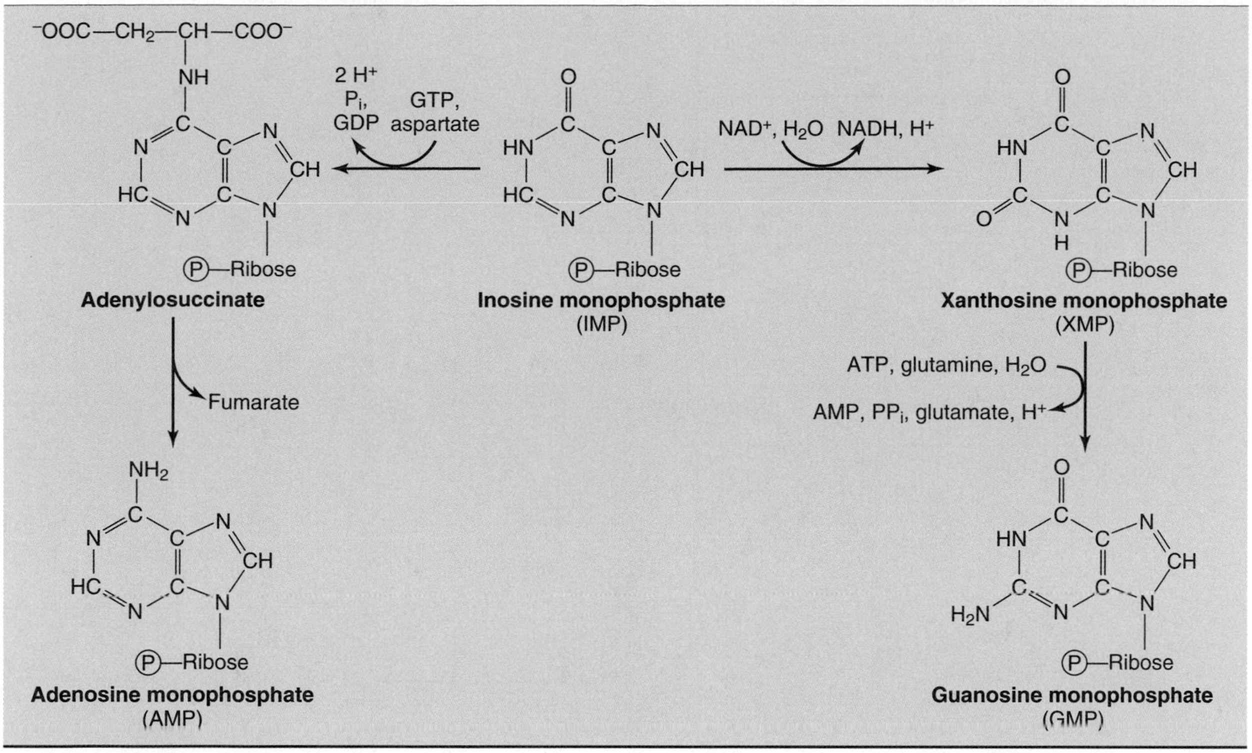

Figure 28.3 Synthesis of AMP and GMP from IMP.

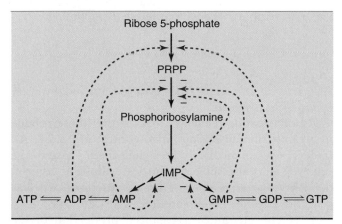

Figure 28.4 Feedback inhibition of de novo purine biosynthesis by nucleotides. *ADP,* Adenosine diphosphate; *AMP,* adenosine monophosphate; *ATP,* adenosine triphosphate; *GDP,* guanosine diphosphate; *GMP,* guanosine monophosphate; *GTP,* guanosine triphosphate; *IMP,* Inosine monophosphate; *PRPP,* 5-phosphoribosyl-1-pyrophosphate.

FREE PURINE BASES CAN BE SALVAGED

As an alternative to degradation, the free bases can be recycled into the nucleotide pool. This requires the PRPP-dependent salvage enzymes **hypoxanthine-guanine phosphoribosyltransferase (HGPRT)** and **adenine phosphoribosyl transferase (APRT):**

$$\text{Hypoxanthine} + \text{PRPP} \xrightarrow{\text{HGPRT}} \text{IMP} + \text{PP}_i$$

$$\text{Guanine} + \text{PRPP} \xrightarrow{\text{HGPRT}} \text{GMP} + \text{PP}_i$$

$$\text{Adenine} + \text{PRPP} \xrightarrow{\text{APRT}} \text{AMP} + \text{PP}_i$$

The salvage reactions are the only source of purine nucleotides for tissues that cannot synthesize the nucleotides de novo. HGPRT is quantitatively by far the more important salvage enzyme because most of the adenine is released as hypoxanthine. HGPRT is competitively inhibited by IMP and GMP, whereas APRT is inhibited by AMP.

PYRIMIDINES ARE SYNTHESIZED FROM CARBAMOYL PHOSPHATE AND ASPARTATE

Most proliferating cells synthesize pyrimidines de novo, whereas quiescent cells synthesize pyrimidine nucleotides from imported bases. Most cancer cells have highly active de novo pyrimidine synthesis.

Unlike the purine ring, the pyrimidine ring is synthesized before the ribose is added (*Fig. 28.6*). The pathway starts with **carbamoyl phosphate** and **aspartate,** and **orotic acid** is formed as the first pyrimidine. Orotic acid is processed to the uridine nucleotides, which are the precursors of the cytidine nucleotides. The enzymes of the pathway are cytosolic except for dihydroorotate dehydrogenase (reaction ④ in *Figure 28.6*), which is on the outer surface of the inner mitochondrial membrane.

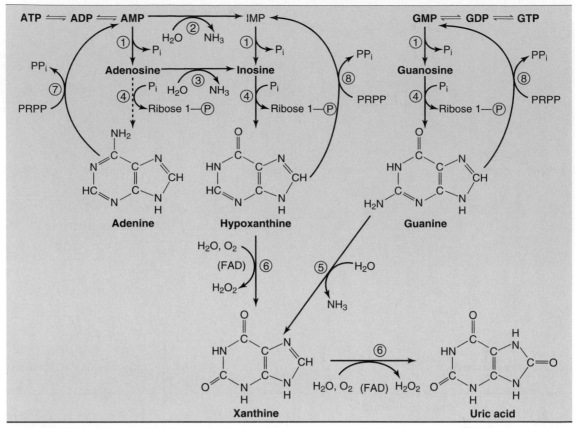

Figure 28.5 Degradation of purine nucleotides to uric acid, and the salvage of purine bases. (1), 5'-Nucleotidase; (2), AMP deaminase; (3), adenosine deaminase; (4), purine nucleoside phosphorylase; (5), guanine deaminase; (6), xanthine oxidase; (7), adenine phosphoribosyltransferase; (8), hypoxanthine-guanine phosphoribosyltransferase. *IMP*, Inosine monophosphate; *PRPP*, 5-phosphoribosyl-1-pyrophosphate.

The carbamoyl phosphate for pyrimidine biosynthesis is synthesized by the cytoplasmic **carbamoyl phosphate synthetase II.** Unlike the mitochondrial enzyme, which makes carbamoyl phosphate for the urea cycle, the cytoplasmic enzyme uses the side chain of glutamine as a source of nitrogen.

The first three enzymes of the pathway, including carbamoyl phosphate synthetase II, aspartate transcarbamoylase, and dihydroorotate dehydrogenase (enzymes 1, 2, and 3 in *Fig. 28.6*), are formed by different domains of a single large polypeptide. Both this multienzyme complex and the CTP synthetase are feedback inhibited by CTP.

An inhibitor of dihydroorotate dehydrogenase, **leflunomide,** blocks pyrimidine biosynthesis. It has been used as an immunomodulatory drug for the treatment of rheumatoid arthritis and psoriatic arthritis.

The pyrimidines are degraded to water-soluble products that are either excreted as such or oxidized to carbon dioxide and water (*Fig. 28.7*).

DNA SYNTHESIS REQUIRES DEOXYRIBONUCLEOTIDES

The synthesis of 2-deoxyribonucleotides from the corresponding ribonucleotides requires two reactions: *reduction of ribose to 2-deoxyribose* and *methylation of uracil to thymine.*

Ribonucleotide reductase reduces the ribose residue in all four ribonucleoside diphosphates (*Fig. 28.8, A*). Its level rises immediately preceding the S phase of the cell cycle. It is also subject to intricate allosteric control. dATP is a negative effector for all reactions, whereas other nucleotides modulate the substrate specificity and thereby guarantee a balanced production of the four deoxyribonucleotides.

Thymine is synthesized by **thymidylate synthase.** In this reaction, the methylene group of tetrahydrofolate is reduced to a methyl group during its transfer to dUMP, and tetrahydrofolate is oxidized to dihydrofolate (see *Fig. 28.8, B*). The active coenzyme form, tetrahydrofolate, has to be regenerated by **dihydrofolate reductase** (see *Fig. 28.8, C*).

MANY ANTINEOPLASTIC DRUGS INHIBIT NUCLEOTIDE METABOLISM

The development of drugs with selective toxicity for cancer cells is difficult because cancer cells are too similar to normal cells. Therefore drugs that kill cancer cells are likely to kill normal cells as well. Cancer cells

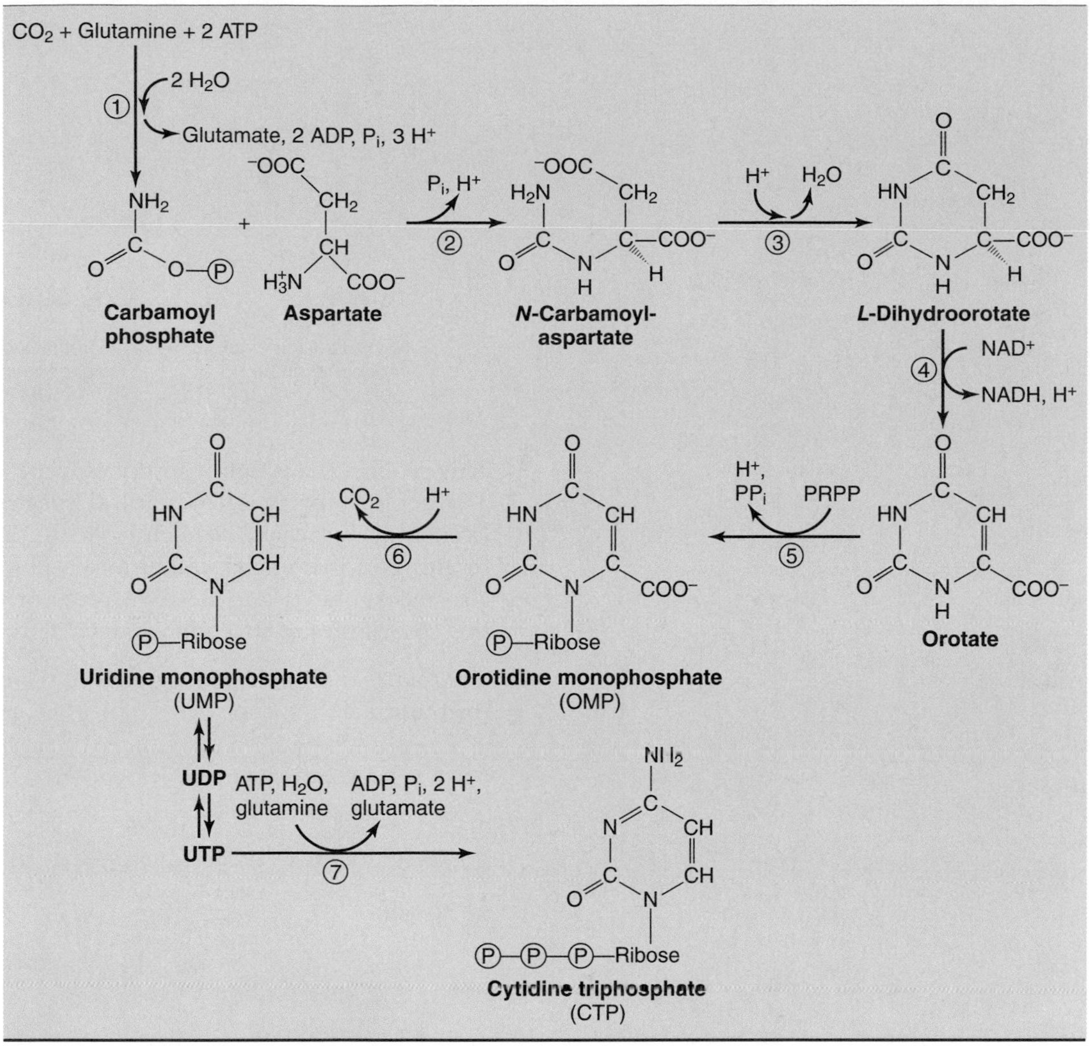

Figure 28.6 Biosynthesis of pyrimidine nucleotides. ①, Carbamoyl phosphate synthetase II; ②, aspartate transcarbamoylase; ③, dihydroorotase; ④, dihydroorotate dehydrogenase; ⑤, orotate phosphoribosyltransferase; ⑥, orotidylate decarboxylase; ⑦, CTP synthetase. *PRPP*, 5-Phosphoribosyl-1-pyrophosphate.

CLINICAL EXAMPLE 28.1: Hereditary Orotic Aciduria

Deficiencies of orotate phosphoribosyltransferase and/or orotidylate decarboxylase (reactions ⑤ and ⑥ in *Figure 28.6*), which are two enzymatic activities of a single protein, lead to hereditary orotic aciduria (*Table 28.1*). This rare condition is characterized by megaloblastic anemia, a crystalline sediment of orotic acid in the urine, and poor growth. The important clinical signs are caused not by orotic acid accumulation but by pyrimidine deficiency. The patients are pyrimidine auxotrophs who can be treated quite effectively with large doses of orally administered uridine.

Orotic aciduria is also seen in some urea cycle enzyme deficiencies, in which carbamoyl phosphate accumulates in liver mitochondria. Some of this leaks into the cytoplasm, where it is converted to orotic acid (see *Clinical Example 26.1*).

Table 28.1 Inherited Disorders of Purine and Pyrimidine Metabolism

Disease	Enzyme Deficiency	Signs and Symptoms
Adenosine deaminase deficiency	Adenosine deaminase	Severe combined immunodeficiency
Purine nucleoside phosphorylase deficiency	Purine nucleoside phosphorylase	Immunodeficiency with T-cell defect
Familial orotic aciduria	Orotate phosphoribosyltransferase	Accumulation of orotic acid in blood and urine, failure to thrive
Lesch-Nyhan syndrome	Hypoxanthine-guanine phosphoribosyltransferase	Mental retardation with self-mutilation, hyperuricemia

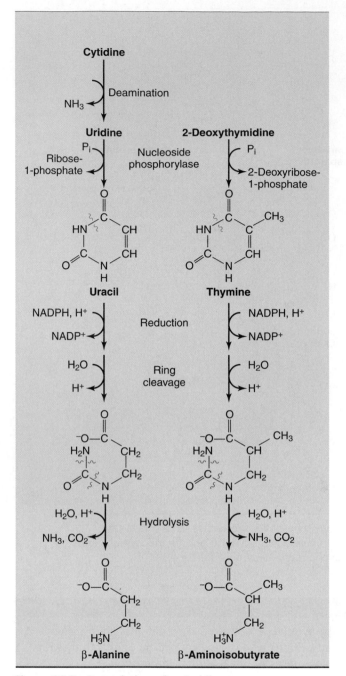

Figure 28.7 Degradation of pyrimidines.

do, however, have a higher mitotic rate than normal cells. Therefore *they have a higher requirement for DNA synthesis and nucleotide synthesis*. With this in mind, drugs have been developed as antagonists of nucleotide synthesis:

1. *Structural analogs of bases or nucleosides* act either as inhibitors of nucleotide biosynthesis or through their incorporation into DNA or RNA. **5-Fluorouracil** is used to treat cancers of the colon, pancreas, stomach, esophagus, and breast. It is processed to fluorodeoxyuridine monophosphate in the body:

5-Fluorodeoxyuridine monophosphate

Deoxyuridine monophosphate (dUMP)

This product binds tightly to thymidylate synthase as a structural analog of its natural substrate dUMP. Eventually it reacts covalently with the enzyme, resulting in irreversible inhibition. 5-Fluorouracil is also incorporated into RNA in place of uracil, and this contributes to its antineoplastic activity.

2. *Antifolates* are best exemplified by **amethopterin (methotrexate):**

Amethopterin (methotrexate)

Folic acid

Methotrexate inhibits dihydrofolate reductase competitively, thereby depleting the cell of tetrahydrofolate. Thymidylate synthase is the only important enzyme that converts a tetrahydrofolate coenzyme to dihydrofolate. Therefore rapidly dividing cells, with their high activity of this enzyme, are most vulnerable to methotrexate.

These anticancer drugs cause collateral damage to rapidly dividing cells in bone marrow, intestinal mucosa, and hair bulbs. Therefore bone marrow depression, diarrhea, and hair loss are common side effects of cancer chemotherapy.

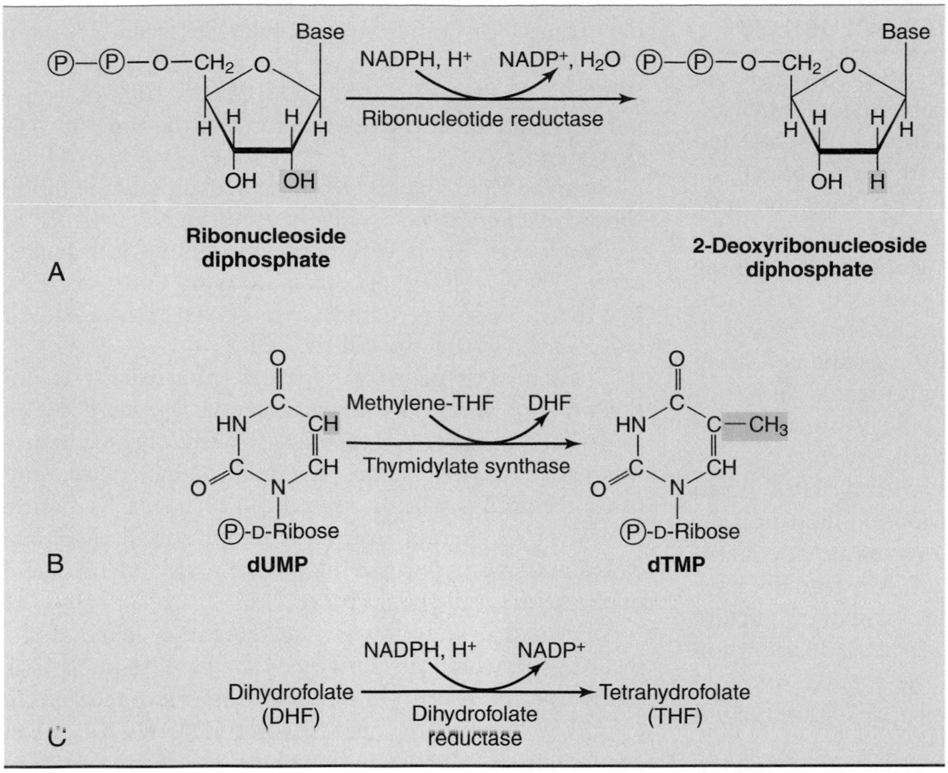

Figure 28.8 Synthesis of 2-deoxyribonucleotides, the precursors for DNA synthesis. *DHF*, Dihydrofolate; *dTMP*, deoxythymidine monophosphate; *dUMP*, deoxyuridine monophosphate; *THF*, tetrahydrofolate.

A **Ribonucleoside diphosphate** → **2-Deoxyribonucleoside diphosphate** (Ribonucleotide reductase; NADPH, H$^+$ → NADP$^+$, H$_2$O)

B **dUMP** → **dTMP** (Thymidylate synthase; Methylene-THF → DHF)

C Dihydrofolate (DHF) → Tetrahydrofolate (THF) (Dihydrofolate reductase; NADPH, H$^+$ → NADP$^+$)

CLINICAL EXAMPLE 28.2: Severe Combined Immunodeficiency

Deficiency of **adenosine deaminase (ADA)** leads to an autosomal recessive form of severe combined immunodeficiency (SCID), a type of disease with combined B-cell and T-cell defects. ADA deaminates adenosine to inosine and deoxyadenosine to deoxyinosine (*Fig. 28.9*).

Both adenosine and deoxyadenosine can also be phosphorylated to the corresponding nucleoside monophosphate. However, whereas AMP can be deaminated to IMP by AMP deaminase, dAMP has no alternative route of degradation. It accumulates, together with its diphosphate and triphosphate derivatives. dATP is thought to cause the immunodeficiency by inhibiting ribonucleotide reductase, thus depriving the cell of precursors for DNA synthesis. We do not know why lymphocytes are more sensitive than other cells to this metabolic defect.

Enzyme replacement therapy with injected bovine adenosine deaminase is possible, but its usefulness is limited by high cost and by immunological reactions to the injected enzyme. Gene therapy is more promising. For gene therapy, hematopoietic stem cells from the patient are treated in vitro with an ADA-containing retroviral vector. After partial destruction of the patient's bone marrow by chemotherapy, the engineered cells are reinserted in the patient. Unencumbered by ADA deficiency, the engineered cells can take over the ecosystem from the unmodified lymphocytes.

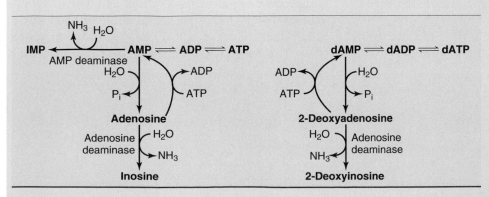

Figure 28.9 Role of adenosine deaminase in the metabolism of adenine nucleotides. The ribonucleotides can be catabolized by AMP deaminase, but the deoxyribonucleotides accumulate in adenosine deaminase deficiency. *dADP*, deoxy-ADP; *dAMP*, deoxy-AMP; *dATP*, deoxy-ATP; *IMP*, inosine monophosphate; *P$_i$*, inorganic phosphate.

URIC ACID HAS LIMITED WATER SOLUBILITY

All purines are catabolized to uric acid. Although not very toxic, uric acid has a serious problem: *low water solubility*. It can form damaging crystals both in the urine and in the tissues. Uric acid is a weak acid, with a pK of 5.7, and its water solubility depends on its ionization state (*Fig. 28.10*).

The protonated form usually is less soluble than the deprotonated form. In urine of pH 5.0, uric acid becomes insoluble at concentrations above 0.9 mmol/L (15 mg/dl). Uric acid stones can form in the collecting ducts, where the urine becomes concentrated and acidified. Between 5% and 10% of all kidney stones consist of uric acid.

In plasma and interstitial fluids, with a pH of 7.3 to 7.4 and a high sodium concentration, sodium urate is the least soluble form. It tends to precipitate at concentrations above 0.4 mmol/L (7 mg/dl). Most adults have serum urate levels between 3 and 7 mg/dl. Therefore *even a moderate rise of the serum urate concentration will exceed the limit of solubility.* The average uric acid level is higher in men than in women by about 1 mg/dl and rises with increasing age.

HYPERURICEMIA CAUSES GOUT

A serum uric acid level above the limit of solubility (**hyperuricemia**) can lead to the formation of sodium urate crystals in the tissues. Focal deposits of sodium urate in subcutaneous tissues, known as **tophi,** are asymptomatic, but sodium urate crystals in the joints trigger the inflammatory response of **gouty arthritis.** Gout is a common disease. In Britain, the prevalence of gout is 1.4% in all men and 7% in men over the age of 65 years. The prevalence is nearly four times higher in men than in women.

Gouty arthritis takes the form of acute attacks of joint pain and inflammation, separated by asymptomatic intervals. The disease has a predilection for small peripheral joints, and the metatarsophalangeal joint of the big toe is initially affected in about half of the patients. This is because the solubility of sodium urate is temperature dependent, and crystals form in the coldest parts of the body first.

Any sustained hyperuricemia is likely to cause gouty arthritis, but uric acid levels are somewhat variable over time. On random sampling, between 2% and 18% of healthy people have uric acid levels above the solubility limit of 7 mg/dl, and 10% to 20% of gouty patients have levels below this limit at the time of their first attack.

Synovial fluid analysis from an acutely inflamed joint shows *needle-shaped optically birefringent crystals of sodium urate,* often within polymorphonuclear leukocytes. These cells phagocytize sodium urate crystals, but the razor-sharp, undigestible crystals damage their lysosomes and thereby kill the cell.

The cause of **primary hyperuricemia** usually is unknown, but **secondary hyperuricemia** is caused by an underlying disease. It is seen in psoriasis, chronic hemolytic anemias, pernicious anemia, malignancies, and other conditions with increased cell turnover. Radiation treatment or chemotherapy for neoplastic diseases can cause massive hyperuricemia, with a risk of **uric acid nephropathy** and renal failure.

Uric acid production is also increased in metabolic disorders in which the activity of the pentose phosphate pathway is increased. In type I glycogen storage disease (von Gierke disease; see Chapter 22), for example, accumulating glucose-6-phosphate is converted into ribose-5-phosphate by the pentose phosphate pathway. Ribose-5-phosphate feeds into purine nucleotide biosynthesis, and the excess nucleotides are degraded to uric acid. Purines cannot be stored in the body; therefore, *any increase in the rate of their de novo synthesis has to be matched by an increased rate of degradation to uric acid.*

Primary hyperuricemia is caused by *overproduction of uric acid, impairment of its renal excretion, or both.* Urinary excretion in excess of 600 mg/day is evidence of uric acid overproduction. From 15% to 25% of patients with primary gout are overproducers; the other 75% to 85% of patients have reduced renal clearance of uric acid. Renal excretion is complex. Uric acid is first reabsorbed and then actively secreted in the tubular system.

Most animals other than the higher primates do not develop gout because they degrade uric acid to water-soluble products. Why do humans use uric acid as the end product of purine metabolism, and why is our uric acid level so high that we are teetering on the brink of gout? One possible reason is that uric acid is an antioxidant that scavenges hydroxyl radicals, superoxide

Figure 28.10 Water solubility of uric acid depends on its ionization state. Its pK value is 5.7.

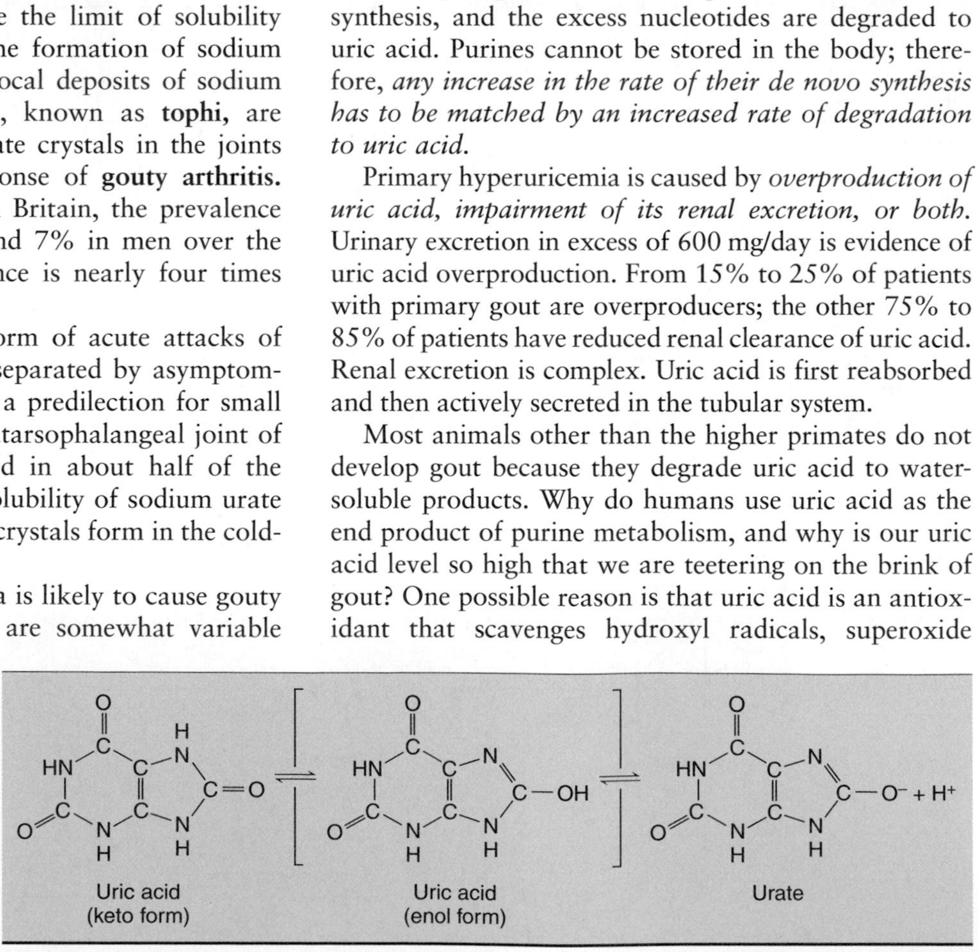

Uric acid (keto form)   Uric acid (enol form)   Urate

radicals, singlet oxygen, and other aggressive oxygen derivatives. It contributes to the body's defenses against oxidative damage.

ABNORMALITIES OF PURINE-METABOLIZING ENZYMES CAN CAUSE GOUT

Abnormalities of two enzymes have been identified in a minority of patients with uric acid overproduction:

1. *Overactivity of PRPP synthetase* increases de novo purine biosynthesis, and purine breakdown must rise in proportion. Elevated levels of IMP, GMP, and AMP from increased de novo biosynthesis inhibit the salvage enzymes and thereby favor uric acid formation over recycling. Hyperuricemia in individuals with an overactive PRPP synthetase shows that this enzyme is normally rate limiting for de novo purine synthesis. The rate of the amidotransferase reaction depends largely on the concentration of its rate-limiting substrate PRPP.
2. *Reduced activity of the salvage enzyme HGPRT* causes hyperuricemia because the substrates of the deficient enzyme accumulate, whereas the levels of its products are reduced:

   - *The cellular levels of the free bases are increased,* thus providing more substrate for uric acid synthesis.
   - *The cellular PRPP level is increased* because of decreased consumption in the salvage reactions, and more substrate is available for the PRPP amidotransferase of the de novo pathway.
   - *The cellular concentrations of the nucleotides are reduced.* This disinhibits the regulated enzymes of the de novo pathway. The result is an increased rate of de novo synthesis, balanced by an equally increased rate of uric acid formation.

Both PRPP synthetase and HGPRT are encoded by genes on the X chromosome, and the enzyme abnormalities are expressed as X-linked recessive traits.

CLINICAL EXAMPLE 28.3: Lesch-Nyhan Syndrome

Partial deficiencies of HGPRT cause only hyperuricemia, but complete deficiency results in **Lesch-Nyhan syndrome.** This rare X-linked recessive disorder is characterized by dystonia, choreoathetosis, spasticity, mental retardation, and bizarre self-mutilating behavior. If unrestrained, the patients chew off their lips and fingers or jam their hands in the spokes of their wheelchairs. The presence of uric acid crystals in the urine is an early sign of the disease, and many patients eventually die of uric acid nephropathy.

The brain disorder, however, is not caused by uric acid overload but by the deficiency of purine nucleotides.

The brain has a very low capacity for de novo purine biosynthesis; therefore, it depends on the salvage enzyme for its purine nucleotides. Although the cause of the neurological symptoms is not known, existing data indicate that there is a loss of the neurotransmitter dopamine in specific neurons in the basal ganglia region of the brain.

GOUT CAN BE TREATED WITH DRUGS

The immediate aim in the treatment of gout is the alleviation of pain and inflammation, but long-term treatment is aimed at reducing the serum uric acid level. The most important drug treatments are as follows:

1. *Antiinflammatory drugs.* **Colchicine** is the classic treatment of the acute attack. It is not very effective in other forms of arthritis; therefore, it can be used for the differential diagnosis of gout. This approach, in which the response to treatment confirms (or refutes) a preliminary diagnosis, is called a diagnosis *ex juvantibus.* Because of gastrointestinal side effects, however, colchicine has been largely replaced by indomethacin, ibuprofen, and other nonsteroidal antiinflammatory drugs.
2. *Uricosuric agents* increase the renal excretion of uric acid. **Probenecid** is an example.
3. *Inhibition of xanthine oxidase* is possible with **allopurinol,** a purine analog that is oxidized to alloxanthine by xanthine oxidase. Alloxanthine remains bound to the enzyme as a competitive inhibitor. As a result, the patient excretes a mix of uric acid, xanthine, and hypoxanthine that is more soluble than uric acid alone. Hypoxanthine and xanthine are turned into IMP and xanthosine monophosphate (XMP), respectively, by HGPRT. These salvage reactions consume PRPP and produce nucleotides that feedback-inhibit the regulated enzymes of the de novo pathway, thereby reducing de novo purine biosynthesis. A new xanthine oxidase inhibitor, **febuxostat,** acts noncompetitively by blocking the channel leading to the active site.

Dietary manipulations are less effective. Dietary purines are degraded to uric acid in the intestinal mucosa. Although much of this uric acid ends up in the stools, in which it is degraded by intestinal bacteria, the consumption of 4 g of yeast RNA per day raises the blood urate to levels typical for gout. On the other hand, eliminating all purines from a typical diet would reduce the serum urate level by only 1 mg/dl.

Alcohol should be avoided because of associated dehydration and because the increased lactate level during alcohol intoxication can impair the renal excretion of uric acid. Acute attacks of gouty arthritis are often triggered by an alcoholic binge.

SUMMARY

Nearly all purines and pyrimidines in the human body are derived from endogenous synthesis. The heterocyclic ring systems are assembled from simple precursors, whereas the ribose portion of the nucleotides comes from PRPP, the activated form of ribose-5-phosphate. The first reactions of the biosynthetic pathways are feedback inhibited by the nucleotides.

The ribonucleotides are the precursors of the corresponding 2-deoxyribonucleotides. Rapidly dividing cells depend on a high rate of nucleotide biosynthesis; therefore, inhibitors of nucleotide biosynthesis can be used for cancer chemotherapy.

Purine nucleotides are catabolized to the free bases, which are either oxidized to the excretory product uric acid or recycled to the corresponding nucleotides in PRPP-dependent salvage reactions. Uric acid is poorly soluble in water. Therefore it can cause kidney stones, and it causes gout when crystals of sodium urate form in the joints.

Further Reading

Aiuti A, Cattaneo F, Galimberti S, et al: Gene therapy for immunodeficiency due to adenosine deaminase deficiency, *N Engl J Med* 360:447–458, 2009.

Alcorn N, Saunders S, Madhok R: Benefit-risk assessment of leflunomide: an appraisal of leflunomide in rheumatoid arthritis 10 years after licensing, *Drug Saf* 32:1123–1134, 2009.

An S, Kumar R, Sheets ED, et al: Reversible compartmentalization of de novo purine biosynthetic complexes in living cells, *Science* 320:103–106, 2008.

Evans DR, Guy HI: Mammalian pyrimidine biosynthesis: fresh insights into an ancient pathway, *J Biol Chem* 279:33035–33038, 2004.

Jinnah HA, Ceballos-Picot I, Torres RJ, et al: Attenuated variants of Lesch-Nyhan disease, *Brain* 133:671–689, 2010.

Riches PL, Wright AF, Ralston SH: Recent insights into the pathogenesis of hyperuricaemia and gout, *Hum Mol Genet* 18:R177–R184, 2009.

Saag KG, Choi H: Epidemiology, risk factors, and lifestyle modifications for gout, *Arthritis Res Ther* 8(Suppl 1):S2, 2006.

Segal NH, Saltz LB: Evolving treatment of advanced colon cancer, *Annu Rev Med* 60:207–219, 2009.

QUESTIONS

1. **Enzyme abnormalities that can lead to hyperuricemia and gout include**

   A. Reduced activity of PRPP synthetase
   B. Reduced activity of xanthine oxidase
   C. Reduced activity of hypoxanthine-guanine phosphoribosyltransferase
   D. Reduced activity of PRPP aminotransferase
   E. Reduced activity of dihydroorotate dehydrogenase

2. **A coenzyme form of tetrahydrofolate is required for**

   A. The de novo synthesis of pyrimidines
   B. The synthesis of thymine-containing nucleotides from uracil-containing nucleotides
   C. The synthesis of xanthine from purine nucleotides
   D. The cleavage of the purine ring in uric acid by an enzyme in the human liver
   E. The reduction of ribonucleotides to 2-deoxyribonucleotides

Chapter 29
VITAMINS AND MINERALS

Traditionally, **vitamins** are divided into water-soluble and fat-soluble vitamins. Most of the water-soluble vitamins are precursors of coenzymes. The fat-soluble vitamins have more diverse functions, for example, as antioxidants or as precursors of hormone-like substances.

Another difference between these two classes of vitamins is their intestinal absorption. Water-soluble vitamins are readily absorbed, but the absorption of fat-soluble vitamins depends on mixed bile salt micelles. Therefore *deficiencies of fat-soluble vitamins are most likely to occur in patients with fat malabsorption.* Supplements of these vitamins are most effective when they are taken with a fatty meal.

Most water-soluble vitamins are transported in the blood as such, but fat-soluble vitamins are transported either as constituents of lipoproteins or bound to specific plasma proteins. Finally, renal excretion of excess water-soluble vitamins is unproblematic, whereas fat-soluble vitamins must be metabolized to water-soluble products before they can be excreted. Therefore *fat-soluble vitamins are more likely to accumulate in the body and cause toxicity.*

Minerals are inorganic nutrients. The **macrominerals** sodium, potassium, calcium, magnesium, phosphate, and chloride are components of the body fluids and the inorganic matrix of bone. They are required in quantities of more than 100 mg/day. The **microminerals,** or **trace minerals,** are required in only small quantities and serve specialized biochemical functions.

The **recommended daily allowance (RDA)** of each nutrient, more recently labeled as **dietary reference intake (DRI)**, is published by the Food and Nutrition Board of the National Academy of Sciences in the United States and by similar agencies in other countries. The DRI defines not a minimal requirement but *a dietary intake that meets the requirements of 97% to 98% of healthy individuals in a category.*

Table 29.1 summarizes the DRIs for adult men and women. Actual requirements depend also on age, body weight, diet, and physiological status. Increases in dietary intake of many nutrients are recommended during pregnancy and lactation.

RIBOFLAVIN IS A PRECURSOR OF FLAVIN MONONUCLEOTIDE AND FLAVIN ADENINE DINUCLEOTIDE

Riboflavin (vitamin B_2) consists of a dimethylisoalloxazine ring covalently bound to the sugar alcohol ribitol (*Fig. 29.1*). *Riboflavin is the dietary precursor*

Table 29.1 Dietary Reference Intakes for Vitamins and Minerals

Nutrient	70-kg Man	55-kg Woman
Water-Soluble Vitamins		
Niacin	16 mg	14 mg
Riboflavin	1.3 mg	1.1 mg
Thiamin	1.2 mg	1.1 mg
Pyridoxine (B_6)	1.3 mg	1.3 mg
Pantothenic acid	5 mg	5 mg
Biotin	30 μg	30 μg
Ascorbic acid	90 mg	75 mg
Folic acid	400 μg	400 μg
Cobalamin (B_{12})	2.4 μg	2.4 μg
Fat-Soluble Vitamins		
Vitamin A	900 μg	700 μg
Vitamin D	5 μg	5 μg
Vitamin K	120 μg	90 μg
Vitamin E	15 mg	15 mg
Macrominerals		
Sodium	1.5 g	1.5 g
Potassium	4.7 g	4.7 g
Calcium	1 g	1 g
Magnesium	420 mg	320 mg
Chloride	2.3 g	2.3 g
Phosphate	700 mg	700 mg
Microminerals		
Iron	8 mg	18 mg
Copper	900 μg	900 μg
Zinc	11 mg	8 mg
Manganese	2.3 mg	1.8 mg
Molybdenum	45 μg	45 μg
Chromium	35 μg	25 μg
Selenium	55 μg	55 μg
Iodide	150 μg	150 μg
Fluoride	4 mg	3 mg

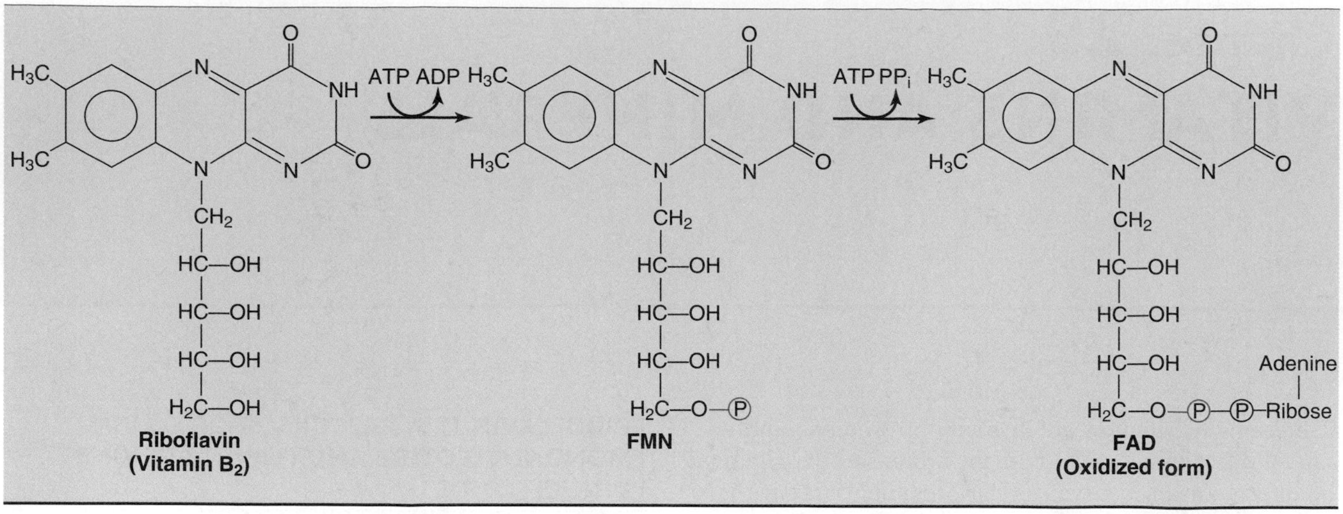

Figure 29.1 Synthesis of flavin mononucleotide (*FMN*) and flavin adenine dinucleotide (*FAD*) from dietary riboflavin.

of flavin adenine dinucleotide (FAD) and flavin mono-nucleotide (FMN), the prosthetic groups of the **flavo-proteins** (from Latin *flavus* meaning "yellow"). Both riboflavin and the flavin coenzymes are yellow in their reduced form, with an absorption band at 450 nm. Although riboflavin and its derivatives are heat stable, they are rapidly degraded to inactive products on exposure to visible light. Therefore riboflavin deficiency can occur in infants receiving phototherapy for hyperbilirubinemia (see Chapter 27), when ribo-flavin as well as bilirubin is destroyed by light in the skin.

Dietary riboflavin is absorbed by an energy-dependent transporter in the upper small intestine and transported to the tissues, where it is converted to the coenzyme forms FMN and FAD. The excess is excreted in the urine or metabolized by microsomal enzymes in the liver.

Good sources of riboflavin include liver, yeast, eggs, meat, enriched bread and cereals, and milk. Riboflavin deficiency usually occurs along with other vitamin deficiencies and is most common in alcoholics. Symptoms include glossitis (magenta tongue), angu-lar stomatitis, sore throat, and a moist (seborrheic) dermatitis of the scrotum and nose. This deficiency may be accompanied by a normochromic normocytic anemia.

Dietary status can be assessed by fluorometric or microbiological determination of urinary riboflavin. Alternatively, the activity of erythrocyte glutathione reductase (see Chapter 22) is determined in freshly lysed red blood cells before and after the addition of its coenzyme FAD. In riboflavin deficiency, the apoenzyme is not completely saturated with its coen-zyme; therefore, the enzymatic activity is increased by added FAD.

NIACIN IS A PRECURSOR OF NAD AND NADP

The term **niacin,** originally applied to nicotinic acid, is often used as a generic term for the vitamin-active pyri-dine derivatives **nicotinic acid** and **nicotinamide:**

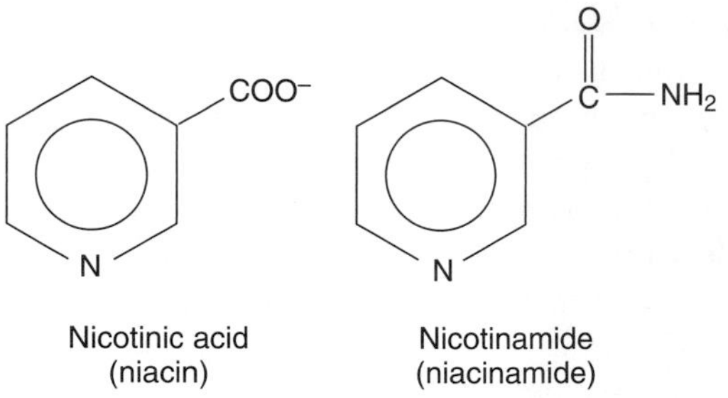

In both the human body and dietary sources, *niacin is present as a constituent of NAD and NADP.* The dietary coenzymes are hydrolyzed in the gastrointesti-nal tract, and free nicotinic acid and nicotinamide are absorbed in the small intestine. After their transport to the tissues, the vitamin forms are incorporated into the coenzymes (***Fig. 29.2***). Excess niacin is readily excreted by the kidneys.

NAD and NADP can be synthesized from dietary tryptophan, but the pathway is inefficient. Sixty milli-grams of tryptophan, which is nutritionally essential itself, is required for the synthesis of 1 mg of niacin. Also, the pathway of endogenous niacin synthesis requires riboflavin, thiamine, and pyridoxine and there-fore is impaired in patients with multiple vitamin defi-ciencies. Most people get about equal amounts of their niacin requirement from dietary tryptophan and from niacin. Good sources of niacin include yeast, meat, liver, peanuts and other legume seeds, and enriched cereals.

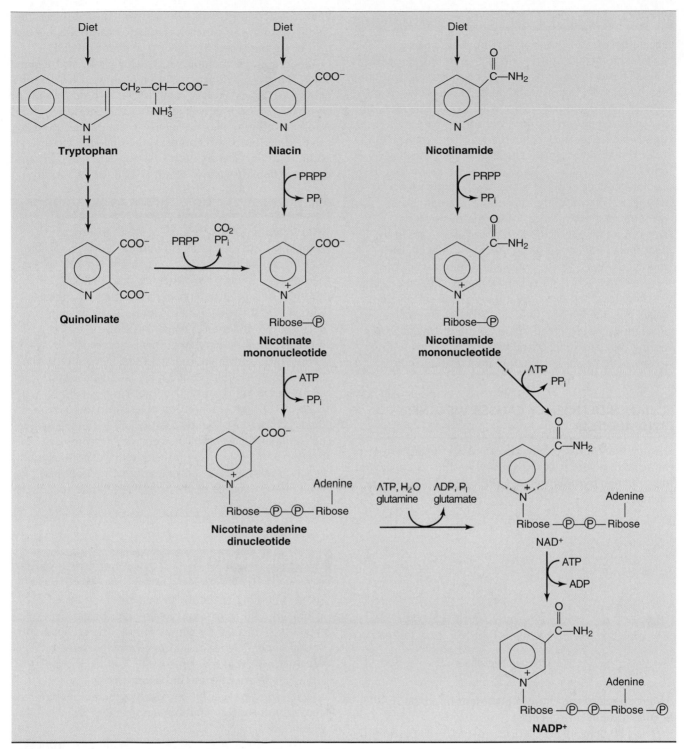

Figure 29.2 Synthesis of nicotinamide adenine dinucleotide (*NAD*) and nicotinamide adenine dinucleotide phosphate (*NADP*). *PRPP*, 5-Phosphoribosyl-1-pyrophosphate.

CLINICAL EXAMPLE 29.1: Pellagra

Niacin deficiency, known as **pellagra** (the name is Italian and means "rough skin"), is seen only in people on a diet low in both niacin and tryptophan. It is often associated with maize-based diets. Maize protein is low in tryptophan, and the niacin, which is actually present in moderate amount, is poorly absorbed because it is tightly bound to other constituents of the grain.

Early deficiency signs include weakness, lassitude, anorexia, indigestion, and a glossitis similar to that in riboflavin deficiency. The signs of severe deficiency are dermatitis, diarrhea, and dementia. The dermatitis presents as a symmetrical erythematous rash on sun-exposed parts of the skin. Diarrhea is caused by widespread inflammation of mucosal surfaces. The mental changes, which initially are quite vague, can progress to a profound encephalopathy with confusion, memory loss, and overt organic psychosis. In severe cases, mental deterioration can become irreversible. Pellagra was widespread in the southern United States during the early years of the twentieth century but now is limited to poverty-stricken regions of the world.

THIAMIN DEFICIENCY CAUSES WEAKNESS AND AMNESIA

Dietary **thiamin** is readily absorbed and transported to the tissues, where it is phosphorylated to its coenzyme form **thiamin pyrophosphate (TPP)** in an ATP-dependent reaction:

Thiamin pyrophosphate
(TPP)

About 30 mg of the vitamin is present in the body, 80% of this in the form of TPP.

The TPP-dependent reactions are *aldehyde transfers* in which the aldehyde is bound covalently to one of the carbons in the thiazole (sulfur-and-nitrogen) ring of the coenzyme. One reaction type, the *oxidative decarboxylation of α-ketoacids,* is catalyzed by mitochondrial multienzyme complexes. Pyruvate dehydrogenase, α-ketoglutarate dehydrogenase (see Chapter 21), branched-chain α-ketoacid dehydrogenase, and α-ketobutyrate dehydrogenase (see Chapter 26) all use the same thiamin-dependent catalytic mechanism.

A different reaction type is encountered in the cytoplasmic *transketolase reaction* (see Chapter 22) in which

TPP transfers a glycolaldehyde from one monosaccharide to another. In general, the major catabolic, energy-producing pathways are most dependent on TPP.

Good sources include yeast, lean pork, and legume seeds. Thiamin deficiency can be evaluated by determination of transketolase activity in whole blood or erythrocytes, both before and after the addition of TPP. Alternatively, the plasma levels of lactate and pyruvate can be determined after an oral glucose load. These acids accumulate in persons with thiamin deficiency because pyruvate dehydrogenase requires TPP for its activity.

CLINICAL EXAMPLE 29.2: Beriberi

Mild thiamin deficiency leads to gastrointestinal complaints, weakness, and a burning sensation in the feet. Moderate deficiency is characterized by peripheral neuropathy, mental abnormalities, and ataxia. Full-blown deficiency, known as **beriberi,** manifests with severe muscle weakness and muscle wasting, delirium, ophthalmoplegia (paralysis of the eye muscles), and memory loss. This is accompanied by peripheral vasodilation and increased venous return to the heart. Myocardial contractility is impaired, and death can result from high-output cardiac failure.

Beriberi became a health problem in parts of Asia at the end of the nineteenth century when the milling and polishing of rice were introduced in these countries. The thiamin in rice is present in the outer layers of the grain, which are removed by polishing; therefore, beriberi became the scourge of poor people who had to subsist mainly on rice.

CLINICAL EXAMPLE 29.3: Wernicke-Korsakoff Syndrome

Today, thiamin deficiency is most common in alcoholics who have poor intestinal absorption in addition to inadequate dietary intake. The combination of thiamin deficiency and alcohol toxicity causes **Wernicke-Korsakoff syndrome.** The acute stage, known as **Wernicke encephalopathy,** is characterized by mental derangements and delirium, ataxia (motor incoordination), and paralysis of the eye muscles.

Wernicke encephalopathy requires immediate treatment with thiamin injections to prevent development of the chronic stage, known as **Korsakoff psychosis.** Patients with Korsakoff psychosis suffer from a severely debilitating anterograde amnesia. They can remember events from the distant past, and their immediate recall is intact, but they cannot transcribe information from short-term to long-term memory.

Korsakoff psychosis is the most common form of amnesia in most countries. The amnesia is attributed to focal lesions in the periventricular areas of the thalamus and

CLINICAL EXAMPLE 29.3: Wernicke-Korsakoff Syndrome—cont'd

hypothalamus, the periaqueductal gray of the midbrain, and the mammillary bodies. The frequent confabulation that distinguishes Korsakoff psychosis from other forms of anterograde amnesia is attributed to concomitant damage in the frontal lobes.

VITAMIN B_6 PLAYS A KEY ROLE IN AMINO ACID METABOLISM

Vitamin B_6 is the generic name for the dietary precursors of the coenzyme **pyridoxal phosphate (PLP)**. They include **pyridoxine, pyridoxal,** and **pyridoxamine** as well as their phosphorylated derivatives (*Fig. 29.3*).

The phosphate is removed by intestinal alkaline phosphatase, and the dephosphorylated forms are absorbed. The total body content of PLP is only 25 mg in adults, and pyridoxal and PLP are the major circulating forms of the vitamin. Synthesis of the coenzyme form is described in *Figure 29.4*.

Several dozen enzymes of amino acid metabolism contain PLP as a tightly bound prosthetic group. In these reactions, the aldehyde group of PLP forms an aldimine derivative with the amino group of the amino acid. The aldimine is stabilized by an intramolecular hydrogen bond with the phenolic hydroxyl group (*Fig. 29.5*).

Liver, fish, whole grains, nuts, legumes, egg yolk, and yeast are good sources of vitamin B_6. Serious deficiency is rare, but when it occurs it is characterized by peripheral neuropathy, stomatitis, glossitis, irritability, psychiatric symptoms, and, especially in children, epileptic seizures. Some of the neurological derangements may result from impaired activity of the PLP-dependent

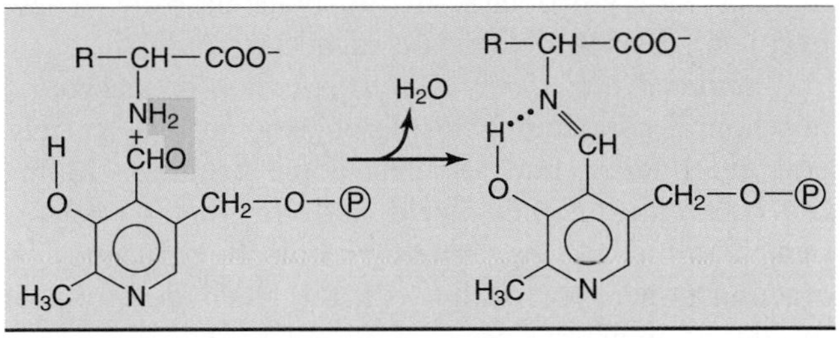

Figure 29.5 In reactions of amino acid metabolism, pyridoxal phosphate forms an aldimine (Schiff base) derivative with the amino group of the amino acid. The further path of the reaction depends on the catalytic specificity of the enzyme.

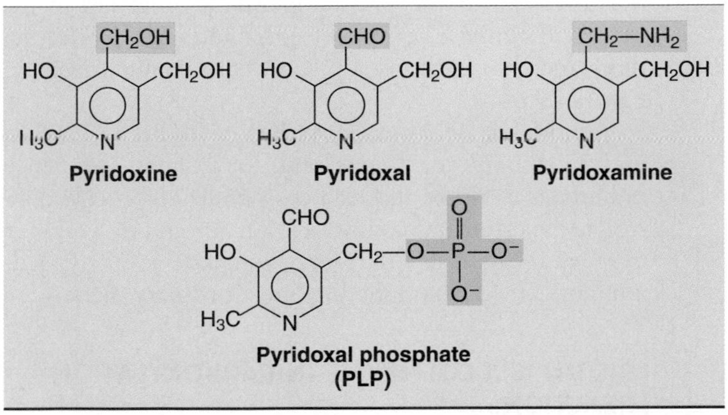

Figure 29.3 Molecular forms of vitamin B_6. All vitamin forms can be converted to the coenzyme form pyridoxal phosphate in the human body.

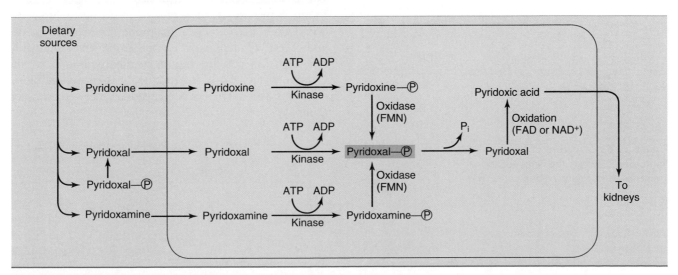

Figure 29.4 Metabolism of vitamin B_6.

enzyme glutamate decarboxylase, which forms the inhibitory neurotransmitter γ-aminobutyric acid (GABA) (see Chapter 16).

Dermatitis, glossitis, and **sideroblastic anemia** are other abnormalities in vitamin B₆ deficiency. Sideroblastic anemia is a microcytic hypochromic anemia, similar to iron deficiency anemia but in the presence of normal serum iron. It is most likely caused by reduced activity of the PLP-dependent aminolevulinic acid (ALA) synthase in the bone marrow and the resulting impairment in heme biosynthesis. Without heme, iron cannot be used for hemoglobin synthesis but accumulates in erythroblasts in the bone marrow. These iron-loaded erythroblasts are called *sideroblasts*.

Vitamin B₆ deficiency is most common in alcoholics, in whom it contributes to sideroblastic anemia, peripheral neuropathy, and seizures. Some drugs, including the tuberculostatic **isoniazid** and the metal chelator **penicillamine**, can precipitate vitamin B₆ deficiency by reacting nonenzymatically with the aldehyde group of pyridoxal or PLP:

Unlike the other water-soluble vitamins, *vitamin B₆ is toxic in high doses*. The daily consumption of more than 500 mg of pyridoxine for several months leads to *peripheral sensory neuropathy*. Doses of 100 to 150 mg/day are used for the symptomatic treatment of carpal tunnel syndrome, a painful nerve entrapment syndrome. The "therapeutic" effect of pyridoxine probably is unrelated to its vitamin function but is related to its toxicity on peripheral nerves.

PANTOTHENIC ACID IS A BUILDING BLOCK OF COENZYME A

Pantothenic acid consists of pantoic acid and β-alanine:

β-Alanine | Pantoic acid

Pantothenic acid

Pantothenic acid functions as *a constituent of coenzyme A (CoA)* and of the phosphopantetheine group in the fatty acid synthase complex (see Chapter 23). The structure and biosynthesis of CoA are summarized in *Figure 29.6*.

Pantothenic acid deficiency has never been observed under ordinary conditions, and an isolated deficiency in humans could be induced only under rigorously controlled experimental conditions. An amount of 5 mg/day is recommended as "safe and adequate intake." This amount is readily supplied by most ordinary diets.

BIOTIN IS A COENZYME IN CARBOXYLATION REACTIONS

Biotin is the prosthetic group of pyruvate carboxylase, acetyl-CoA carboxylase, propionyl-CoA carboxylase, and other *ATP-dependent carboxylases*. These multisubunit enzymes contain biotin covalently bound to the ε-amino group of a lysine residue. In the reaction, biotin functions as a carrier of a bicarbonate-derived carboxyl group:

Isoniazid   Pyridoxal

H₂O

Hydrazone derivative

Figure 29.6 Structure of coenzyme A. Pantothenic acid is the only nutritionally essential component of this coenzyme.

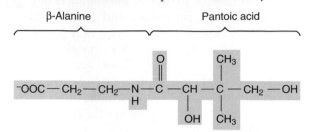

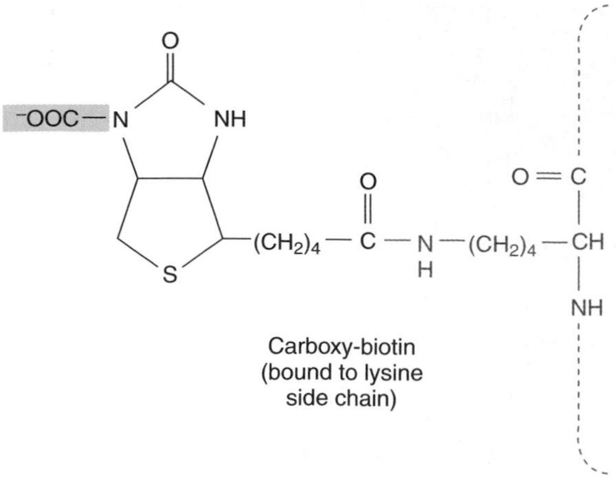

Carboxy-biotin
(bound to lysine
side chain)

Yeast, liver, eggs, peanuts, milk, chocolate, and fish are good sources of biotin, and intestinal bacteria make a sizeable contribution. Humans need only 30 µg of biotin per day, and the only way to induce biotin deficiency is to eat at least 20 raw egg whites per day. Egg white contains the protein **avidin,** so called because it binds biotin avidly, preventing its intestinal absorption.

FOLIC ACID DEFICIENCY CAUSES MEGALOBLASTIC ANEMIA

Folic acid consists of pteroic acid (pteridine + para-aminobenzoic acid [PABA]) and one to seven γ-linked glutamate residues. Dietary polyglutamate forms of folic acid are hydrolyzed to pteroyl monoglutamate in the intestinal lumen:

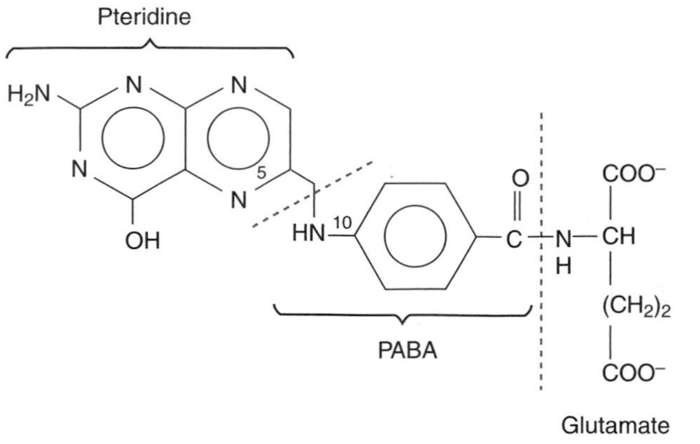

Pteroyl-monoglutamate
(the absorbed form of folic acid)

The monoglutamate is absorbed and reduced to the active coenzyme form **tetrahydrofolate (THF)** by **dihydrofolate reductase** in the intestinal mucosa. The monoglutamate conjugate of methyl-THF is the major circulating form of THF, but intracellular THF is present in the form of polyglutamate conjugates.

THF is a carrier of one-carbon units, which are bound to one or both of the nitrogen atoms N-5 and N-10 (*Fig. 29.8*):

CLINICAL EXAMPLE 29.4: Biotinidase Deficiency

The proteolytic degradation of biotin-containing enzymes, both in the intestinal lumen and in the tissues, produces the biotin-lysine conjugate **biocytin** (*Fig. 29.7*). Biotin is released from biocytin by **biotinidase**. *Biotinidase deficiency causes nondietary biotin deficiency.* Affected infants present with hypotonia, seizures, optic atrophy, dermatitis, and conjunctivitis. This condition can be cured easily with biotin supplements. *Biotinidase deficiency is often included in newborn screening programs,* along with other treatable congenital diseases. It can be diagnosed by enzyme assay in fresh serum or, as a screening test, on a strip of blood-soaked filter paper.

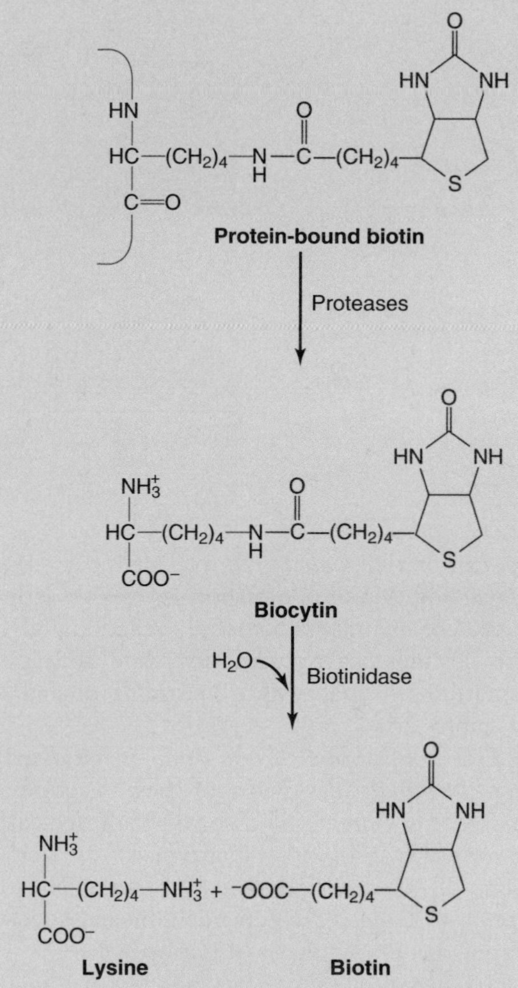

Figure 29.7 Recycling of biotin. These reactions are required both for the utilization of dietary biotin and for the recycling of biotin during the degradation of biotin-containing carboxylase enzymes in the tissues.

Figure 29.8 Tetrahydrofolate (*THF*) as a carrier of one-carbon units. *FIGLU,* Formiminoglutamate (formed during histidine degradation).

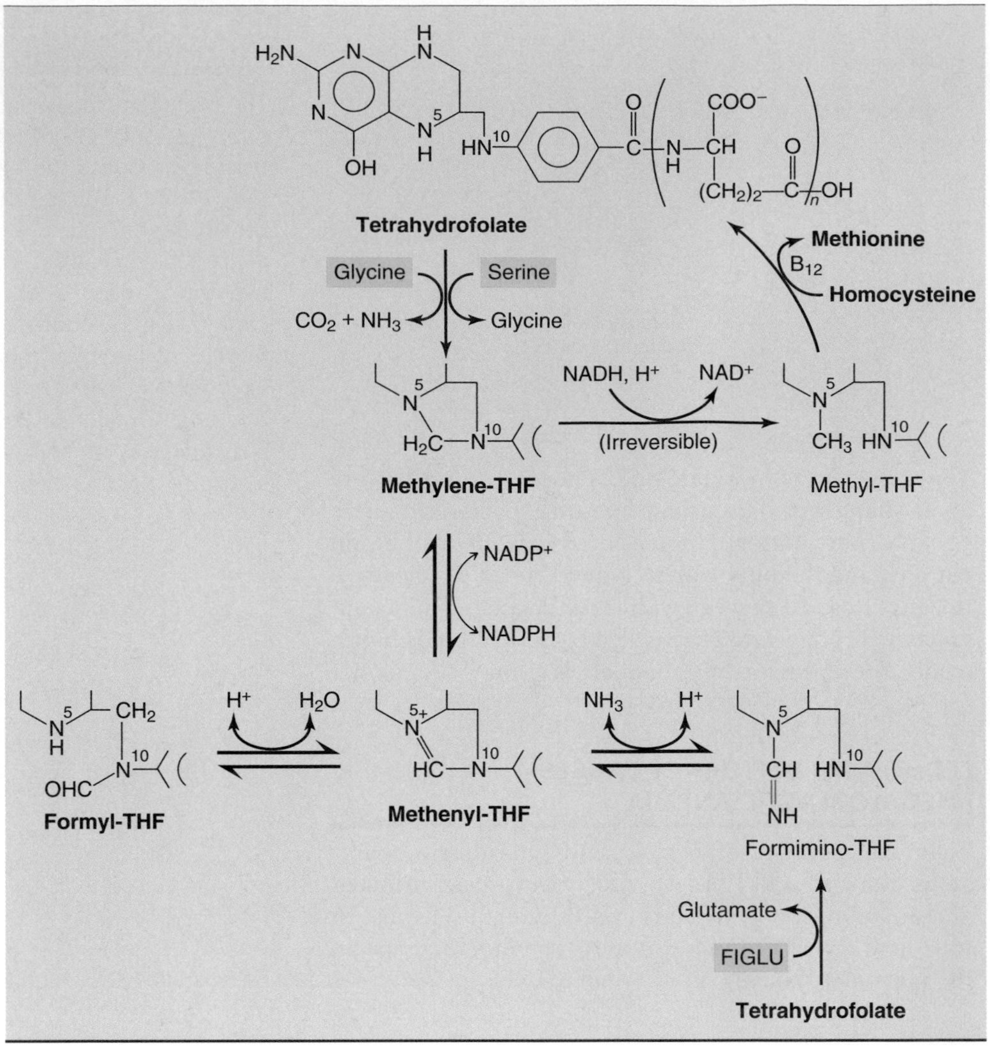

1. *A one-carbon unit is acquired by THF during a catabolic reaction.* Major one-carbon sources are serine in the hydroxymethyl transferase reaction, glycine in the glycine cleavage reaction, and formiminoglutamate in the pathway of histidine degradation (see Chapter 26).

2. *The THF-bound one-carbon unit is oxidized or reduced enzymatically.* Most of these reactions are reversible. They create an assortment of one-carbon units for use by biosynthetic enzymes.

3. *The one-carbon unit is transferred from THF to an acceptor molecule.* THF-dependent biosynthetic processes include the synthesis of purine nucleotides, the thymidylate synthase reaction, and the methylation of homocysteine to methionine.

Folate deficiency leads to impaired DNA replication in dividing cells because of reduced synthesis of purine nucleotides and thymine. In the bone marrow, hemoglobin is synthesized normally and the cytoplasm grows at a normal rate, but cell division is delayed. Therefore the production of mature cells slows down, and the cells that are formed are oversized. The result is called **megaloblastic anemia** or **macrocytic anemia.** Megaloblasts are oversized erythrocyte precursors in the bone marrow, and macrocytes are oversized erythrocytes in the blood.

Good dietary sources include yeast, liver, some fruits, and green vegetables (from Latin *folium* meaning "leaf"). However, folate is heat labile, and losses during food processing can be extensive. The RDA is 400 µg, and total body stores are 5 to 10 mg. Low levels of serum folate are often encountered in late pregnancy, and *megaloblastic anemia can be precipitated by pregnancy.* Alcoholism and intestinal malabsorption syndromes can also cause folate deficiency.

Folate levels can be determined in serum and erythrocytes. In subacute deficiency, the serum "folate" (actually methyl-THF) declines within days, followed much later by a decrease of red blood cell folate. Deficiency signs appear only when the intracellular stores are depleted.

CLINICAL EXAMPLE 29.5: Sulfonamides

Unlike humans, most bacteria make their own folate from pteridine and PABA (***Fig. 29.9***). Therefore their growth can be inhibited with drugs that block folate synthesis. The **sulfonamides** are structural analogs of PABA that inhibit the synthesis of pteroic acid in bacteria. Although they do not kill the bacteria immediately, they prevent their growth. They are bacteriostatic, not bactericidal.

Trimethoprim is an inhibitor of bacterial but not human dihydrofolate reductase. It is frequently combined with the sulfonamide **sulfamethoxazole** for treatment of bacterial infections.

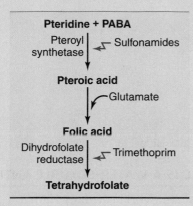

Figure 29.9 Pharmacological inhibition of tetrahydrofolate synthesis in bacteria. *PABA,* Para-aminobenzoic acid.

CLINICAL EXAMPLE 29.6: Prevention of Neural Tube Defects

Neural tube defects are among the most serious birth defects. They include anencephaly (absence of the brain) and spina bifida (incomplete closure of the lumbar spine). Although the reasons for these rather common malformations (1:400 births) are not well understood, folate supplements are known to be effective in their prevention. The current recommendation is that all women who might become pregnant should consume at least 400 µg of folic acid per day. Because many women failed to heed this advice, the United States instituted compulsory fortification of flour and other grain products with folic acid in 1998, and most other countries followed. It is estimated that this program has reduced the incidence of neural tube defects by 46%.

VITAMIN B$_{12}$ REQUIRES INTRINSIC FACTOR FOR ITS ABSORPTION

Vitamin B$_{12}$, or **cobalamin,** is chemically the most complex of all vitamins (***Fig. 29.10***). It is also the rarest of all vitamins. B$_{12}$ is synthesized only by some microorganisms,

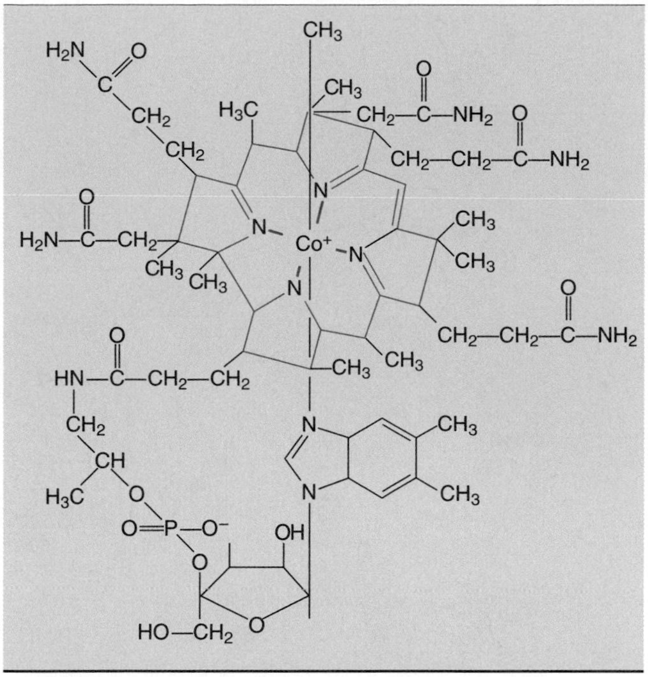

Figure 29.10 Structure of methylcobalamin.

but not by plants. A small amount is synthesized by colon bacteria, but its absorption is negligible.

Specialized mechanisms are required to absorb and retain the 2.4 µg of vitamin B$_{12}$ that is considered the daily requirement. B$_{12}$ absorption requires **intrinsic factor,** a 50-kD glycoprotein secreted by the parietal cells of the stomach (***Fig. 29.11***). Vitamin B$_{12}$ binds tightly to intrinsic factor, and in this form it is absorbed from the ileum. In the blood it binds tightly to **transcobalamin II** and other plasma proteins. Protein binding prevents its renal excretion, and the cobalamin-transcobalamin II complex is taken up into the cells by receptor-mediated endocytosis.

Only two reactions are known to require cobalamin coenzymes in human tissues. The cytoplasmic *methylation of homocysteine to methionine* (see Chapter 26) requires methylcobalamin, and the mitochondrial *methylmalonyl-CoA mutase reaction* (see Chapter 23) requires deoxyadenosylcobalamin.

Because essentially all dietary vitamin B$_{12}$ is derived from animal products, *vegans are at risk for vitamin B$_{12}$ deficiency.* Between 1 and 10 mg of vitamin B$_{12}$ is stored in the body, most of this in the liver. Therefore a sudden switch to a vitamin B$_{12}$–free diet will cause serious deficiency only after more than a decade.

However, between 1 and 10 µg of vitamin B$_{12}$ is secreted into the bile every day, and most of this is reabsorbed with the help of intrinsic factor. Therefore *impaired intestinal absorption causes deficiency within 2 to 4 years* (***Clinical Example 29.7***).

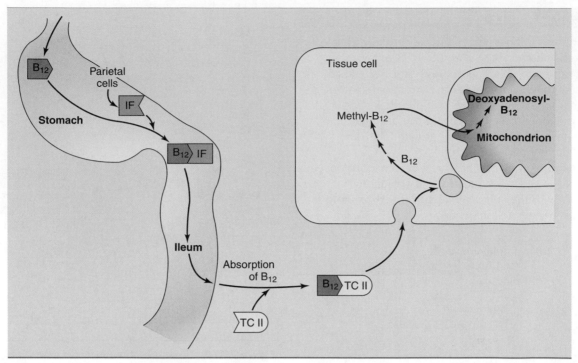

Figure 29.11 Absorption, transport, and tissue utilization of vitamin B_{12}. *IF,* Intrinsic factor; *TC II,* transcobalamin II.

CLINICAL EXAMPLE 29.7: Pernicious Anemia

Most cases of B_{12} deficiency are not caused by dietary deficiency but by malabsorption. Pernicious anemia is an autoimmune disease that destroys the parietal cells in the stomach and thereby deprives the patient of intrinsic factor. Neither dietary nor biliary vitamin B_{12} can be absorbed. This disease was invariably fatal until 1926, when the oral administration of liver extracts was found to be curative. Even in the absence of intrinsic factor, 0.1% to 1% of orally administered vitamin B_{12} is absorbed by nonspecific mechanisms, and the large amount of vitamin B_{12} in the liver extracts was sufficient to correct the deficiency. Pernicious anemia now is treated with either large oral vitamin B_{12} supplements or monthly injections of more moderate doses.

Pernicious anemia shows two types of abnormalities: *megaloblastic anemia* similar to folate deficiency, and *neurological dysfunction* with demyelination in peripheral nerves and spinal cord. The demyelination is not seen in folate deficiency.

The megaloblastic anemia is explained by the **methyl folate trap** hypothesis. During the metabolism of one-carbon units, a small amount of methylene-THF is irreversibly reduced to methyl-THF (see *Fig. 29.8*). Because it is useless for the synthesis of purines and thymine, methyl-THF must be converted back to the other coenzyme forms. *This can be done only by the B_{12}-dependent methylation of homocysteine to methionine, which regenerates free THF.* Therefore methyl-THF accumulates in vitamin B_{12} deficiency, to the detriment of the other coenzyme forms. This mechanism explains the megaloblastic anemia of vitamin B_{12} deficiency, but the cause of the demyelination is unknown.

VITAMIN C IS A WATER-SOLUBLE ANTIOXIDANT

The structure of ascorbic acid, or vitamin C, resembles a monosaccharide (*Fig. 29.12*), and most animals can synthesize it in one of the minor pathways of carbohydrate metabolism (see Chapter 22). Only primates, guinea pigs, and some fruit bats have lost the ascorbate-synthesizing enzyme.

Ascorbic acid is a reducing agent and a scavenger of free radicals (see *Fig. 29.12*). As an antioxidant, it suppresses the formation of carcinogenic nitrosamines from dietary nitrite and nitrate in the gastrointestinal tract, and it protects lipoproteins from oxidative damage. Protective effects against atherosclerosis and some cancers have been postulated, but such effects have been difficult to demonstrate in controlled studies.

Many iron- and copper-containing enzymes require ascorbic acid to keep their metal in the reduced state. Some ascorbate-dependent processes are as follows:

1. *Hydroxylation of prolyl and lysyl residues in procollagen* requires ascorbate (see Chapter 14). Impairment of these reactions accounts for the prominent connective tissue abnormalities of scurvy.
2. *Carnitine synthesis* (see Chapter 26) requires two Fe^{2+}-containing, ascorbate-dependent oxygenases. Carnitine deficiency may contribute to the fatigue and lassitude that are characteristic of scurvy.
3. *Dopamine synthesis* requires the ascorbate-dependent copper enzyme dopamine β-hydroxylase (see Chapter 16).
4. *Bile acid synthesis* is regulated at the level of the ascorbate-dependent enzyme 7α-hydroxylase (see Chapter 24).

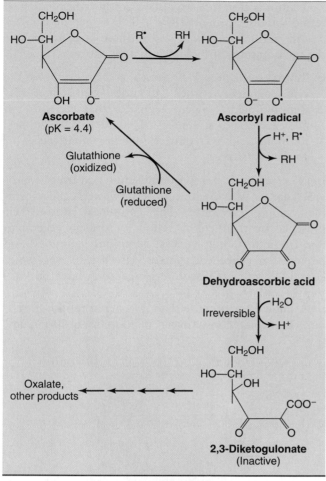

Figure 29.12 Structure and antioxidant action of ascorbic acid (vitamin C). The standard reduction potential of ascorbate/dehydroascorbate is +0.08 V and that of glutathione is -0.23 V. R•, Free radical.

Dietary vitamin C is absorbed by a sodium-dependent transporter in the intestine. This saturable carrier can absorb only a maximum of 1 to 2 g of ascorbic acid per day. Thus megadoses are incompletely absorbed. The plasma level is almost linearly related to the dietary intake up to intakes of about 150 mg/day, but it levels off at higher daily intakes. A plasma level of 1.0 mg/dl is typical on a 100-mg/day diet. The total body pool reaches 20 mg per kilogram of body weight on a 150-mg/day diet and is only slightly higher in people consuming megadoses of more than 1 g/day. About 3% of the vitamin C in the body is excreted in the urine every day, some as unchanged ascorbic acid and some after metabolism to other water-soluble products, including oxalic acid.

Fresh fruits and vegetables are the major dietary sources. Vitamin C is not very stable under neutral or alkaline conditions and is easily oxidized to inactive products by boiling in the presence of oxygen and catalytic amounts of heavy metal ions.

The benefits of megadoses of vitamin C were popularized by the late Linus Pauling, whose name is forever linked not only to the structure of the α-helix but also

to the claim that high doses of vitamin C can prevent the common cold. Recent reviews of the evidence indicate that the incidence of colds is barely reduced by high-dose vitamin C prophylaxis, but the duration and severity of the episodes are somewhat reduced. Phagocytes and lymphocytes concentrate vitamin C to levels up to 100 times higher than in plasma, and it is possible that this reduces collateral damage when phagocytes form oxygen-derived free radicals for the purpose of intracellular killing of ingested microorganisms. Although the advisability of very large doses still is controversial, Pauling lived to the age of 97 years, consuming several grams of vitamin C per day for his last 40 years.

CLINICAL EXAMPLE 29.8: Scurvy

During recorded history, scurvy has been one of the most frequently mentioned nutritional deficiencies. It was a disease of seafarers and explorers until the eighteenth century, when lemon juice was found to be curative.

The first signs of scurvy appear 2 to 3 months after a sudden switch to a vitamin C–free diet, when the total body pool is reduced to 300 mg. *Cutaneous petechiae and purpura* (small and medium-sized hemorrhages) appear, along with *follicular hyperkeratosis* (gooseflesh). Dry mouth and eyes, decaying peeling gums, and loose teeth are seen in more advanced cases. Wound healing and scar formation are disrupted, and bleeding from old scars can occur. The patient experiences weakness and lethargy, sometimes accompanied by joint pain and aching of the legs. A daily intake of 20 to 50 mg vitamin C is sufficient to cure scurvy.

RETINOL, RETINAL, AND RETINOIC ACID ARE THE ACTIVE FORMS OF VITAMIN A

The biologically active forms of vitamin A are the **retinoids**:

All-*trans*-retinol

All-*trans*-retinal

All-*trans*-retinoic acid

Foods of animal origin contain most of their vitamin A in the form of *esters between retinol and a long-chain fatty acid*. The retinol esters are hydrolyzed by a pancreatic enzyme in the small intestine, and free retinol is absorbed with an efficiency of 60% to 90% (*Fig. 29.13*).

β-Carotene, the orange pigment of carrots and many other vegetables, is the major vitamin A precursor in plants. It is cleaved by **β-carotene dioxygenase** in the cytoplasm of the intestinal mucosal cell (*Fig. 29.14*). Absorption and cleavage are not very efficient, and 6 mg of β-carotene is needed to produce 1 mg of retinal. Carotenes other than β-carotene can be processed to retinal, but the yield is even lower.

Retinal is in equilibrium with retinol through a reversible, NADH-dependent reaction. A small amount is irreversibly oxidized to **retinoic acid** (see *Fig. 29.13*). The intestinal mucosa esterifies most of the retinol with fatty acids and exports the retinol esters as constituents of chylomicrons. Chylomicron remnants bring the retinol esters to the liver (see Chapter 25), which stores up to 100 mg of retinol esters in the stellate cells (see *Fig. 29.13*).

Retinol is exported from the liver in tight binding to **retinol-binding protein (RBP)**. The target tissues can oxidize retinol to retinal and retinoic acid, which are the most important biologically active forms:

- **Retinal** is the *prosthetic group of the rhodopsins,* the visual pigments of rods and cones (see Chapter 17).
- **Retinoic acid** is a gene regulator that acts through nuclear receptors, similar to the steroid hormones. Retinoic acid is required for the *maintenance of epithelial tissues.*

Liver, meat, eggs, dairy products, and cod liver oil provide vitamin A in the form of retinol esters, and vegetables supply carotenes. The carotenes betray their presence by their color. Yellow or orange vegetables and fruits, including carrots, pumpkins, mangoes, and papayas, are excellent sources. Green leafy vegetables contain carotenes. Uncolored vegetables have no vitamin A activity.

A single dose of more than 200 mg of retinol or retinal, or chronic consumption of more than 40 mg/day,

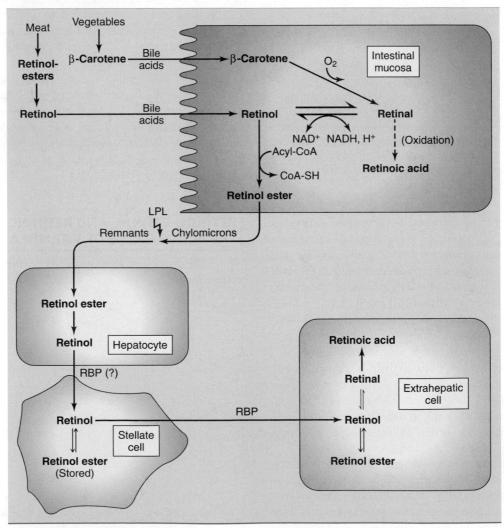

Figure 29.13 Transport and metabolism of retinoids. Retinol is esterified by two different enzymes that use acyl-coenzyme A (acyl-CoA) and lecithin, respectively, as a source of the fatty acid. *LPL,* Lipoprotein lipase; *RBP,* retinol-binding protein.

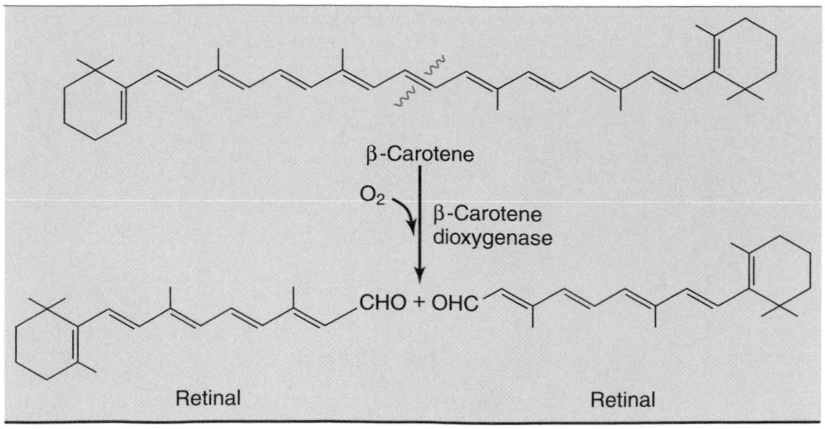

Figure 29.14 The β-carotene dioxygenase reaction cleaves one molecule of dietary β-carotene into two molecules of retinal.

causes nonspecific signs of toxicity. More important is that retinoic acid is a gene regulator during early fetal development. *Both vitamin A deficiency and vitamin A excess are teratogenic.* Vitamin A preparations are used for treatment of skin diseases, including common acne, and all it takes for major complications is an acne-plagued teenage girl who is taking high doses of retinoids and unexpectedly becomes pregnant.

Vitamin A status can be evaluated by determination of serum retinol. Values between 0.7 and 3.0 μmol/L are considered normal. Lower and higher values suggest vitamin A deficiency and toxicity, respectively.

Carotenes are not toxic, but they can accumulate in lipid-rich structures of the body. The skin of babies who are overfed with carrot juice can turn orange, and the adipose tissue of some cadavers in the anatomy laboratory has a yellow tint from dietary carotenes. The presence of dietary carotenes in the skin can reduce sunburn, probably because carotenes absorb some of the damaging ultraviolet radiation.

Both the retinoids and the carotenes are effective antioxidants at the low oxygen partial pressures in the tissues. Unlike the water-soluble vitamin C, the carotenoids and retinoids are present in membranes and other lipid-rich structures, in which they can help in the control of lipid peroxidation.

CLINICAL EXAMPLE 29.9: Vitamin A Deficiency

Vitamin A deficiency is one of the most common nutritional deficiencies in developing countries. It presents mainly with epithelial changes. Columnar epithelia are transformed into heavily keratinized squamous epithelia, a process known as **squamous metaplasia**. Follicular hyperkeratosis (gooseflesh) is an early sign, together with night blindness. In the most advanced cases, the conjunctiva of the eye loses its mucus-secreting cells and becomes keratinized, and the glycoprotein content of the tears is reduced as well. These changes disrupt the fluid film that normally bathes the cornea.

This condition, known as **xerophthalmia** ("dry eyes"), is often complicated by bacterial or chlamydial infection, which results in perforation of the cornea and blindness. Other abnormalities in vitamin A deficiency include microcytic anemia, susceptibility to infections, and impairment of reproductive function in both men and women.

Worldwide, 3 million to 10 million children become xerophthalmic every year, and between 250,000 and 500,000 of these children go blind. Another one million die of infections that they would have survived had they not had vitamin A deficiency.

VITAMIN D IS A PROHORMONE

Vitamin D is not a true vitamin because it is not required for people who have adequate sun exposure. *Vitamin D is synthesized photochemically in the skin* by the action of ultraviolet radiation on the minor membrane steroid 7-dehydrocholesterol (*Fig. 29.15*).

The product of this reaction, **cholecalciferol** (vitamin D_3), has no biological activity. It must first be hydroxylated to **25-hydroxycholecalciferol** in the liver, followed by hydroxylation to **1,25-dihydroxycholecalciferol** (**calcitriol**) in the kidney. All forms of vitamin D are tightly bound to a specialized binding protein in the plasma.

25-Hydroxylation in the liver is fast, and 25-hydroxycholecalciferol is the major circulating form of the vitamin. 1α-Hydroxylation in the kidney is the slow, rate-limiting step, and it is tightly regulated. It is stimulated by parathyroid hormone (PTH), hypocalcemia, and hypophosphatemia. Calcitriol is far less abundant than 25-hydroxycholecalciferol, but it is nearly 1000 times more potent. The half-life of cholecalciferol is approximately 2 months, of 25-hydroxycholecalciferol is 15 days, and of calcitriol is 12 to 24 hours.

Calcitriol is a hormone-like substance. Its receptor is a ligand-regulated transcription factor that resembles the receptors for retinoic acid, steroid hormones, and thyroid hormones. Along with PTH, calcitriol regulates the disposition of calcium and phosphate in the body.

Calcium is required for the functioning of excitable tissues; therefore, its plasma level must be tightly

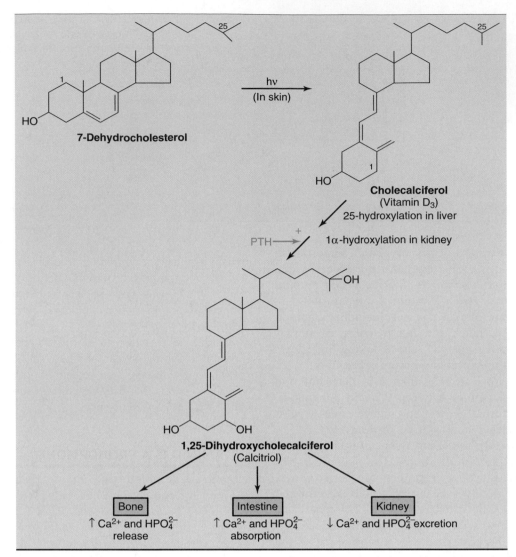

7-Dehydrocholesterol

hν
(In skin)

Cholecalciferol
(Vitamin D$_3$)
25-hydroxylation in liver

PTH →

1α-hydroxylation in kidney

1,25-Dihydroxycholecalciferol
(Calcitriol)

Bone	Intestine	Kidney
↑ Ca^{2+} and HPO$_4^{2-}$ release	↑ Ca^{2+} and HPO$_4^{2-}$ absorption	↓ Ca^{2+} and HPO$_4^{2-}$ excretion

Figure 29.15 Synthesis of calcitriol, the active form of vitamin D, from 7-dehydrocholesterol. *PTH,* Parathyroid hormone.

regulated. *PTH maintains the plasma calcium level constant on a minute-to-minute basis.* It does so primarily by activating osteoclasts and mobilizing calcium from the bones as soon as the plasma calcium level drops too low. This effect is mediated by cyclic AMP (cAMP) and therefore is fast.

The most important effect of vitamin D is the stimulation of intestinal calcium absorption. Thus *vitamin D regulates the calcium level in the body.* Acting mainly through protein synthesis, its effect is long term.

Vitamin D is present in only a few natural foodstuffs, including liver, egg yolk, and saltwater fish (cod liver oil) as well as in fortified foods. The synthesis of cholecalciferol in the skin is affected by skin color. White skin produces about five times more vitamin D than does black skin. Protection from rickets (*Clinical Example 29.10*) is the reason why white skin evolved in human races that lived in cloudy climates.

Calcitriol can be used for treatment of **osteoporosis,** a common cause of pathological fractures in the elderly. It may actually be involved in the etiology of this ailment. The calcitriol receptor occurs in two common allelic variants (B and b) in the population, and homozygosity for the B allele has been claimed to be a risk factor for osteoporosis.

CLINICAL EXAMPLE 29.10: Rickets

Vitamin D deficiency is called **rickets** in children and **osteomalacia** in adults. The immediate effect is reduced intestinal calcium absorption, which tends to reduce the plasma calcium concentration. Maintenance of the blood calcium level has top priority, so PTH is released. Even in long-term vitamin D deficiency, plasma calcium can be maintained at a near-normal level by PTH but at the expense of the bones, which are gradually drained of their mineral content. As a result, affected children have soft cartilaginous bones that bend easily, and affected adults have brittle bones that break easily. Rickets was common in England and other cloudy countries but now is rare.

Hypervitaminosis D, which is caused by overuse of vitamin D supplements, leads to rampant hypercalcemia, hypercalciuria, and metastatic calcification (abnormal calcification of soft tissues). The toxic state persists for a few months after the offending agent is discontinued if the condition was caused by cholecalciferol but for only about 1 week in the case of calcitriol.

VITAMIN E IS AN ANTIOXIDANT

At least eight closely related substances with vitamin E activity occur in nature, but **α-tocopherol** is the most potent (**Fig. 29.16**). In the presence of bile salts, between 30% and 70% of α-tocopherol is absorbed from the small intestine. The liver obtains all forms of vitamin E from chylomicrons and other lipoproteins but selectively secretes α-tocopherol back into the plasma while excreting other tocopherols into the bile. Being lipid soluble, vitamin E associates with plasma lipoproteins, membranes, and storage fat.

Vitamin E is an antioxidant and scavenger of free radicals. It protects membranes, fat depots, and lipoproteins from lipid peroxidation (see Chapter 23). The inactive oxidized derivatives of vitamin E formed in these reactions are reduced back to the active forms by reducing agents, including ascorbate and glutathione (see *Fig. 29.16*).

Unlike most other vitamins, vitamin E was not discovered by the observation of a deficiency disease in humans but as a result of animal experiments. Human deficiency is rare. It can be seen in premature infants who are born with low tissue stores and who have poor intestinal absorption for several weeks after birth, and in fat malabsorption syndromes at all ages. Typical deficiency signs include neurological abnormalities and fragility of red blood cells. The most serious form of vitamin E deficiency occurs in patients with abetalipoproteinemia (see Chapter 25), who develop neuropathic and myopathic changes in addition to hemolysis.

Being an antioxidant, vitamin E has a reputation for reducing the risk of cancer, coronary heart disease, and age-related degenerative diseases, but both epidemiological studies and intervention studies with high doses of the vitamin have produced mixed results.

Good sources include vegetable oils, various oil seeds, and wheat germ. Although vitamin E is a popular

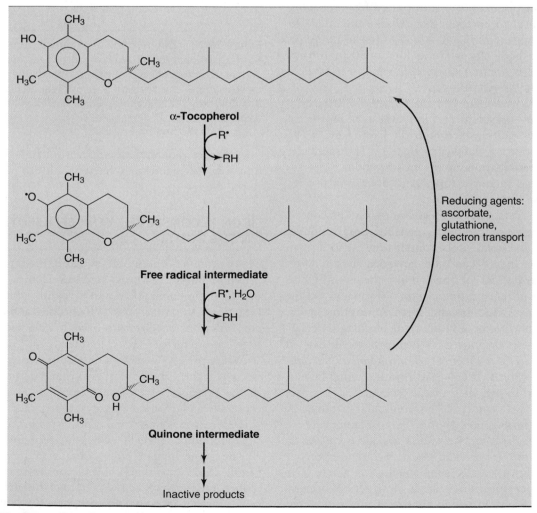

Figure 29.16 The action of α-tocopherol as a scavenger of free radicals. R•, Free radical.

object of abuse by health food enthusiasts, the dangers of overdosage are minimal. Unlike vitamins A and D, vitamin E is nontoxic in doses up to 50 times higher than the recommended intake of 15 mg/day.

VITAMIN K IS REQUIRED FOR BLOOD CLOTTING

The name vitamin K is derived from "koagulation" because a clotting disorder is the only abnormality in vitamin K deficiency. The naturally occurring forms of the vitamin are isoprenoids containing a quinoid ring structure. Phylloquinone is the most common form of the vitamin in plants:

Structurally similar forms of vitamin K, known as menaquinones, are produced by bacteria, including intestinal bacteria. Vitamin K has no specific binding protein in the plasma but is transported from the intestine to the liver in chylomicrons. Unlike the other fat-soluble vitamins, *vitamin K is not stored to any great extent.* Total body stores are as low as 50 to 100 μg, so *vitamin K is the first fat-soluble vitamin to be deficient in acute fat malabsorption.*

Vitamin K participates in the enzymatic carboxylation of glutamyl residues during synthesis of prothrombin and other clotting factors in the liver (*Fig. 29.17*). The only important deficiency sign is a clotting disorder, and determination of the prothrombin time (see Chapter 15) is the most important laboratory test for evaluation of vitamin K status.

Vitamin K deficiency is most common in newborns. Tissue stores are low at birth, intestinal flora is not yet established, and breast milk contains only 1 to 2 μg of vitamin K per liter. Because the newborn has a requirement of 5 μg/day (3 L of breast milk), the levels of vitamin K–dependent clotting factors normally decline during the first 2 to 3 days after birth. At this time in perhaps 1:400 newborns, an abnormal bleeding tendency develops that is diagnosed as **hemorrhagic disease of the newborn.** *This is the most common nutritional deficiency in newborns.* It can lead to intracranial hemorrhages with lasting neurologic sequelae. Therefore prophylaxis with oral or intramuscular vitamin K shortly after birth is now routine in most countries.

Vitamin K deficiency in adults usually is caused by fat malabsorption. For example, it is common practice to administer vitamin K supplements for a few days before surgery for biliary tract obstruction because these patients have impaired vitamin K absorption and possibly impaired blood clotting.

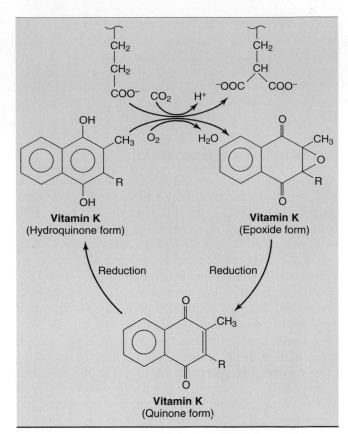

Figure 29.17 Carboxylation of glutamate residues during posttranslational modification of clotting factors in the endoplasmic reticulum of the liver. Unlike other carboxylations, this reaction does not require biotin and ATP; it is driven by the exergonic oxidation of the vitamin K cofactor. *R,* Variable side chain.

A dietary requirement is hard to define because vitamin K made by intestinal bacteria adds to the vitamin K in the diet.

IRON IS CONSERVED VERY EFFICIENTLY IN THE BODY

Many proteins contain iron, either in the form of a heme group or bound to amino acid side chains. The ferrous heme iron in hemoglobin and myoglobin binds molecular oxygen, and the iron in cytochromes and other redox enzymes transfers electrons by switching back and forth between the ferrous (Fe^{2+}) and ferric (Fe^{3+}) states.

When present in excess or in the wrong place, *iron is toxic.* It forms reactive hydroxyl and peroxide radicals in the presence of molecular oxygen. Ferrous iron is especially dangerous as a catalyst of free radical reactions. Therefore iron is stored and transported in the ferric state, tightly bound to specialized binding proteins.

The adult human body contains 3 to 4 g of iron (*Table 29.2*). Two thirds of this iron is present in hemoglobin, and much of the rest is storage iron in liver, spleen, bone marrow, intestinal mucosa, pancreas, myocardium, and other tissues. The amount of stored iron is highly

Table 29.2 Distribution of Body Iron in a "Typical" 70-kg Man and 55-kg Woman

Protein	Amount (g) in	
	70-kg Man	**55-kg Woman**
Hemoglobin	2.50	1.70
Myoglobin	0.15	0.10
Enzymes, cytochromes, iron-sulfur proteins	0.15	0.10
Storage iron		
Ferritin	0.50	0.30
Hemosiderin	0.50	0.10
Transferrin	0.003	0.002
Total	3.8	2.3

variable. It is near zero in many children and menstruating women but is more than 1 g in some older men.

Iron is stored in the cells as **ferritin**. This protein forms a shell of 24 polypeptides, made from two slightly different polypeptide chains (molecular weights 19 kD and 21 kD). This shell of apoferritin, with an external diameter of 13 nm and an internal cavity 6 nm across, is riddled with pores that allow the entry and exit of ionized iron. The hollow core can accommodate up to 4500 ferric iron atoms in the form of ferric oxide hydroxide ($FeOOH$) crystals but actually rarely contains more than 3000.

Hemosiderin is a partially denatured derivative of ferritin. Ferritin is the more abundant storage form when the tissue stores are low, and hemosiderin predominates when tissue stores are high. The abnormal accumulation in tissues is called **hemosiderosis**. A small amount of ferritin, consisting mainly of apoferritin with little bound iron, is present in the blood. This ferritin is released during normal cell turnover in the liver and other organs.

Transferrin is the iron transport protein in the plasma (see Chapter 15). It has two binding sites that bind ferric iron with extremely high affinity. *Almost all iron in the plasma is bound to transferrin.* In the laboratory, the transferrin concentration is measured as **total iron binding capacity (TIBC)**, and the percentage of high-affinity binding sites that is occupied by iron is expressed as the **iron saturation**. An iron saturation between 10% and 60% is considered normal.

Cells acquire transferrin-bound iron through a **transferrin receptor** in the plasma membrane. The receptor binds iron-loaded transferrin in preference to apotransferrin, and receptor binding is followed by endocytosis. Endocytosed iron dissociates from transferrin in the acidic environment of the endosome and is reduced to the ferrous state and then transferred to the cytoplasm. Transferrin is recycled into the blood (***Fig. 29.18***).

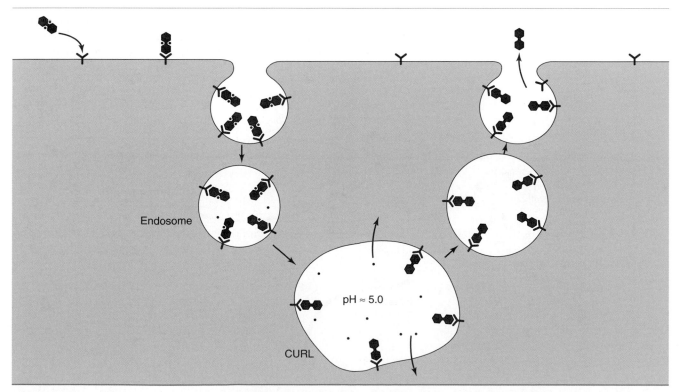

pH ≈ 5.0

Endosome

CURL

Figure 29.18 Utilization of transferrin-bound iron by receptor-mediated endocytosis. In this variation of the endocytic pathway, the endosome is acidified to a pH of approximately 5.0. In this acidified organelle, known as *CURL* (compartment of uncoupling of receptor and ligand), iron is released from transferrin. Whereas iron is transported into the cytoplasm, the receptor-bound apotransferrin is returned to the cell surface. ⬢⬢, Apotransferrin; •, Fe^{3+}; Υ, transferrin receptor.

IRON ABSORPTION IS TIGHTLY REGULATED

Most people consume between 10 and 20 mg of iron per day. Much of this is derived not from the foodstuffs but from the cooking utensils used for food preparation. Therefore the replacement of iron cooking ware by aluminum products and the increasing use of Teflon-coated pots and pans can promote iron deficiency.

Iron is absorbed in the ferrous form, mainly in the duodenum. Although both intracellular storage and transport in the blood are in the ferric form, *only ferrous iron is transported across membranes*. The reduction of ferric iron in food is favored by the low pH in the stomach and the presence of reducing substances, especially ascorbic acid. Therefore *iron absorption is enhanced by vitamin C–rich fruit juices and reduced by achlorhydria* (lack of gastric acid) and after gastrectomy (surgical removal of the stomach).

Iron absorption is reduced by tannins, oxalate, phytate (inositol hexaphosphate), large quantities of inorganic phosphate, and phosphate-containing antacids that form insoluble or nonabsorbable iron complexes. The absorption of nonheme iron varies between 0.8% (rice) and 10% (soybeans) but can double in response to iron deficiency. *Any anemic state, regardless of its cause, enhances intestinal iron absorption.* Heme iron, which accounts for a significant portion of iron in meat, is absorbed by separate mechanisms and with an efficiency of 20% to 25%.

Dietary nonheme iron is reduced with the help of reductases on the apical surface of the intestinal mucosal cell. The ferrous iron is absorbed into the cell with the help of a divalent metal transporter (**DMT1**) in the apical membrane. Heme-bound iron is absorbed by a different transporter. The absorbed iron either binds to ferritin in the cell or is transported across the basolateral membrane by the iron carrier **ferroportin.** After transport by ferroportin, the iron is oxidized to the ferric state before binding to transferrin.

Iron is excreted as well as absorbed by the intestinal mucosa. The cells take up iron from transferrin and store it as ferritin. This iron is excreted when the mucosal cell is sloughed off into the intestinal lumen at the end of its 2- to 6-day lifespan. Virtually no iron is present in urine, sweat, bile, and digestive secretions. Therefore *the intestine is the only important route of iron excretion.* In a healthy adult man, intestinal iron absorption and excretion are expected to be equal. The amount of absorbed or secreted iron is minimal compared to the amount that is recycled from destroyed blood cells in spleen and liver (*Fig. 29.19*).

Iron absorption is controlled mainly by the liver. When iron is plentiful, the liver releases the 25-amino-acid peptide **hepcidin** into the blood. In intestine and other tissues, hepcidin binds to the iron transporter ferroportin and induces its internalization and degradation. This is the major mechanism reducing intestinal iron absorption and preventing iron overload when body iron stores are sufficient.

The cells adjust their iron uptake by regulating the number of their transferrin receptors. They achieve this by adjusting the stability of the transferrin receptor mRNA (*Fig. 29.20*). This mRNA has a set of stem-loop structures in its 3′-untranslated region that function as **iron response elements (IREs)**. IREs bind **iron regulatory proteins (IRPs)** in the iron-depleted state. When

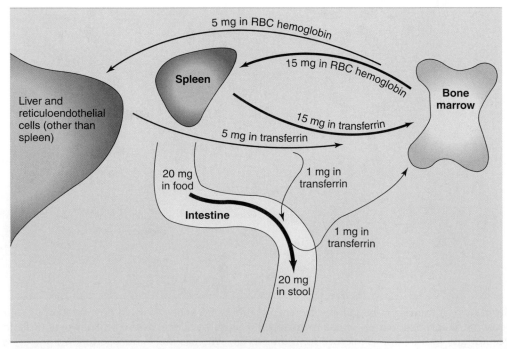

Figure 29.19 Daily transport of iron in the body. *RBC,* Red blood cell.

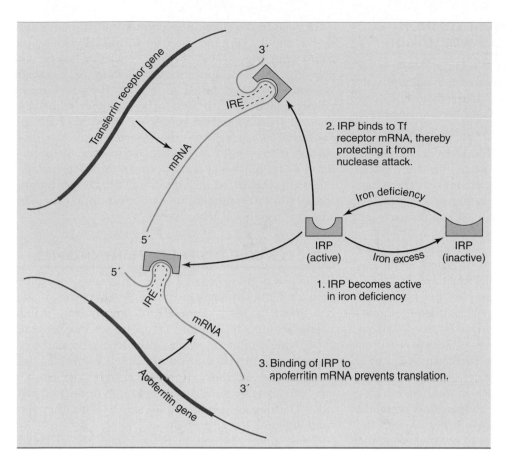

2. IRP binds to Tf receptor mRNA, thereby protecting it from nuclease attack.

Iron deficiency

IRP (active)

Iron excess

IRP (inactive)

1. IRP becomes active in iron deficiency

3. Binding of IRP to apoferritin mRNA prevents translation.

Figure 29.20 Cellular adaptations in the iron-deficient state. More transferrin (*Tf*) receptors are synthesized to acquire iron from circulating transferrin, and the synthesis of apoferritin is inhibited. The iron response element (*IRE*) is a regulatory sequence of approximately 30 nucleotides in the mRNAs for transferrin receptor and apoferritin. In iron deficiency, the iron regulatory protein (*IRP*) is converted to an active form that binds the IREs with high affinity.

an IRP binds to the IREs, it prolongs the lifespan of the mRNA by protecting it from nucleases. In consequence, *the cell makes more transferrin receptors when it needs more iron.* The intestinal iron transporters DMT1 and ferroportin appear to be regulated in the same way. Through iron response elements in their mRNAs, their synthesis is stimulated directly when iron stores in the enterocyte are running low.

Ferritin mRNA has an IRE not in the 3'-untranslated region but in the 5'-untranslated region near the cap. When an IRP binds this IRE in the iron-deficient state, it prevents the initiation of translation. Therefore *apoferritin is synthesized only when iron is abundant.*

CLINICAL EXAMPLE 29.11: Hemochromatosis

Hemochromatosis is an iron overload syndrome with progressive hemosiderosis and resulting organ damage. It can lead to liver cirrhosis and liver cancer, diabetes mellitus, cardiomyopathy, hyperpigmentation of the skin, endocrine disorders, and joint pain. Accumulating the 10 to 40 g of iron needed to produce symptoms takes some decades, and women are protected by menstruation and childbearing. Therefore iron overload is seen mainly in older men.

In people of European descent, the condition is associated with homozygosity for a mutation in the HFE gene, whose protein product participates in iron sensing

by the liver. The most important mutation is a missense mutation replacing a cysteine in position 282 of the polypeptide by tyrosine. This mutation reduces the amount of hepcidin released by the liver. The relative deficiency of hepcidin up-regulates ferroportin in the intestine and increases iron absorption. The hemochromatosis mutation originated in northwestern Europe sometime during the past 5000 years. It now is common in this population, with the highest frequency in Scandinavian countries, Great Britain, and Ireland. About 1:400 white Americans is homozygous for this gene, and 10% are heterozygous.

Fewer than 5% of the homozygotes are said to develop clinical signs of iron overload. However, iron overload can contribute to common diseases such as liver damage, diabetes, and arthritis, and its role often remains unrecognized. Elevated iron levels are common in liver biopsy samples of patients with "alcoholic cirrhosis," and whether iron overload is the cause or the result of liver disease is not always clear.

Symptomatic hemochromatosis is treated by repeated phlebotomy. Because leeches are out of fashion, weekly blood donations for up to 1 or 2 years are the best option.

Because there is only one major hemochromatosis mutation in northern European populations, genetic screening is fairly easy. If the genotype is ascertained early in life, iron overload in genetically predisposed individuals can be prevented by occasional blood donations.

IRON DEFICIENCY IS THE MOST COMMON MICRONUTRIENT DEFICIENCY WORLDWIDE

When iron becomes scarce in the body, *storage iron is mobilized first*. Next, impairment of hemoglobin synthesis causes anemia. Finally, multiple cellular functions suffer when iron-containing enzymes become impaired. Iron deficiency is seen in the following contexts:

1. *Acute massive hemorrhage.* Blood loss of 1 L drains approximately 500 mg of iron from the body. Most people have enough storage iron to make up for a loss of this magnitude, and the hematocrit returns to normal within 1 or 2 weeks. Iron supplements are required only if the iron stores of the body are low.

2. *Chronic blood loss.* During each menstrual period, most women lose 20 to 40 ml of blood containing 10 to 20 mg of iron (0.35–0.7 mg/day). "Occult" blood loss is caused not by vampires but by chronic hemorrhage into the alimentary canal from esophageal varices, peptic ulcer, hemorrhoids, blood-sucking intestinal parasites, or tumors. Unexplained iron deficiency anemia in men can be the first sign of a malignancy.

3. *Growth.* Adults need to absorb iron only to balance iron excretion, but growing children must maintain a positive iron balance as the blood volume expands. The iron content of breast milk is low; therefore, the blood hemoglobin concentration normally declines from 18% to 20% at birth to 10% to 14% at 5 months. Oxygen delivery is not much affected by this decline because fetal hemoglobin is replaced by adult hemoglobin during this time period, and adult hemoglobin is the better oxygen carrier after birth. Iron supplements are sometimes given at this time to prevent a decline below 10%, which can be considered the lower limit of the "normal" range.

4. *Pregnancy and lactation.* From 250 to 300 mg of iron is transferred to the fetus during pregnancy. An additional 80 to 400 mg is lost in the placenta and umbilical cord and in blood loss at birth. Another 100 to 180 mg is lost during lactation. The drain is minimal during the first months of pregnancy, but up to 5 mg/day is transferred to the fetus during the third trimester. Because many women have negligible iron stores, supplements are routinely given during late pregnancy.

Iron deficiency is the most common cause of *microcytic hypochromic anemia*. (*Microcytic* means "small red blood cells," and *hypochromic* means low hemoglobin content per cell.) Pallor, weakness, and lassitude are typical manifestations of iron deficiency.

Iron deficiency anemia is treated with iron supplements, usually in the form of ferrous sulfate combined with ascorbic acid. Treatment is given for several months and should be continued for some months after hematological improvement to allow for the formation of adequate tissue stores.

Depending on diagnostic criteria, nutritional habits in the population, and the iron fortification of staple foods, the prevalence of iron deficiency anemia in growing children and in menstruating or pregnant women is often reported as 2% to 15% in affluent countries and 10% to 50% in poor countries. Worldwide, 0.5 to 0.6 billion people are affected. *With the exception of protein-calorie malnutrition, iron deficiency is the most prevalent nutritional deficiency worldwide.* Biochemical indices of iron deficiency anemia are summarized in *Table 29.3*. Serum ferritin and transferrin saturation are the two most important measures in the clinical laboratory.

ZINC IS A CONSTITUENT OF MANY ENZYMES

With total body stores of 1.5 to 2.5 g, zinc is the most abundant trace mineral in the body after iron. It is a *constituent of the zinc metalloenzymes,* which include carbonic anhydrase, the cytoplasmic (copper-zinc) superoxide dismutase, alcohol dehydrogenase, carboxypeptidases A and B, DNA and RNA polymerases, and many others. In the *zinc finger proteins,* it serves a structural role by stabilizing small loops in the polypeptide. The human genome is known to code for more than 300 zinc finger proteins.

Some zinc is bound to the storage protein **metallothionein** in the tissues. This protein also binds copper and many other heavy metals, thereby reducing their toxicity. Its synthesis is induced by zinc, cadmium, bismuth, arsenic, and other metals.

Zinc is absorbed incompletely in the small intestine. It is also present in pancreatic juice, and excess zinc is

Table 29.3 Biochemical Indices of Iron Deficiency and Iron Overload

Index	Normal	Changes in Iron Deficiency	Changes in Iron Overload
Hematocrit			
Male	43%–49%	Decreased	Normal
Female	41%–46%		
Blood hemoglobin			
Male	14%–18%	Decreased	Normal
Female	12%–16%		
Total plasma iron	50-160 µg/dl	Decreased	Increased
Total iron binding capacity	250-400 µg/dl	Increased	Increased
Transferrin saturation	20%–55%	Decreased	Increased
Serum ferritin			
Male	5-30 µg/dl	Decreased	Increased
Female	1.2-10 µg/dl		

excreted in the stools. Transport in the blood is in association with serum albumin. Only small amounts are lost in urine (0.5 mg/day), sweat (0.2 to 2.0 mg/day), and seminal fluid (up to 1 mg per ejaculate). Meat, nuts, beans, and wheat germ are good dietary sources of zinc. The adult male RDA is 15 mg/day.

Zinc deficiency leads to dermatitis and poor wound healing, hair loss, neuropsychiatric impairments, decreased taste acuity, and, in children, poor growth and testicular atrophy. **Acrodermatitis enteropathica** is a rare recessively inherited disease with dermatitis, diarrhea, and alopecia (hair loss) caused by impaired intestinal zinc absorption. High doses of orally administered zinc are curative.

COPPER PARTICIPATES IN REACTIONS OF MOLECULAR OXYGEN

The adult human body contains 80 to 110 mg of copper. Its major function is as a cofactor of enzymes that use either molecular oxygen or an oxygen derivative as one of their substrates. Examples include cytochrome oxidase, dopamine β-hydroxylase, monoamine oxidase, tyrosinase, Δ^9-desaturase, lysyl oxidase, and the cytoplasmic superoxide dismutase.

The dietary requirement is between 1 and 3 mg/day, and the major route of copper excretion is the bile. Of the copper in the serum, 60% is tightly bound in **ceruloplasmin,** and the rest is loosely bound to albumin or complexed with histidine.

Copper deficiency is characterized by a microcytic hypochromic anemia, leukopenia, hemorrhagic vascular changes, bone demineralization, hypercholesterolemia, and neurological problems. It is uncommon and has been seen mainly in patients receiving total parenteral nutrition and in infants being fed copper-deficient formulas.

Menkes syndrome is a rare X-linked recessive disorder caused by the deficiency of an ATP-dependent membrane transporter for copper. The transfer of copper from the intestinal mucosal cells to the blood is blocked, and its intracellular transport is abnormal as well. This fatal disease is characterized by growth retardation, mental deficiency, seizures, arterial aneurysms, bone demineralization, and brittle hair. It can be treated by administration of the copper-histidine complex, but affected children nevertheless die during the first years of life.

Wilson disease (hepatolenticular degeneration) is a rare recessively inherited deficiency of a different copper transporter. The intestinal absorption of copper is intact, but its biliary excretion is blocked. This leads to copper accumulation in liver and brain, with resulting liver damage, neurological degeneration, or both. This disease can manifest at any time during the lifespan. It is treated with D-penicillamine, which forms a soluble, excretable copper complex.

SOME TRACE ELEMENTS SERVE VERY SPECIFIC FUNCTIONS

Some other trace minerals serve highly specialized functions in the body. They include the following:

- *Manganese.* This metal stimulates the activity of many enzymes but can, in most cases, be replaced by magnesium. An adequate intake is 2 to 5 mg/day. Excess manganese is toxic, causing psychosis and parkinsonism ("manganese madness").
- *Molybdenum.* This metal occurs in a few oxidase enzymes, including xanthine oxidase.
- *Selenium.* In the form of selenocysteine, this element occurs in about 20 human proteins, including the important antioxidant enzyme glutathione peroxidase. Both selenium deficiency and toxicity have been described. **Keshan disease** is an endemic cardiomyopathy in parts of China that is caused by the low selenium content of locally grown foodstuffs. The selenium content of the soil varies widely in different parts of the world and is reflected in the selenium content of the food plants grown on these soils.
- *Iodine.* This halogen is needed only for the synthesis of thyroid hormones.
- *Fluorine.* The fluoride ion can be incorporated in the inorganic substance of bones and teeth. Although not absolutely essential, it strengthens teeth and bones. It may even have some protective effect in osteoporosis.

SUMMARY

Vitamins are essential micronutrients that serve specialized functions in metabolism. Most of the water-soluble vitamins are precursors of coenzymes. For example, riboflavin is required for the synthesis of the flavin coenzymes: niacin for NAD and NADP, thiamine for TPP, pantothenic acid for CoA, and folic acid for THF.

Other vitamins, notably vitamins A, D, and E, are antioxidants that scavenge destructive free radicals. They suppress lipid peroxidation, and they may have antimutagenic properties.

Other vitamins are precursors of hormone-like products. Vitamin A is converted to retinoic acid, and vitamin D is converted to calcitriol. These vitamin derivatives are gene regulators, with mechanisms of action similar to the steroid hormones.

Macrominerals are bulk constituents of the body fluids that are required in fairly large quantities in the diet. Microminerals serve specialized functions and are required only in small quantities. Iron, in particular, is required as a constituent of heme proteins and iron-sulfur proteins.

Nutritional deficiencies of individual vitamins and minerals cause distinctive deficiency states that are related to the metabolic functions of the missing nutrient. For example, vitamin C deficiency (scurvy) causes connective tissue problems because of impaired collagen synthesis, and iron deficiency causes anemia because of impaired hemoglobin synthesis. Although the incidence of severe nutritional deficiencies has declined in affluent countries, vitamin and mineral nutrition is still a major public health concern for at-risk groups, including infants, pregnant women, alcoholics, and the elderly.

Further Reading

Batts KP: Iron overload syndromes and the liver, *Mod Pathol* 20:S31–S39, 2007.

Beutler E: Hemochromatosis: genetics and pathophysiology, *Annu Rev Med* 57:331–347, 2006.

Brewer GJ: Iron and copper toxicity in diseases of aging, particularly atherosclerosis and Alzheimer's disease, *Exp Biol Med* 232:323–335, 2007.

Camaschella C: BMP6 orchestrates iron metabolism, *Nat Genet* 41:386–388, 2009.

Cappellini MD, Pattoneri P: Oral iron chelators, *Annu Rev Med* 60:25–38, 2009.

Combet E, El Mesmari A, Preston T, et al: Dietary phenolic acids and ascorbic acid: influence on acid-catalyzed nitrosative chemistry in the presence and absence of lipids, *Free Radic Biol Med* 48:763–771, 2010.

Cousins RJ, Liuzzi JP, Lichten LA: Mammalian zinc transport, trafficking, and signals, *J Biol Chem* 281:24085–24089, 2006.

De Bie P, Muller P, Wijmenga C, et al: Molecular pathogenesis of Wilson and Menkes disease: correlation of mutations with molecular defects and disease phenotypes, *J Med Genet* 44:673–688, 2007.

Douglas RM, Hemilä H: Vitamin C for preventing and treating the common cold, *PLoS Med* 2(6):e168, 2005.

Gloth FM: The ABD's of long-term care: a review of the use of some vitamin supplements in the LTC setting, *Ann Long-Term Care* 16(2):28–32, 2008.

Hemilä H, Chalker E, Douglas B: Vitamin C for preventing and treating the common cold, *Cochrane Database Syst Rev* 2007(3):CD000980, 2007.

Jones G: Pharmacokinetics of vitamin D toxicity, *Am J Clin Nutr* 88:582S–586S, 2008.

Kaplan JH, Lutsenko S: Copper transport in mammalian cells: special care for a metal with special needs, *J Biol Chem* 284:25461–25465, 2009.

Kawaguchi R, Yu J, Honda J, Hu J, et al: A membrane receptor for retinol binding protein mediates cellular uptake of vitamin A, *Science* 315:820–825, 2007.

Khanal RC, Nemere I: Regulation of intestinal calcium transport, *Annu Rev Nutr* 28:179–196, 2008.

Kiokias S, Varzakas T, Oreopoulou V: In vitro activity of vitamins, flavonoids, and natural phenolic antioxidants against the oxidative deterioration of oil-based systems, *Crit Rev Food Sci Nutr* 48:78–93, 2008.

Lichtenstein AH: Nutrient supplements and cardiovascular disease: a heartbreaking story, *J Lipid Res* 2009: S429–S433, 2009.

Lu J, Holmgren A: Selenoproteins, *J Biol Chem* 284:723–727, 2009.

Mock DM: Marginal biotin deficiency is common in normal human pregnancy and is highly teratogenic in mice, *J Nutr* 139:154–157, 2009.

Muckenthaler MU, Galy B, Hentze MW: Systemic iron homeostasis and the iron-responsive element/iron-regulatory protein (IRE/IRP) regulatory network, *Annu Rev Nutr* 28:197–213, 2008.

Obican SG, Finnell RH, Mills JL, et al: Folic acid in early pregnancy: a public health success story, *FASEB J* 24: 4167–4174, 2010.

Traber MG: Vitamin E regulatory mechanisms, *Annu Rev Nutr* 27:347–362, 2007.

Tümer Z, Møller LB: Menkes disease, *Eur J Hum Genet* 18:511–518, 2010.

Turski ML, Thiele DJ: New roles for copper metabolism in cell proliferation, signaling, and disease, *J Biol Chem* 284:717–721, 2009.

Wolf G: Identification of a membrane receptor for retinol-binding protein functioning in the cellular uptake of retinol, *Nutr Rev* 65:385–388, 2007.

Zempleni J, Hassan YI, Wijeratne SSK: Biotin and biotinidase deficiency, *Expert Rev Endocrinol Metab* 2008:715–724, 2008.

Zhang A-S, Enns CA: Iron homeostasis: recently identified proteins provide insight into novel control mechanisms, *J Biol Chem* 284:711–715, 2009.

Ziouzenkova O, Plutzky J: Retinoid metabolism and nuclear receptor responses: new insights into coordinated regulation of the PPAR-RXR complex, *FEBS Lett* 582:32–38, 2008.

QUESTIONS

1. **A finding that would support a diagnosis of iron deficiency anemia in a 25-year-old woman with a hematocrit of 28% is**

   A. Presence of oversized erythrocytes
   B. Low iron saturation of transferrin
   C. Reduced serum transferrin concentration
   D. Increased level of serum ferritin
   E. Reduced level of metallothionein in a liver biopsy sample

2. **Retinoic acid in high doses is sometimes used for the treatment of skin diseases, including common acne. Retinoic acid can cause many toxic effects at high doses. The *most important* of these toxic effects is**

   A. Bone demineralization, which leads to pathological fractures
   B. Connective tissue weakness with multiple small subcutaneous hemorrhages

C. Teratogenic effects during the first trimester of pregnancy

D. Peripheral neuropathy

E. Amnesia

3. **Vitamin D can be produced by the action of sunlight on 7-dehydrocholesterol in the skin, but it has to be converted to its biologically active form by hydroxylation reactions in**

A. Lungs and brain

B. Endothelium and intestines

C. Skeletal muscle and adrenal cortex

D. Adipose tissue and bone

E. Liver and kidneys

4. **Some vitamins have antioxidant properties and therefore are considered promising for the prevention of atherosclerosis, cancer, and age-related degenerative diseases. Antioxidant properties have been demonstrated for all of the following vitamins *except***

A. Thiamine (vitamin B_1)

B. α-Tocopherol (vitamin E)

C. Ascorbic acid (vitamin C)

D. Retinol (vitamin A)

5. **Thiamine deficiency can cause both acute encephalopathy and irreversible memory impairment. These problems are most often seen in thiamine-deficient**

A. Newborns

B. Alcoholics

C. Diabetics

D. Vegetarians

E. Medical students

Chapter 30

INTEGRATION OF METABOLISM

For the individual cell, the most immediate challenge is the safeguarding of its own energy supply. Beyond the imperative of self-preservation, however, cells and organs must cooperate unselfishly for the common good of the body. Together they must master the everyday challenges of overeating, fasting, and muscular activity and the less routine challenges of infectious illnesses and environmental toxins.

These challenges require the organism-wide coordination of metabolic pathways. This coordination is provided by nervous and hormonal signals that reach every part of the body. This chapter discusses the metabolic adaptations to environmental challenges and varying physiological needs. It describes the hormonal mechanisms of metabolic regulation and some clinical conditions in which these regulatory mechanisms are deranged.

INSULIN IS A SATIETY HORMONE

After a hearty meal, the body is flooded with monosaccharides, amino acids, and triglycerides. Not all of this bounty can be oxidized immediately, and *excess nutrients have to be stored as glycogen and fat.*

Insulin is the hormone of the well-fed state. Its synthesis and release are powerfully stimulated by glucose, and this effect is potentiated by amino acids. Therefore *the plasma level of insulin is highest after a carbohydrate-rich meal.* The list of insulin effects given in *Table 30.1* shows that insulin stimulates the *utilization of dietary*

Table 30.1 Metabolic Effects of Insulin

Tissue	Affected Pathway	Affected Enzyme
Liver	↑ Glucose phosphorylation	Glucokinase
	↑ Glycolysis	Phosphofructokinase-1,* pyruvate kinase[†]
	↓ Gluconeogenesis	PEP-carboxykinase, fructose-1,6-bisphosphatase,* glucose-6-phosphatase
	↑ Glycogen synthesis	Glycogen synthase[†]
	↓ Glycogenolysis	Glycogen phosphorylase[†]
	↑ Fatty acid synthesis	Acetyl-CoA carboxylase,[†] ATP-citrate lyase, malic enzyme
	↑ Pentose phosphate pathway	Glucose-6-phosphate dehydrogenase
Adipose tissue	↑ Glucose uptake	Glucose carrier
	↑ Glycolysis	Phosphofructokinase-1
	↑ Pentose phosphate pathway	Glucose-6-phosphate dehydrogenase
	↑ Pyruvate oxidation	Pyruvate dehydrogenase[†]
	↑ Triglyceride utilization (from lipoproteins)	Lipoprotein lipase
	↑ Triglyceride synthesis	Glycerol-3-phosphate acyl transferase
	↓ Lipolysis	Hormone-sensitive lipase[†]
Skeletal muscle	↑ Glucose uptake	Glucose carrier
	↑ Glycolysis	Phosphofructokinase-1
	↑ Glycogen synthesis	Glycogen synthase[†]
	↓ Glycogenolysis	Glycogen phosphorylase[†]
	↑ Protein synthesis	Translational initiation complex

*Insulin acts indirectly by promoting the dephosphorylation of phosphofructokinase-2/fructose-2,6-bisphosphatase, thereby increasing the level of fructose-2,6-bisphosphate.
[†]Insulin acts by promoting the dephosphorylation of the enzyme.
Most of the other insulin effects included here are actions on the rate of synthesis or degradation of the affected enzyme.
PEP, Phosphoenolpyruvate.

nutrients, including glucose, amino acids, and triglycerides. It diverts excess nutrients into the synthesis of glycogen, fat, and protein.

In skeletal muscle and adipose tissue, glucose uptake into the cell through glucose transporter-4 (GLUT4) carriers is the rate-limiting step of glucose metabolism. This step is stimulated 10-fold to 20-fold by insulin.

In the liver, glucose uptake by the insulin-insensitive GLUT2 transporter is not rate limiting, but *the glucose-metabolizing enzymes are stimulated by insulin.* Insulin induces the synthesis of glycolytic enzymes and represses the synthesis of gluconeogenic enzymes on a time scale of many hours to several days.

On a minute-by-minute time scale, insulin dephosphorylates metabolic and regulatory enzymes, thereby stimulating glycolysis and glycogen synthesis while inhibiting gluconeogenesis and glycogenolysis (see Chapter 22).

Glucose metabolism in brain and erythrocytes is not insulin dependent. These tissues are inept at metabolizing alternative fuels. Therefore they must keep consuming glucose even in the fasting state, when the insulin level is low.

Insulin regulates the metabolism of fat and protein as well as of carbohydrate. It induces the conversion of excess carbohydrate to fat by stimulating glycolysis and fatty acid synthesis. At the same time, it promotes fat synthesis in adipose tissue while inhibiting fat breakdown. Insulin stimulates protein synthesis rather nonselectively, in large part by actions at the level of translation. Thus excess nutrients are used for the synthesis of glycogen, fat, and body protein.

GLUCAGON MAINTAINS THE BLOOD GLUCOSE LEVEL

The secretion of glucagon from the pancreatic α-cells is increased twofold to threefold by hypoglycemia and reduced to half of the basal release by hyperglycemia. Acting through its second messenger cyclic AMP (cAMP), *glucagon up-regulates the blood glucose level when dietary carbohydrate is in short supply.* Its actions on the pathways of glucose metabolism are opposite to those of insulin (*Table 30.2*), but, unlike insulin, *glucagon acts almost exclusively on the liver;* it has negligible effects on adipose tissue, muscle, and other extrahepatic tissues.

CATECHOLAMINES MEDIATE THE FLIGHT-OR-FIGHT RESPONSE

Norepinephrine is the neurotransmitter of postganglionic sympathetic neurons, and both epinephrine and norepinephrine are released from the adrenal medulla in response to acetylcholine released by preganglionic sympathetic neurons. *These catecholamines are stress hormones.* They are released during physical exertion and cold exposure and also in response to psychological stress (e.g., during a biochemistry examination).

The catecholamines can raise the cellular cAMP level through β-adrenergic receptors, and the calcium level through α_1-adrenergic receptors. Muscle and adipose tissue have mainly β receptors, and the liver has both β and α_1 receptors.

The metabolic actions of the catecholamines are summarized in *Table 30.3*. These actions, which appear within seconds, are part of the **flight-or-fight response.** Most important is the *mobilization of fat and glycogen reserves for use by the muscles.* In muscle tissue itself, the major effects are *stimulation of glycogen degradation and glycolysis.*

The regulatory metabolite fructose-2,6-bisphosphate activates phosphofructokinase-1 in muscle, as it does in the liver (see Chapter 22). However, the phosphofructokinase-2/fructose-2,6-bisphosphatase of skeletal muscle

Table 30.2 Metabolic Effects of Glucagon on the Liver*

Effect on Pathway	Affected Enzyme	Enzyme Induction/Repression	Enzyme Phosphorylation	Other
↓ Glycolysis	Glucokinase	+		
	Phosphofructokinase-1			+†
	Pyruvate kinase	+		
↑ Gluconeogenesis	PEP-carboxykinase	+		
	Fructose-1,6-bisphosphatase	+		+†
	Glucose-6-phosphatase	+		
↓ Glycogen synthesis	Glycogen synthase		+	
↑ Glycogenolysis	Glycogen phosphorylase		+	
↓ Fatty acid synthesis	Acetyl-CoA carboxylase	+	+	
↑ Fatty acid oxidation	Carnitine-palmitoyl transferase-1	+		

*Both the enzyme phosphorylations and the effects on gene expression are mediated by cyclic AMP (cAMP).
†Mediated by the cAMP-dependent phosphorylation of phosphofructokinase-2/fructose-2,6-bisphosphatase and a decreased cellular concentration of fructose-2,6-bisphosphate.
CoA, Coenzyme A; *PEP*, phosphoenolpyruvate.

Table 30.3 Metabolic Effects of Norepinephrine and Epinephrine

Tissue	Affected Pathway	Affected Enzyme	Second Messenger
Adipose tissue	↑↑↑ Lipolysis	Hormone-sensitive lipase*	
	↓ Triglyceride utilization (from lipoproteins)	Lipoprotein lipase‡	cAMP
Liver	↓ Glycolysis	Phosphofructokinase-1†	
	↑ Gluconeogenesis	Fructose-1,6-bisphosphatase†	cAMP
	↓↓ Glycogen synthesis	Glycogen synthase*	
	↑↑↑ Glycogenolysis	Glycogen phosphorylase*	Ca²⁺, cAMP
	↓ Fatty acid synthesis	Acetyl-CoA carboxylase*	cAMP
Skeletal muscle	↑↑↑ Glycolysis	Phosphofructokinase-1†	
	↓↓ Glycogen synthesis	Glycogen synthase*	
	↑↑↑ Glycogenolysis	Glycogen phosphorylase*	cAMP
	↑ Triglyceride utilization (from lipoproteins)	Lipoprotein lipase	?

↑ and ↓, Weak or inconsistent effect; ↑↑ and ↓↓, moderately strong effect; ↑↑↑ and ↓↓↓, strong effect.
*Effects mediated by enzyme phosphorylation.
†Mediated indirectly by phosphorylation of phosphofructokinase-2/fructose-2,6-bisphosphatase.
‡Decreased translation.
cAMP, Cyclic adenosine monophosphate.

is different from the liver enzyme. Its kinase activity is not inhibited but is stimulated by cAMP-induced phosphorylation. Therefore the catecholamines, acting through β receptors and cAMP, stimulate rather than inhibit glycolysis in skeletal muscle.

The catecholamines are functional antagonists of insulin that raise the blood levels of glucose and free fatty acids. They are not very important for blood glucose regulation under ordinary conditions, but *their release is potently stimulated by hypoglycemia.* Therefore hypoglycemic episodes in metabolic diseases are always accompanied by signs of excessive sympathetic activity, including pallor, sweating, and tachycardia.

GLUCOCORTICOIDS ARE RELEASED IN CHRONIC STRESS

Stress, especially chronic stress, stimulates cortisol secretion from the adrenal cortex through corticotropin-releasing factor from the hypothalamus and adrenocorticotropic hormone (ACTH) from the anterior pituitary gland. The metabolic actions of cortisol and other glucocorticoids (*Table 30.4*) can best be understood as adaptations to life in a dangerous world.

By and large, the glucocorticoids are synergistic with epinephrine, but there is an important difference. Epinephrine works through the second messengers cAMP and calcium, whereas the glucocorticoids are primarily gene regulators. Therefore epinephrine induces its effects in a matter of seconds, but most glucocorticoid effects are cumulative over many hours to days.

The glucocorticoids prepare the body for the action of epinephrine. They stimulate the synthesis of the hormone-sensitive lipase and the adipose tissue triglyceride lipase. They also increase gluconeogenesis from amino acids by causing net protein breakdown in peripheral

Table 30.4 Important Metabolic Actions of Cortisol and Other Glucocorticoids*

Tissue	Affected Pathway	Affected Enzyme
Adipose tissue	↑ Lipolysis	Lipases
Muscle tissue	↑ Protein degradation	?
Liver	↑ Gluconeogenesis	Enzymes of amino acid catabolism, PEP-carboxykinase
	↑ Glycogen synthesis	Glycogen synthase

*The glucocorticoid effects are mediated by altered rates of enzyme synthesis.
PEP, Phosphoenolpyruvate.

tissues and inducing phosphoenolpyruvate (PEP) carboxykinase in the liver. Excess glucose-6-phosphate produced by gluconeogenesis is diverted into glycogen synthesis, thus providing more substrate for epinephrine-induced glycogenolysis.

It now is apparent how cortisol and epinephrine cooperate in a stressful situation. During an extended hunting expedition by a stone-age caveman, cortisol induced the lipases in his adipose tissue and built up the glycogen stores in his liver. As soon as the hunter was attacked by a cave bear, epinephrine immediately stimulated the release of fatty acids from adipose tissue and of glucose from the liver. Thanks to the supply of these fuels to his muscles, the caveman managed to dodge the cave bear's attack and kill the animal with his club. This gave him the chance to transmit his metabolic regulator genes to us, his descendants.

For the caveman's degenerate descendants today, the stress hormones are troublemakers rather than lifesavers. Patients suffering from infections, autoimmune diseases, malignancies, injuries, surgery, or psychological upheaval have elevated levels of glucocorticoids and catecholamines. Cortisol-induced protein breakdown leads to *negative nitrogen balance and muscle wasting.* Because the stress hormones oppose the metabolic effects of insulin, *seriously ill patients have insulin resistance and poor glucose tolerance.* The insulin requirement of insulin-dependent diabetic patients rises substantially during otherwise harmless infections or other illnesses.

Some **cytokines,** which are released by white blood cells during infections and some other diseases, have metabolic effects similar to the stress hormones. **Interleukin-1** stimulates proteolysis in skeletal muscle, and **tumor necrosis factor** promotes lipolysis in adipose tissue. These mediators contribute to the weight loss that is common in patients with malignancies or chronic infections.

ENERGY MUST BE PROVIDED CONTINUOUSLY

The basal metabolic rate (BMR) is the amount of energy that a resting person consumes in the "postabsorptive" state, 8 to 12 hours after the last meal. It is calculated with predictive formulas, for example, the **Harris-Benedict equation:**

$$BMR\male = 66.5 + (13.75 \times Weight) + (5.00 \times Height) - (6.76 \times Age)$$

$$BMR\female = 655.1 + (9.56 \times Weight) + (1.85 \times Height) - (5.68 \times Age)$$

or the Mifflin-St. Jeor equation:

$$BMR = Constant + (9.99 \times Weight) + (6.25 \times Height) - (4.92 \times Age)$$

where Constant = 5 for males and −161 for females.

In these equations, BMR is calculated as kilocalories per day. Weight is measured in kilograms, height in centimeters, and age in years.

BMR depends on body composition. Men tend to have a higher BMR per body weight than do women because men have relatively more muscle than fat (*Table 30.5*). Women need more fat as an energy reserve for pregnancy, and men traditionally needed more muscle to fight over the women.

On top of the BMR, additional energy is spent for **postprandial thermogenesis** (additional energy expenditure after a meal). Postprandial thermogenesis is produced by metabolic interconversions after a meal and by increased futile cycling in metabolic pathways. It depends on the size and composition of the meal. The digestion, absorption, and storage of fat require only 2% to 4% of the fat energy, but the conversion of carbohydrate to storage fat requires 24% of the energy content of the carbohydrate.

Muscular activity is the most variable item in the energy budget but is generally less than 1500 kcal/day except in people who engage in very strenuous physical labor all day long.

Multipliers are used to calculate the caloric expenditure (and dietary requirement) for different physiological states:

Long-term fasting : BMR × 0.8

Sedentary lifestyle : BMR × 1.2

Lightly active : BMR × 1.375

Moderately active : BMR × 1.55

Very active : BMR × 1.725

Extremely active : BMR × 1.9

Table 30.5 Metabolic Rates of Various Organs and Tissues

Organ	Organ Metabolic Rate (kcal/ kg/day)	Tissue or Organ Weight (kg)			Percent of Body Weight			Metabolic Rate (% of Total)		
		Male	Female	Child (6 Months)	Male	Female	Child (6 Months)	Male	Female	Child (6 Months)
Liver	200	1.8	1.4	0.26	2.57	2.41	3.51	21	21	14
Brain	240	1.4	1.2	0.71	2.00	2.07	9.51	20	21	44
Heart	440	0.33	0.24	0.04	0.47	0.41	0.53	9	8	4
Kidneys	440	0.31	0.28	0.05	0.44	0.47	0.71	8	9	6
Muscle	13	28	17	1.88	40	29.3	25	22	16	6
Adipose tissue	4.5	15	19	1.50	21.4	32.8	20	4	6	2
Others	12	23.2	18.9	3.06	33.1	32.6	40.7	16	19	24
Total		70	58	7.50	100	100	100	100*	100†	100‡

Data from Kinney JM, Tucker HN: *Energy metabolism,* New York, 1992, Raven Press.
*1680 kcal/day.
†1340 kcal/day.
‡390 kcal/day.

Table 30.6 Energy Reserves of the "Textbook" 70-kg Man

Stored Nutrient	Tissue	Amount Stored (kg)	Energy Value (kcal)
Triglyceride	Adipose tissue	10–15	90,000–140,000
Glycogen	Muscle	0.3	1200
	Liver	0.08*	320*
Protein	Muscle	6–8	30,000–40,000

*After a meal. Liver glycogen is approximately 20% to 30% of this value after an overnight fast of 12 hours.

Energy is spent round the clock, but most people eat in well-spaced meals. An ample supply is available only for 3 to 4 hours after a typical meal. For the rest of the day, we depend on stored energy reserves that were laid down after meals.

The fat in adipose tissue contains almost 100 times more energy than do the combined glycogen stores of liver and muscle (*Table 30.6*). Therefore only fat can keep us alive during prolonged fasting. It is easy to calculate that with fat stores of 16 kg and BMR of 1500 kcal/day, people can survive for about 100 days on tap water and vitamin pills alone, actually 125 days if we assume that the metabolic rate in prolonged fasting is 20% below BMR. The time to death on a hunger strike depends on the fat reserves, but survival times near 100 days are typical.

Glycogen is rapidly depleted. It is a checking account from which withdrawals are made on an hour-by-hour basis, whereas fat is a savings account. Indeed, only liver glycogen supplies energy for the whole body. Muscle glycogen is earmarked strictly for muscular activity.

Unlike fat and glycogen, protein is not a specialized energy storage form. Still, much of the protein in muscle and other tissues can be mobilized during fasting. Only the protein in brain, liver, kidneys, and other vital organs is taboo, even during prolonged starvation.

During long-term fasting, net protein breakdown is required to supply amino acids for gluconeogenesis. Because even-chain fatty acids are not substrates of gluconeogenesis, only amino acids are available in sufficient quantity to cover the glucose requirement during fasting. Therefore *the loss of protein from muscle and other tissues is inevitable during prolonged fasting.*

Figure 30.1 shows some of the changes in blood chemistry during the transition from the well-fed state to starvation. The most important hormonal factor is *the balance between insulin and its antagonists,* especially glucagon. During fasting, the plasma level of insulin falls, whereas first epinephrine, then glucagon, and finally cortisol levels rise.

During the first few days on a zero-calorie diet of tap water and vitamin pills, between 70 and 150 g of body protein is lost per day. The rate of protein loss then declines in parallel with the rising use of ketone bodies. Nevertheless, 1 kg of protein is lost within the first 15 days of starvation.

Adding 100 g of glucose to the zero-calorie diet reduces the need for gluconeogenesis and cuts the protein loss by 40%. The addition of 55 g of protein per day to the zero-calorie diet cannot prevent a negative nitrogen balance initially, but many subjects regain nitrogen equilibrium after about 20 days.

ADIPOSE TISSUE IS THE MOST IMPORTANT ENERGY DEPOT

The blood glucose level declines only to a limited extent even during prolonged fasting, but free fatty acid levels rise fourfold to eightfold, and the levels of ketone

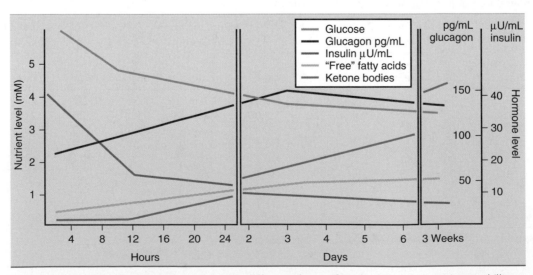

Figure 30.1 Plasma levels of hormones and nutrients at different times after the last meal. *mM,* mmol/liter.

bodies (β-hydroxybutyrate and acetoacetate) rise up to 100-fold.

Plasma free fatty acids are low after a carbohydrate meal because lipolysis in adipose tissue is inhibited by insulin, and fat synthesis is stimulated. Insulin also stimulates the lipoprotein lipase in adipose tissue but not in muscle after a meal, thus routing the dietary triglycerides in chylomicrons to adipose tissue (*Fig. 30.2*).

During fasting, fat synthesis in adipose tissue is reduced, whereas lipolysis is stimulated by the combination of the low insulin level and the high levels of insulin antagonists. Adipose tissue is very sensitive to insulin, and *lipolysis is inhibited even at moderately high insulin levels* during the early stages of fasting.

THE LIVER CONVERTS DIETARY CARBOHYDRATES TO GLYCOGEN AND FAT AFTER A MEAL

Being devoid of lipoprotein lipase, *the liver is not a major consumer of triglycerides after a meal*. It obtains only a small amount of dietary triglyceride from chylomicron remnants. However, the liver metabolizes approximately one third of the dietary glucose after a carbohydrate-rich meal. Because of the high Michaelis constant (K_m) of glucokinase for glucose, *hepatic glucose utilization is controlled by substrate availability*. Insulin induces the synthesis of glucokinase, but this effect becomes maximal only after 2 or 3 days on a high-carbohydrate diet.

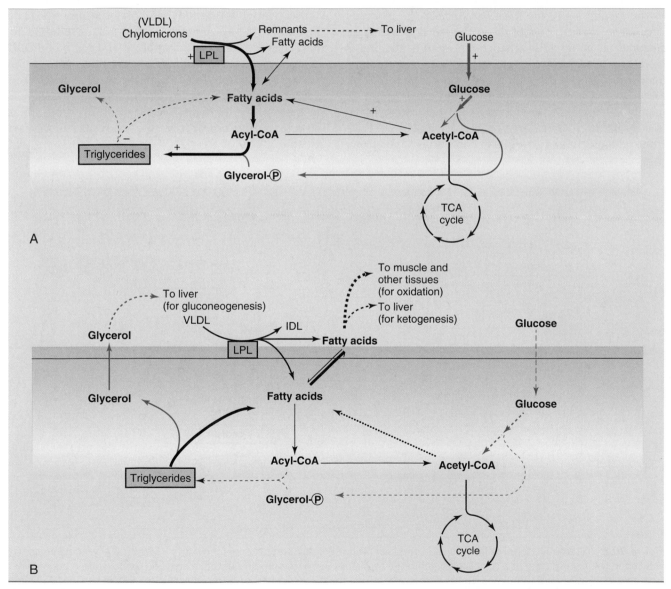

Figure 30.2 Metabolism of adipose tissue after a mixed meal containing all major nutrients and during fasting. **A,** After a meal. Insulin-stimulated or insulin-inhibited steps are marked by + or −, respectively. **B,** During fasting. *CoA*, Coenzyme A, *IDL*, intermediate-density lipoprotein (VLDL remnant); *LPL*, lipoprotein lipase; *TCA*, tricarboxylic acid, *VLDL*, very-low-density lipoprotein.

The liver converts at least two thirds of its glucose allotment into glycogen after a meal. Most of the rest is metabolized by glycolysis, but amino acids rather than glucose provide most of the liver's energy needs after a mixed meal. Much of the acetyl coenzyme A (acetyl-CoA) from glycolysis is channeled into the synthesis of fatty acids and triglycerides. *In the liver, glycolysis is the first step in the conversion of carbohydrate to fat.* Triglycerides and other lipids from endogenous synthesis in the liver are exported as constituents of very-low-density lipoprotein (VLDL). Insulin coordinates this process by stimulating both glycolysis and fatty acid biosynthesis (*Fig. 30.3*).

THE LIVER MAINTAINS THE BLOOD GLUCOSE LEVEL DURING FASTING

In the fasting state, *the liver has to feed the glucose-dependent tissues.* The brain is the most demanding customer. It is the most aristocratic organ in the body; therefore, it requires a large share of the communally owned resources. Although it accounts for only 2% of the body weight in the adult, it consumes approximately 20% of the total energy in the resting body (see *Table 30.5*). This large energy demand is covered from glucose under ordinary conditions and from glucose and ketone bodies during prolonged fasting. The brain oxidizes 80 g of glucose per day in the well-fed state and 30 g during long-term fasting.

Three to four hours after a meal, the liver becomes a net producer of glucose. After this time liver glycogen is the major source of blood glucose until 12 to 16 hours after the last meal, when gluconeogenesis becomes the major and finally the only source of glucose. This switch is required because *liver glycogen stores are almost completely exhausted after 48 hours.* More than half of the glucose produced in gluconeogenesis is from amino acids. Other substrates are glycerol from adipose tissue and lactic acid from erythrocytes and other anaerobic cells (*Fig. 30.4*).

Most tissues switch from glucose oxidation to the oxidation of fatty acids and ketone bodies during the transition from the well-fed to the fasting state. Consequently, total body glucose consumption falls (*Fig. 30.5*). Only tissues that depend on glucose for their energy needs, including brain and red blood cells, do not respond to insulin. They continue to consume glucose even during long-term fasting. The switch from glucose oxidation to fat oxidation leads to a decline of the **respiratory quotient** (see Chapter 21) from about 0.9 after a mixed meal to slightly above 0.7 in the fasting state.

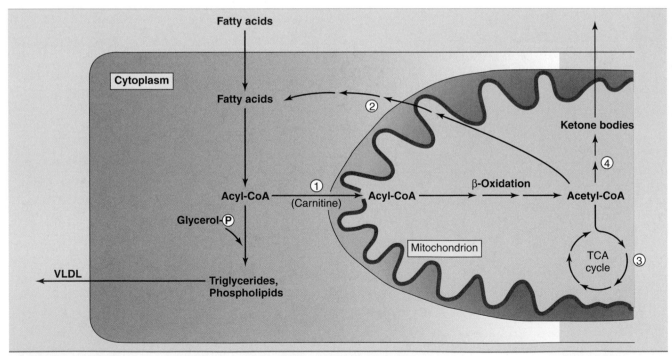

Figure 30.3 Alternative fates of fatty acids in the liver. The regulated steps are as follows: ① Carnitine acyl transferase-1 is induced in the fasting state. It also is acutely inhibited by malonyl-CoA, the product of the acetyl-CoA carboxylase reaction when fatty acid biosynthesis is stimulated after a carbohydrate-rich meal. ② Acetyl-CoA carboxylase is induced in the well-fed state. It is inhibited in the fasting state by high levels of acyl-CoA, low levels of citrate (direct allosteric effects), and a high glucagon/insulin ratio (leading to phosphorylation and inactivation). ③ The tricarboxylic acid (*TCA*) cycle is inhibited when alternative sources supply ATP and NADH. Therefore a high rate of β-oxidation reduces its activity. ④ The ketogenic enzymes are induced during fasting. *VLDL,* Very-low-density lipoprotein.

KETONE BODIES PROVIDE LIPID-BASED ENERGY DURING FASTING

The fasting liver spoon-feeds the other tissues with **ketone bodies** as well as with glucose. In theory, both carbohydrates and fatty acids can be converted into ketone bodies through acetyl-CoA. Actually, however, *the liver forms ketone bodies from fatty acids during fasting but not from carbohydrates after a meal.*

The liver has only a moderately high capacity for glycolysis, and much of the glycolyzed glucose is converted into fat. Therefore very little is left for ketogenesis. However, the liver has a very high capacity for fatty acid oxidation. Over a wide range of plasma levels, about 30% of incoming fatty acids is extracted and metabolized. This means that *hepatic fatty acid utilization is controlled by substrate availability.* It rises during fasting,

when adipose tissue supplies large amounts of free fatty acids.

The fasting liver has two options for the metabolism of these fatty acids (see *Fig. 30.3*). One option is *esterification into triglycerides and other lipids for export in VLDL,* which is released by the liver at all times. The fatty acids of VLDL lipids are made from dietary carbohydrate after a meal but come from adipose tissue during fasting.

The second option is *uptake into the mitochondrion followed by β-oxidation.* Carnitine-palmitoyltransferase-1, which controls the transport of long-chain fatty acids into the mitochondrion, is induced by glucagon through its second messenger cAMP and by fatty acids through the nuclear fatty acid receptor peroxisome proliferator-activated receptor-α (PPAR-α).

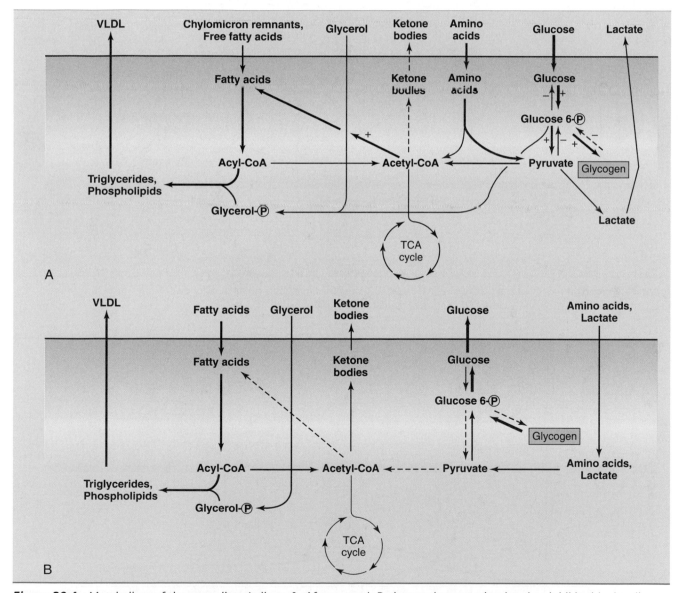

Figure 30.4 Metabolism of the yoyo dieter's liver. **A,** After a meal. Pathways that are stimulated or inhibited by insulin are marked by + or −, respectively. **B,** Twelve hours after the last meal.

Continued

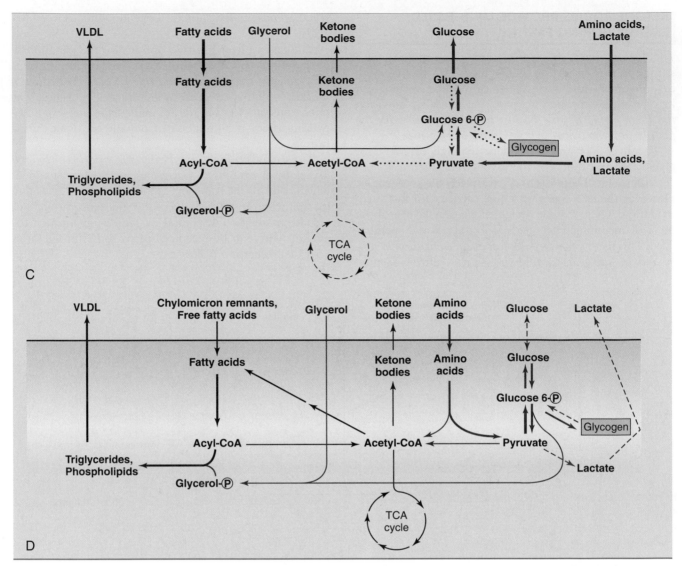

Figure 30.4—cont'd **C,** Four days after the last meal. **D,** After the first good meal that follows 4 days of fasting. *CoA,* Coenzyme A; *TCA,* tricarboxylic acid; *VLDL,* very-low-density lipoprotein.

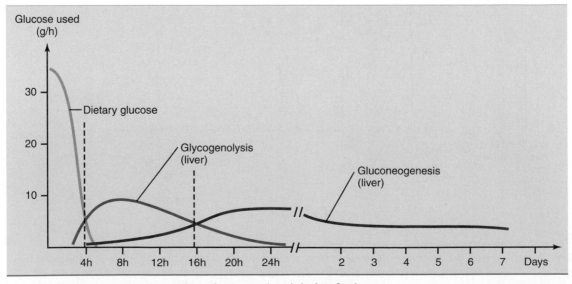

Figure 30.5 Total body glucose consumption after a meal and during fasting.

In the well-fed state, carnitine-palmitoyltransferase-1 is inhibited by malonyl-CoA, the product of the acetyl-CoA carboxylase reaction in fatty acid biosynthesis. During fasting, however, acetyl-CoA carboxylase is switched off by high levels of acyl-CoA, low levels of citrate, and a high glucagon/insulin ratio. Malonyl-CoA is no longer formed, and an increased fraction of acyl-CoA can be transported into the mitochondrion for β-oxidation.

The acetyl-CoA that is formed in β-oxidation must be partitioned between the tricarboxylic acid (TCA) cycle and ketogenesis. The activity of the TCA cycle depends on the cell's need for ATP. It is inhibited by ATP and a high [NADH]/[NAD$^+$] ratio (see Chapter 21). β-oxidation produces NADH and, indirectly, ATP. By inhibiting the TCA cycle, these products divert acetyl-CoA from TCA cycle oxidation to ketogenesis.

Ketogenesis amounts to an incomplete oxidation of fatty acids. Whereas the complete oxidation of one molecule of palmitoyl-CoA produces 131 molecules of ATP (see Chapter 23), its conversion to acetoacetate and β-hydroxybutyrate produces 35 and 23 molecules of ATP, respectively. The conversion of 50 g of fatty acids to acetoacetate during a hungry day supplies enough energy to synthesize 190 g of glucose from lactic acid without any need for the TCA cycle.

Why does the liver convert fatty acids to ketone bodies when carbohydrates are in short supply? The main reason is that *the brain can oxidize ketone bodies but not fatty acids.* Although the brain obtains almost all of its energy from glucose under ordinary conditions, it covers up to two thirds of its energy needs from ketone bodies during prolonged fasting, when ketone body levels are very high. This reduces the need for gluconeogenesis and thereby spares body protein. Liver metabolism in different nutritional states is summarized in *Figure 30.4.*

The nutrient flows in the body change dramatically in different nutritional states. *Figure 30.6* shows the flow of nutrients after different kinds of meal. *Figure 30.7* shows the changes during the transition from the well-fed state to prolonged fasting. The intestine provides for all of the body's needs after a mixed meal, but adipose tissue and liver assume this role during fasting.

The refeeding of severely starved patients can be problematic. The levels of glycolytic enzymes in the liver are very low, and patients show profound carbohydrate intolerance. Therefore *refeeding should be started slowly,* especially in advanced cases.

OBESITY IS THE MOST COMMON NUTRITION-RELATED DISORDER IN AFFLUENT COUNTRIES

Obesity is the most visible medical problem in modern societies. Its prevalence depends on the definitions used. One convenient measure, the **body mass index (BMI)**, is defined as follows:

$$BMI = Weight/Height^2$$

BMI of 20 to 24.9 kg/m^2 is considered normal, BMI between 25 and 29.9 signifies overweight, and BMI of 30 or greater indicates obesity. The prevalence of overweight and obesity in different population groups in the United States during the early 1990s is listed in *Table 30.7.* The problem has worsened since then. In the United States, 31.1% of adult men and 33.2% of adult women were found to be obese (BMI ≥30) in 2003 and 2004.

Body weight tends to change over the lifespan. In affluent countries, women tend to gain weight between the ages of 20 and 60 years. Men tend to gain weight more slowly from age 20 to age 50 years and to get thinner again after age 60. However, even with constant weight, the amount of lean body mass declines slowly with advancing age whereas fat rises.

Until the early years of the twentieth century, body weight was related to social class, with rich people being heavier than poor people. Socioeconomic status (SES) still is important today, but now poor people are fatter than rich people. A study in the United States found that 30% of low-SES women, 16% of middle-SES women, but only 5% of upper-SES women were obese. A similar but weaker relationship was seen in men.

Actuarial tables of life insurance companies typically show that mortality is lowest in people who are considered 10% underweight. Overweight and obese people, but also those who are severely underweight, are more likely to die. Only among the elderly are slightly overweight people less likely to die than are underweight people, probably because weight loss is an effect (rather than a cause) of aging as well as of many chronic diseases.

By and large, however, obesity is unhealthy. For every 10% rise in relative weight, systolic blood pressure rises by 6.5 mmHg, cholesterol by 12 mg/dl, and fasting blood glucose by 2 mg/dl in men. These associations are only a bit weaker in women. Nevertheless, there is no evidence that weight reduction reduces the mortality of the ex-obese compared to those who remained obese.

Obesity is inevitable when energy intake exceeds energy consumption. After adjustment for age, sex, weight, and lean body mass versus fat, obese people have virtually the same metabolic rate as lean people. This implies *that individual variations in appetite control, rather than metabolic rate, are the important cause of obesity.* Several rare monogenic forms of obesity are known in humans. Most of them incriminate brain-expressed genes or genes whose products act on the brain. The same seems to be the case for obesity-associated

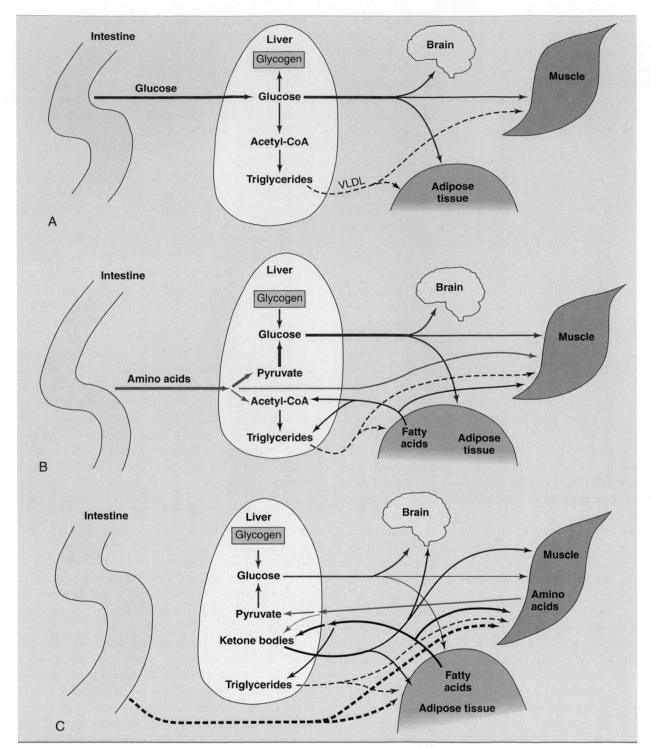

Figure 30.6 Disposition of nutrients after different types of meals. **A,** After a carbohydrate meal (insulin high, glucagon low). **B,** After a protein meal (insulin moderately high, glucagon high). **C,** After a fat meal (insulin low, glucagon high). *CoA,* Coenzyme A; *VLDL,* very-low-density lipoprotein.

polymorphisms that have been pinpointed in genome-wide association studies.

Appetite is controlled by chemical signals that inform the brain about the nutrient status of the body. High levels of blood glucose, insulin, and fatty acids signal nutrient abundance and suppress appetite. The gastric hormone **ghrelin,** which is released by the empty but not the filled stomach, stimulates appetite; and the hormone **leptin,** which is released from adipose tissue when the adipose cells are "filled," suppresses appetite. Deficiency of either leptin or the leptin receptor causes morbid obesity both in mouse mutants and in some humans.

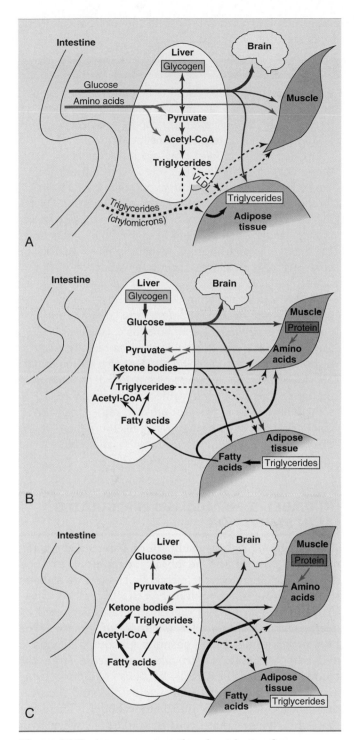

Figure 30.7 Interorgan transfer of nutrients after a mixed meal and during fasting. **A,** After a mixed meal. **B,** Postabsorptive state, 12 hours after the last meal. **C,** One week after the last meal. *CoA,* Coenzyme A; *VLDL,* very-low-density lipoprotein.

Normally, the number of adipocytes increases fivefold between the ages of 2 and 22 years. Only 10% of adipocytes are renewed per year during adult life, and a common concern is that overeating, especially at a young age, leads to adipose tissue hyperplasia that is difficult to reverse.

Table 30.7 Prevalence of Overweight and Obesity among Adults 20 Years and Older in Different Population Groups in the United States, 2003–2004

	Male	Female
Overweight or Obese (BMI ≥25)		
White	70.6	58.0
Black	69.1	81.6
Mexican	76.1	75.4
Obese (BMI ≥30)		
White	31.1	30.2
Black	34.0	53.9
Mexican	31.6	42.3

Data from Kuczmarski RJ, Flegal KM, Compbell SM, et al: Increasing prevalence of overweight among US adults. The National Health and Nutrition Surveys, 1960 to 1991, *JAMA* 272:205-211, 1994. *BMI,* Body mass index.

Table 30.8 Typical Features of the Two Major Types of Diabetes Mellitus

Parameter	Type 1	Type 2
Age at onset (years)	≤20	>20
Lifetime incidence	0.2%–0.4%	5%–10%
Heritability	≈50%	≈80%
Pancreatic β-cells	Destroyed	Initially normal
Circulating insulin	Absent	Normal, high, or low
Tissue response to insulin	Normal	Reduced (most patients)
Fasting hyperglycemia	Severe	Variable
Metabolic complications	Ketoacidosis	Nonketotic hyperosmolar coma
Treatment	Insulin	Diet, oral antidiabetics, or insulin

Typically, the metabolic rate of obese people drops by 15% to 20% during weight loss and remains reduced when weight is stabilized at a lower level. Thus the ex-obese have to live permanently with a metabolic rate that is otherwise typical for serious starvation. This is a likely reason why 80% to 85% of weight-reduced obese patients quickly regain until they reach their previous weight. We do not know whether sustained weight reduction for at least a decade leads to a reduced number of adipocytes.

DIABETES IS CAUSED BY INSULIN DEFICIENCY OR INSULIN RESISTANCE

Diabetes mellitus is caused by a relative or absolute deficiency of insulin action. **Hyperglycemia** (abnormally elevated blood glucose) is the biochemical hallmark of diabetes mellitus, but the pathways of all major nutrients are deranged. The two major primary forms of diabetes are type 1 and type 2 (*Table 30.8*).

Type 1 diabetes typically starts in childhood or adolescence. It is an autoimmune disease that leads to the

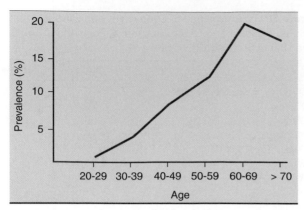

Figure 30.8 Prevalence of diabetes mellitus in the United States in 2001. The large majority of cases are type 2 diabetes.

destruction of pancreatic β-cells. Without endogenous insulin production, patients depend on insulin injections for life. Being a protein, insulin is not orally active because it is destroyed by digestive enzymes. Type 1 diabetes afflicts perhaps 1:400 individuals, and its incidence is not strongly related to lifestyle.

Type 2 diabetes is a disease of middle-aged and older individuals (*Fig. 30.8*). It is far more common than type 1, is less severe, and has more complex origins. The pancreatic β-cells are intact, and the plasma level of insulin is normal, reduced, or elevated. The problem is either *reduced insulin secretion* or *insulin resistance* of the target tissues, or a combination of both. Two hundred million people are affected worldwide, and the prevalence rises steeply with rising affluence. In the United States, the prevalence of diabetes among adults rose from 6.3% in 1991 to 8.8% in 2001, and the cost of the disease is estimated at more than $100 billion per year.

Most patients with poorly controlled type 1 diabetics are thin, but most type 2 diabetics are obese. Their obesity is not a consequence of their diabetes but precedes the onset of diabetes by many years or even decades.

Obese patients with type 2 diabetes are invariably insulin resistant. Even nondiabetic obese individuals have higher insulin levels than do thin people, and their tissue responsiveness is proportionately reduced. A reduced number of insulin receptors is a frequent finding, but overall, defects in intracellular insulin signaling are more important than is reduced receptor number. The nature of the molecular link between obesity and insulin resistance is not known. Most obese type 2 diabetics are insulin resistant even before they develop hyperglycemia, and they become diabetic only when β-cells become dysfunctional. The reasons for this "burnout" of β-cells are incompletely known (*Clinical Example 30.1*). In most obese type 2 diabetics, a balanced weight-reduction diet restores tissue responsiveness and corrects the metabolic derangements. Because not all patients comply with this cruel and unreasonable treatment, insulin or oral antidiabetic drugs are often required.

CLINICAL EXAMPLE 30.1: Islet Amyloid

Most obese type 2 diabetics are insulin resistant even before they develop fasting hyperglycemia, and they become diabetic only after developing β-cell dysfunction and/or reduced β-cell mass.

The deposition of **islet amyloid** in the islets of Langerhans appears to play a role in the "burnout" of the β-cells. Islet amyloid is an abnormally folded form of the hormone **amylin**, which is secreted by the β-cells together with insulin and C peptide after a meal. Amylin inhibits insulin secretion and has hormonal effects that are synergistic with those of insulin. It delays gastric emptying, and it reduces appetite by an action in the brain.

Unlike human amylin, mouse amylin has no propensity for amyloid formation, and laboratory mice do not become diabetic spontaneously. However, transgenic mice whose own amylin has been replaced by human amylin do develop diabetes that is frequently but not always accompanied by amyloid deposition in the islets. The diabetogenic effect is attributed to soluble oligomers of the islet amyloid rather than the insoluble deposits. Whether transgenic humans expressing the gene for mouse amylin would be resistant to type 2 diabetes is unknown.

IN DIABETES, METABOLISM IS REGULATED AS IN STARVATION

The decline of blood insulin during extended fasting mediates most of the metabolic adaptations to food deprivation. Therefore the metabolic changes of diabetes resemble those of starvation (*Fig. 30.9*).

The hyperglycemia of diabetes mellitus is caused by *overproduction and underutilization of glucose.* The liver makes rather than consumes glucose, and muscle and adipose tissue fail to take up glucose from the blood. There is also *excessive lipolysis in adipose tissue.* The levels of plasma free fatty acids rise, and the liver turns excess fatty acids into ketone bodies. These are the same changes that occur in starvation, when liver and adipose tissue must keep the other organs alive by doling out glucose, fatty acids, and ketone bodies.

The oversupply of fatty acids reduces glucose catabolism in liver and skeletal muscle. For example, ATP generated by fatty acid oxidation reduces glycolysis by inhibiting phosphofructokinase. A more specific effect is inhibition of insulin release from the pancreatic β-cells by acyl-CoA. Because of these effects, *an oversupply of dietary fat is as detrimental as is an oversupply of dietary carbohydrate.*

In addition to inhibiting glucose oxidation and insulin release, fatty acids promote triglyceride synthesis and

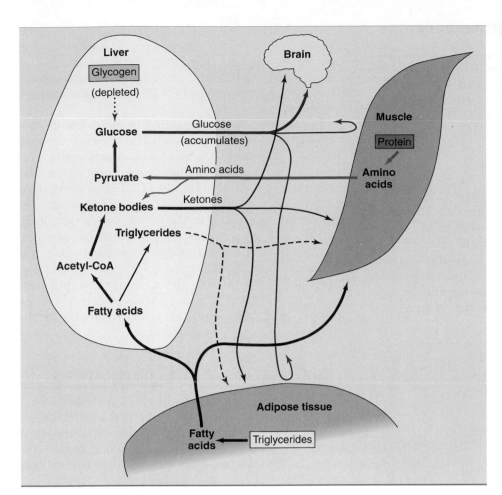

Figure 30.9 Disposition of the major nutrients in diabetes mellitus (postabsorptive state).

the accumulation of fat in liver and muscle. The triglyceride content of muscle and liver is directly related to the degree of hyperglycemia.

VLDL is elevated in many diabetics because the oversupply of fatty acids promotes triglyceride synthesis in the liver, whereas the activity of lipoprotein lipase in adipose tissue is reduced. Elevated VLDL and plasma triglycerides contribute to the accelerated development of atherosclerosis and coronary heart disease in diabetes.

The acute complications of diabetes include **diabetic ketoacidosis** in type 1 diabetes (*Clinical Example 30.2*) and **nonketotic hyperosmolar coma** in elderly patients with type 2 diabetes. The latter is caused by excessive glucosuria with osmotic diuresis. If the patient forgets to drink, the resulting dehydration can become sufficiently severe to affect the central nervous system.

Overtreatment of diabetes with insulin or oral antidiabetic drugs leads to **hypoglycemic shock.** It presents with dizziness, sweating, tachycardia, and pale skin and can proceed to loss of consciousness. These signs are caused by brain dysfunction and by compensatory hyperactivity of the sympathetic nervous system. Therefore *patients must be educated to time their insulin injections with their meals.* Increasingly, insulin pumps with adjustable flow rate are used by diabetic patients.

CLINICAL EXAMPLE 30.2: Diabetic Ketoacidosis

The complete absence of insulin in type 1 diabetes leads to diabetic ketoacidosis. Acidosis is present because the ketone bodies that are overproduced (acetoacetic acid and β-hydroxybutyric acid) are acids that are formed from a nonacidic precursor (triglycerides). Ketosis is accompanied by blood glucose levels that can be as high as 1000 mg/dl. Large amounts of glucose and ketone bodies are lost in the urine, and osmotic diuresis causes dehydration and electrolyte imbalances. The coma is caused by dehydration, electrolyte disturbances, and acidosis. Hyperglycemia as such is not acutely damaging to the brain. *Untreated ketoacidosis is fatal.* Proper treatment includes fluid replacement, correction of the acidosis, and generous insulin injections.

In persons without diabetes, hypoglycemic episodes sometimes are caused by an **insulinoma,** a rare insulin-secreting tumor of pancreatic β-cells. The diagnosis of insulinoma is established by the measurement of elevated levels of insulin or C-peptide (see Chapter 16).

DIABETES IS DIAGNOSED WITH LABORATORY TESTS

Urinalysis is a quick screening test for diabetes mellitus. *Whenever the blood glucose level exceeds 9 to 10 mmol/L (160–180 mg/dl), glucose appears in the urine.* Ketone bodies are also excreted in the urine. There is no true renal threshold for ketone bodies, but ordinarily only trace amounts are excreted. Only in uncontrolled diabetes are ketone bodies excreted in substantial quantity.

Determination of the *fasting blood glucose level* is the most important laboratory test for diabetes. A blood glucose concentration greater than 7.8 mmol/L (140 mg/dl) on two different occasions can be used as a diagnostic cutoff. Borderline cases can be evaluated with the **glucose tolerance test.** It involves repeated measurements of blood glucose both immediately before and at different intervals after ingestion of a glucose solution (*Fig. 30.10*). Both the fasting blood

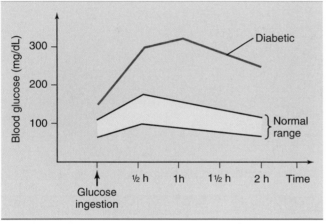

Figure 30.10 Glucose tolerance test. Blood glucose is measured at different time intervals after oral ingestion of a flavored glucose solution (75 g of glucose). In normal individuals, but not in diabetic patients, the blood glucose returns to the fasting level within 2 hours.

glucose concentration and, to a far greater extent, the glucose tolerance test show wide variations among healthy individuals. Therefore the diagnostic cutoff between "normal" and "diabetic" is as arbitrary as that between "pass" and "fail" on a biochemistry examination.

Hemoglobin A$_{1C}$ is measured to assess the quality of long-term metabolic control in treated diabetic patients. This product is formed by nonenzymatic glycosylation of the terminal amino groups in the α-chains and β-chains (*Fig. 30.11*). *The concentration of glycosylated hemoglobin is proportional to the blood glucose level.* It is 4% to 5.9% in normal individuals and greater than 6% in diabetic patients. Target values of less than 6.5% or less than 7.0% are variously recommended for diabetic patients. Because hemoglobin has a lifespan of 4 months, this test provides information about the average severity of hyperglycemia during the last weeks to months before the test.

DIABETES LEADS TO LATE COMPLICATIONS

In the course of many years, diabetic patients develop accelerated atherosclerosis, nephropathy, retinopathy, cataracts, and peripheral neuropathy. Diabetes is an important cause of blindness, renal failure, and atherosclerosis. Two biochemical mechanisms have been proposed for these delayed complications:

1. *Nonenzymatic glycosylation of terminal amino groups* (see *Fig. 30.11*) interferes with the normal function or turnover of proteins. This mechanism has been suggested for the thickening of basement membranes that is observed in the renal glomeruli of diabetic patients.

2. *Increased formation of sorbitol and fructose by the polyol pathway* (see Chapter 22) is favored by hyperglycemia:

Figure 30.11 Nonenzymatic glycosylation of the terminal amino groups in proteins. A stable fructose derivative is formed in these reactions. Hemoglobin A$_{1c}$ and glycosylated albumin are formed this way.

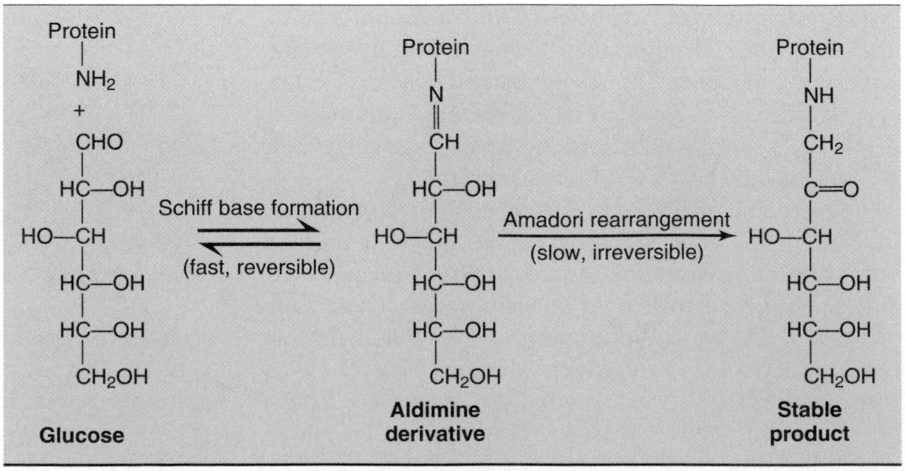

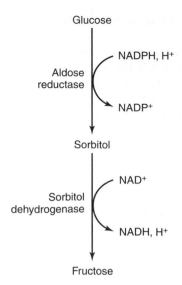

The K_m of aldose reductase for glucose is near 200 mmol/L, which is 40 times higher than the normal blood glucose level. Therefore the reaction rate depends directly on the glucose concentration. Sorbitol and fructose not only are osmotically active but also can interfere with the metabolism of inositol. Aldose reductase is abundant in Schwann cells of peripheral nerves, papillae of the kidney, and lens epithelium, sites that are affected in patients with diabetes.

In diabetic patients, the intracellular glucose concentration is not elevated in muscle and adipose tissue, whose glucose uptake is insulin dependent. However, nerve sheaths, blood vessels, kidneys, and the retina have insulin-independent glucose uptake. These tissues are most vulnerable to diabetes.

CONTRACTING MUSCLE HAS THREE ENERGY SOURCES

During contraction, the energy expenditure of skeletal muscle can rise 50-fold above the resting level. The energy is supplied by three metabolic systems.

Creatine Phosphate

During vigorous contraction, all ATP would be hydrolyzed to ADP and phosphate within 2 to 4 seconds. In this situation, ATP can be regenerated quickly in the reversible **creatine kinase** reaction (*Fig. 30.12*). The reaction equilibrium ($\Delta G^{0'} = -3.0$ kcal/mol for ATP formation) favors ATP and creatine. The concentration of creatine phosphate in resting muscle is at least 20 mmol/kg, whereas the ATP concentration is only 5 to 6 mmol/kg (*Table 30.9*).

During contraction, creatine phosphate is utilized while the ATP concentration is only slightly reduced from its resting level. This system requires neither oxygen nor external nutrients, but *it can supply ATP for only 6 to 20 seconds of vigorous exercise.* It is the main energy source for weight lifting and during a 100-m sprint.

Table 30.9 Concentrations of Some Phosphate Compounds in the Quadriceps Femoralis Muscle at Rest

Compound	Muscle Tissue (mmol/kg)
ATP	5.85
ADP	0.74
AMP	0.02
Creatine phosphate	24*
Creatine	5*

*Determined in situ, by nuclear magnetic resonance. In biopsy samples, the ratio of phosphocreatine/creatine is approximately 3:2.

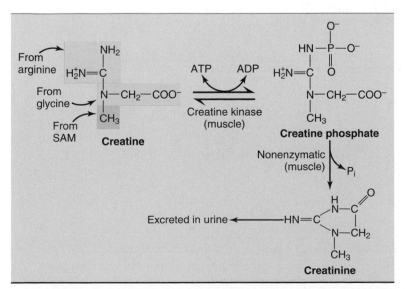

Figure 30.12 Creatine and the creatine kinase reaction. *SAM,* S-adenosylmethionine.

Creatine is not degraded enzymatically, but creatine phosphate cyclizes spontaneously to **creatinine**. Because the creatinine concentration in the plasma is more or less constant and creatinine is neither secreted nor reabsorbed to any great extent in the kidney tubules, it is used routinely for determination of the glomerular filtration rate ("creatinine clearance").

Anaerobic Glycolysis

Stored glycogen $(Glc)_n$ is the major substrate for glycolysis in skeletal muscle:

$$(Glc)_n + 3\ ADP + 3\ P_i$$
$$\downarrow$$
$$(Glc)_{n-1} + 2\ Lactate + 3\ ATP + 2\ H_2O$$

This system requires no oxygen, but *it is limited by the accumulation of lactic acid*, which acidifies the tissue and inhibits phosphofructokinase (*Fig. 30.13*). Anaerobic glycolysis is the most important energy source between 20 seconds and 2 minutes after onset of vigorous exercise.

Oxidative Metabolism

Oxidative metabolism produces at least 10 times more ATP than does anaerobic glycolysis from glycogen, but *it is limited by the oxygen supply*. Muscle can oxidize glycogen, glucose, fatty acids, ketone bodies, and amino acids. Resting muscle relies mainly on fatty acid oxidation during the postabsorptive state, although glucose is important after a carbohydrate meal. Fatty acids are still the major fuel during mild to moderate physical activity, but vigorously contracting muscle depends in large part on carbohydrate oxidation (*Fig. 30.14*).

To some extent, the muscle fibers are metabolic specialists. **Fast-twitch fibers** ("white" fibers) have large glycogen stores, an abundance of glycolytic enzymes, and few mitochondria. They depend on anaerobic metabolism of their stored glycogen and are specialized for rapid, vigorous, short-lasting contractions. **Slow-twitch fibers** ("red" fibers), in contrast, are well equipped with mitochondria and can maintain their activity for prolonged periods. Human muscles consist of a mix of fast-twitch and slow-twitch fibers in variable proportions.

CATECHOLAMINES COORDINATE METABOLISM DURING EXERCISE

Anaerobic exercise (e.g., weight lifting) impairs the blood supply of the muscle. It does not require the supply of external fuels; it relies on creatine phosphate and the anaerobic metabolism of stored glycogen.

In **aerobic exercise** (e.g., running, swimming), however, blood flow to the active muscles is increased because lactic acid and other local mediators relax vascular smooth muscle. Therefore oxidative metabolism can function as the major energy source. Both stored glycogen and external nutrients are oxidized (*Figs. 30.14* and *30.15*), and *the combined use of all nutrients is necessary for maximum performance*.

The nutrient supply to exercising muscle is under neural and hormonal control. The plasma insulin concentration decreases during strenuous exercise. Glucagon initially

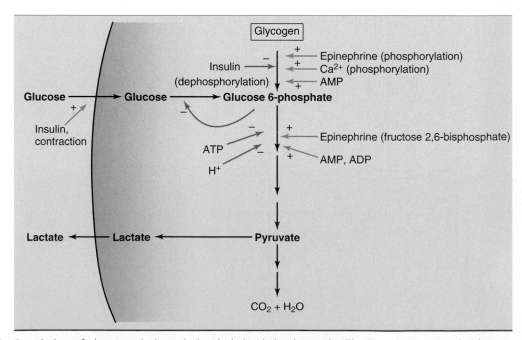

Figure 30.13 Regulation of glycogenolysis and glycolysis in skeletal muscle. The important control points are glycogen phosphorylase, phosphofructokinase, and the glucose carrier in the plasma membrane.

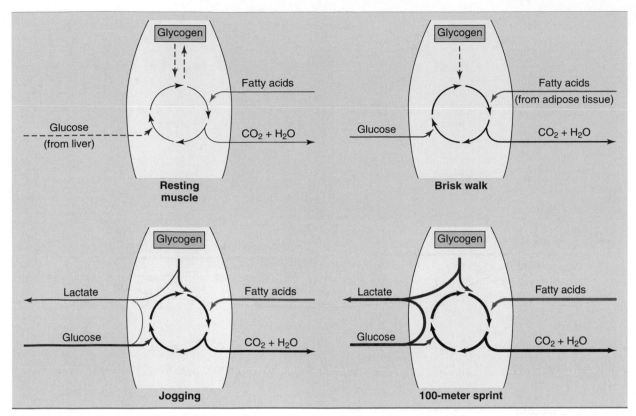

Figure 30.14 Muscle metabolism during exercise.

is unchanged but tends to rise with prolonged vigorous activity. Most important, however, are norepinephrine and epinephrine. The plasma levels of these two catecholamines rise 10-fold to 20-fold during strenuous physical activity.

In skeletal muscle itself, the catecholamines *stimulate glycogen degradation and glycolysis* (see *Fig. 30.13*). These effects are mediated by β-adrenergic receptors and cAMP.

In adipose tissue, *the catecholamines stimulate fat breakdown* through β-adrenergic receptors and cAMP; in the liver, *they stimulate glycogen degradation*. This latter effect is mediated by α_1-adrenergic receptors and inositol-1,4,5-trisphosphate (IP_3) and by β-adrenergic receptors and cAMP. cAMP also stimulates gluconeogenesis. The liver supplies substantial amounts of glucose during exercise, most of it derived from glycogen.

Gluconeogenesis becomes important only during prolonged vigorous exercise (see *Fig. 30.15*). Most of the substrate for gluconeogenesis is actually supplied by the muscles. Lactate is transported from active muscle to the liver in the **Cori cycle** and alanine in the **alanine cycle** (*Fig. 30.16*).

The plasma levels of glucose, fatty acids, and ketone bodies are only mildly elevated during physical exercise. Although these fuels are produced in quantity by adipose tissue and liver, they are rapidly consumed by the muscles. *The uptake of circulating glucose, which is insulin dependent in resting muscle, is stimulated by active contraction without the need for insulin.* This is the reason why physical exercise is recommended for diabetics. Stimulation of glucose uptake by physical exercise appears to be mediated by the AMP-activated protein kinase (see Chapter 23), whereas insulin stimulation of glucose transport depends on the insulin-stimulated protein kinase B (also known as Akt).

PHYSICAL ENDURANCE DEPENDS ON OXIDATIVE CAPACITY AND MUSCLE GLYCOGEN STORES

Regular strenuous exercise leads to important adaptive changes. Endurance athletes have increased capillary density in their trained muscles, and their muscle mitochondria are increased in size and number. The activities of enzymes for fatty acid and ketone body oxidation are increased, and the amounts of the lactate transporter and GLUT-4 are increased as well. Glucose uptake by GLUT-4 is the rate-limiting step in muscle glucose metabolism.

Muscle mass can also increase in response to physical exercise. This increase results from increased mass per fiber rather than from the formation of new muscle fibers. During a bout of vigorous exercise, muscle actually loses mass because of increased protein breakdown. This is followed by a period of up to 48 hours when the muscle is inclined to bulk up by increasing net protein synthesis, *but only if amino acid substrates are in ample supply.*

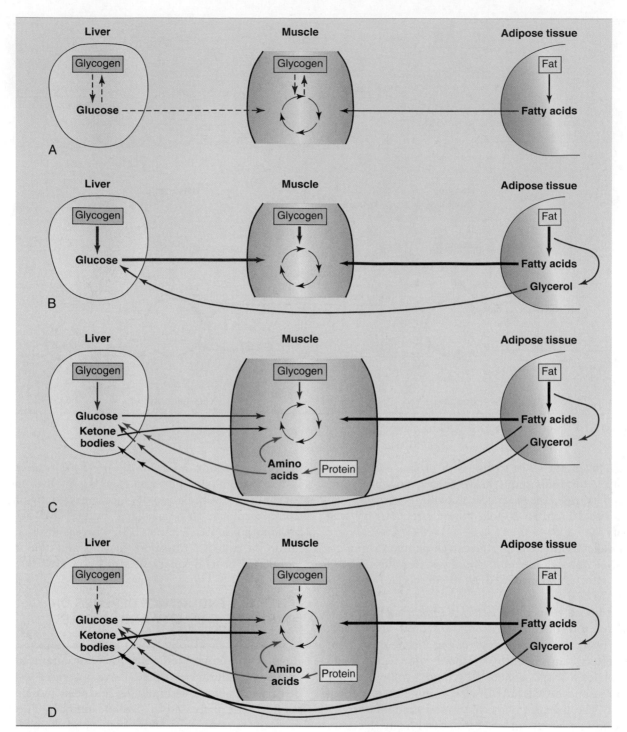

Figure 30.15 Marathoner's plight. **A,** Resting. **B,** After 10 minutes, muscle glycogen and glucose from liver glycogen are the most important fuels. **C,** After 2 hours, glycogen reserves in muscle and liver are seriously reduced. Fatty acids become more important. **D,** At the finish line, both liver and muscle glycogen are depleted. Runner drops from exhaustion.

Exercise combined with low protein intake is unlikely to increase muscle mass. The current recommendation for athletes and body builders is to consume at least 20 g of protein within a few hours after a bout of vigorous muscular activity.

Muscle mass depends on two antagonistic signaling cascades:

1. Stimulation of muscle protein synthesis is mediated by the protein kinase mammalian target of rapamycin (**mTOR**), which was introduced in Chapter 18. mTOR increases protein synthesis by actions at the ribosomal level (see *Fig. 18.17*). Signals from several sources converge on this protein kinase. They include insulin and insulin-like growth factor 1

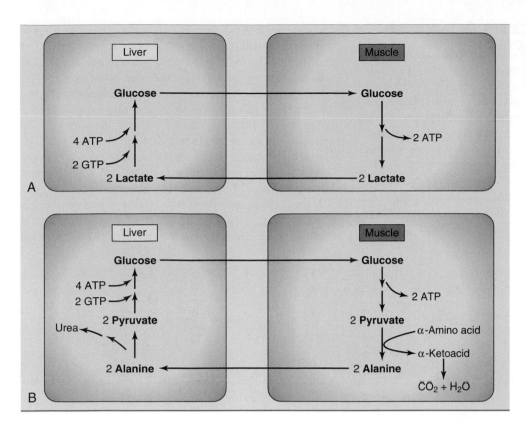

(IGF-1), which work mainly through protein kinase B (Akt) and the tuberous sclerosis (hamartin-tuberin) complex as shown in *Figure 18.17*. IGF-1 is derived from the liver, and its release into the blood is stimulated by growth hormone. Amino acids not only are substrates for mTOR-stimulated protein synthesis; they also provide a signal to mTOR. The mechanism of amino acid sensing by muscle tissue is poorly understood.

2. **Myostatin** is a hormone-like protein that is released by muscle tissue and circulates in the blood. Its major effect is *inhibition of protein synthesis in skeletal muscle*. It does so by triggering a signaling cascade similar to that of transforming growth factor β (TGF-β) described in Chapter 18 (see *Fig. 18.24*). The main targets of this cascade are nuclear transcription factors in the muscle fibers. Myostatin-inhibiting drugs and monoclonal antibodies potentially can be used for treatment of muscular dystrophies.

CLINICAL EXAMPLE 30.3: Carbohydrate Loading

Prolonged severe exercise (e.g., during a marathon race) depends on muscle glycogen. Glycogen is metabolized both aerobically and anaerobically, and its depletion leads to severe exhaustion. This occurs when, 2 or 3 hours into a marathon, the runner encounters the dreaded "wall" (see *Fig. 30.15*). *The amount of muscle glycogen depends on the carbohydrate content of the diet.*

For this reason, methods of **carbohydrate loading** have been devised to build up large glycogen stores before an important athletic contest. Typically, the athlete is placed on a 70% to 80% carbohydrate diet for 3 to 4 days before the event.

CLINICAL EXAMPLE 30.4: Myostatin Mutations

Farm animals that are genetically deficient in myostatin have at least twice the muscle mass of other breeds, combined with low adipose tissue mass. The first human case of a myostatin-deficient boy was reported in 2004 in Germany. The patient was evaluated at birth for myoclonus and unusual muscle mass. He was found to be homozygous for a splice site mutation in the myostatin gene that left him with no functional myostatin.

The boy's mother had been a professional athlete, and several family members had been unusually strong. Thus a null mutation in the myostatin gene appears to be sufficient to increase muscle mass in heterozygotes, with a far greater effect in the rare homozygotes.

A boy with similar appearance who had intact myostatin was described in the United States. This boy was homozygous for a null mutation in the myostatin receptor. When a boy with one of these mutations is asked why he is so strong, he can say "because I'm a mutant." Isn't that cool?

LIPOPHILIC XENOBIOTICS ARE METABOLIZED TO WATER-SOLUBLE PRODUCTS

Along with useful nutrients, humans ingest useless chemicals that must be removed from the body. These **xenobiotics** include a wide variety of plant metabolites, not all of them harmless, and a vast number of synthetic products, such as drugs, intoxicants, food additives, industrial and agricultural chemicals, and pyrolysis products in cigarette smoke and in fried, roasted, and smoked foods.

Water-soluble products can be excreted in urine or bile, but lipophilic xenobiotics cannot be easily excreted. They tend to accumulate in adipose tissue and other lipid-rich structures. For example, a substantial amount of $\triangle^1$-tetrahydrocannabinol (THC), the active constituent of marijuana, still is present in the body several days after inhalation. *Lipophilic xenobiotics must be metabolized to water-soluble products* before they can be excreted.

The most important organs of xenobiotic metabolism are liver, intestines, and lungs. The lungs metabolize airborne pollutants, and liver and intestines guard against food-borne products. Xenobiotics are metabolized in two phases. In **phase 1 reactions,** the substance is oxidized, usually by the attachment of one or more hydroxyl groups. In some cases, these reactions detoxify a toxic substance or terminate the effect of a drug. In other cases, however, an otherwise innocuous substance is converted into a toxin (*Fig. 30.17*), or an

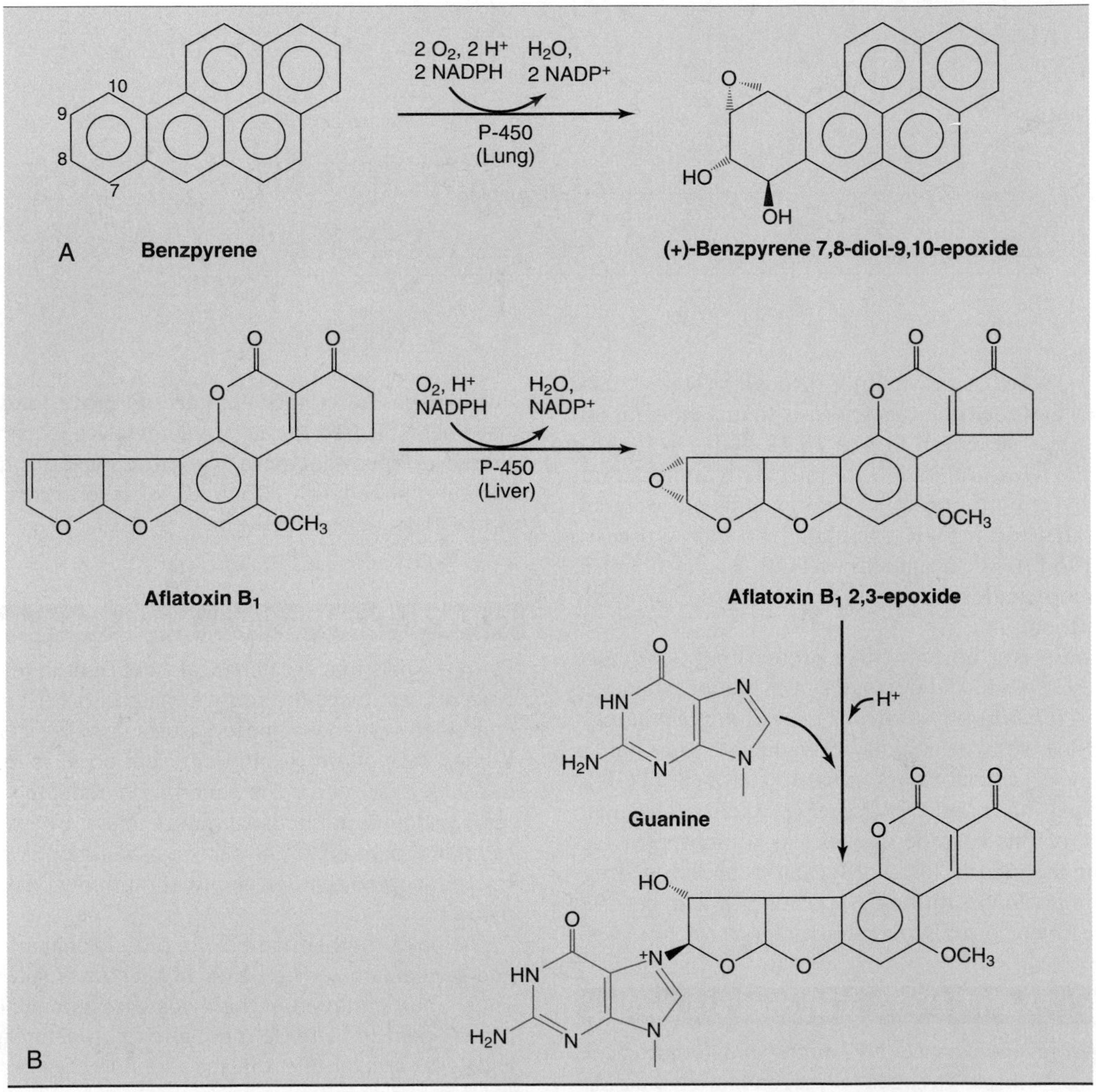

Figure 30.17 Metabolic activation of carcinogens. **A,** Metabolic activation of benzpyrene, a polycyclic hydrocarbon in cigarette smoke. Although benzpyrene itself is innocuous, the epoxide reacts spontaneously with DNA bases, causing point mutations. Individuals with a genetically determined high activity of the activating cytochrome P-450 have an increased risk of lung cancer if they smoke. **B,** Activation of aflatoxin B_1, a toxin of the mold *Aspergillus flavus*. The resulting epoxide reacts spontaneously with guanine residues in DNA, causing point mutations. Besides hepatitis B virus, aflatoxins are a major risk factor for liver cancer. The offending mold thrives under hot and humid conditions; thus, liver cancer is common in many tropical countries.

inactive prodrug is processed to a pharmacologically active metabolite.

In **phase 2 reactions,** the foreign substance or its metabolite is conjugated with a hydrophilic molecule, such as glucuronic acid, sulfate, glycine, glutamine, or glutathione (***Fig. 30.18***). The products of these conjugation reactions not only are water soluble and excretable but also have lost the biological activities of the parent compounds.

XENOBIOTIC METABOLISM REQUIRES CYTOCHROME P-450

The oxidative reactions in phase 1 metabolism are *monooxygenase reactions* that require **cytochrome P-450** as an electron carrier. This cytochrome is also found in the steroid-producing endocrine glands, in which it participates in hydroxylation and side chain cleavage reactions (see Chapter 16). The balance of these hydroxylation reactions is as follows:

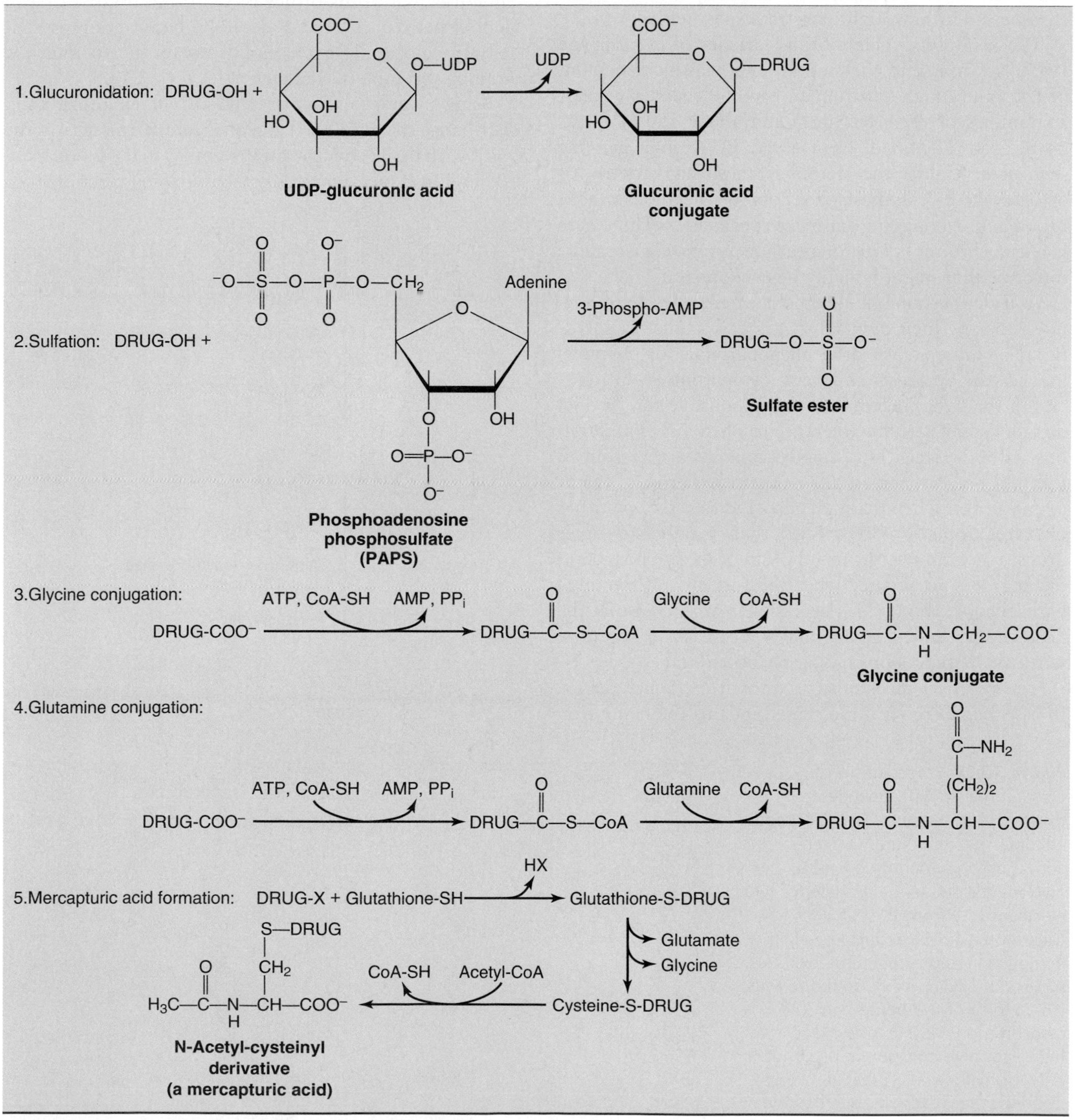

Figure 30.18 Conjugation reactions of drugs (*DRUG*) and other xenobiotics used in phase 2 of xenobiotic metabolism. Most of these reactions take place in the liver, and the water-soluble products are excreted in bile or urine.

$$\text{Substrate-H} + O_2 + \text{NADPH} + H^+$$
$$\downarrow$$
$$\text{Substrate-OH} + H_2O + \text{NADP}^+$$

Cytochrome P-450 is not a single protein but a whole superfamily of heme-containing proteins. They are membrane bound in the endoplasmic reticulum ("microsomes") or in the inner mitochondrial membrane. Approximately a dozen of them participate in normal lipid metabolism, including the synthesis of steroid hormones (see Chapter 16) and the ω-oxidation of fatty acids (see Chapter 23). These species of cytochrome P-450 have tight substrate specificities.

The xenobiotic-metabolizing varieties of cytochrome P-450 are found in the smooth endoplasmic reticulum of liver and lungs. The human genome encodes at least 14 families of these enzymes, and about 150 isoforms have been identified from their RNA and genome sequences. Unlike the steroid-synthesizing varieties of cytochrome P-450, those of xenobiotic metabolism have broad and overlapping substrate specificities. Thus there is a cytochrome P-450 for nearly every foreign organic molecule that might possibly be encountered.

As a rule, xenobiotic-metabolizing enzymes are inducible either by their own substrates or by other xenobiotics. The antiepileptic drug phenobarbital, for example, induces the synthesis of several cytochrome P-450 species in the liver, including those responsible for its own metabolism. Therefore tolerance to phenobarbital develops within 1 week, and this necessitates a threefold to fourfold dosage increase to maintain the original therapeutic effect. Phenobarbital also induces the synthesis of cytochrome P-450 species that metabolize other drugs. For example, the metabolism of the anticoagulant dicumarol is accelerated when the patient is also treated with phenobarbital. This necessitates an increase in the dose of the anticoagulant and a decrease in the dose when the patient stops taking phenobarbital.

The reaction mechanism is shown in *Figure 30.19*. In essence, an oxygen molecule binds to the heme iron and becomes activated by an electron transfer. This highly reactive oxygen molecule attacks the substrate, depending on the substrate specificity of the enzyme. The activating electron is derived from NADPH and is transmitted to the iron by a flavoprotein.

ETHANOL IS METABOLIZED TO ACETYL-CoA IN THE LIVER

Ethanol is not only an intoxicant but also a nutrient with an energy value of 7.1 kcal/g. Therefore a drinker can cover half of his or her BMR from 100 to 120 g of alcohol per day. Distilled alcoholic beverages represent "empty calories," so alcoholics are prone to multiple vitamin and mineral deficiencies.

Being a water-miscible organic solvent, ethanol rapidly distributes through the aqueous compartments of the body, with tissue concentrations similar to the blood alcohol level. It is metabolized by the following reactions:

$H_3C\text{-}CH_2OH$
Ethanol

NAD$^+$
Alcohol dehydrogenase (cytosol)
NADH, H$^+$

$H_3C\text{-}CHO$
Acetaldehyde

NAD$^+$, H$_2O$
Aldehyde dehydrogenase (mitochondrion)
NADH, 2H$^+$

$H_3C\text{-}COO^-$
Acetate

Figure 30.19 Mechanism of cytochrome P-450–dependent hydroxylation reactions in the smooth endoplasmic reticulum. Oxygen activation by cytochrome P-450 involves the sequential transfer of two electrons (e$^-$) from the NADPH–cytochrome P-450 reductase. As in hemoglobin and cytochrome oxidase, molecular oxygen binds to the ferrous (Fe^{2+}) form of the heme iron. The cytochrome P-450–bound oxygen is highly reactive and can be used not only for hydroxylation reactions but also for other reactions, such as the formation of epoxides (see *Fig. 30.17*).

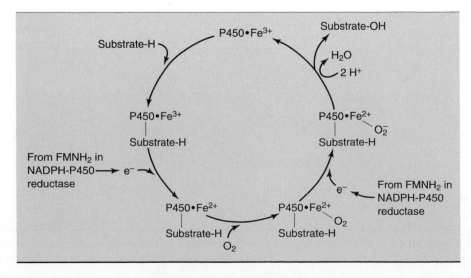

These reactions take place in the liver and, to a lesser extent, in the stomach wall, but most of the acetate is released into the blood and oxidized by other tissues. **Alcohol dehydrogenase (ADH)** catalyzes the rate-limiting step, but *availability of NAD$^+$ is another limiting factor* for alcohol metabolism. The K_m of ADH for ethanol is near 1 mmol/L (46 mg/L). Therefore the enzyme is essentially saturated after only one drink, and *alcohol metabolism follows zero-order kinetics*. Most people metabolize about 10 g of alcohol per hour, and the blood alcohol level decreases by about 0.15 g/L every hour. These calculations are important when a blood sample from a drunken driver has been obtained some hours after an accident.

Genetic variants of alcohol-metabolizing enzymes contribute to individual differences in alcohol tolerance. Three genetic variants of ADH have been described with different pH optima and maximal reaction rate (V_{max}). The most interesting polymorphism, however, affects the mitochondrial aldehyde dehydrogenase that oxidizes acetaldehyde to acetate. This enzyme normally is not rate limiting, and because of its low K_m of 10 μmol/L for acetaldehyde, this intermediate does not accumulate to any great extent. A drunken man's blood alcohol level is between 20 and 50 mmol/L and his acetic acid level is between 1 and 2 mmol/L, but his acetaldehyde level remains less than 20 μmol/L.

Many East Asians have an atypical aldehyde dehydrogenase with a single amino acid substitution (Glu→Lys) in position 487 of the polypeptide. This genetic variant behaves as a "dominant negative" mutation. This means that even heterozygotes, who still produce the normal enzyme in addition to the defective one, have near-zero enzyme activity, possibly because the mutant enzyme forms inactive oligomers with the normal one. In these individuals, acetaldehyde is oxidized by a cytosolic aldehyde dehydrogenase whose K_m for acetaldehyde is close to 1 mmol/L. Therefore *toxic acetaldehyde accumulates to high levels after only one or two drinks.*

The result is the **oriental flush** response, with vasodilation, facial flushing, and tachycardia. These effects are so unpleasant that affected individuals rarely become alcoholics. From 30% to 40% of Chinese, Japanese, Mongolians, Koreans, Vietnamese, and Indonesians and many South American Indians have the atypical aldehyde dehydrogenase.

The mitochondrial aldehyde dehydrogenase can be inhibited pharmacologically by **disulfiram (Antabuse)**. This drug is used for treatment of alcoholism, but its use requires strict medical supervision. Fatal reactions have occurred when the drug was mixed into an unsuspecting alcoholic's drink.

Alcohol is also metabolized by the cytochrome P-450 system:

$$H_3C\text{-}CH_2OH + O_2 + NADPH + H^+ \text{ (Ethanol)}$$
$$\downarrow$$
$$H_3C\text{-}CHO + NADP^+ + 2\,H_2O \text{ (Acetaldehyde)}$$

This reaction accounts for only a small percentage of total alcohol metabolism in most people, but, unlike ADH, cytochrome P-450 synthesis is induced by alcohol. Therefore an increased proportion of the alcohol is metabolized by this route in alcoholics.

The alcohol-induced cytochrome P-450 enzymes metabolize barbiturates and many other drugs in addition to alcohol. Therefore the sober alcoholic is not very responsive to these drugs, which can cause problems for the induction of surgical anesthesia. However, alcohol restores responsiveness to the drug because it competes with the drug for the drug-metabolizing enzyme. Fatal reactions have occurred when barbiturates and alcohol were used at the same time.

LIVER METABOLISM IS DERANGED BY ALCOHOL

Unlike carbohydrate and fatty acid oxidation, alcohol metabolism is not subject to negative controls. Therefore *alcohol oxidation takes precedence over the oxidation of other nutrients*. The reactions of alcohol metabolism evolved presumably for the detoxification of the small amount of alcohol that is normally formed by bacterial fermentation in the colon. Thus the lack of feedback inhibition was no handicap before the invention of fermented beverages.

Alcohol metabolism produces large quantities of acetyl-CoA, NADH, and ATP. These products inhibit glucose metabolism at the level of phosphofructokinase and pyruvate dehydrogenase (*Fig. 30.20*). Fatty acid oxidation is impaired by the depletion of NAD$^+$. The TCA cycle is inhibited by high levels of ATP and NADH and by the depletion of NAD$^+$. The TCA cycle is dispensable for the drunken liver because the respiratory chain oxidation of the NADH generated in the oxidation of ethanol to acetic acid is more than sufficient to provide for the energy needs of the cell.

Rather than being oxidized, the fatty acids are esterified into triglycerides for export as VLDL. Therefore VLDL tends to be elevated in alcoholics.

Despite high levels of ATP and NADH, gluconeogenesis from pyruvate and oxaloacetate is inhibited by alcohol because the high [NADH]/[NAD$^+$] ratio drives the reversible lactate dehydrogenase and malate dehydrogenase reactions in the "wrong" direction:

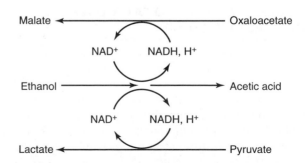

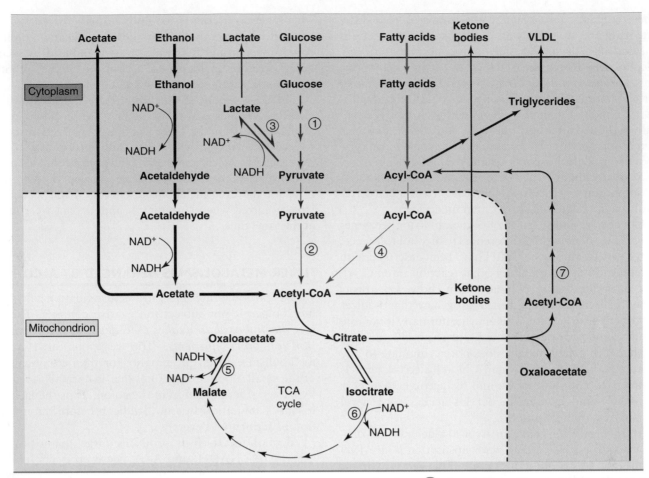

Figure 30.20 Effects of alcohol on liver metabolism. Important control points: ① phosphofructokinase: inhibited by high energy charge; ② pyruvate dehydrogenase: inhibited by high energy charge, high NADH/NAD$^+$ ratio, and high acetyl-coenzyme A (*CoA*); ③ lactate dehydrogenase: high NADH/NAD$^+$ ratio favors lactate formation; ④ β-oxidation: slowed down because of low NAD$^+$; ⑤ malate dehydrogenase: high NADH/NAD$^+$ ratio favors malate formation, oxaloacetate is depleted; ⑥ isocitrate dehydrogenase: inhibited by high energy charge and high NADH/NAD$^+$ ratio; and ⑦ acetyl-CoA carboxylase: may be stimulated by high citrate (accumulates because isocitrate dehydrogenase is inhibited). *TCA*, Tricarboxylic acid; *VLDL*, very-low-density lipoprotein.

As a result, the gluconeogenic substrates pyruvate and oxaloacetate are depleted, whereas the blood level of lactate is increased. *Alcohol can precipitate hypoglycemia when liver glycogen is depleted.* A marathoner must never consume an alcoholic drink after a race. Alcohol itself is not a substrate for gluconeogenesis. It is ketogenic but not glucogenic.

ALCOHOLISM LEADS TO FATTY LIVER AND LIVER CIRRHOSIS

The liver synthesizes triglycerides at all times, not for storage but for export in VLDL. A **fatty liver** develops as a result of *increased triglyceride synthesis, reduced VLDL formation,* or both (*Table 30.10*). Fatty liver causes no functional impairment, and it is reversible. Alcohol is the most common cause of fatty liver. It does not prevent VLDL formation but increases fat synthesis.

Fatty liver is most likely in alcoholics who also suffer from protein deficiency because protein deficiency impairs VLDL formation.

In **liver cirrhosis,** hepatocytes degenerate and are replaced by fibrous connective tissue. Cirrhosis is the final outcome of many liver diseases, but in industrialized countries, 60% to 70% of cases are associated with alcoholism. *Table 30.11* summarizes some of the abnormalities in patients with liver cirrhosis.

MOST "DISEASES OF CIVILIZATION" ARE CAUSED BY ABERRANT NUTRITION

The disease patterns in industrialized countries changed dramatically during the twentieth century. Infectious diseases have given way to cardiovascular disease and cancer as the leading causes of death (*Table 30.12*). Even more "ancient" patterns of mortality and morbidity

Table 30.10   Conditions Leading to Fat Accumulation in the Liver

Condition	Examples	Mechanism
Increased triglyceride synthesis	Starvation	Increased supply of fatty acids from adipose tissue
	Diabetes mellitus	
	Alcoholism	Decreased fatty acid oxidation; possibly increased intrahepatic fatty acid synthesis
Decreased formation of VLDL	Protein deficiency	Decreased synthesis of VLDL apolipoprotein
	Essential fatty acid deficiency	Decreased phospholipid synthesis
	Toxic liver damage	VLDL formation impaired to greater extent than triglyceride synthesis

VLDL, Very-low-density lipoprotein.

Table 30.11   Biochemical Abnormalities in Advanced Liver Cirrhosis

Abnormality	Impaired Function
Fasting hypoglycemia	Glycogenolysis, gluconeogenesis
Prolonged clotting time	Synthesis of clotting factors
Edema	Albumin synthesis*
Hyperammonemia	Urea cycle
"Fetid" breath	Metabolism of sulfhydryl compounds formed by intestinal bacteria
Alcohol intolerance	Alcohol metabolism
Jaundice	Bilirubin metabolism

*Impaired lymph flow is another cause of abdominal edema (ascites).

Table 30.12   Top 10 Causes of Death in the United States, 1900 and 1998

Rank	Cause of Death	Percent of All Deaths
	1900	
1	Pneumonia	12
2	Tuberculosis	11
3	Diarrhea and enteritis	8
4	Heart disease	8
5	Chronic nephritis	5
6	Accidents	4
7	Stroke	4
8	Diseases of infancy	4
9	Cancer	4
10	Diphtheria	2
	1998	
1	Heart disease	31
2	Cancer	23
3	Stroke	7
4	Lung diseases	5
5	Pneumonia and influenza	4
6	Accidents	4
7	Diabetes	3
8	Suicide	1
9	Kidney diseases	1
10	Liver diseases	1

have been described in simple agricultural and preagricultural societies, but *infectious diseases have always been the leading cause of death.*

Thanks to better hygiene and antibiotics, most people now escape the ravages of infectious diseases. In preindustrial societies, infant and childhood mortality hovered near 40%, and life expectancy at birth was in the range from 25 to 40 years. Because more people today survive to an advanced age, age-related diseases, including cancer and cardiovascular disease, have become more prevalent.

However, why do nearly half of all people die of cardiovascular disease rather than, for example, kidney or brain disease? Why do 5% of all adults in industrialized societies suffer from diabetes mellitus rather than some other endocrine disorder? Why are so many people overweight rather than underweight? And why do 20% of adults suffer from hypertension, whereas hypotension is rare?

"Diseases of civilization" are prevalent today because human beings, like all other creatures, are adapted to their environment by mutation and selection. Therefore we have inherited those genetic variants that enabled early humans to reproduce in the environments in which they lived.

Ancestral environments were very different from the conditions under which people are living today. Levels of physical activity were high, and food was sometimes scarce. Therefore humans had to evolve a ravenous appetite and a preference for foods with high caloric density, especially those rich in fat or sugar. They also had to store as much energy as possible in their adipose tissue to maximize the chance of survival during bad seasons.

The ancient food preferences are still wired into human brains today, and people still store excess energy in adipose tissue. This programming, evolved under conditions of frequent food shortages, is the reason for near-universal obesity in affluent societies.

Until less than 10,000 years ago, all humans lived by hunting and gathering rather than farming. Human metabolic and physiologic systems evolved under these Paleolithic conditions. *Table 30.13* compares the typical nutrient intakes under these conditions with the

Table 30.13 Nutrient Intake during Paleolithic Period Compared with Current Nutrient Intake in the United States and Recommended Intakes

	Paleolithic Intake	Current U.S. Intake	Recommended Intake
Macronutrients			
% Protein	37	14	12
% Carbohydrate	41	50	
Sugars	3	21	
% Fat	22	36	
Saturated	6	14	<10
Trans-unsaturated	0	3	
Monounsaturated	7.5	13.5	
Polyunsaturated	8.5	5.5	
Cholesterol (mg)	480	450	<300
Vitamins (mg/day)			
Riboflavin	6.5	1.7	1.7
Folic acid	0.4	0.18	0.2
Thiamin	3.9	1.4	1.5
Ascorbic acid	604	100	60
Vitamin A	3.8	1.8	1
Vitamin E	32.8	9	10
Minerals (mg/day)			
Iron	87.4	11	10
Zinc	43.4	13	15
Sodium	768	4000	500–2400
Potassium	10,500	2500	3500
Fiber (g/day)	104	10–20	20–30

typical modern American diet and the recommended daily allowances set by experts.

Contrary to common prejudice, ancestors of today's humans were not vegetarians; rather, they covered about one third of their energy needs from meat. Meat supplied most of their dietary protein. Whereas modern Americans typically consume 100 g of protein per day, human ancestors consumed closer to 250 g per day. As a result, typical early humans were at least as tall as the tallest populations in modern industrialized countries, muscular, and lean.

Dietary carbohydrate was as abundant in Paleolithic times as in the modern diet. However, modern carbohydrate consists of easily digestible starch and refined sugar. Today, sugars alone contribute 21% of the daily energy intake. Most of the carbohydrate in the Paleolithic diet was in the form of complex carbohydrates with a low **glycemic index.** The glycemic index is a measure of the extent to which the carbohydrate raises the blood glucose after a meal. Even people who are genetically predisposed to type 2 diabetes would rarely ever develop diabetes if they were on a Paleolithic diet.

People who are genetically predisposed to type 2 diabetes are known to have reduced postprandial thermogenesis. They have a *thrifty genotype* that reduces energy wastage after an ample meal. This genetic predisposition used to be advantageous because it made the conversion of excess food into storage fat more efficient. It became maladaptive only in a world in which people gorge themselves on sugary junk food.

Fat was less abundant in the Paleolithic diet than in modern diets. Wild game animals are always lean. Unlike farm animals, they cannot afford excess fat stores that would compromise running speed. Thus most of the fat in human ancestral diets was derived from oily seeds and nuts. Saturated fat, which is considered the main dietary risk factor for coronary heart disease, made up only 6% of the energy content in the typical Paleolithic diet, as opposed to 13% or 14% in the modern American diet.

Interestingly, the plasma total cholesterol levels measured in hunter-gatherers averaged only 125 mg/dl even though the cholesterol content of their diet was quite high. The average level of the modern American is 205 mg/dl. This difference is attributed to the different types of fat consumed and to the deficiency of fiber in modern diets. Modern Americans consume, on average, less than 20 g of dietary fiber per day, but the "natural" diet of Paleolithic humans contained more than 100 g of fiber per day.

The term **metabolic syndrome** is applied to a constellation of obesity, poor glucose tolerance, and an atherogenic lipid profile. The reason these abnormalities are often found combined in the same person is that they all have the same underlying cause: overeating foods with high caloric density.

Another reason for the high incidence of cardiovascular disease in modern societies is the aberrant pattern of mineral consumption. Humans are adapted to a diet that contains almost 14 times more potassium than sodium (see *Table 30.13*). Today, potassium intake has dropped to one third and sodium intake has risen almost sixfold. Of the sodium consumed today, 75% is bought in processed foods.

A high sodium intake is the principal risk factor for hypertension because it tends to expand the blood volume, at least in people whose kidneys are slow to excrete the excess. In one major study, the average blood pressure of human groups that do not use added salt was 102/62 mmHg. The average for the groups that did use salt was 119/74. There is a linear relationship between blood pressure and the complications of hypertension even in the "normal" range. The "low" blood pressure typical for no-salt human groups is healthier than the blood pressure that is considered "normal" in modern societies.

Unlike the Paleolithic diet, the diets of traditional farmers often are deficient in protein, vitamins, and minerals. When human groups made the transition from hunting and gathering to agriculture, they typically became shorter, and their skeletal remains show signs of nutritional deficiencies. These nutritional deficiencies are still seen in traditional farmers from the less industrialized parts of the world.

Can humans adapt genetically to the conditions of civilized life? One common observation is that in affluent societies, type 2 diabetes is most common among groups whose ancestors either were nonagricultural or were exposed to frequent famine. For example, type 2 diabetes is twice as common in acculturated Australian aborigines than in white Australians, and in the United States, Pima Indians are at least three times more likely to develop diabetes than are white people. Apparently, populations with a long history of carbohydrate-rich diets in traditional agricultural economies did become genetically less susceptible to type 2 diabetes. Similarly, hypertension seems to be most common in populations whose ancestors had no access to salt.

AGING IS THE GREATEST CHALLENGE FOR MEDICAL RESEARCH

Old age is the deadliest of all diseases, with a mortality of 100%. Although the *average* lifespan has increased through advances in medicine, the *maximal* lifespan has remained the same. Several mechanisms have been postulated as contributors to the aging process:

1. *Accumulation of somatic mutations.* Somatic mutations are believed to contribute to age-related functional decline, especially in tissues that cannot replace defective cells. However, the extent to which somatic mutations are responsible for the cell loss that occurs in these tissues with advancing age is not known.
2. *Damage by reactive oxygen species.* Reactive oxygen species, including the superoxide radical, hydrogen peroxide, and hydroxyl radicals, damage our cells by causing somatic mutations, lipid peroxidation, and other cellular damage.
3. *Mitochondrial dysfunction.* The mutation rate is higher in mitochondrial DNA than in nuclear DNA. This results from the abundance of reactive oxygen species in this organelle and probably also from less efficient DNA repair. Deletions in mitochondrial DNA are especially likely to accumulate, probably because the shortened DNA molecules are replicated faster than is full-length DNA. Declines in oxidative capacity are commonly observed in aging tissues. Terminally differentiated cells, in particular, tend to accumulate abnormal oversized mitochondria that are inefficient at ATP synthesis but still produce reactive oxygen species.
4. *Telomere shortening.* In most tissues, telomerase is no longer expressed after birth. As a result, telomeres tend to shorten in tissues whose cells keep dividing throughout life. Shortened telomeres can trigger apoptosis.
5. *Accumulation of garbage.* Aged lysosomes of nondividing cells accumulate an undegradable yellow product called **lipofuscin** that is derived from oxidized lipids and cross-linked denatured proteins. Extracellular garbage accumulates in the form of insoluble **amyloid** (see Chapter 2).
6. *Collateral damage.* Because infections were the leading cause of death until the twentieth century, humans evolved a vigilant immune system that responds to the slightest provocation. In allergies, immune responses are mounted against harmless environmental materials; in autoimmune diseases, they are mounted against components of the body. Most age-related diseases have an inflammatory component, and collateral damage can be caused by abortive immune responses to abnormal stimuli (e.g., deposits of cholesterol esters in arterial walls).
7. *Hormonal mechanisms.* Animal experiments have shown that the signaling system represented by insulin and insulin-like growth factor 1 (IGF-1) in humans shortens life in addition to stimulating growth and metabolism. Mice with reduced numbers of IGF-1 receptors and mice that lack insulin receptors in adipose tissue have a prolonged lifespan. Whether transgenic humans with similar changes also live longer remains to be seen.

But why have humans not evolved more effective ways of counteracting these threats to their continued existence? Aging and age-related diseases are explained by the theory of **antagonistic pleiotropy**. In essence, mortality from infections, accidents, and homicide was so high in ancestral populations that few people ever became very old. There would be little selective advantage for a genetic variant that offered better health or continued reproductive capacity at an old age because most of the potential beneficiaries never reached that age. Worse, any genetic variant that offers a great advantage to the old but at the cost of a slight disadvantage for the young will be selected out of the gene pool. Thus we must expect that our defenses against aging and age-related diseases are less than optimal. Only genetic engineering can change this sorry state of affairs.

Short of genetic engineering, the most effective life-prolonging intervention is caloric restriction. Rats that are kept at 70% of free-feeding weight live 20% longer than do those with an unlimited food supply. Even rhesus monkeys live longer when their caloric intake is restricted. This life-prolonging effect is accompanied by a reduced metabolic rate and therefore most likely a reduced formation of reactive oxygen derivatives. However, the effect of caloric restriction is not duplicated with antioxidants. Caloric restriction also reduces the level of insulin and IGF-1, and this may well be the mechanism of its life-prolonging effect.

For most people, a life-prolonging pill would be more attractive than caloric restriction to 70% of free-feeding weight. Animal experiments have shown at least two effective drugs. One is **rapamycin,** an inhibitor of the protein kinase mTOR (see *Fig. 18.17*). This is one branch of the signaling cascades that is initiated by insulin, IGF-1, other growth factors, and nutrients.

The other effective drug appears to be **resveratrol,** a constituent of red wine and an activator of **sirtuins.** The sirtuins are protein deacetylases whose activity depends on a sufficiently high level of NAD^+ in the cell. An elevated $NAD^+/NADH$ ratio is typical for starvation. Therefore sirtuins are activated during starvation and conceivably can mediate the effects of caloric restriction. Resveratrol from red wine is poorly absorbed, and most of the absorbed resveratrol is metabolized in the liver as a first-pass effect; however, more potent, metabolically stable sirtuin activators are being developed.

One of the more interesting effects of sirtuins is the stimulation of **macroautophagy** (see Chapter 8). Macroautophagy is involved in the defense against intracellular parasites (see *Clinical Example 8.2*) but also has a more general function in the removal of defective mitochondria and of insoluble protein deposits that may have formed in the cell.

Whether any life-prolonging drug proves suitable for human use remains to be seen. In the meantime, quitting smoking and drinking would not be a bad idea either.

SUMMARY

The major metabolic pathways must adapt to the nutrient supply. After a meal, insulin stimulates glucose utilization by enhancing glucose uptake in muscle and adipose tissue and by stimulating glucose-metabolizing enzymes in most tissues. It also directs dietary triglycerides to adipose tissue for storage and promotes the conversion of excess carbohydrate into fat.

Fatty acids from adipose tissue are the main energy source during fasting. The fatty acids are oxidized either directly or after their initial conversion to ketone bodies by the liver. A few tissues, including brain and erythrocytes, require glucose even during fasting. The liver supplies these tissues with glucose, initially by glycogen degradation and later by gluconeogenesis from amino acids, lactate, and glycerol. These processes are stimulated by glucagon, the main insulin antagonist in the liver.

During stress and physical exertion, epinephrine and norepinephrine mobilize stored fat and glycogen for use by the muscles. These effects are potentiated by the other important type of stress hormone, the glucocorticoids.

"Diseases of civilization" are caused by the prevalent dietary habits in modern societies. Obesity and type 2 diabetes are caused by overeating, whereas hypertension is caused to a large extent by excessive salt consumption. Alcohol is detoxified in the liver, but this process can lead to liver damage. Other drugs, food additives, and environmental toxins are also handled by detoxifying systems in liver and other organs, but damage by these agents cannot always be prevented.

Further Reading

Anderson KA, Means AR: Central control of feeding, *Biol Rep* 1:10, 2009.

Anderson RM, Weindruch R: Metabolic reprogramming, caloric restriction and aging, *Trends Endocrinol Metab* 21:134–141, 2010.

Andrali SS, Sampley ML, Vanderford NL, et al: Glucose regulation of insulin gene expression in pancreatic beta-cells, *Biochem J* 415:1–10, 2008.

Attie AD, Scherer PE: Adipocyte metabolism and obesity, *J Lipid Res* 2009:S395–S399, 2009.

Banks J, Marmot M, Oldfield Z, et al: Disease and disadvantage in the United States and in England, *JAMA* 295:2037–2045, 2006.

Barger JL, Kayo T, Vann JM, et al: A low dose of dietary resveratrol partially mimics caloric restriction and retards aging parameters in mice, *PLoS ONE* 3(6):e2264, 2008.

Cahill GF: Fuel metabolism in starvation, *Annu Rev Nutr* 26:1–22, 2006.

Colman VJ, Anderson RM, Johnson SC, et al: Caloric restriction delays disease onset and mortality in rhesus monkeys, *Science* 325:201–204, 2009.

DeFronzo RA: Overview of newer agents: where treatment [of type 2 diabetes] is going, *Am J Med* 123:S38–S48, 2010.

Dupuis J, Langenberg C, Prokopenko I, et al: New genetic loci implicated in fasting glucose homeostasis and their impact on type 2 diabetes risk, *Nat Genet* 42:105–116, 2010.

Edinger AL: Controlling cell growth and survival through regulated nutrient transporter expression, *Biochem J* 406:1–12, 2007.

Erion DM, Shulman GI: Diacylglycerol-mediated insulin resistance, *Nat Med* 16:400–402, 2010.

Finkel T, Deng C-X, Mostoslavsky R: Recent progress in the biology and physiology of sirtuins, *Nature* 460:587–591, 2009.

Flachsbart F, Caliebe A, Kleindorp R, et al: Association of FOXO3A variation with human longevity confirmed in German centenarians, *Proc Natl Acad Sci U S A* 106: 2700–2705, 2009.

Forsum E, Löf M: Energy metabolism during human pregnancy, *Annu Rev Nutr* 27:277–292, 2007.

Foster KG, Fingar DC: Mammalian target of rapamycin (mTOR): conducting the cellular signaling symphony, *J Biol Chem* 285:14071–14077, 2010.

Friedman JM: Causes and control of excess body fat, *Nature* 459:340–342, 2009.

Fukui H, Moraes CT: Mechanisms of formation and accumulation of mitochondrial DNA deletions in aging neurons, *Hum Mol Genet* 18:1028–1036, 2009.

Gesta S, Tseng Y-H, Kahn CR: Developmental origin of fat: tracking obesity to its source, *Cell* 131:242–256, 2007.

Ghosh HS, McBurney M, Robbins PD: SIRT1 negatively regulates the mammalian target of rapamycin, *PLoS ONE* 5(2): e9199, 2010.

Goberdhan DCI, Ögmundsdóttir MH, Kazi S, et al: Amino acid sensing and mTOR regulation: inside or out? *Biochem Soc Trans* 37:248–252, 2009.

Gregg EW, Cheng YJ, Narayan KMV, et al: The relative contributions of different levels of overweight and obesity to the increased prevalence of diabetes in the United States: 1976–2004, *Prevent Med* 45:348–352, 2007.

Haataja L, Gurlo T, Huang CJ, et al: Islet amyloid in type 2 diabetes, and the toxic oligomer hypothesis, *Endocr Rev* 29:303–316, 2008.

Harrington M, Gibson S, Cottrell RC: A review and meta-analysis of weight loss on all-cause mortality risk, *Nutr Res Rev* 22:93–108, 2009.

Harrison DE, Strong R, Sharp ZD, et al: Rapamycin fed late in life extends lifespan in genetically heterogeneous mice, *Nature* 460:392–395, 2009.

Illig T, Gieger C, Zhai G, et al: A genome-wide perspective of genetic variation in human metabolism, *Nat Genet* 42:137–141, 2010.

Kaeberlein M: Resveratreol and rapamycin: are they anti-aging drugs? *Bioessays* 32:96–99, 2010.

Kenyon CJ: The genetics of ageing, *Nature* 464:504–512, 2010.

Kwon H-S, Ott M: The ups and downs of SIRT1, *Trends Biochem Sci* 33:517–525, 2008.

Lusis AJ, Attie AD, Reue K: Metabolic syndrome: from epidemiology to systems biology, *Nat Rev Genet* 9:819–830, 2008.

Madsen L, Kristiansen K: The importance of dietary modulation of cAMP and insulin signaling in adipose tissue and the development of obesity, *Ann N Y Acad Sci* 1190:1–14, 2010.

Mainous AG, Baker R, Koopman RJ, et al: Impact of the population at risk of diabetes on projections of diabetes burden in the United States: an epidemic on the way, *Diabetologia* 50:934–940, 2007.

Marchetti P, Dotta F, Lavro D, et al: An overview of pancreatic beta-cell defects in human type 2 diabetes: implications for treatment, *Regul Pept* 146:4–11, 2008.

Minich DM, Bland JS: Dietary management of the metabolic syndrome beyond macronutrients, *Nutr Rev* 66:429–444, 2008.

Narkar VA, Downes M, Yu RT, et al: AMPK and PPARδ agonists are exercise mimetics, *Cell* 134:405–415, 2008.

Nolan CJ, Prentki M: The islet β-cell: fuel responsive and vulnerable, *Trends Endocrinol Metab* 19:285–291, 2008.

Ogden CL, Carroll MD, Curtin LR, et al: Prevalence of overweight and obesity in the United States, 1999–2004, *JAMA* 295:1549–1555, 2006.

O'Rahilly S: Human genetics illuminates the paths to metabolic disease, *Nature* 462:307–314, 2009.

Powell K: The two faces of fat, *Nature* 447:525–527, 2007.

Prokopenko I, McCarthy MI, Lindgren CM: Type 2 diabetes: new genes, new understanding, *Trends Genet* 24:613–621, 2008.

Ranganathan G, Pokrovskaya I, Ranganathan S, et al: Role of A kinase anchor protein in the tissue-specific regulation of lipoprotein lipase, *Mol Endocrinol* 19:2527–2534, 2005.

Richter EA, Ruderman NB: AMPK and the biochemistry of exercise: implications for human health and disease, *Biochem J* 418:261–275, 2009.

Schuelke M, Wagner KR, Stolz LE, et al: Myostatin mutation associated with gross muscle hypertrophy in a child, *N Engl J Med* 350:2682–2688, 2004.

Selivanov VA, de Atauri P, Centelles JJ, et al: The changes in the energy metabolism of human muscle induced by training, *J Theor Biol* 252:402–410, 2008.

Spalding KL, Arner E, Westermark PO, et al: Dynamics of fat cell turnover in humans, *Nature* 453:783–787, 2008.

Spriet LL, Perry CGR, Talanian JL: Legal pre-event nutritional supplements to assist energy metabolism, *Essays Biochem* 44:27–43, 2008.

Starck CS, Sutherland-Smith AJ: Cytotoxic aggregation and amyloid formation by the myostatin precursor protein, *PLoS ONE* 5(2):e9170, 2010.

Stipanuk MH: Leucine and protein synthesis: mTOR and beyond, *Nutr Rev* 65:122–129, 2007.

Taubes G: Prosperity's plague, *Science* 325:256–260, 2009.

Tomlinson DR, Gardiner NJ: Glucose neurotoxicity, *Nat Rev Neurosci* 9:36–45, 2008.

Vijg J, Campisi J: Puzzles, promises and a cure for ageing, *Nature* 454:1065–1071, 2008.

Wackerhage H, Ratkevicius A: Signal transduction pathways that regulate muscle growth, *Essays Biochem* 44:99–108, 2008.

Wahren J, Ekberg K: Splanchnic regulation of glucose production, *Annu Rev Nutr* 27:329–345, 2007.

Wang PYT, Caspi L, Lam CKL, et al: Upper intestinal lipids trigger a gut-brain-liver axis to regulate glucose production, *Nature* 452:1012–1016, 2008.

Weiss MA: Proinsulin and the genetics of diabetes mellitus, *J Biol Chem* 284:19159–19163, 2009.

QUESTIONS

1. How can you best describe the function of cytochrome P-450 in xenobiotic metabolism?

A. It transfers an electron to adrenodoxin.
B. It binds a water molecule, thereby activating it for a nucleophilic attack on the substrate.
C. It accepts two electrons and a proton from NADPH for transfer to the substrate.
D. It activates an oxygen molecule.
E. It acts as an ATPase.

2. The brain produces most of its energy by the oxidation of glucose; during long-term fasting, however, it can cover more than half of its energy needs from

A. Anaerobic glycolysis
B. Oxidation of its stored glycogen
C. Oxidation of free fatty acids
D. Oxidation of amino acids
E. Oxidation of ketone bodies

3. When an insulin-dependent diabetic patient undergoes surgery (any surgery), you should monitor his or her blood glucose level extra carefully because

A. Stress hormones antagonize insulin, and the patient may therefore require extra insulin
B. Stress reduces insulin release from the pancreas, a condition known as insulin shock
C. Insulin can inhibit the blood clotting system
D. Any physical or psychological stress is likely to cause hypoglycemia

4. During long-term fasting, the liver produces acetyl-CoA by the β-oxidation of fatty acids. What is the major metabolic fate of this acetyl-CoA?

A. Fatty acid biosynthesis
B. Gluconeogenesis
C. Amino acid biosynthesis
D. Ketogenesis
E. Oxidation in the TCA cycle

5. The catecholamines epinephrine and norepinephrine adjust metabolic activity throughout the body to satisfy the energy demands of the working muscles. All of the following catecholamine effects are important during physical activity *except*

A. Stimulation of glycogenolysis in the liver
B. Stimulation of glycogenolysis in skeletal muscle
C. Inhibition of glycolysis in skeletal muscle
D. Inhibition of glycolysis in the liver
E. Stimulation of lipolysis in adipose tissue

6. When you get up in the morning, 12 hours after dinner, what is the main source of your blood glucose?

A. Dietary glucose
B. Liver glycogen
C. Muscle glycogen
D. Gluconeogenesis from lactate
E. Gluconeogenesis from amino acids

ANSWERS TO QUESTIONS

Chapter 1
1. D
2. C
3. A

Chapter 2
1. C
2. D
3. D
4. D
5. C
6. E

Chapter 3
1. B
2. B
3. A

Chapter 4
1. E
2. C
3. E
4. A
5. D
6. B

Chapter 5
1. E
2. D
3. A

Chapter 6
1. B
2. D
3. C
4. E
5. B

Chapter 7
1. B
2. C
3. E
4. C
5. D
6. E
7. A

Chapter 8
1. A
2. D

Chapter 9
1. E
2. B
3. D
4. C
5. B

Chapter 10
1. A
2. E

Chapter 11
1. E
2. E
3. C
4. D
5. D
6. A
7. C
8. C
9. A
10. E
11. D

Chapter 12
1. D
2. D
3. D
4. A

Chapter 13
1. E
2. B
3. C
4. A

Chapter 14
1. A
2. E
3. B
4. D
5. A

Chapter 15
1. A
2. D
3. D
4. A
5. C

Chapter 16
1. E
2. B
3. C
4. E

Chapter 17
1. D
2. C
3. A
4. E
5. D

Chapter 18
1. C
2. B
3. D
4. C
5. C
6. B
7. E
8. A
9. D

Chapter 19
1. C
2. D

Chapter 20
1. D
2. B

Chapter 21
1. A
2. E
3. C
4. B
5. C
6. D
7. E

Chapter 22
1. B
2. E
3. A
4. E
5. C

Chapter 23
1. D
2. C
3. B
4. A

Chapter 24
1. B
2. D
3. B

Chapter 25
1. E
2. D
3. B
4. E

Chapter 26
1. D
2. A
3. B
4. E
5. C

Chapter 27
1. D
2. B

Chapter 28
1. C
2. B

Chapter 29
1. B
2. C
3. E
4. A
5. B

Chapter 30
1. D
2. E
3. A
4. D
5. C
6. B

GLOSSARY

Abetalipoproteinemia An inherited inability to form chylomicrons and very-low-density lipoprotein (VLDL).

Acetyl-CoA carboxylase The rate-limiting enzyme of fatty acid biosynthesis.

Acetylcholinesterase An extracellular acetylcholine-degrading enzyme in cholinergic synapses.

Achondroplasia A dominantly inherited form of dwarfism caused by constitutive activation of a growth factor receptor.

Acid A proton donor.

Acid phosphatase A marker for prostatic cancer.

Acidosis Abnormally low blood pH.

Acrodermatitis enteropathica A disease caused by an inherited defect of intestinal zinc absorption.

Actin A globular protein that polymerizes into microfilaments.

Actinomycin D An inhibitor of transcription that binds to double-stranded DNA.

Active site The place on the enzyme protein to which the substrate binds and where catalysis takes place.

Acute intermittent porphyria A hepatic porphyria, with abdominal pain and neurological symptoms.

Acute-phase reactants Plasma proteins whose levels are elevated or reduced within 1 to 2 days of an acute stress.

Acyl-CoA The activated form of a fatty acid.

Adenomatous polyposis coli (APC) An inherited cancer susceptibility syndrome.

Adenosine deaminase deficiency A cause of severe combined immunodeficiency.

Adenosine triphosphate (ATP) The "energetic currency" of the cell.

S-Adenosylmethionine (SAM) A cosubstrate that supplies an activated methyl group.

Adenylate cyclase The cyclic adenosine monophosphate (cAMP)-synthesizing enzyme, located in the plasma membrane.

Adrenergic receptors Receptors for epinephrine and norepinephrine.

Adrenodoxin A mitochondrial iron-sulfur protein that participates in hydroxylation reactions of steroids.

Adrenogenital syndrome Inherited defects of corticosteroid synthesis that lead to overproduction of adrenal androgens.

Aggrecan A large, aggregating proteoglycan in cartilage.

Agonist A stimulatory ligand for a receptor.

Akinesia Poverty of spontaneous movement.

Alanine cycle Cycling of alanine and glucose between muscle and liver during fasting.

Alanine transaminase A liver enzyme; its serum level is elevated in liver diseases.

Albumin A plasma protein that accounts for approximately 60% of the total plasma protein.

Alcohol dehydrogenase A cytosolic liver enzyme that oxidizes ethanol to acetaldehyde.

Aldose Monosaccharide with an aldehyde group.

Alkaline phosphatase A diagnostically useful enzyme in bones and biliary system.

Alkalosis Abnormally high blood pH.

Alkaptonuria A rare inborn error of tyrosine metabolism, with accumulation of homogentisate.

Allele-specific oligonucleotide probes Probes that can distinguish between different alleles (variants) of a gene.

Allelic heterogeneity Different disease-causing mutations in the same gene.

Allopurinol An inhibitor of xanthine oxidase, used to treat gout.

Allosteric effector A ligand that affects the equilibrium between the alternative conformations of an allosteric protein.

Allosteric protein A protein that can exist in alternative conformations.

Alport syndrome Genetic disorder of type IV collagen leading to kidney failure.

Alu sequences A large family of short interspersed elements.

Alzheimer disease The most common type of age-related dementia.

α-Amanitine A mushroom poison that inhibits RNA polymerase II.

Aminoacyl-tRNA A transfer RNA (tRNA) with an amino acid covalently bound to its 3′ terminus.

Aminoacyl-tRNA synthetases Cytoplasmic enzymes that attach an amino acid to a tRNA.

γ-Aminobutyric acid (GABA) An inhibitory neurotransmitter in the brain, synthesized from glutamate.

Aminolevulinic acid (ALA) synthase The regulated enzyme of heme biosynthesis.

Amphipathic Containing hydrophilic and hydrophobic portions in the same molecule.

α-Amylase A starch-degrading endoglycosidase in saliva and pancreatic juice.

Amylin A hormone that can form amyloid deposits in the endocrine pancreas.

Amyloid Abnormally folded, insoluble proteins with β-pleated sheet structure.

Amyloidogenic Amyloid-forming.

Anabolic pathway Biosynthetic pathway.

Anaerobic Oxygen deficient.

Anaplerotic reactions Reactions that result in the net production of a tricarboxylic acid (TCA) cycle intermediate.

Anchorage dependence The inability of cultured cells to grow in the absence of a solid support.

Androgen insensitivity syndrome (testicular feminization) Sex reversal caused by the absence of functional androgen receptor in a genotypic male.

Androgens Male sex steroids derived from progestins by a side-chain cleavage reaction.

Anemia Abnormal decrease of the blood hemoglobin concentration.

Aneuploidy Deficiency or excess of a chromosome.

Angiotensin II The active form of the vasoconstrictor angiotensin.

Angiotensin-converting enzyme (ACE) An enzyme of angiotensin synthesis; important drug target.

Anion Negatively charged ion.

Annealing Formation of a double strand from two complementary nucleic acid strands.

Anomers Monosaccharides that differ only in the orientation of substituents around their carbonyl carbons.

Antagonist An inhibitory ligand for a receptor.

Anticodon The base triplet of the tRNA that base pairs with the codon during protein synthesis.

Antigen-antibody complex A noncovalent aggregate between antigen and antibody.

Antimycin A An inhibitor of electron flow through the QH_2-cytochrome c reductase complex.

Antiport The coupled membrane transport of two substrates in opposite directions.

α₁-Antiprotease A circulating protease inhibitor, deficiency of which causes lung emphysema.

Antithrombin III A circulating inhibitor of thrombin and some other activated clotting factors.

AP endonuclease An endonuclease that cleaves a phosphodiester bond formed by a baseless ("apurinic") nucleotide in DNA.

Aplastic anemia Anemia caused by bone marrow failure.

ApoA-I, apoA-II The major apolipoproteins of high-density lipoprotein (HDL).

ApoB-100 The major apolipoprotein of very-low-density lipoprotein (VLDL) and low-density lipoprotein (LDL).

ApoB-48 The major apolipoprotein of chylomicrons.

ApoC-II An apolipoprotein that activates lipoprotein lipase.

ApoC-III An apolipoprotein that inhibits lipoprotein lipase.

ApoE An apolipoprotein that mediates the endocytosis of remnant particles by binding to hepatic apo-E receptors.

Apolipoprotein Protein component of a lipoprotein.

Apoprotein The polypeptide component of a conjugated protein.

Apoptosis Programmed cell death.

Apoptosome A cytoplasmic protein complex that activates caspases, causing apoptosis.

Arachidonic acid A 20-carbon polyunsaturated fatty acid, precursor of prostaglandins and leukotrienes.

Arginase The urea-forming enzyme of the urea cycle.

Aromatase The enzyme that converts androgens to estrogens.

Arrestin A cytoplasmic protein that binds to activated hormone receptors, inactivating them and marking them for endocytosis.

Arsenate A poison that competes with phosphate in many phosphate-dependent reactions.

Arsenite An inhibitor of pyruvate dehydrogenase that binds to dihydrolipoic acid.

Ascorbic acid Vitamin C, a water-soluble antioxidant.

Asialoglycoprotein Glycoprotein that has lost the terminal sialic acid residues from its oligosaccharides; undergoes endocytosis by the liver.

Ataxia-telangiectasia A syndrome that is caused by impaired repair of DNA double-strand breaks.

Atheromatous plaque The defining lesion of atherosclerosis.

Atrial natriuretic factor A hormone from the heart that stimulates a membrane-bound guanylate cyclase.

Autophagy A process leading to the lysosomal destruction of defective organelles and intracellular bacteria.

Autosome Non–sex chromosome.

Avidin A biotin-binding protein in egg white.

B lymphocyte A type of lymphocyte that produces membrane-bound immunoglobulin.

Bacteriophage "Phage"; bacteria-infecting virus.

Basal metabolic rate The energy consumed in the absence of physical activity.

Basal mutation rate Mutation rate in the absence of mutagens.

Base A proton acceptor.

Base excision repair Removal of an abnormal base by a DNA glycosylase.

Base pairing The specific interaction between two bases in opposite strands of a double-stranded nucleic acid.

Base stacking The noncovalent interaction between successive bases within a nucleic acid strand.

Basement membrane An extracellular matrix structure beneath single-layered epithelia.

Bence Jones protein Immunoglobulin light chains overproduced by some patients with multiple myeloma (a malignant plasma cell dyscrasia).

Beriberi   Thiamin deficiency, with severe neuromuscular weakness.

Bile acids   Emulsifiers in bile; required for lipid absorption.

Bilirubin   A yellow pigment formed from biliverdin.

Biliverdin   A green pigment formed from heme.

Biotin   The prosthetic group of carboxylase enzymes.

2,3-Bisphosphoglycerate (BPG)   An allosteric effector that reduces the oxygen affinity of hemoglobin.

Blood group substances   Polymorphic constituents of the erythrocyte membrane.

Blood urea nitrogen   A measure for the accumulation of urea in uremia.

Body mass index   Weight/height^2.

Bohr effect   Decreased oxygen-binding affinity of hemoglobin at low pH.

Bortezomib   A proteasome inhibitor that is effective against some cancers.

BRCA1, BRCA2   Two tumor suppressor genes associated with inherited susceptibility to breast and ovarian cancers.

Bromouracil   An analog of thymine that causes mutations after being incorporated in DNA.

Brush border enzymes   Enzymes on the luminal surface of intestinal mucosal cells.

Buffer   A solution whose pH value is stabilized by the presence of ionizable groups.

Burkitt lymphoma   A B-cell malignancy in which the *myc* proto-oncogene has been translocated to an immunoglobulin locus.

C-peptide   A biologically inactive fragment of proinsulin that is released together with insulin.

C-reactive protein   The most sensitive acute-phase reactant.

Cadherins   Membrane-spanning cell adhesion proteins in the zonula adherens.

Calcitriol   1,25-Dihydroxycholecalciferol, the active form of vitamin D.

Calcium channel blockers   Drugs that block voltage-gated calcium channels in excitable cells.

Calmodulin   A calcium-dependent enzyme activator.

cAMP response element-binding protein (CREB)   Protein that mediates effects of cyclic AMP on gene transcription.

Cap   A methylguanosine-containing structure at the 5' end of eukaryotic messenger RNA.

Capsid   The protein coat of the virus particle.

Carbamino hemoglobin   Hemoglobin with carbon dioxide covalently bound to its terminal amino groups.

Carbamoyl phosphate   An intermediate in the synthesis of urea and pyrimidines.

Carbohydrate loading   A procedure aimed at the buildup of large muscle glycogen stores in endurance athletes.

α-Carbon   The carbon next to the carboxyl carbon.

Carbon monoxide   A competitive inhibitor of oxygen binding to hemoglobin and myoglobin.

Carbonic anhydrase   An enzyme that establishes equilibrium among carbon dioxide, water, and carbonic acid.

γ-Carboxyglutamate   A posttranslationally formed amino acid in prothrombin and factors VII, IX, and X.

Carboxypeptidases A and B   Two pancreatic carboxypeptidases.

Carcinoma   Cancer of epithelial tissues.

Cardiolipin   A phosphoglyceride in the inner mitochondrial membrane.

Cardiotonic steroids   A class of drugs that inhibit the sodium-potassium ATPase.

Carnitine   A coenzyme that carries long-chain fatty acids into the mitochondrion.

Carnosine   The dipeptide β-alanyl-histidine; used as a pH buffer in muscle tissue.

Carotenes   Dietary precursors of vitamin A in vegetables.

Caspases   Proteases whose activation triggers apoptosis.

Catabolic pathway   Degradative pathway.

Catabolite repression   Repression of catabolic operons in the presence of glucose.

Catalase   A hydrogen peroxide-degrading enzyme.

Catalytic rate constant   The rate constant k_{cat} that describes the rate of product formation from the enzyme substrate complex.

Catecholamines   Tyrosine-derived; biogenic amines dopamine, norepinephrine, epinephrine.

Catechol-O-methyltransferase (COMT)   A catecholamine-inactivating enzyme.

Cation   Positively charged ion.

cDNA library   A collection of complementary DNA (cDNA)-containing bacterial clones.

Centromere   The region of the chromosome that interacts with microtubules during mitosis.

Ceramide   A lipid consisting of sphingosine and a fatty acid.

Cerebrosides   Sphingolipids containing a monosaccharide.

Ceruloplasmin   A copper-containing plasma protein.

Chaperone   A protein that assists in the folding of other proteins.

Chelators   Small molecules that bind a metal with high affinity.

Chirality   Optical isomerism, created by alternative configurations of substituents around an asymmetrical carbon.

Cholecalciferol   The form of vitamin D that is made photochemically in the skin.

Cholera toxin   The enterotoxin of *Vibrio cholerae*. Causes cAMP accumulation in the intestinal mucosa by covalent modification of the G_s protein.

Cholestasis Lack of bile flow.

Cholesterol The only important membrane steroid in humans.

Cholesterol ester transfer protein A protein that transfers cholesterol esters from high-density lipoprotein (HDL) to other lipoproteins.

Cholesterol esters Esters of cholesterol with a fatty acid.

Cholestyramine A bile acid-binding resin that is used as a cholesterol-lowering agent.

Choline-acetyltransferase The acetylcholine-synthesizing enzyme in nerve terminals.

Cholinesterase A serum enzyme that participates in the metabolism of some drugs.

Choluric jaundice Jaundice accompanied by the urinary excretion of bilirubin diglucuronide.

Chondrodysplasias A group of skeletal deformity syndromes, often caused by abnormal cartilage collagens.

Chondroitin sulfate The most abundant glycosaminoglycan (GAG) in many connective tissues.

Chromatin DNA complexed with histones.

Chylomicrons Lipoproteins that carry dietary lipids from the intestine to other tissues.

Chymotrypsin A serine protease from the pancreas.

Ciprofloxacin An antibiotic that inhibits bacterial topoisomerases.

Cirrhosis Fibrous degeneration of the liver.

Class switching A change in the class of the immunoglobulin expressed by a B lymphocyte.

Clathrin The protein that forms the coat of coated vesicles.

Clonal selection Selective growth stimulation by an antigen of a B-cell clone carrying a matching surface antibody.

Clone A population of genetically identical cells that are descended from the same ancestral cell.

Cloning vector A plasmid, bacteriophage or artificial chromosome containing foreign DNA.

Cobalamin Vitamin B_{12}.

Cockayne syndrome Neurological degeneration and early senility caused by inherited defects of transcription-coupled nucleotide excision repair.

Coding strand (sense strand) The strand of a gene whose base sequence corresponds to the base sequence of the RNA transcript.

Codon A base triplet on messenger RNA that specifies an amino acid.

Coenzyme A (CoA) A cosubstrate that forms energy-rich thioester bonds with many organic acids.

Coiled coil Two or three α-helices coiled around each other.

Colchicine An alkaloid that inhibits the formation of microtubules.

Collagen A family of fibrous proteins in the extracellular matrix, with a characteristic triple-helical structure.

Colloid-osmotic pressure The osmotic pressure of macromolecules.

Committed step The first irreversible reaction unique to a metabolic pathway.

Comparative genomic hybridization A method for the detection of copy number variations (deletions, duplications) in DNA.

Competitive inhibition Inhibition by an agent that binds noncovalently to the active site of the enzyme.

Complementary DNA (cDNA) The double-stranded DNA copy of a single-stranded RNA.

Compound heterozygote Person who carries two different mutations in different copies of the same gene.

Condensation reaction Bond formation with release of a water molecule.

Conformation The noncovalent higher-order structure of a protein.

Congenital Present at birth. The opposite of *congenital* is *acquired*.

Conjugation Transfer of a self-transmissible plasmid from one cell to another.

Conjugation reactions Reactions in which a hydrophilic molecule becomes covalently linked to a chemical.

Connexin A channel-forming transmembrane protein in gap junctions.

Consensus sequence The sequence of the most commonly encountered bases in a functionally defined nucleic acid sequence.

Constitutive proteins Proteins that are synthesized at all times.

Contact inhibition Inhibition of cell proliferation by contact with neighboring cells.

Contact-phase activation The very first reactions in the intrinsic pathway of blood clotting.

Cooperativity Interactions between multiple binding sites for the same ligand in an allosteric protein.

Copper A trace mineral; present in many enzymes that use molecular oxygen as a substrate.

Cori cycle The shuttling of glucose and lactate between muscle and liver during physical exercise.

Corticosteroids Glucocorticoids and mineralocorticoids; C-21 steroids that are derived from progestins by hydroxylation reactions.

Cortisol The most important glucocorticoid; a stress hormone.

Coumarin-type anticoagulants Vitamin K antagonists; inhibit the posttranslational formation of γ-carboxyglutamate in some clotting factors.

Covalent bond Strong chemical bond formed by a binding electron pair.

Covalent catalysis A catalytic mechanism that involves the formation of a covalent bond between enzyme and substrate.

Cre recombinase An integrase from a bacteriophage, used for highly selective splicing reactions in recombinant DNA technology.

Creatine A metabolite in muscle that forms the energy-rich compound creatine phosphate.

Creatine kinase An enzyme whose level is elevated in the serum of patients with muscle diseases and acute myocardial infarction.

Cretinism The result of untreated congenital hypothyroidism; characterized by mental deficiency and growth retardation.

Creutzfeldt-Jacob disease A sporadic or inherited prion disease.

Crigler-Najjar syndrome Inherited defect of bilirubin conjugation.

Crohn disease A type of inflammatory bowel disease.

Crossing-over The exchange of DNA between homologous chromosomes during meiosis and (rarely) mitosis.

Cryoprecipitate A plasma protein preparation enriched in some clotting factors.

Curare An arrow poison that blocks acetylcholine receptors in the neuromuscular junction.

Cyanide A poison that prevents the reduction of molecular oxygen by cytochrome oxidase.

Cyanosis In hypoxia, blue discoloration of mucous membranes that is caused by deoxyhemoglobin.

Cyclic adenosine monophosphate (cAMP) A second messenger of many hormones.

Cyclic guanosine monophosphate (cGMP) Another second messenger in many cells.

Cyclin-dependent kinases (CDKs) Positive regulators of cell cycle progression.

Cyclins Activators of cyclin-dependent protein kinases.

Cyclooxygenase The key enzyme for the synthesis of prostaglandins, prostacyclin, and thromboxane.

Cystic fibrosis A genetic disease cause by malfunction of a chloride channel in secretory epithelia.

Cystinuria An inherited defect in the transport of dibasic amino acids in kidney and intestine; causes kidney stones.

Cytochrome oxidase Complex IV in the respiratory chain, transfers electrons to O_2.

Cytochrome P-450 A large family of heme-containing proteins that participate in monooxygenase reactions.

Cytochromes Heme proteins that function as electron carriers.

Cytokines Biologically active proteins released by activated lymphocytes and monocytes/macrophages.

Death receptors Receptors for extracellular ligands; their activation triggers apoptosis.

7-Dehydrocholesterol A steroid that is photochemically cleaved to cholecalciferol (vitamin D_3) in the skin.

Dehydrogenase reactions Hydrogen transfer reactions.

Dementia Loss of mental capacities.

Denaturation Destruction of a protein's or nucleic acid's higher-order structure.

Desaturases Enzymes that introduce double bonds into fatty acids.

Desmolase The rate-limiting enzyme for the synthesis of steroid hormones.

Desmosine A covalent cross-link in elastin.

Desmosomes Spot welds that hold neighboring cells together.

1,2-Diacylglycerol A second messenger formed by phospholipase C.

Dialysis Removal of small molecules and inorganic ions through a semipermeable membrane.

Diastereomers Geometric isomers.

Dideoxyribonucleotides Nucleotide analogs that are used for chain termination in DNA sequencing.

Dihydrofolate reductase An enzyme that reduces dihydrofolate to tetrahydrofolate.

Dihydrotestosterone A potent androgen formed from testosterone by 5α-reductase in androgen target tissues.

Dioxygenases Enzymes that incorporate both oxygen atoms of O_2 in their substrate.

Dipalmitoyl phosphatidylcholine The main constituent of lung surfactant.

Diphtheria toxin A bacterial toxin that inactivates an elongation factor of eukaryotic protein synthesis.

Dipole A structure with asymmetrical distribution of electric charges.

Dipole-dipole interaction Attraction force between the components of two polarized bonds.

Dissociation constant (K_D) A measure for the affinity between a protein and its ligand.

Disulfide bond A covalent bond formed by an oxidative reaction between two sulfhydryl groups.

Disulfiram Antabuse; an aldehyde dehydrogenase inhibitor used for treatment of alcoholism.

DNA fingerprinting DNA-based methods for the identification of persons in criminal cases.

DNA glycosylases Enzymes that remove abnormal bases from DNA.

DNA ligase An enzyme linking two DNA strands.

DNA methylation A covalent modification of DNA that suppresses transcription.

DNA microarray "DNA chip" used for studies of gene expression or genetic variation.

DNA polymerases DNA-synthesizing enzymes.

Dolichol phosphate A lipid that participates in the synthesis of N-linked oligosaccharides in glycoproteins.

Dominant Determining the phenotype in the heterozygous (as well as the homozygous) state.

Dopamine neurons Neurons that use dopamine as a neurotransmitter.

Dot blotting A rapid screening method for mutations and DNA polymorphisms.

Doxorubicin An anticancer drug that inhibits human topoisomerases.

Duchenne muscular dystrophy A severe inherited muscle disease caused by defects of the structural protein dystrophin.

Dynein The ATPase that moves cilia and flagella.

E2F A transcription factor that is negatively regulated by the retinoblastoma protein.

E6, E7 The oncogenes of the human papillomavirus; they bind and inactivate p53 and pRB, respectively.

Edema Abnormal fluid accumulation in the interstitial tissue spaces.

Ehlers-Danlos syndrome A group of genetic diseases characterized by stretchy skin and loose joints.

Elastase An endopeptidase from pancreas and other sources.

Elastin The major component of elastic fibers.

Electrogenic transport Net transport of electrical charges across a membrane.

Electronegativity The tendency of an atom to attract electrons.

Electrophoresis Separation of molecules in an electrical field.

Electrostatic interaction "Salt bond"; the attraction force between oppositely charged ions.

Emphysema A lung disease, characterized by degeneration of the alveolar walls.

Enantiomers Isomers that are mirror images.

Endergonic reaction Reaction with positive ΔG.

Endocytosis Cellular uptake of soluble macromolecules or particles through an endocytic vesicle.

Endorphins Peptides that activate opiate receptors.

Endosome An organelle derived from endocytic vesicles.

Endosymbiont hypothesis The hypothesis that mitochondria (and chloroplasts) are derived from symbiotic prokaryotes.

Energy charge A measure for the energy status of a cell.

Energy-rich bonds Bonds whose hydrolysis releases an unusually large amount of energy.

Enhancers DNA sequences that increase the rate of transcription by binding regulatory proteins.

Enterohepatic circulation The cycling of bile acids (and other compounds) through liver and intestine.

Enteropeptidase An enzyme that activates trypsinogen in the duodenum.

Enthalpy The energy content of a molecule.

Entropy The randomness of a thermodynamic system.

Envelope A membrane, acquired from the host cell, that surrounds many animal viruses.

Enzyme-substrate complex Enzyme with a noncovalently bound substrate.

Epidermal growth factor (EGF) A growth factor that is mitogenic for epithelial cells.

Epidermolysis bullosa Inherited skin-blistering diseases caused by abnormalities of proteins in the dermal-epidermal junction.

Epimers Monosaccharides differing in the configuration of substituents around one of their asymmetrical carbons.

Epinephrine Synonym for adrenaline, a stress hormone from the adrenal medulla.

Equilibrium constant A thermodynamic constant that is defined as product concentration(s) divided by substrate concentration(s) at equilibrium.

Erythropoietin A kidney-derived growth factor that stimulates erythropoiesis in the bone marrow.

Escherichia coli **(E. coli)** An intestinal bacterium.

Estrogens 18-Carbon steroids, synthesized from androgens by the aromatization of ring A.

Euchromatin A dispersed, transcriptionally active form of chromatin.

Eukaryotes Cells with a membrane-bounded nucleus.

Exergonic reaction Reaction with negative ΔG.

Exocytosis Secretion of water-soluble substances by fusion of an exocytic vesicle with the plasma membrane.

Exons The parts of the gene that are represented in the mature RNA.

Expression vector A cloning vector from which the cloned cDNA can be transcribed.

Extracellular Outside the cells.

Extracellular signal-regulated kinases (ERKs) Serine/threonine kinases of the mitogen-activated protein (MAP) kinase family.

F factor A self-transmissible plasmid in *Escherichia coli*.

Fab The antigen-binding fragment of immunoglobulins.

Facilitated diffusion A passive type of carrier-mediated transport.

Familial combined hyperlipoproteinemia A genetic predisposition to type II and type IV hyperlipoproteinemia.

Familial hypercholesterolemia Inherited deficiency of low-density lipoprotein (LDL) receptors.

Fatty liver A reversible lesion caused by increased hepatic triglyceride synthesis or impaired very-low-density lipoprotein (VLDL) formation.

Fatty streak Accumulation of cholesterol esters in arterial walls.

Fc The crystallizable fragment of immunoglobulins, formed from the carboxyl-terminal halves of the heavy chains.

Feedback inhibition   Inhibition of a metabolic pathway by its end product.

Feedforward stimulation   Stimulation of a metabolic pathway by its substrate.

Ferritin   The principal intracellular iron storage protein; trace amounts are present in the plasma.

α-Fetoprotein   A fetal plasma protein, levels of which are elevated in serum of patients with liver cancer and in amniotic fluid if the fetus has an open neural tube defect.

Fibrate drugs   Lipid-lowering drugs that activate peroxisome proliferator-activated receptor-α (PPAR-α).

Fibrillin   Protein in microfibrils that is defective in Marfan syndrome.

Fibrinogen   The circulating precursor of fibrin.

Fibronectin   A glycoprotein that binds to cell surfaces and extracellular matrix constituents.

First-order reaction   Reaction whose velocity is proportional to the concentration of a substrate.

Flavin adenine dinucleotide (FAD)   A hydrogen-transferring prosthetic group of flavoproteins.

Flavoproteins   Proteins containing a flavin coenzyme (either flavin mononucleotide [FMN] or flavin adenine dinucleotide [FAD]) as a prosthetic group; participate in hydrogen transfer reactions.

Fluid-mosaic model   A model of membrane structure that assumes globular proteins embedded in a lipid bilayer.

Fluorescent in situ hybridization (FISH)   Method for the detection of DNA sequences in a chromosome spread.

Fluorouracil   A base analog used in cancer chemotherapy.

Foam cell   A macrophage filled with droplets of cholesterol esters.

Follicular hyperkeratosis   Gooseflesh; occurs in deficiency of vitamin C and vitamin A.

Frameshift mutation   Insertion or deletion that changes the reading frame of the messenger RNA.

Free energy   The "useful" energy in chemical reactions.

Fructokinase   The major fructose-metabolizing enzyme.

Fructose-1,6-bisphosphatase   An important regulated enzyme of gluconeogenesis.

Fructose-2,6-bisphosphate   A regulatory metabolite that mediates hormonal effects on phosphofructokinase and fructose-1, 6-bisphosphatase.

Fructose intolerance   Hereditary disorders caused by deficiency of a fructose-metabolizing enzyme.

Furanose ring   Five-member ring in monosaccharides.

Futile cycle   Simultaneous activity of two opposing metabolic reactions, leading to ATP hydrolysis.

G proteins   GTP-binding signal transducing proteins that mediate most hormone effects.

G_0 phase   The nondividing state of a cell.

G_1 phase   The time between mitosis and S phase.

G_2 phase   The time between S phase and mitosis.

Galactokinase   The enzyme that phosphorylates galactose to galactose-1-phosphate.

Galactosemia   A hereditary disease caused by the deficiency of a galactose-metabolizing enzyme.

β-Galactosidase   A lactose-hydrolyzing enzyme.

Gallstones   Calculi formed from cholesterol or other poorly soluble substances in the biliary system.

Gangliosides   Sphingolipids containing an acidic oligosaccharide.

Gap junction   A small aqueous channel connecting the cytoplasm of neighboring cells.

Gas gangrene   A severe type of wound infection caused by collagenase-producing anaerobic bacteria.

Gaucher disease   A lipid storage disease in which glucocerebroside accumulates.

Gelatin   Denatured collagen.

Gene   A length of DNA directing the synthesis of a polypeptide or a functional RNA.

Gene families   Structurally related genes with a common evolutionary origin.

Gene therapy   The introduction of a functional gene into the patient's cells.

Genome-wide association study   A study that relates a large number of DNA variants to a disease or other phenotype.

Genomic library   A collection of bacterial clones containing fragments of genomic DNA.

Germline mutation   Mutation arising in the cell lineage that gives rise to gametes.

Gilbert syndrome   Benign hyperbilirubinemia caused by a promoter mutation in the gene for bilirubin-UDP-glucuronyl transferase.

Glitazone drugs   Pharmacological activators of peroxisome proliferator-activated receptor-γ (PPAR-γ) that sensitize cells to insulin.

Glucagon   A pancreatic hormone that stimulates the glucose-producing pathways of the liver.

Glucogenic   Glucose forming.

Glucokinase   The liver isoenzyme of hexokinase.

Gluconeogenesis   Synthesis of glucose from noncarbohydrates.

Glucose oxidase test   An enzymatic method for the selective determination of glucose in the clinical laboratory.

Glucose-6-phosphatase   The glucose-producing enzyme in gluconeogenic tissues and glucose-transporting epithelia.

Glucose-6-phosphate dehydrogenase   The first enzyme in the oxidative branch of the pentose phosphate pathway.

Glucose-6-phosphate dehydrogenase deficiency A common enzyme deficiency that leads to hemolysis after exposure to certain drugs.

Glucose tolerance test A laboratory test that determines the effect of glucose ingestion on the blood glucose level.

Glucose transporter 4 (GLUT-4) An insulin-dependent glucose carrier in muscle and adipose tissue.

Glutamate dehydrogenase An enzyme that catalyzes the oxidative deamination of glutamate and the reductive amination of α-ketoglutarate.

Glutaminase A hydrolytic enzyme that releases ammonia from glutamine.

Glutathione A tripeptide with reducing properties.

Glutathione reductase An NADPH-dependent enzyme that keeps glutathione in the reduced state.

Glycemic index A measure for the extent to which a food raises the blood glucose level.

Glycerol phosphate shuttle The transfer of electrons from cytoplasmic NADH to the respiratory chain.

Glycogen phosphorylase The enzyme that cleaves glycogen to glucose-1-phosphate.

Glycogen synthase The enzyme that synthesizes glycogen from UDP-glucose.

Glycolipid Carbohydrate-containing lipid.

Glycoprotein A protein containing covalently bound carbohydrate.

Glycosaminoglycans (GAGs) Polysaccharides containing an amino sugar in every other position.

Glycosidases Enzymes that cleave glycosidic bonds.

Glycosidic bond Bond formed by the anomeric carbon of a monosaccharide.

Glycosyl transferases Biosynthetic enzymes that use activated monosaccharides.

Goiter Enlargement of the thyroid gland; seen in some forms of hypothyroidism and hyperthyroidism.

Gouty arthritis Arthritis caused by sodium urate deposits in the joints.

Graves disease An autoimmune disease leading to hyperthyroidism.

Growth factors Soluble extracellular proteins that stimulate the proliferation or differentiation of cultured cells.

Guanylate cyclases Cyclic GMP-synthesizing enzymes.

Half-life The time that it takes for half of the substrate molecules to react in a first-order reaction.

Haptoglobin A hemoglobin-binding protein in serum.

Hartnup disease An inherited defect in the renal and intestinal transport of large neutral amino acids, with pellagra-like symptoms.

Hashimoto disease Autoimmune thyroiditis, the most common cause of hypothyroidism.

Heat shock proteins Chaperones that are induced by heat exposure.

Heinz bodies Abnormal protein aggregates in erythrocytes.

Helicases Enzymes separating the strands of double-stranded DNA.

α-Helix A compact secondary structure in proteins that is stabilized by intrachain hydrogen bonds between peptide bonds.

Hematin An oxidized derivative of heme containing a ferric iron.

Hematocrit The percentage of the blood volume that is occupied by blood cells.

Hemochromatosis An iron overload syndrome.

Hemodialysis The major procedure for treatment of renal failure.

Hemoglobin A_{1c} Hemoglobin A modified by a reaction between terminal amino groups and glucose.

Hemoglobin Bart A γ_4 tetramer, in patients with α-thalassemia.

Hemoglobin H A β_4 tetramer, in patients with α-thalassemia.

Hemoglobin S Sickle cell hemoglobin.

Hemoglobinopathies Genetic diseases caused by abnormalities of hemoglobin structure or synthesis.

Hemolysis Destruction of erythrocytes.

Hemopexin A heme-binding protein in serum.

Hemophilia A group of inherited clotting disorders; the most common is factor VIII deficiency.

Hemorrhagic disease of the newborn A neonatal bleeding disorder caused by vitamin K deficiency.

Hemosiderin A partially denatured form of ferritin.

Hemosiderosis Abnormal accumulation of hemosiderin.

Henderson-Hasselbalch equation The equation that relates protonation states to pK and pH.

Heparan sulfate A glycosaminoglycan (GAG) in many cell surface and connective tissue proteoglycans.

Heparin A sulfated glycosaminoglycan (GAG) made by mast cells and basophils.

Hepatic encephalopathy Brain dysfunction caused by hyperammonemia and other aberrations in patients with liver cirrhosis.

Hepatic lipase An extracellular enzyme in the liver that hydrolyzes triglycerides and phospholipids in remnant particles and high-density lipoprotein (HDL).

Hereditary fructose intolerance Inherited defect in hepatic fructose metabolism.

Hereditary nonpolyposis colon cancer (HNPCC) An inherited cancer susceptibility syndrome caused by defects of postreplication mismatch repair.

Hereditary persistence of fetal hemoglobin γ-Chain production in an adult.

Heterochromatin A condensed, transcriptionally inactive form of chromatin.

Heteroplasmy Presence of both normal and pathogenic mitochondrial DNA.

Heterozygote advantage   Improved survival and/or reproduction of heterozygous mutation carriers.

Heterozygous   Carrying two different variants of a gene.

Hexokinase   The enzyme that phosphorylates glucose to glucose-6-phosphate.

Hexose   Six-carbon sugar.

High-density lipoprotein   A protein-rich lipoprotein that transports cholesterol to the liver.

Histidinemia   A relatively benign inborn error of histidine metabolism.

Histones   Small, basic proteins that are tightly associated with DNA in chromatin.

Homocysteine   An amino acid derived from methionine; possible risk factor for atherosclerosis.

Homocystinuria   An inborn error in the metabolism of the sulfur amino acids, causing skeletal deformities and mental deficiency.

Homologous recombination   Reciprocal exchange of DNA between two DNA molecules of related sequence.

Homozygous   Carrying two identical variants of a gene.

Hormone-sensitive lipase   An enzyme in adipose cells that hydrolyzes stored triglycerides.

Human artificial chromosomes   Vectors for germline genetic engineering.

Huntington disease   An inherited neurodegenerative disease caused by expansion of a trinucleotide repeat.

Hutchinson-Gilford progeria   Premature aging caused by inherited defects in nuclear lamins.

Hyaluronic acid   A large, unsulfated glycosaminoglycan (GAG), not bound to a core protein.

Hybridization   Annealing of nucleic acids from different sources.

Hydrogen bond   Dipole-dipole interaction involving a hydrogen atom.

Hydrogen peroxide   A toxic product of some oxidative reactions.

Hydrolase   Enzyme catalyzing hydrolytic cleavage reactions.

Hydrolysis   Cleavage of a bond by the addition of water.

Hydrophobic interactions   Interactions between hydrophobic groups, resulting from reduction of the aqueous-nonpolar interface.

3-Hydroxy-3-methylglutaryl-coenzyme A (HMG-CoA) reductase   The regulated enzyme of cholesterol synthesis.

Hydroxyapatite   The major inorganic component of bone.

Hydroxyl radical   An extremely reactive and highly toxic byproduct of oxidative metabolism.

Hydroxylase   Enzyme that introduces a hydroxyl group in its substrate.

7α-Hydroxylase   The regulated enzyme of bile acid synthesis.

Hyperammonemia   Too much ammonia in the blood.

Hyperbaric oxygen   Oxygen applied under increased pressure.

Hyperbilirubinemia   Too much bilirubin in the blood.

Hyperlipidemia   Too much lipid in the blood.

Hyperuricemia   Too much uric acid in the blood.

Hypervariable regions   The most variable parts of the variable domains in the immunoglobulins; sites of contact with the antigen.

Hypochromia   Reduced hemoglobin content of erythrocytes.

Hypoglycemia   Too little blood glucose, resulting in brain dysfunction.

Hypoxanthine   A deamination product of adenine.

Hypoxanthine-guanine phosphoribosyltransferase (HGPRT)   The most important salvage enzyme for purine bases.

Hypoxia   Oxygen deficiency.

I-cell disease   A lysosomal storage disease caused by misrouting of lysosomal enzymes.

Imprinting   Silencing of specific genes in the germline, usually by DNA methylation.

Indels   Insertions and deletions.

Induced-fit model   A model that assumes a flexible substrate-binding site in the enzyme.

Inducible proteins   Proteins whose synthesis is regulated.

Inosine   A nucleoside containing hypoxanthine and ribose.

Inositol 1,4,5-trisphosphate (IP$_3$)   A second messenger formed by phospholipase C; releases calcium from the endoplasmic reticulum.

Insertion sequence   A mobile element in prokaryotes that contains a gene for transposase.

Insulinoma   An insulin-secreting tumor of pancreatic β-cells.

Integral membrane proteins   Proteins that are embedded in the lipid bilayer.

Integrases   Enzymes that catalyze site-specific recombination.

Integrins   Integral membrane proteins that function as receptors for components of the extracellular matrix.

Intermediate filament   A type of cytoskeletal fiber formed from proteins in a coiled coil conformation.

International unit (IU)   The enzyme activity that converts 1 μmol of substrate to product per minute.

Interspersed elements   Repetitive, mobile DNA sequences in eukaryotic genomes.

Intracellular   Inside the cells.

Intrinsic factor   A glycoprotein from parietal cells in the stomach, required for efficient vitamin B$_{12}$ absorption.

Introns   The parts of a gene that do not appear in the mature, functional RNA product.

Ion channel A pore in the membrane that is selectively permeable for specific ions.

Ion-dipole interaction Attraction force between an ion and a component of a polarized bond.

Ionizing radiation Energy-rich radiation that forms free radicals in the body.

Iron-sulfur proteins Nonheme iron proteins that participate in electron transfer reactions.

Irreversible inhibition Inhibition by the formation of a covalent bond with the enzyme.

Irreversible reaction A reaction that proceeds in only one direction under physiological conditions.

Ischemia Interruption of the blood supply.

Isoelectric point The pH value at which the number of positive charges on the molecule equals the number of negative charges.

Isoenzymes Enzymes catalyzing the same reaction but composed of different polypeptides.

Isomerase Enzyme that interconverts isomers.

Isomers Alternative molecular forms with identical composition.

Isoniazid A tuberculostatic that can induce vitamin B_6 deficiency.

Isoprenoids Lipids synthesized from branched-chain five-carbon units.

J chain A polypeptide in polymeric immunoglobulins.

J gene A small gene that participates in the assembly of an immunoglobulin gene in developing B lymphocytes.

Janus kinase (JAK) A type of tyrosine kinase that associates with activated receptors for cytokines, growth hormone, prolactin, and erythropoietin.

Jaundice Yellow discoloration of skin and sclera in patients with hyperbilirubinemia.

Junk DNA Noncoding DNA of unknown function.

Kartagener syndrome A recessively inherited condition with immotile cilia, male infertility, and situs inversus.

Keratin A type of intermediate filament protein in epithelial cells.

Kernicterus Brain damage caused by deposition of bilirubin in the basal ganglia.

Ketoacidosis A metabolic emergency in insulin-dependent diabetics, with hyperglycemia, acidosis, dehydration, and electrolyte imbalances.

Ketogenesis Synthesis of ketone bodies.

Ketogenic Ketone body forming.

Ketone bodies Acetoacetate, β-hydroxybutyrate, and acetone.

Ketose Monosaccharide with a keto group.

Kinase An enzyme that transfers a phosphate group from a nucleotide.

Kinetics The description of reaction rates.

Kinetochore A proteinaceous structure on the centromere to which spindle fibers attach.

Knockout mouse A mouse in which a gene has been disrupted by genetic manipulations.

Kuru A now extinct prion disease transmitted by cannibalism.

β-Lactamase Penicillinase; an enzyme that inactivates penicillin and related antibiotics.

Lactate dehydrogenase The enzyme that interconverts pyruvate and lactate.

Lactic acidosis Decrease of the blood pH resulting from lactic acid accumulation.

Lactose intolerance Digestive disturbances after the ingestion of milk or milk products, caused by low activity of intestinal lactase.

Lactose operon An operon in *Escherichia coli* that codes for enzymes of lactose metabolism.

Lagging strand The strand that is synthesized piecemeal during DNA replication.

Lamin A type of intermediate filament protein in the nucleus.

Laminin A glycoprotein in basement membranes.

LDL receptor A lipoprotein receptor that mediates the endocytosis of low-density lipoprotein (LDL).

Leading strand The strand that is synthesized continuously during DNA replication.

Leber hereditary optic neuropathy Adult-onset blindness caused by mutations in mitochondrial DNA.

Lecithin Synonym for phosphatidylcholine, a phosphoglyceride.

Lecithin-cholesterol acyltransferase (LCAT) An enzyme in high-density lipoprotein (HDL) that converts free cholesterol into cholesterol esters.

Leprechaunism A serious disorder caused by congenital absence of functional insulin receptors.

Leptin A polypeptide hormone from overfed adipose cells that reduces appetite.

Lesch-Nyhan syndrome A neurological disorder caused by complete deficiency of hypoxanthine-guanine phosphoribosyltransferase (HGPRT).

Leucine zipper A structural feature of some DNA-binding proteins, required for dimerization.

Leukotrienes Biologically active products formed in asthma and other allergic diseases.

Lewy bodies Intracellular inclusions of insoluble proteins in neurons, found in some neurodegenerative diseases.

Li-Fraumeni syndrome A cancer susceptibility syndrome caused by germline mutations of the *p53* gene.

Ligand A small molecule that binds noncovalently to a protein.

Ligand-gated ion channels Ion channels that are regulated by the binding of a neurotransmitter.

Ligase A type of enzyme that forms a bond while hydrolyzing a high-energy phosphate.

Lineweaver-Burk plot A double-reciprocal plot that describes the relationship between substrate concentration and reaction rate.

Linoleic acid An ω_6-polyunsaturated fatty acid.

Linolenic acid An ω_3-polyunsaturated fatty acid.

Lipase   Triglyceride-degrading enzyme.

Lipids   Substances with strong hydrophobic properties.

Lipofuscin   "Age pigment," formed from partially oxidized lipids and partially denatured proteins.

Lipoic acid   A prosthetic group of pyruvate dehydrogenase.

Lipolysis   Triglyceride hydrolysis.

Lipoproteins   Noncovalent aggregates of protein and lipid.

α-Lipoprotein   High-density lipoprotein (HDL).

β-Lipoprotein   Low-density lipoprotein (LDL).

Lipoprotein(a)   A form of low-density lipoprotein (LDL) that promotes atherosclerosis.

Lipoprotein lipase   An endothelial enzyme that hydrolyzes triglycerides in chylomicrons and very-low-density lipoprotein (VLDL).

Lipoxygenases   Enzymes that produce leukotrienes and other biologically active products from polyunsaturated fatty acids.

Lock-and-key model   A model that assumes a rigid substrate-binding site in the enzyme.

Locus heterogeneity   A situation where mutations in more than one gene can lead to the same disease.

Long terminal repeats   The terminal repeat sequences of retroviral cDNAs.

Low-density lipoprotein (LDL)   The lipoprotein that delivers cholesterol to the cells.

LoxP site   Recognition site for the DNA-splicing enzyme Cre recombinase.

Lung surfactant   A lipid secretion that reduces the surface tension in the lung alveoli.

Lyase   An enzyme that removes a group nonhydrolytically from its substrate.

Lysogenic bacterium   A bacterium that harbors a prophage.

Lysogenic pathway   A reproductive strategy of some bacteriophages that involves the integration of the viral DNA into the host-cell chromosome.

Lysophosphoglyceride   A phosphoglyceride with one fatty acid missing.

Lysozyme   An enzyme that cleaves the peptidoglycan in bacterial cell walls.

Lysyl oxidase   An enzyme that produces allysyl residues in collagen; required for crosslinking.

Lytic pathway   The reproductive strategy of bacteriophages that destroy their host cell.

α₂-Macroglobulin   A circulating protease inhibitor, with a very high molecular weight (725,000 D).

Malate-aspartate shuttle   The reversible shuttling of hydrogen, in the form of malate, across the inner mitochondrial membrane.

Malondialdehyde   A chemically reactive product formed during lipid peroxidation.

Maple syrup urine disease   An inborn error of branched-chain amino acid metabolism, causing mental and neurological deficits.

Marfan syndrome   Dominantly inherited disorder caused by abnormalities of the connective tissue protein fibrillin.

McArdle disease   Deficiency of glycogen phosphorylase in muscle, causing muscle weakness.

Mdm2   A protein that inactivates the p53 protein.

Mediator   A large nuclear protein complex involved in transcriptional regulation.

Medium-chain acyl-CoA dehydrogenase deficiency   An inherited defect of β-oxidation that causes fasting hypoglycemia.

Megaloblastic anemia   A type of anemia characterized by oversized red blood cells, caused by impaired DNA synthesis.

Melanin   The dark pigment of skin and hair.

Melatonin   A pineal hormone derived from serotonin.

Menkes disease   An inherited defect of copper absorption.

Messenger RNA (mRNA)   Specifies the amino acid sequence during protein synthesis.

Metabolic syndrome   The abnormalities seen in people who eat more than they can metabolize.

Metallothionein   A protein that binds heavy metals.

Metastable   Stable kinetically but not thermodynamically.

Metastatic calcification   Abnormal calcification of soft tissues.

Metformin   An antidiabetic drug that activates the AMP-dependent protein kinase.

Methemoglobin   A nonfunctional hemoglobin in which the heme iron is oxidized to the ferric state.

Methemoglobinemia   Methemoglobin in the blood (suffix *–emia* means "in the blood"; suffix *–uria* means "in the urine").

Methotrexate   An anticancer drug that inhibits dihydrofolate reductase.

Methylation reaction   Transfer of a methyl group from one molecule (often *S*-adenosyl methionine [SAM]) to another.

Methylmalonic aciduria   Excretion of methylmalonic acid in the urine, caused by an inherited enzyme deficiency or by vitamin B_{12} deficiency.

Methylxanthines   Caffeine and related purines, inhibit many phosphodiesterases.

Micelle   Small globule or sheet formed from amphipathic lipids.

Michaelis constant (K_m)   The substrate concentration at which the rate of an enzymatic reaction is half maximal.

Microcytosis   Presence of abnormally small erythrocytes.

Micro-RNA (miRNA)   A type of small RNA that inhibits mRNA translation.

Microfilaments   Cytoskeletal fibers formed by the polymerization of actin.

Microsatellites   Very small tandem repeats.

Microsomes Fragments of the endoplasmic reticulum obtained by cell fractionation.

Microtubules Cytoskeletal fibers formed by the polymerization of tubulin.

Minisatellites Small tandem repeats.

Mismatch repair A repair system that corrects replication errors.

Missense mutation Mutation leading to a single amino acid substitution.

Mitogen Mitosis-inducing agent.

Mitogen-activated protein (MAP) kinases A family of protein kinases that are activated in response to growth factors or stress.

Monoamine oxidase (MAO) An enzyme that inactivates catecholamines and serotonin.

Monoclonal gammopathy Overproduction of a single immunoglobulin by a plasma cell clone.

Monooxygenases Enzymes that incorporate a single oxygen atom from O_2 in their substrate.

Monosaccharide Polyalcohol containing a carbonyl group.

Monounsaturated fatty acid Fatty acid with one carbon-carbon double bond.

Mucopolysaccharidoses Lysosomal storage diseases caused by deficiencies of glycosaminoglycan (GAG)-degrading enzymes.

Muscarinic receptors G protein-linked receptors for acetylcholine.

Mutagen Mutation-inducing agent.

Mutarotation Spontaneous interconversion of anomeric forms in a monosaccharide.

Mutation Heritable change in DNA structure.

Mutation-selection balance The balance between new mutations and purifying selection that determines the prevalence of pathogenic mutations.

Mutational load "Genetic garbage" that accumulates from generation to generation.

MYC An oncogene or proto-oncogene coding for a nuclear transcription factor, amplified in many spontaneous cancers.

Myoglobin An oxygen-binding protein in muscle tissue.

Myosin The protein of the thick filaments in muscle.

Myosin light-chain kinase A calcium-calmodulin activated protein kinase that induces contraction in smooth muscle.

Myxedema Hypothyroidism in adults.

N-Acetylglutamate An activator of mitochondrial carbamoyl phosphate synthetase.

N-Acetylneuraminic acid Sialic acid; an acidic sugar derivative in glycolipids and glycoproteins.

N-Linked oligosaccharides Oligosaccharides bound to asparagine side chains in glycoproteins.

Natural selection The process of differential survival and reproduction that changes allele frequencies from generation to generation.

Neoplasia Abnormal growth of either a benign or a malignant nature.

Nephrotic syndrome A type of kidney disease with massive proteinuria.

Niacin Nicotinic acid; also used as a generic name for nicotinic acid and nicotinamide.

Nicotinamide adenine dinucleotide (NAD), nicotinamide adenine dinucleotide phosphate (NADP) Two cosubstrates that accept or donate electrons (+ proton) in many dehydrogenase reactions.

Nicotinic receptors Acetylcholine-operated cation channels.

Nitric oxide (NO) An unstable, diffusible messenger molecule produced in endothelial cells and some other tissues.

Nitrogen balance The difference between ingested nitrogen and excreted nitrogen.

Nitroglycerin A vasodilator drug that is metabolized to nitric oxide.

Nitrous acid The acid form of the nitrites, causes mutations by deaminating DNA bases.

Noncompetitive inhibition Inhibition by an agent that binds the enzyme noncovalently outside its active site.

Nonketotic hyperglycinemia An inborn error of glycine metabolism causing brain damage and early death.

Nonketotic hyperosmolar coma A metabolic emergency in patients with type 2 diabetes, with hyperglycemia and dehydration but no acidosis.

Nonsense mutation A mutation that creates a stop codon.

Nonsteroidal antiinflammatory drugs (NSAIDs) Drugs that inhibit cyclooxygenase.

Nonviral retroposons DNA sequences produced by the reverse transcription of a cellular RNA.

Northern blotting A method for the identification of RNA after gel electrophoresis, using a probe.

Nucleases Enzymes cleaving phosphodiester bonds in a nucleic acid.

Nucleocapsid The particle formed from viral nucleic acid and protein coat.

Nucleoside A structure formed from a pentose sugar and a base.

Nucleosome The structural unit of chromatin, formed from DNA and histones.

Nucleotide A structure formed from pentose sugar, base, and a variable number of phosphate groups.

Nucleotide excision repair A DNA repair system for bulky lesions.

O-Linked oligosaccharides Oligosaccharides bound to hydroxyl groups in proteins.

Okazaki fragments Pieces of DNA synthesized in the lagging strand during DNA replication.

Oleic acid A C-18 monounsaturated fatty acid.

Oligomycin An inhibitor of the mitochondrial ATP synthase.

Oncogene A growth-promoting gene in cancer cells.

Operator A repressor-binding regulatory DNA sequence in bacterial operons.

Operon The unit of promoter, operator, and structural genes in bacteria.

Opsonization Stimulation of phagocytosis by an antibody or other protein bound to the surface of a particle.

Organophosphates Irreversible inhibitors of acetylcholinesterase, used as pesticides and as nerve gases.

Oriental flush Hypersensitivity to alcohol, caused by deficiency of a mitochondrial aldehyde dehydrogenase in many Asians.

Orotic acid An intermediate of pyrimidine biosynthesis.

Orphan receptors Proteins that resemble known receptors but whose natural ligands are unknown.

Osteogenesis imperfecta Disorder characterized by brittle bones, caused by inherited defects of type I collagen.

Osteomalacia Rickets in adults.

Osteoporosis Brittle, fragile bones in elderly people.

Oxalic acid A component of kidney stones that can be formed from glycine.

α-Oxidation A minor catabolic pathway that shortens fatty acids by one carbon.

β-Oxidation The major pathway of fatty acid oxidation.

ω-Oxidation Oxidation of the last carbon in a medium-chain fatty acid.

Oxidoreductase Enzyme catalyzing oxidation-reduction reactions.

Oxygenation Reversible binding of oxygen.

Palindrome A type of symmetrical DNA sequence.

Palmitic acid A saturated C-16 fatty acid.

Pancreatic lipase The major enzyme of fat digestion.

Pantothenic acid A nutritionally essential constituent of coenzyme A.

Papillomavirus A DNA virus associated with cervical cancer.

Para-aminobenzoic acid (PABA) A constituent of folic acid.

Paracrine signaling The action of an extracellular messenger on neighboring cells within its tissue of origin.

Parkinson disease Age-related degeneration of dopamine neurons, causing a motor disorder.

Passive diffusion Nonsaturable diffusion across a membrane.

Pellagra Niacin deficiency; symptoms include dermatitis, diarrhea, and dementia.

Penicillamine A metal chelator used to treat Wilson disease and rheumatoid arthritis.

Pentachlorophenol A wood preservative that uncouples oxidative phosphorylation.

Pentose Five-carbon sugar.

Pepsin An endopeptidase in gastric juice.

Peptidases Enzymes that cleave peptide bonds in polypeptides.

Peptide bond Amide bond between two amino acids.

Peptidoglycan The major bacterial cell wall polysaccharide.

Peptidyl transferase The enzymatic activity of the large ribosomal subunit that forms the peptide bond.

Peripheral membrane proteins Proteins that are attached to the surface of the membrane.

Pernicious anemia Megaloblastic anemia and neuropathy caused by vitamin B_{12} malabsorption.

Peroxidases Enzymes that consume hydrogen peroxide or organic peroxides.

Peroxidation The nonenzymatic, free radical–mediated oxidation of polyunsaturated fatty acids.

Peroxisome proliferator-activated receptors (PPARs) Nuclear receptors that regulate lipid and carbohydrate metabolism.

Peroxisomes Catalase-rich organelles that contain oxidative enzymes.

Pertussis toxin A toxin produced by *Bordetella pertussis*; causes cyclic AMP accumulation by inactivation of the G_i protein.

pH Value The negative logarithm of the hydrogen ion concentration.

λ Phage A temperate bacteriophage of *Escherichia coli*.

Phagocytosis "Cell eating"; the cellular uptake of a solid particle.

Phenylketonuria (PKU) Inherited deficiency of phenylalanine hydroxylase, causing mental retardation.

Phenylpyruvate A phenylalanine-derived metabolite in phenylketonuria (PKU).

Pheochromocytoma Endocrine tumor secreting catecholamines.

Philadelphia chromosome A chromosomal translocation in patients with chronic myelogenous leukemia.

Phorbol esters Tumor promoters from croton oil; stimulate protein kinase C.

Phosphatase-1 The enzyme that dephosphorylates glycogen synthase, glycogen phosphorylase, and phosphorylase kinase.

Phosphatidic acid Glycerol + two fatty acids + phosphate.

Phosphoadenosine phosphosulfate (PAPS) The "activated sulfate" used for sulfation reactions.

Phosphodiester bond Bond between phosphate and two hydroxyl groups.

Phosphodiesterases Enzymes that hydrolyze cyclic AMP, cyclic GMP, or both.

Phosphoenolpyruvate (PEP) An energy-rich intermediate of glycolysis and gluconeogenesis.

Phosphoenolpyruvate (PEP) carboxykinase A gluconeogenic enzyme that is induced by glucagon and glucocorticoids.

Phosphofructokinase The enzyme that catalyzes the committed step of glycolysis.

Phosphoglycerides Lipids structurally related to phosphatidic acid.

Phosphoinositide 3-kinase A lipid kinase that mediates effects of growth factors and insulin.

Phospholipase C A type of enzyme that cleaves phosphoglycerides between glycerol and phosphate.

Phospholipases Phosphoglyceride-hydrolyzing enzymes.

Phospholipids Lipids with phosphate in their hydrophilic head group.

Phosphopantetheine A prosthetic group of fatty acid synthase.

Phosphoprotein A protein containing covalently bound phosphate.

Phosphoribosyl pyrophosphate (PRPP) The precursor of the ribose in purine and pyrimidine nucleotides.

Phosphorylase A type of enzyme that cleaves a bond by the addition of phosphate.

Phosphorylase kinase A protein kinase that phosphorylates glycogen phosphorylase.

Phosphorylation reactions Reactions in which a phosphate group becomes covalently attached to an acceptor molecule.

Phototherapy Treatment by exposure to light, used for hyperbilirubinemia in newborns.

Physiological jaundice The common jaundice of newborns.

Phytosterols Steroids from plants.

Pinocytosis Nonselective uptake of fluid droplets into the cell.

pK value The negative logarithm of the dissociation constant for an acid.

Plasma cells Immunoglobulin-producing cells in blood and lymphatic tissues.

Plasmalogens Phosphoglycerides containing an α,β-unsaturated fatty alcohol.

Plasmids Circular, double-stranded DNAs that function as "accessory chromosomes" in bacteria.

Plasmin The principal fibrin-degrading enzyme.

Platelet activation A change in shape and membrane structure of platelets, accompanied by the release of various mediators.

Platelet-activating factor (PAF) A soluble, biologically active phosphoglyceride released from white blood cells.

Platelet-derived growth factor (PDGF) Released from activated platelets during blood clotting.

β-Pleated sheet An extended secondary structure in proteins stabilized by hydrogen bonds between polypeptides.

Point mutation Change in a single base pair.

Poly-A tail A structure at the 3′ end of eukaryotic messenger RNA.

Polyadenylation signal A conserved sequence (AAUAAA) at the 3′ end of eukaryotic genes.

Polycistronic mRNA A messenger RNA (mRNA) that has been transcribed from more than one gene.

Polyclonal gammopathy Nonspecific overproduction of immunoglobulins.

Polygenic diseases Diseases caused by interactions between multiple genes and the environment.

Polymerase chain reaction (PCR) A method for amplifying selected DNA sequences.

Polymorphism Sequence variation in DNA.

Polyol pathway A pathway that synthesizes fructose from glucose.

Polyp A benign tumor of mucous membranes.

Polypeptide Polymer of amino acids.

Polysaccharide Polymer of monosaccharides.

Polyunsaturated fatty acids Fatty acids containing more than one C=C double bond.

Pompe disease A systemic glycogen storage disease causing death in childhood.

Porphyria cutanea tarda A porphyria characterized by cutaneous photosensitivity.

Porphyrias Diseases caused by impairment of heme biosynthesis, with accumulation of biosynthetic intermediates.

Porphyrin A type of pigment containing four pyrrole rings.

Postprandial thermogenesis Metabolic heat production in response to food intake.

Posttranscriptional processing Chemical modification of RNA.

Posttranslational processing Chemical modification of proteins.

Preimplantation genetic diagnosis Diagnosis of genetic diseases in the early embryo after in vitro fertilization.

Prenatal diagnosis The diagnosis of diseases in the fetus during early pregnancy.

Pre-procollagen The earliest precursor of collagen.

Primary bile acids Bile acids that are synthesized by the liver.

Primary structure The covalent structure of a protein.

Primase A specialized RNA polymerase that synthesizes a primer during DNA replication.

Probe A labeled oligonucleotide or polynucleotide that is used to identify a specific base sequence in DNA.

Processed pseudogenes Nonviral retroposons derived by the reverse transcription of a messenger RNA.

Processivity The ability of a DNA or RNA polymerase to synthesize long strands without interruption.

Progestins A class of steroid hormones that are precursors for the other steroid hormones.

Prohormone   The inactive or less active biosynthetic precursor of an active hormone.

Prokaryote   A cellular organism without a nucleus.

Proliferating cell nuclear antigen (PCNA)   A clamp protein that holds the DNA template during eukaryotic DNA replication.

Promoter   A regulatory DNA sequence at the upstream end of a gene or an operon.

Proopiomelanocortin   A prohormone in the anterior pituitary gland.

Propeptides   The N- and C-terminal extensions in procollagen.

Prophage   Bacteriophage DNA that has been integrated into the host-cell chromosome.

Prostate-specific antigen (PSA)   A marker for prostatic cancer.

Prosthetic group   A nonpolypeptide component in a protein.

Proteasome   A particle that destroys worn-out cellular proteins.

Protein kinase A   The cyclic AMP activated protein kinase.

Protein kinase B (Akt)   A protein kinase that mediates effects of growth factors and insulin.

Protein kinase C   The diacylglycerol-activated protein kinase.

Protein kinase G   The cyclic GMP activated protein kinase.

Proteoglycans   Products consisting of core protein and covalently bound sulfated glycosaminoglycans (GAGs).

Proteome   The totality of proteins made by a particular cell at a particular time.

Prothrombin time   A clotting test that detects deficiencies in the extrinsic and final common pathways.

Protonation/deprotonation   Reversible binding and release of a proton by an ionizable (acidic or basic) group.

Protoporphyrin IX   The organic portion of the heme group.

Proximal histidine   A histidine residue in hemoglobin and myoglobin that is bound to the heme iron.

Pseudogene   Degenerate, nonfunctional gene that is related to a functional gene.

Pseudohypoparathyroidism   Reduced responsiveness to parathyroid hormone.

PTEN   A lipid phosphatase that hydrolyzes 3-phosphorylated phosphoinositides; the product of an important tumor suppressor gene.

Purifying selection   A form of natural selection that removes detrimental mutations from the gene pool.

Pyranose ring   Six-member ring in monosaccharides.

Pyridoxal phosphate   The coenzyme form of vitamin B_6, used as prosthetic group in many enzymes of amino acid metabolism.

Pyrimidine dimer   A DNA lesion caused by ultraviolet radiation.

Pyruvate carboxylase   The mitochondrial enzyme that turns pyruvate into oxaloacetate.

Pyruvate dehydrogenase   The mitochondrial enzyme complex that turns pyruvate into acetyl-CoA.

Pyruvate kinase   The glycolytic enzyme that turns phosphoenolpyruvate (PEP) into pyruvate.

Q_{10} value   The factor by which the reaction rate increases in response to a 10°C rise in the temperature.

Quaternary structure   The subunit interactions of an oligomeric protein.

R factor   A plasmid that carries genes for antibiotic resistance.

Radioimmunoassay (RIA)   A highly sensitive analytical method used for the determination of hormone levels.

RAS   A (proto)oncogene coding for the Ras protein, a membrane-associated, mitogen-activated G protein.

Rate constant   A measure for the rate of a reaction.

Reading frame   The frame in which the codons on the messenger RNA are translated.

Receptor   A cellular protein that causes physiological effects after binding an extracellular agent.

Recessive   Determining the phenotype in the homozygous but not the heterozygous state.

Recombinational repair   Repair of DNA double-strand breaks guided by the homologous DNA sequence.

Recommended daily allowance   Dietary reference intake, the dietary intake considered optimal under ordinary conditions.

Redox reaction   Electron transfer reaction.

Reduction potential   A measure for the tendency of a redox couple to donate electrons in a redox reaction.

Refsum disease   Inherited defect in α-oxidation, causing neurological degeneration.

Remnant particles   Lipoproteins that are produced by the action of lipoprotein lipase on very-low-density lipoprotein (VLDL) or chylomicrons.

Renin   The rate-limiting enzyme of angiotensin synthesis.

Repressor   A DNA-binding protein that prevents transcription.

Respiratory chain   A system of electron carriers in the inner mitochondrial membrane.

Respiratory distress syndrome   Dyspnea with cyanosis, resulting from insufficient lung surfactant in newborns.

Respiratory quotient   The ratio of respiratory CO_2 produced to O_2 consumed.

Response element   A regulatory DNA sequence that mediates the effects of a hormone, second messenger, nutrient, or metabolite on gene transcription.

Restriction endonucleases Bacterial enzymes that cleave specific palindromic sequences in double-stranded DNA.

Restriction fragment DNA fragment produced by a restriction endonuclease.

Restriction site polymorphism DNA sequence variation that changes the cleavage site of a restriction endonuclease.

Retinoblastoma A rare tumor of immature retinal cells in children; can be either sporadic or inherited.

Retinoblastoma protein (pRB) The "guardian of the G_1 checkpoint," encoded by the retinoblastoma (*RB1*) tumor suppressor gene.

Retinol-binding protein A plasma protein that carries retinol from the liver to other tissues.

Retrovirus A type of virus that inserts a double-stranded DNA copy of its RNA genome into the host cell genome.

Rett syndrome A neurodevelopmental disorder caused by mutations in a methylcytosine-binding protein.

Reverse cholesterol transport The transport of cholesterol from extrahepatic tissues to the liver.

Reverse transcriptases Enzymes that transcribe RNA into a double-stranded DNA.

Rhodopsin The light-sensing protein in retinal rod cells.

Riboflavin Vitamin B_2, a constituent of flavin adenine dinucleotide (FAD) and flavin mononucleotide (FMN).

Ribonucleotide reductase The enzyme that reduces ribose to 2-deoxyribose in the nucleoside diphosphates.

Ribozyme Catalytic RNA.

Rickets Bone demineralization caused by vitamin D deficiency in children.

Rifampicin An inhibitor of bacterial RNA polymerase.

Rigor Stiffness of skeletal muscles.

RNA editing Enzymatic modification of a base in messenger RNA.

RNA interference Selective destruction of a messenger RNA after exposure to the corresponding double-stranded RNA.

RNA polymerases RNA-synthesizing enzymes.

RNA replicase A viral enzyme that synthesizes RNA on an RNA template.

RNase H An enzyme that degrades the RNA strand in a DNA-RNA hybrid.

Rotenone A fish poison that inhibits electron flow through NADH-Q reductase.

Rous sarcoma virus A retrovirus that causes sarcomas in chickens.

S phase The phase of DNA replication.

Salvage reactions Reactions that convert free bases to nucleotides.

Sarcoma Malignant connective tissue tumor.

Sarcomere A functional compartment of the muscle fiber.

Sarcoplasmic reticulum The endoplasmic reticulum of muscle cells, a specialized calcium-storage organelle.

Saturated fatty acids Fatty acids without $C=C$ double bond.

Scavenger receptors Lipoprotein receptors with broad substrate specificity that mediate the uptake of low-density lipoprotein (LDL) by macrophages.

Schizophrenia A group of severe psychiatric diseases in which new mutations are frequently observed.

Scurvy Disease caused by vitamin C deficiency, with impaired collagen synthesis and connective tissue abnormalities.

Second messengers Small, diffusible molecules that mediate many effects of hormones.

Secondary active transport Transport that dissipates an ATP-dependent ion gradient.

Secondary bile acids Bile acids that are synthesized from the primary bile acids by intestinal bacteria.

Secondary structure The repetitive folding pattern of a polypeptide.

Secretory pathway The organelles through which secreted proteins are processed: endoplasmic reticulum, Golgi apparatus, and secretory vesicles.

Segmental duplications DNA duplications that have become a normal feature of the human genome.

Selectable marker A gene that permits the selective survival of genetically modified cells.

Semiconservative replication The mechanism of DNA replication that leads to a daughter molecule with one old strand and one new strand.

Serotonin 5-Hydroxytryptamine (5-HT), the major indolamine.

Serum Blood plasma from which clotting factors have been removed.

Severe combined immunodeficiency Inherited diseases with combined B-cell and T-cell defects.

SH2 domain A domain of many signal transducing proteins that binds to phosphotyrosine groups on proteins.

Shine-Dalgarno sequence A ribosome-binding sequence in the 5' untranslated region of bacterial mRNAs.

Sickle cell trait Heterozygosity for hemoglobin S.

Sideroblastic anemia A microcytic anemia in the presence of high iron stores; seen in vitamin B_6 deficiency.

Signal peptidase An enzyme in the endoplasmic reticulum that cleaves off the signal sequence.

Signal recognition particle A cytoplasmic ribonucleoprotein that binds the signal sequence.

Signal sequence An amino acid sequence at the amino end of secreted proteins that directs them to the endoplasmic reticulum.

Sildenafil (Viagra) A phosphodiesterase inhibitor that prevents the degradation of cyclic GMP in the corpora cavernosa.

Silencers DNA sequences that reduce the rate of transcription by binding regulatory proteins.

Single-nucleotide polymorphism (SNP) The most common type of polymorphism in the human genome.

Site-directed mutagenesis The production of specific mutations in the test tube.

7SL RNA A component of the signal recognition particle and the grandfather of the Alu sequences.

Small interfering RNA (siRNA) Small double-stranded RNAs that inhibit translation and/or cause degradation of the messenger RNA.

Small nuclear ribonucleoproteins (snRNPs, pronounced "snurps") Components of the spliceosome.

Sodium cotransport A symport system that brings a substrate into the cell together with a sodium ion.

Sodium-potassium ATPase The sodium-potassium pump in the plasma membrane of all cells.

Sodium urate The poorly soluble uric acid salt that deposits in the joints of patients with gout.

Somatic mutation Mutation in a somatic (nongermline) cell.

Sorbitol A sugar alcohol formed by aldose reductase, intermediate in fructose biosynthesis.

Southern blotting A method for the identification of DNA fragments after gel electrophoresis, using a probe.

Spectrin A membrane-associated cytoskeletal protein in erythrocytes.

Spectrin repeat A three-stranded coiled-coil module in spectrin and dystrophin.

Spherocytosis Inherited defects in the membrane skeleton of erythrocytes, leading to spherical shape of the cells.

Sphingolipidosis Lipid storage disease, a type of disease caused by the deficiency of a sphingolipid-degrading lysosomal enzyme.

Sphingomyelin A phosphosphingolipid.

Sphingosine A long-chain, hydrophobic amino alcohol.

Spike proteins Viral proteins associated with the viral envelope.

Splice site mutation Mutation causing aberrant intron-exon splicing.

Spliceosomes Nuclear ribonucleoproteins that remove introns from primary transcripts.

Spongiform encephalopathies Rapidly progressive neurodegenerative diseases caused by misfolded prion protein.

Spot desmosome A spotlike cell-cell adhesion that is linked to intermediate filaments.

SRC A (proto)oncogene coding for a nonreceptor tyrosine protein kinase.

Standard conditions Conditions with 1 mol/L concentrations of all reactants at a pH of 7.

Statins Lipid-lowering drugs that inhibit 3-hydroxy-3-methylglutaryl-coenxzme A (HMG-CoA) reductase.

Steady state A state in which the rate of synthesis equals the rate of degradation.

Stearic acid A saturated C-18 fatty acid.

Steatorrhea Fatty stools.

Steroids Lipids containing a cyclopentanoperhydrophenanthrene ring system.

Sterol response element binding protein A cholesterol-regulated transcription factor.

Storage disease A type of inborn error of metabolism in which a nonmetabolizable macromolecule accumulates.

Streptokinase A plasmin-activating bacterial protein.

Streptomycin An antibiotic that binds to the small (30S) subunit of bacterial ribosomes.

Stress fibers Actin microfilaments underlying the plasma membrane.

Structural gene Gene coding for a functional, nonregulatory protein product.

Substrate The starting material for an enzymatic reaction.

Substrate-level phosphorylation The use of an energy-rich metabolic intermediate for the synthesis of ATP or GTP.

σ Subunit A subunit of bacterial RNA polymerase required for promoter recognition.

Sulfonamides Bacteriostatic agents that inhibit bacterial folate synthesis.

Superoxide dismutase An enzyme that turns superoxide into oxygen and hydrogen peroxide.

Superoxide radical A free radical formed by the transfer of a single electron to molecular oxygen.

Supertwisting Overwinding or underwinding of double-helical DNA.

Symport Coupled membrane transport of two substrates in the same direction.

T-cell receptor The antigen-binding receptor on the surface of T lymphocytes.

T lymphocytes Lymphocytes possessing no surface antibody but an antigen-recognizing T-cell receptor.

Tandem repeats Head-to-tail repeat sequences in eukaryotic genomes.

Tangier disease An inherited disease with near absence of high-density lipoprotein (HDL).

Taq polymerase A heat-stable DNA polymerase used for polymerase chain reaction (PCR).

TATA box A sequence motif in some eukaryotic promoters.

Tau protein An axonal protein that is misfolded in many neurodegenerative diseases.

Tay-Sachs disease A lipid storage disease caused by deficiency of a ganglioside-degrading lysosomal enzyme.

Telomerase An RNA-containing enzyme that extends the telomeres.

Telomere   The end piece of the eukaryotic chromosome.

Template strand   The DNA strand complementary to a newly synthesized DNA or RNA.

Tenase complex   The complex of clotting factors VIII and IX that activates factor X.

Tertiary structure   The overall folding of a polypeptide.

Tetrahydrobiopterin   A coenzyme for the hydroxylation of aromatic amino acids.

Tetrahydrofolate   The coenzyme form of folic acid; acts as a carrier of one-carbon units.

Thalassemia   Underproduction of hemoglobin α-chains (α-thalassemia) or β-chains (β-thalassemia).

Thermodynamics   The description of reaction equilibria and free energy changes.

Thermogenin   A mitochondrial uncoupling protein in brown adipose tissue.

Thiamin   The dietary precursor of thiamin pyrophosphate.

Thiamin pyrophosphate   A prosthetic group that transfers carbonyl compounds.

Thioester bond   An energy-rich bond between a sulfhydryl group and a carboxyl group.

Thrombin   An activated serine protease in the blood clotting system that acts on fibrinogen and on factors V, VII, VIII, XI, and XIII.

Thrombomodulin   An anticoagulant protein on endothelial cells.

Thromboxane   A prostaglandin-related product made by platelets.

Thrombus   A clot formed in an intact blood vessel.

Thymidylate synthase   The folate-dependent enzyme that methylates uracil to thymine in deoxyuridine monophosphate.

Thyroglobulin   A glycoprotein secreted into the thyroid follicle; precursor of the thyroid hormones.

Thyroperoxidase   The key enzyme of thyroid hormone synthesis.

Thyroxine-binding globulin   The main binding protein for thyroid hormones in the blood.

Tight junction   Beltlike cell-cell adhesion in epithelial tissues that impairs the diffusion of extracellular solutes and of membrane constituents.

Tissue factor   A glycoprotein in the plasma membrane of nonendothelial cells that activates factor VII.

Tissue-type plasminogen activator   A fibrin-binding protease that activates plasminogen to plasmin.

Titration   Treatment of a weak acid or base with a strong base or acid, respectively.

α-Tocopherol   The most active form of vitamin E; an important lipid-soluble antioxidant.

Tophi   Subcutaneous deposits of sodium urate in gouty patients.

Topoisomerases   Enzymes that regulate the supertwisting of double-helical DNA.

TP53   A tumor suppressor gene encoding the p53 protein; mutated in at least half of all spontaneous cancers.

Transaminases   Enzymes catalyzing the reversible, vitamin B_6–dependent transfer of an amino group from an amino acid to an α-keto acid.

Transcortin   A cortisol-binding protein in plasma.

Transcription   Synthesis of RNA on a DNA template.

Transcription factors   DNA-binding proteins that are required for transcription or that increase the rate of transcription.

Transcriptome   The totality of RNAs transcribed in a particular cell at a particular time.

Transcytosis   Vesicular transport across a single-layered epithelium.

Transducin   A G protein in retinal rod cells that mediates the effects of light exposure on a cyclic GMP-specific phosphodiesterase.

Transduction   The cell-to-cell transfer of DNA by a bacteriophage.

Transfection   Virus-mediated gene transfer for gene therapy.

Transferase   Enzyme that transfers a group between substrates.

Transferrin   The iron transport protein in the blood.

Transformation   Nonselective uptake of foreign DNA by a cell.

Transgenic mouse   Mouse with an artificially inserted gene.

Transglutaminase   Clotting factor XIII_a, a fibrin-crosslinking enzyme.

Transition state   The most unstable intermediate in a chemical reaction.

Translation   Ribosomal protein synthesis.

Translocation   (1) Movement of the ribosome along the messenger RNA. (2) Transfer of DNA from one chromosome to another.

Transmembrane helix   A membrane-spanning, hydrophobic α-helix in integral membrane proteins.

Transposase   An enzyme that catalyzes the movement of an insertion sequence or transposon.

Transposon   A mobile element in prokaryotes that contains a gene for transposase and other genes.

Transthyretin ("Prealbumin")   A plasma protein that binds thyroxine and retinol-binding protein.

Tremor   Trembling.

Trimethylamine   A fish-smelling product of bacterial glycine degradation.

Triose   Three-carbon sugar.

Tropocollagen   The collagen molecule.

Tropomyosin   A long, thin, fibrous protein associated with actin microfilaments.

Troponin   A calcium-sensing regulatory protein on the thin filaments of striated muscle.

Trypsin   A serine protease from the pancreas.

Tryptophan operon   An operon in *Escherichia coli* that codes for enzymes of tryptophan biosynthesis.

Tubulin   A globular protein that polymerizes into microtubules.

Tumor necrosis factor   An apoptosis-inducing cytokine.

Tumor progression   The progressive accumulation of oncogenic mutations in neoplastic cells.

Tumor suppressor gene   A growth-inhibiting gene in normal cells, whose inactivation contributes to neoplasia.

Turnover number   The number of substrate molecules converted to product by one enzyme molecule per second.

Tyrosinase   An enzyme in melanocytes that is required for melanin synthesis.

Tyrosine hydroxylase   The enzyme catalyzing the committed step of catecholamine synthesis.

Ubiquinone   Coenzyme Q, a lipid that carries hydrogen in the inner mitochondrial membrane.

Ubiquitin   A ubiquitous protein that marks worn-out cellular proteins for destruction by the proteasome.

Ubiquitin ligases   Enzymes that transfer ubiquitin to cellular proteins.

Urea   The major nitrogen-containing waste product in urine.

Urease   An enzyme in some bacteria and plants that cleaves urea to carbonic acid and ammonia.

Uremia   Retention of nitrogenous wastes in patients with kidney failure.

Uric acid   The end product of purine degradation.

Uric acid nephropathy   Kidney damage caused by urate deposits.

Urinalysis   Semiquantitative determination of urinary metabolites.

Urobilinogens   Uncolored products formed from bilirubin by intestinal bacteria.

Urobilins   Colored products formed from bilirubin by intestinal bacteria.

Uronic acid pathway   The pathway of glucuronic acid metabolism.

Valinomycin   A potassium ionophore.

van der Waals forces   Nonspecific attractive and repulsive forces between molecules.

Very-low-density lipoprotein (VLDL)   The lipoprotein that carries triglycerides from the liver to other tissues.

Viral retroposons   The remnants of retroviral genomes.

Virion   The virus particle.

Vitamin K   A fat-soluble vitamin that is required for the synthesis of blood clotting factors.

Voltage-gated ion channels   Ion channels that open in response to membrane depolarization.

von Gierke disease   Deficiency of glucose-6-phosphatase, causing hepatomegaly and severe fasting hypoglycemia.

von Willebrand factor   A plasma protein that mediates the binding of platelets to collagen.

Watson-Crick double helix   The principal higher-order structure of double-stranded DNA.

Wernicke-Korsakoff syndrome   Encephalopathy and amnesia caused by thiamin deficiency in alcoholic persons.

Western blotting   A method for the identification of separated proteins, with the use of antibodies.

Wild-type allele   The normal form of a gene.

Wilson disease   An inherited copper transport defect, with abnormal copper accumulation in liver and brain.

Wobble   Freedom of base-pairing between the third codon base and the first anticodon base.

Xanthine oxidase   A flavoprotein enzyme that produces uric acid.

Xanthoma   Visible subcutaneous lipid deposit.

Xenobiotics   Foreign substances without nutritive value.

Xeroderma pigmentosum   An inherited defect of nucleotide excision repair, characterized by cutaneous photosensitivity.

Xerophthalmia   Dry eyes, in vitamin A deficiency.

Zero-order reaction   Reaction whose velocity is independent of the substrate concentration.

Zeta-associated protein 70 (ZAP-70)   A protein kinase in T lymphocytes, activated by antigen binding to the T-cell receptor.

Zinc   A trace mineral in the body; constituent of many enzymes.

Zinc finger protein   A type of DNA-binding protein.

Zonula adherens   "Belt desmosome" that holds the cells of single-layered epithelia together.

Zwitterion   A molecule that contains at least one positive and at least one negative charge.

Zymogen   The catalytically inactive precursor of an enzyme.

CREDITS

Figure 2.6 Based on illustration © Irving Geis from Dickerson RE, Geis I: *The structure and action of proteins,* New York: 1969, WA Benjamin & Co. Permission from the estate of Irving Geis.

Figure 2.7 Redrawn from Pauling L: *The nature of the chemical bond,* ed 3, Ithaca, NY, 1960, Cornell University Press. Used with permission of the publisher, Cornell University Press.

Figure 2.9 Redrawn from Richardson JS: The anatomy and taxonomy of protein structure, *Adv Protein Chem* 34:264-265, 1981.

Figure 3.2 Redrawn from Dickerson RE: *The proteins,* ed 2, New York, 1964, Academic Press.

Figure 6.8 Redrawn from Devlin TM: *Textbook of biochemistry with clinical correlations,* ed 4. © 1997 Wiley-Liss. Redrawn with permission of Wiley-Liss, Inc., a subsidiary of John Wiley & Sons, Inc.

Figure 6.26 Redrawn with permission from Quigley GJ, Rich A: Structural domains of transfer RNA molecules, *Science* 194:797, 1976. ©1976 American Association for the Advancement of Science.

Figure 7.1 A, Adapted from Kornberg A: *DNA replication.* © 1980 WH Freeman and Company. Used with permission. **B,** Adapted from Devlin TM: *Textbook of biochemistry,* ed 4. © 1997 Wiley-Liss. Reprinted with permission of Wiley-Liss, Inc., a subsidiary of John Wiley & Sons, Inc.

Figure 7.13 © Elsevier Trends Journals, 1991. **C,** Modified from Lamb P, McKnight SL: Diversity and specificity in transcriptional regulation: the benefits of heterotypic dimerization, *Trends Biochem Sci* 16(11):421, 1991.

Figure 9.1 From Behrman RE: *Nelson textbook of pediatrics,* ed 17, 2004, Elsevier, p 385.

Figure 9.10 Courtesy of M. L. Levy, Baylor College of Medicine and Texas Children's Hospital, Houston,

from Nussbaum: *Thompson & Thompson genetics in medicine,* ed 7, 2007, Elsevier.

Figure 11.11 From Khan J, Simon R, Bittner ML, et al: Gene expression profiling of alveolar rhabdomyosarcoma with cDNA microarrays, *Cancer Res* 58:5009, 1998.

Figure 13.13 Modified from Stryer L: *Biochemistry,* ed 4, New York, 1995, WH Freeman, p 406.

Figure 14.13 From Bowman W: *Phil Trans R Soc Lond Biol Sci* 130:457, 1840.

Figure 15.9 Redrawn from Stites PP, Terr AI, Parslow TG: *Basic and clinical immunology,* ed 8, New York, 1994, Appleton & Lange.

Figure 15.10 A, Modified from Branden C, Tooze J: *Introduction to protein structure,* New York, 1991, Garland Publishing, p 185. **B,** Modified from Silverton EW, Navia MA, Davies DR: Three-dimensional structure of an intact human immunoglobulin, *Proc Natl Acad Sci U S A* 74:5142, 1977.

Figure 15.12 Redrawn from Stites PP, Terr AI, Parslow TG: *Basic and clinical immunology,* ed 8, New York, 1994, Appleton & Lange.

Figure 15.13 Redrawn from Stites PP, Terr AI, Parslow TG: *Basic and clinical immunology,* ed 8, New York, 1994, Appleton & Lange.

Figure 17.3 Redrawn from Unwin N: Neurotransmitter action: opening of ligand-gated ion channels, *Cell* 72 (suppl):31-41, 1993. © 1993 Cell Press.

Case Study: Viral Gastroenteritis Adapted from Montgomery R, Conway T, Spector A, et al: *Biochemistry: a case-oriented approach,* ed 16, St Louis, 1996, Mosby-Year Book.

Case Study: A Mysterious Death Adapted with permission from Hoffman M: Scientific sleuths solve a murder mystery, *Science* 254:931, 1991. © 1991 American Association for the Advancement of Science.

INDEX